The Art of Breastfeeding

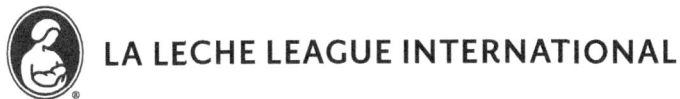 LA LECHE LEAGUE INTERNATIONAL

The Art *of* Breastfeeding

COMPLETELY REVISED AND UPDATED 9TH EDITION

PREVIOUS EDITION PUBLISHED AS
THE WOMANLY ART OF BREASTFEEDING

Bibiana Moreno Carranza,
Jayne Joyce, Teresa Pitman,
and Anna Swisher

No book can replace the diagnostic expertise and medical advice of a trusted physician. Please be certain to consult with your doctor before making any decisions that affect your health, particularly if you suffer from any medical condition or have any symptom that may require treatment.

As of the time of initial publication, the URLs displayed in this book link or refer to existing websites on the Internet. Pinter & Martin Limited is not responsible for, and should not be deemed to endorse or recommend, any website other than its own or any content available on the Internet (including without limitation at any website, blog page, information page) that is not created by Pinter & Martin Limited.

This edition first published in the UK 2024 by Pinter & Martin, published by arrangement with Ballantine Books, an imprint of Random House, a division of Penguin Random House, LLC.

Copyright © 1958, 1963, 1981, 1987, 1991, 1992, 2004, 2010
by La Leche League International
Copyright renewed © 1986, 1991 by La Leche League International

All rights reserved.

This work was originally published as *The Womanly Art of Breastfeeding* in 1958 by La Leche League.

Revised editions of the work were published in 1963, 1981, 1987, 1991, 1992, 2004, and 2010.

The authors have asserted their moral right to be identified as the authors of this work in accordance with the Copyright, Designs and Patents Act of 1988.

ISBN 978-1-78066-810-9

Also available in ebook and audio formats

British Library Cataloguing-in-Publication Data
A catalogue record for this book is available from the British Library.

This book is sold subject to the condition that it shall not, by way of trade and otherwise, be lent, resold, hired out, or otherwise circulated without the publisher's prior consent in any form or binding or cover other than that in which it is published and without a similar condition being imposed on the subsequent purchaser.

Printed in Poland by Hussar Books

pinterandmartin.com

Book design by Mary A. Wirth, Cover by Blok Graphic
Cover photographs (front) Paola Frias Prince (back, left to right) Itzul Bayardo, anonymous, Nikoesi Lisane (back) Matilda Macmillan

*To all the families who have shared their stories with us,
not only for the book but over our years as La Leche League Leaders,
thank you*

FOREWORD

Breastfeeding has been unequivocally shown to prevent maternal, child, and infant morbidity and mortality, serving as a critical factor in saving lives around the world. In both the Global South and the Global North, it can mean the difference between life and death.

Breastfeeding protects, enhances, and improves the health of women and children. It decreases the risk and duration of diseases such as diarrhoea and respiratory infection, reduces the risk of cancers for both children and mothers, and even lowers the risk of Alzheimer's disease. The longer a mother breastfeeds, the more significant the risk reduction.

Moreover, breastfeeding prevents malnutrition in all its forms, including obesity, underweight, wasting, and stunting. It has also been shown to relieve physical pain and promote maternal and child psychosocial well-being. It is nurturing care for both mother and child. The feel-good hormones released through breastfeeding reduce stress and depression and enable connection and bonding. It is on the mother's breast that babies learn love and compassion. Breastfeeding is a beautiful, living art.

As if its myriad of miracles wasn't enough, breastfeeding also has far-reaching effects on a family's and nation's economics, education, and environment. It transforms mere survival into thriving, demonstrating its significance as a cornerstone of human health, well-being, and development.

I'm deeply humbled to have been asked to write this foreword. My appreciation for La Leche League runs deep. I'll always be grateful that LLL answered my urgent call for help protecting, promoting, and supporting breastfeeding in Botswana back in 2014. At that time, as part of the compassion movement, I was working on maternal child health and nutrition for deprived communities in Jwaneng, a mining town, where the squatter camps stood next to the richest diamond mine in the world.

I've learned that compassion is an action, a verb. Mostly it is tender, but sometimes, it's fierce. True power has always been you and your incredible body. Breastfeeding enables us to reclaim our power. Breastfeeding empowers!

La Leche League saves lives, one mother and one child at a time. Thanks to LLL's peer support, we are restoring our sense of community and creating a village that provides vital help and evidence-based information, free from commercial interests. Most important, we are empowering people.

This book is needed now more than ever. Enjoy *The Art of Breastfeeding*!

With all my LLLove,
Magdalena Whoolery, PhD
Maternal Child Health and Infant Young Child Feeding Emergency Response Consultant, Breastfeeding International

CONTENTS

FOREWORD BY MAGDALENA WHOOLERY   vii

WOULD YOU LIKE TO . . . ?   xi

INTRODUCTION   xiii

ONE • Preparing   3

TWO • Connecting   21

THREE • Birth!   39

FOUR • Latching and Attaching   71

FIVE • The First Few Days: Hello, Baby . . .   97

SIX • Four to Fourteen Days: Milk!   131

SEVEN • Two to Six Weeks: Finding Your Way   167

EIGHT • Six Weeks to Four Months: Hitting Your Stride   205

NINE • Four to Nine Months: In the Zone   237

TEN • Nine to Eighteen Months: On the Move   263

ELEVEN • Nursing Toddlers and Beyond: Moving On   283

TWELVE • Sleeping Like a Baby   303

THIRTEEN • Beginning Family Foods   337

FOURTEEN • When You're Away from Your Baby   361

FIFTEEN • Milk to Go   397

SIXTEEN • Everybody Weans   423

SEVENTEEN • Alternate Routes		461
EIGHTEEN • A–Z "Tech Support" Tool Kit		507
ACKNOWLEDGEMENTS		571
NOTES		575
PICTURE CREDITS		615
INDEX		617

WOULD YOU LIKE TO . . . ?

- Explore the topics in this book in more detail
- Read more stories from parents all around the world
- Find up-to-date information on a huge range of breastfeeding issues
- Connect with La Leche League in your area or language
- Learn more about the history of LLL and what we're doing now
- Find out about becoming an LLL Leader
- Donate to support our volunteer work

Head over to our website:
www.llli.org

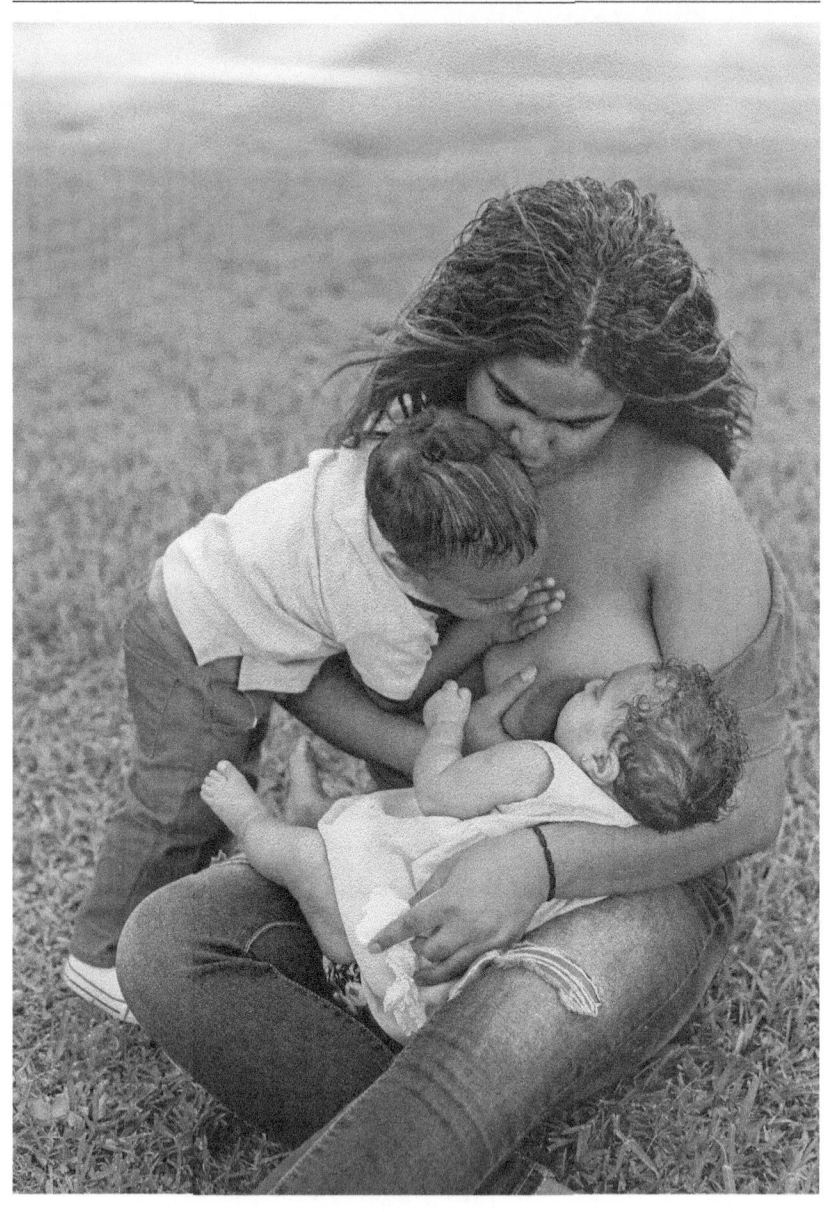

INTRODUCTION

Welcome to the ninth edition of La Leche League's "meeting in a book" – the world's bestselling guide to breastfeeding since it was first published in 1958.

The seven extraordinary women who founded La Leche League (LLL) in 1956 were swimming against the tide, nursing their babies in a time and place where most people didn't. They wondered whether what they'd learned might be useful to others. They started by reaching out to their friends and neighbours, offering local meetings and providing breastfeeding help by phone and sending handwritten letters (some people reading this have probably never received one of those!). It turned out that what they had to share – real-life experience, backed up by sound science – was pretty useful. Today, La Leche League volunteers can be found in more than eighty countries worldwide.

La Leche League is like a group of singers. We began as a small choir of women, living in the same city, with similar backgrounds and families. As the organisation has grown, families from around the world have joined the chorus, adding harmonies in their own languages and styles. It's our great privilege here to present the myriad voices of La Leche League in its seventh decade.

If you're familiar with previous editions of the book, you'll notice that we've included *a lot* more stories in this one. (To fit in as many as we can, we've used mostly short excerpts. You can find a selection of longer stories at www.llli.org, "Art of Breastfeeding" tab). They're the heart of the book, enabling you to hear directly from families across the LLL community in their own words. We'll tell you where each story comes from, as the contributors chose the wording for their locations. You'll probably relate to some of these stories, while others may feel less familiar or useful. As we say in our meetings, "Feel free to take what works for you, and leave the rest behind." We hope that everyone who picks up this book will find some reflection of their own experience, and know that there is a warm welcome for *you* in La Leche League.

So, what's new this time? The breastfeeding information has been updated, of course – there's been lots of exciting new research. Check out the Notes at the end of the book if you'd like to see some of these new studies. We've used the same structure as the eighth edition: following the breastfeeding journey from pregnancy to weaning (chapters 1–16), with separate chapters on sleep and family foods (solids). "Alternate Routes" (Chapter 17) is for those who've had a more complicated or unusual breastfeeding journey. Chapter 18 is our "A–Z 'Tech Support' Tool Kit," with key information on some common questions and challenges. This chapter is really only a taste – you can find much more information on LLL websites (either llli.org or your country-specific LLL website) and of course from our volunteer Leaders.

The stories in this edition come from all over the world. Previous editions included stories sourced mainly from North America, where LLL started. But after almost seventy years, LLL is truly international. You'll find stories from parents living everywhere from Canada to Chile, and every continent except Antarctica. (If you've breastfed in Antarctica, we'd love to hear from you. And if your experience isn't well represented in this edition, please consider writing your story *now*, in time for the tenth edition!) We don't assume, as previous editions did – to our shame – that your skin is white. We collected stories in eight languages; please forgive us if your voice doesn't come across quite as you intended in this English translation. Huge thanks to everyone who generously shared their stories, and to our team of volunteer translators. You can find the names of all our story contributors in the index, so you can locate your own or your friend's story, or follow a single story contributor through the book – we've used pieces from some stories in several different chapters.

Some of the language we use in this edition is new, too, reflecting the diversity of families who nurse and feed their babies human milk. *Chestfeeding* was barely on our radar in 2010, when the last edition was written; now it's an established term that some nursing parents, especially those who are trans or nonbinary, prefer. We use the word *parents* as well as *mothers* to acknowledge these members of our community, as well as the many fathers and co-mothers who play a vital role in the upbringing of their children. Breastfeeding rarely happens in isolation. We've written some sections especially for co-parents and supporters, and for the first time, we've included stories from fathers and grandmothers.

If this book is an old friend, you'll probably have noticed that the word *womanly* is gone from the title. *Womanly* was an off-putting old-fashioned word for many younger readers. Some of the eleven languages that the previous editions were translated into didn't have a word for *womanly,* so their titles have always been some version of *The Art of Breastfeeding.* We also want to acknowledge that not everyone who nurses a baby wants to be called a woman. This approach *isn't* about erasing or eliminating mothers or women. The vast majority of those who give birth and breastfeed will of course be women and mothers, and many (including ourselves) feel a real sense of pride in those titles. We honour you – and trust you will understand why it's also important to honour those who are proud to use other names as they give birth to and feed their babies.

Often, we use *nursing* as our preferred term for direct breastfeeding. We love it because it includes the idea of *nurturing,* not just delivering milk. The term isn't so well known in some versions of English (such as British English), but we hope you might come to appreciate it! *Breastfeeding,* of course, is still used throughout the book. But even that word has evolved. Since the last edition was published, feeding babies expressed milk – either your own milk or milk shared by someone else – has become much more common. We think it's a hugely encouraging sign that more families are recognising the importance of human milk for their babies, even when direct breastfeeding isn't possible or their milk supply is low. We've included more about this topic, including sections for EP (exclusively pumping) mothers. Their dedication is astonishing and deserves to be more widely seen and celebrated. Informal milk sharing – a practice as old as breastfeeding itself – has become more widespread with the advent of the internet and the availability of new kinds of pumps. We've included more on this practice, too, along with some deeply moving stories.

At times, our language might come across as a bit clumsy; language changes fast, and we're learning all the time. We appreciate your patience. Another note on language: people who breastfeed come in all shapes and sizes, and language is evolving in this area, too. It can be difficult to find descriptive words that don't have negative connotations. We have chosen to talk about people *having* (rather than *being*) overweight, or *having obesity,* to reflect new understanding and language about size and health.

This edition has more illustrations, tables, and bullet points than its predecessors. We hope this will make the information more accessible if you're reading it in a language that's not your first (or second or third!), as well as if you are neurodivergent or have a more visual learning style.

Like earlier editions of the book, we expect this one to be around for several years. Web links and resources included in books can quickly become outdated or may be contradicted by newer research. If you want to explore a topic further, you can find a "Want to know more?" section for each chapter at www.llli.org, "Art of Breastfeeding."

Whether you're reading this book cover to cover or just looking up one topic, we hope you will take time to read the heartfelt stories from families who are more like you than you might imagine, as well as from those who are completely different. You will find that we all have the same hopes, dreams, fears, and joys when it comes to nursing our babies and desiring to provide them with the best possible start in life. *The Art of Breastfeeding* is dedicated to helping you achieve your breastfeeding goals, whatever they may be.

With LLLove,
The Writing Team
9TH EDITION

The Art of Breastfeeding

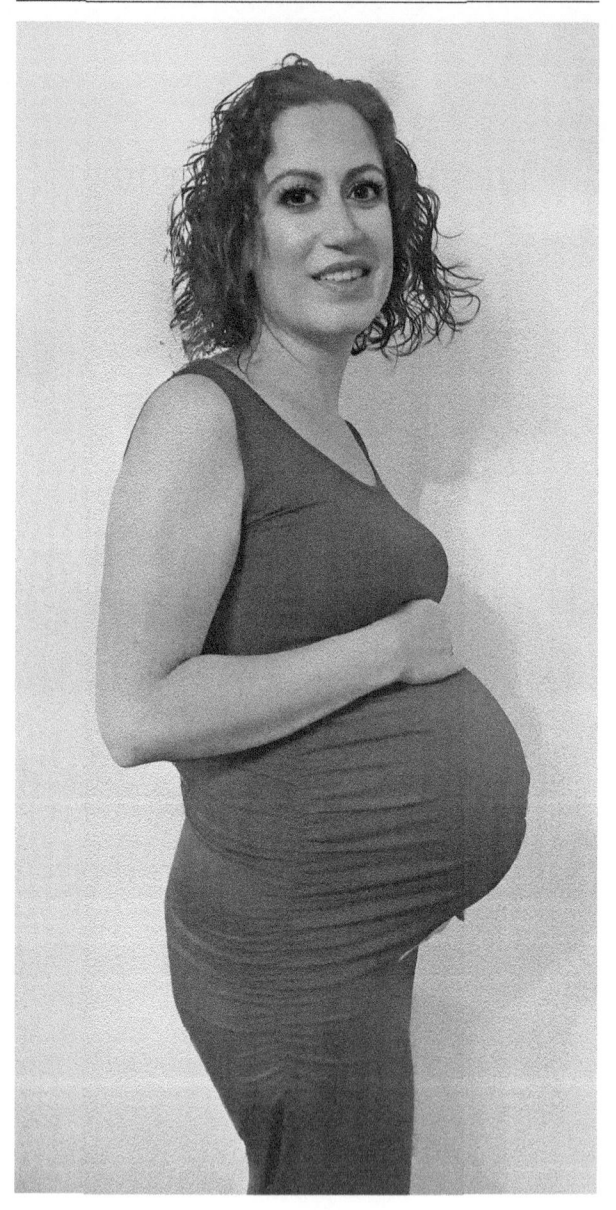

ONE

Preparing

Hello, nice to meet you, welcome to our meeting!
Refreshments are on the table. You're welcome to sit anywhere you'd like.
Oh, you're expecting a baby? That's wonderful! You probably have
lots of questions – and we're happy to help.

Whether you're pregnant, adopting, or working with a surrogate, congratulations! Maybe you can't wait to have your baby in your arms – but you still have lots of questions. Maybe you are feeling a mix of emotions: along with excitement, you're wondering how a baby will affect your relationships or you're concerned about how your career path will change.

Maybe an earlier pregnancy ended in a miscarriage or stillbirth, so you find it hard to even look ahead to holding a baby in your arms. Some of us have been there, too. We hope you have supportive friends, family, or counsellors to help.

Perhaps you've breastfed before and nursing didn't go well. That's what happened to Kirsten:

> I have breastfed twice, and each time was completely different. The first time, breastfeeding was tough, painful, and frustrating because I didn't have enough milk. This time I prepared myself much better by reading a few books about breastfeeding and talking to other mothers who have successfully breastfed. This made a huge difference. This time I could really enjoy breastfeeding.
>
> – Kirsten, from the Netherlands, living in Austria

As you research baby names, parental leave, and other issues, you're probably also thinking about how to feed your baby. Today, most expectant mothers choose breastfeeding – for very good reasons. You might be wondering what you need to do to prepare. We have some ideas for that!

Preparing to Breastfeed

Here's the good news: your body has already done a lot of preparation. In fact, it started even before you were born.

As your body developed inside your mother's womb, tiny ducts for carrying milk formed in your chest, under your nipples.

During puberty, as your breasts grew, these ducts developed branches.

Once you started menstruating, more branches grew during each cycle. Milk-making tissue started to grow as well, and you may have noticed some breast sensitivity before each period.

During the first three months of pregnancy, the ducts and milk-making cells grow more quickly. You may have noticed breast tenderness, a change in your bra size, and maybe blue veins or stretch marks on your breasts. Your *areolae,* the darker brown or pink circles around your nipples, may get darker and larger. Small bumps, *Montgomery glands,* may form on your areolae. They secrete tiny amounts of oil and milk to keep your nipples clean and moisturised. These are all good signs that your body is getting ready to nourish your baby!

The insides of your breasts are like maps of small towns connected by roads and highways. Your breasts grow tiny clusters of milk-making cells called *alveoli.* These alveoli are hollow, surrounded by thin muscle bands. Milk collects in the hollow centres, is squeezed out by those muscles, and follows the ducts to your nipple. Other ducts join along the way, so that milk flows out at the nipple through four to eighteen nipple holes (pores).

During the middle three months of pregnancy, breast growth continues. Between the twelfth and sixteenth weeks, your breasts start to produce colostrum, your baby's first milk.

During the last three months of pregnancy, you might leak drops of colostrum. If you don't leak at this point, no worries – your breasts are still getting ready to feed your baby.

If you've always felt that your breasts look different, or if you haven't experienced any tenderness or changes at all, talk to your healthcare provider, and for tips to get breastfeeding off to the best possible start, see Chapter 17.

Extra Breastfeeding Challenges

At the start, you might need extra help with breastfeeding if you have or have had

- diabetes of any kind
- scant breast tissue that hasn't grown during pregnancy
- bariatric surgery
- a thyroid disorder
- polycystic ovary syndrome (PCOS)
- breast surgery of any kind
- infertility issues
- other pregnancy or postnatal complications

If you are expecting multiples or if you know your baby is likely to need special care because he'll be born early or with health issues, you might also need extra help with breastfeeding at the start. Check out chapters 17 and 18 and consider contacting a La Leche League (LLL) Leader, an International Board Certified Lactation Consultant (IBCLC), or a healthcare provider with breastfeeding expertise.

Expressing Colostrum

The last few weeks of pregnancy may be a good time to learn how to express milk using your hands. Don't expect more than drops at first, but it will add up!

Trevor, a trans man who'd had chest masculinisation surgery, collected an impressive amount of colostrum (the first milk), a little at a time:

> I began painstakingly collecting my precious liquid. By the end of the pregnancy, I had forty or fifty syringes . . . a total of 20 or 25 ml.
> — *Trevor, Manitoba, Canada*

You can freeze any colostrum you get. This first milk is packed with immune factors to protect your newborn – if your baby needs any extra milk after birth, it's the best possible choice.

Don't worry, for each drop you express, you'll make more to replace it. So if you feel like expressing your colostrum and your healthcare provider agrees, go ahead! For how to do this, see Chapter 15.

A Different Way

Are you adopting, or is your baby being carried by a surrogate? Is breastfeeding a possibility? How do you prepare?

Yes, breastfeeding may well be possible! Some mothers who are adopting take hormones to encourage breast growth. Some others simply put the baby to the breast often and use a breast pump as well. Aren't breasts amazing? Results vary – you might make a small amount of milk – or a lot! For more on this alternate route for breastfeeding, see Chapter 17.

The Baby Is Born and Breastfeeding Begins!

After birth, the hormonal "wall" that held back milk production comes down when your placenta is delivered. The alveoli secrete colostrum (the first milk) for the first few days. Then, the volume increases and you begin producing mature milk. For what to expect in the early days after birth, see chapters 4 and 5.

You probably have lots of questions. Here are common ones asked at LLL meetings.

What About Emotional Preparation?

Just as pregnancy causes changes in your breasts and uterus, it changes your brain. Although science says that any parent caring for a child experiences changes, pregnancy and breastfeeding give you a head start. Milk-making hormones help you be more responsive and nurturing when your baby is born. You might forget things – mostly those that have nothing to do with taking care of your baby. The old connections in your brain make room for new ones that help you tune in to your baby.

How Important Is Breastfeeding, Really?

Extremely! There is almost nothing you can do for your child in her whole life that will affect her both emotionally and physically as profoundly as breastfeeding. You've probably heard that breastfeeding is good for your baby's health. But the impact of how babies are fed goes far beyond their health, as Ivannia learned:

> I am the mother of two teenagers and a preteen. I breastfed all three because I always knew it was the best way to protect them. I was, however, unaware that I was also protecting myself from postnatal stress and expensive medical bills.
> – Ivannia, Costa Rica

This would be a *much* longer book if we described all the ways that breastfeeding is valuable for you, your baby, your family, the healthcare system, and our planet. And research keeps finding more. Here are a few highlights.

The Impact on Your Baby

Your milk provides the appropriate nutrition for your baby's healthy growth and development. Human milk is packed with vitamins, minerals, healthy sugars and fats, proteins, and living cells, all working together to help your baby grow and develop, especially her brain. Your milk protects her from infections, both bacterial and viral – everything from ear infections to diarrhoea, pneumonia, and much more. At the same time, your milk helps your baby's immune system develop and become strong.

And that's just the milk. The act of nursing at the breast helps your baby develop strong jaw muscles and a wide palate, leading to straighter teeth and less risk of later problems such as sleep apnoea and snoring.

The impact continues long after your baby stops breastfeeding. Even as an adult, someone who was not breastfed is at higher risk for many diseases: type 1 and type 2 diabetes, heart disease, obesity, Crohn's disease, ulcerative colitis, certain cancers, and depression, among others.

The Impact on You

Mothers who don't breastfeed tend to have more trouble losing pregnancy weight. Without breastfeeding, the uterus takes longer to return to its normal size. If you breastfeed exclusively and your baby nurses often, including at least once during the night, your periods probably won't return for at least six months (see Chapter 9). Mothers who don't breastfeed are more likely to get pregnant again sooner and more likely to become anaemic.

Not breastfeeding increases your risk for hypertension, heart disease, diabetes, osteoporosis, and autoimmune diseases such as rheumatoid arthritis. Mothers who don't breastfeed also have higher rates of breast, uterine, and cervical cancers.

Oxytocin and *prolactin* are the main hormones that make breastfeeding happen, and they have amazing effects. Every time you nurse your baby, these hormones surge through your body. Mothers who don't breastfeed tend to be less responsive, more stressed, and less confident about caring for their baby. The closeness of breastfeeding helps build a strong connection between your baby and you, as Alison discovered:

> When I was pregnant with my son, a woman I met asked me if I planned to breastfeed. I told her, "Yes, that's my plan." She said, "Oh good! I loved it! You'll love it, too!" I walked away thinking, *What a strange thing to say*. At that time, I only understood breastfeeding as a way to nourish your child; I had no idea how much it would nourish my heart.
>
> – Alison, Canada

Many nursing mothers are surprised by the strength of the connection they feel with their babies. Lilly had planned to go back to work a few weeks after her daughter was born. She didn't think it would be worth initiating breastfeeding because she'd have to wean when she began working again. Then a colleague loaned her a previous edition of this book, and Lilly learned more about breastfeeding while working. She decided to give it a try. What surprised her was not just how well it went, but how deeply attached she was to her nursing baby. In the end, she didn't return to work until her baby was fourteen months old. For how to combine breastfeeding and working, see Chapter 14.

The Wider Impact

Of course, babies who are breastfed can still get ear infections or pneumonia, struggle in school, or have other issues. The risks are higher, however, for babies who are not breastfed. One review found that if almost all babies around the world were breastfed, the deaths of 823,000 babies would be prevented and there would be 20,000 fewer deaths from breast cancer each year.

Formula-feeding increases the burden on healthcare systems and the environmental impact of having a child. Formulas need manufacturing, packaging, and transporting, as well as the advertising and marketing industries to encourage people to use them. All this causes pollution, waste, and depletion of natural resources.

Breastfeeding promotes normal brain development. A baby who is not breastfed averages several points lower in intelligence, fewer years of schooling, and lower income. Breastfeeding benefits our whole society.

But Aren't Formulas Now Almost the Same as Human Milk?

Not really! Have you seen the list of components in human milk? It's so long we'd need several pages to name them all – and researchers are discovering new ones every year.

Not only that, your milk is a living fluid that *changes* all the time. Your milk differs, depending on your baby's age, what you're eating, the bacteria or viruses you and your baby have been exposed to, and the time of day (for instance, you make "sleepy milk" at night). Your milk even changes from the beginning to the end of each feeding (there's more fat later in the feed – dessert!). It's impossible for a standardised, ultra-processed product like formula to do any of this.

If breastfeeding did not already exist, someone who invented it today would deserve a dual Nobel Prize in medicine and economics.
– *Keith Hansen, Vice President for Human Development at the World Bank*

Understanding Breastfeeding Research

The formula industry claims that breastfeeding has benefits when compared to their products. And you might see lists of the benefits of breastfeeding from health authorities. But (are you sitting down?) breastfeeding doesn't have "benefits"; it's just the biologically normal way to feed a baby. We've been thinking about it backward.

Here's why. Let's say we're testing a new drug. We focus on the people who get the drug and compare them with a group of ordinary people. That's how we know what the drug does and whether it makes things better or worse. Now think about most of the research on breastfeeding. Exactly. It's research on *breastfeeding*! Most studies have treated formula as the standard and breastfeeding as the unusual thing. This approach makes the high rates of formula-fed illness seem like expected baby health, and the outcomes of breastfeeding seem like bonus points.

Breastfeeding or feeding your baby human milk doesn't reduce the risk of infection, illness, and disease. It doesn't add IQ points. Using the same information from the same studies – defining formula-fed babies as the actual experimental group – we can say that babies are at increased risk for all those short-term and long-term illnesses and diseases when they *don't* get human milk.

Researchers have minimised formula problems by stating the benefits of human milk and nursing – as if nursing a baby is a nice but unnecessary extra. Fortunately, that perspective is changing. More studies now use breastfed babies as the starting point and look at what happens to babies when their systems are altered. This can be a scary way to look at infant feeding – to see a list of risks instead of a list of benefits. But it's a more honest, accurate approach. Breastfeeding doesn't give you nice extras. Anything else adds risk.

Is It Right for Me?

Of course we want to say, "Yes, breastfeeding is right for you and for everyone!" But we acknowledge that everyone is different. There are millions of babies in our world and millions of ways to parent. Maybe you come from a culture where breastfeeding is not the norm and you feel uncomfortable at the thought of nursing. Maybe you've always thought of your breasts as sexual parts of your body, so the idea of milk coming out of them or having a baby attached to them seems strange. Maybe you are focused on your career or other parts of your life and you think breastfeeding will take too much time and energy. Or maybe you have previous experiences (perhaps abuse or trauma) or health concerns that make breastfeeding difficult or problematic. (We touch on some of these issues in chapters 3, 17, and 18.) If you are interested in providing your baby with your milk, even for a short time, we're here to support you.

Nursing is the way you're naturally designed to care for your new baby. So why doesn't it always come naturally? Lots of reasons! Friends may have told you all about their tough experiences. Maybe your mother or grandmother couldn't breastfeed and you wonder if you'll have trouble, too. The great news is that we've learned a lot since your mother or grandmother tried. We've learned more about understanding and respecting the instincts that you and your baby both have. We've learned that the fewer interventions you have during birth, the easier these instincts are to tap into. And La Leche League is always here to help you work through any issues that come up.

You might want to breastfeed because you know it's good for your baby's health – and yours. It might just feel right to you. All these reasons are good enough. And there might be practical reasons, too. After the early weeks, when nursing has become second nature, you'll find you can gentle your baby out of almost anything – hunger, tiredness, overstimulation, fear, pain – with a little nursing. Nursing stops being a feeding device and becomes an all-purpose parenting tool.

You might have heard that formula-feeding is easier and more practical. Marketing is powerful. But nursing means no cans of formula or bottles. No washing, sterilising, or storing. No measuring, spilling, heating. No planning, equipment, or leftovers. Your milk is always available, always the right temperature, and never spoiled, no matter how hot or cold it is outside. The money that you don't spend on formula in a year could pay for a major appliance. And – this is a big one – in an emergency of any kind, from a minor problem to a natural disaster involving formula shortages or no clean water, nursing your baby ensures you'll always have a safe way to feed your child. For more about feeding in emergencies, see Chapter 18.

> The headlines were stark – the hurricane was headed our way. This time we had a baby with us – it was time to evacuate. The drive took hours and hours as our car sat in traffic. But no matter how long it took, no matter whether we had water or electricity, no matter how stressed everyone around us was, I was able to feed Katherine.
> – *Helen, from the United States, living in the UK*

We're not saying nursing is free, because it isn't. It costs your time. It will reduce your income if you leave your job or take a longer maternity leave, and you may need to buy a pump and containers if you pump while at work. Overall, though, there are many important reasons to nurse your baby.

What if you aren't sure if nursing is for you? You're not committing yourself if you just give it a go. You may be surprised! You might find you and your baby both love it. You can stop any time if you change your mind. It's much easier to switch from breastfeeding to formula than the other way around. If feeding at the breast doesn't seem like it will work for you, expressing milk for your baby is the next best thing, and we can also support you with that (see Chapter 17, Exclusive Pumping).

Will My Breasts Work? Will I Have Enough Milk?

Good news: breastfeeding can almost always work! Yes, there are some people who require extra support, especially at first, but the odds of making enough milk are very good for most of us.

The most common early reasons for babies not getting enough milk – complicated or premature births and latching problems – are usually fixed with time, patience, and help if you need it. We will cover these in chapters 3, 4, and 17.

Ali had a tough birth that made starting breastfeeding harder:

> Labour with my first child was long, and I lost a lot of blood. I was finding it hard to lift her and try to breastfeed as my arms were so weak. It turned out afterwards that no one had looked at my blood count results and I was so anaemic I needed a blood transfusion. For a day or so I struggled to latch, feeling more and more desperate and scared that my daughter wasn't really feeding – I hadn't slept for several days by that point.
>
> Eventually a midwife looked at the state of me, sobbing and shaking in bed, and strongly advised giving formula. My husband and I agreed. After that, my daughter and I both had a sleep. When I woke up, I felt refreshed. We tried again, and this time, my daughter took it and I started breastfeeding. After that, although it was by no means smooth, I managed to establish breastfeeding and went on to breastfeed her for eighteen months.
>
> – Ali, England

For more about how to use extra milk and feeding tools to support breastfeeding, see Chapter 18, Supplementing.

Maybe you have other reasons to worry about making enough

milk. Perhaps this is a subsequent baby and your previous breastfeeding experience didn't go well. Or you have one or more of the issues that can affect milk production.

It's important to know two things. First, you never know how much milk you can make until you give it a try. Having a particular "risk factor" doesn't guarantee you'll have problems. And second, breasts get better at making milk over time. Many of us find that we make more milk with our later babies than we did with our first, because more milk-making tissue grows during each pregnancy. Breasts that have had surgery can heal over time, too. And if you've breastfed before, chances are that you'll be quicker to reach out for help – which can make a big difference.

You'll find tips for breastfeeding with all kinds of breasts and breastfeeding issues in Chapter 18, our "A–Z 'Tech Support' Tool Kit." Whatever your issue, we've probably seen it before. And even if we haven't, we'll be happy to help you figure it out or find someone who can!

One last thought: the only person who gets to say what your breastfeeding journey should look like or decide its value is *you*. Any amount of nursing and human milk is valuable for your baby, and we think it deserves to be celebrated. Jeanie put it beautifully:

> I had a breast reduction a year before Marceline was born.... The knowledge given to me by LLL made a huge difference. Don't ever wonder if you did enough. You are enough. Give it your best. Even if all you have that day is 40 percent, if you give your baby that 40 percent, then that's 100 percent of what you have available.
>
> – Jeanie, Michigan, United States

Will My Baby Latch?

Breastfeeding is a survival skill for babies! Your baby has all the reflexes required to nurse, even if birth has been challenging or there are other issues.

The good news is that it's not all up to you to make this work. Search online and you'll find videos of newborns placed on their mothers' bodies, crawling to the breast, and latching with minimal help. Your baby is built for this, and your own breastfeeding instincts will guide you to provide the support your baby needs.

It's also true that there are babies who "can't get their act together" for a while, often because of a difficult labour or birth or because they were born prematurely or have health issues. In all these situations, the key is to keep your milk supply high (by expressing your milk), keep your baby fed (ideally with that expressed milk), and be patient. For more on these situations, see Chapter 4.

Will My Nipples Work?

Many mothers worry that their nipples are too big, too small, or too inverted for breastfeeding, but almost all of them can work just fine – sometimes with a little "tech support." For more detailed help, see Chapter 18, Nipple Diversity.

Montserrat shares her experience of breastfeeding with flat nipples:

> My youngest daughter was born superhealthy, but I couldn't feed her with my flat nipple – she could not grab the nipple until [I used] nipple shields. Thanks to them, I was able to breastfeed. I had a very nice connection with her, she looked at me with eyes of love, she caressed my breast every time she took her milk. I was happy to be able to do it, because with my two older children I didn't do it, and with her I did. Without a doubt it was something wonderful.
>
> – *Montserrat, Querétaro, Mexico*

While Montserrat found nipple shields helpful, not everyone does, so be sure to talk to a breastfeeding helper for ideas to fit your situation (see Chapter 18, Nipple Shields).

What about a nipple that is too big for your baby's mouth? This is another situation requiring some patience! You may need to express milk until your baby grows enough to manage your large nipples. Fortunately, babies grow quickly, so this is usually a short-term problem.

Will Nursing Hurt?

When a mother cat feeds her kittens, she's not thinking about how much milk each kitty is getting, or what the latch looks like. She just lies there (usually purring!) and lets them nurse. If it hurts, though, the mother cat reacts. She moves her body a little, nudges the kitten with her nose, or gets up, shakes the kitten off, and starts over.

The same is true for humans. Nipple sensitivity is common in the first couple of weeks (see Chapter 18, Sore Nipples). But if nursing really *hurts*, that's your body's signal to change something.

Pain is the body's way of guiding us to find a more comfortable position. If you get a pebble in your sandal, you don't keep walking on the pebble. You'll stop to do something, maybe shake your foot, to get the pebble out. If that doesn't work, you'll intuitively do something else so you can walk comfortably. More comfort for you means more milk for your baby.
– Christina Smillie, MD, United States physician
and breastfeeding specialist

For more about latching and attaching – making nursing truly comfortable (and efficient) – see Chapter 4. And the best way to work on pain is usually to find a breastfeeding helper. The difference that help makes can be dramatic.

How Long Will I Be Doing This?

The short answer is, as long as you and your baby want. Based on research, the World Health Organization and many other experts advise exclusive breastfeeding (no other drinks or solid foods) for about six months, with family foods gradually added and breastfeeding continuing for at least two years. Many nurse longer.

Can't imagine nursing a two-year-old? Not many of us can when we have a new baby; for that matter, it's hard to imagine what it's like taking care of a two-year-old when you've never done it. For now, focus on feeding your new baby and getting help if you need it. Then when breastfeeding is going smoothly, you can decide when you want to stop, instead of stopping because you had no choice. When you're ready to think about weaning, see Chapter 16.

How Can I Be Sure I'm Prepared?

There's no way to *fully* prepare for any part of becoming a parent, including breastfeeding. But gathering information, finding support, and being determined are hugely helpful. Reading this book is a great first step! What else can you do? Talk to friends and relatives who breastfed. Hang out with anyone you know who's currently nursing. If you can, check out a La Leche League meeting, either in person or virtually. You'll pick up tips and tricks that will help later. To learn how to build your support network, see Chapter 2.

> I am a single mother. . . . I had a C-section with my first son and couldn't breastfeed because I was too uninformed. That wasn't going to happen to me with my second child! I attended LLL breastfeeding preparation courses during my pregnancy, read books, and looked for a breastfeeding consultant. Thanks to good preparation and good information, we are fully breastfeeding.
> – *Rafaela, Austria*

What Stuff Do I Need?

There are many products on the market for breastfeeding families, yet a nursing baby doesn't need much. Here are our thoughts on some of the most common ones.

Nursing Clothes? It depends

Clothes made especially for nursing, with hidden flaps and openings, are nice but not necessary. It's easy to nurse in normal clothes, especially if you're wearing

- a top that's loose or stretchy enough to pull up from the bottom
- a shirt or dress that you can unbutton
- two layers: one underneath that you pull down, and one over it that you pull up

Nursing bras have flaps that open for easy access. The size you wore in your last trimester will probably fit after your baby's born, although your cup size may be bigger for the first couple of months. A regular bra that's stretchy enough to pull the cup down or up to breastfeed might work fine. It's a good idea to avoid underwires and any bra that's tight enough to leave marks on your skin. If you're happy braless, stay braless. Nursing doesn't mean you need to start wearing bras if you don't want to!

Breast (Nursing) Pads? Maybe

Some breasts never leak – that's perfectly normal. Leaking has nothing to do with milk supply. However, if you do leak, pads might be helpful. Both disposable and washable brands are available. Be careful to change a disposable pad whenever it gets soaked to keep your skin comfortable and healthy. If you don't need pads between feeds, you might leave a cloth nappy or muslin around the house to catch any drips that happen while you're nursing.

Breast Pump? Not Always

If you won't be separated from your baby often, you probably don't need a pump. If you want to express milk for any reason, there are many options. You might find you can express all the milk you need using your hands, or a good-quality manual pump may be all you need. If you'll be pumping frequently, an electric pump might be a better option. For the whole range of expression methods, see Chapter 15. It's often best to wait and see what you need when the time comes.

You might find yourself in a situation where you need a hospital-grade pump – perhaps because your newborn is too ill or weak to nurse at the breast. No need to prepare in advance, though – if your hospital or midwife can't provide a pump, your local breastfeeding helper or support group can help you find one.

Nursing Furniture? Not Necessarily

If you nurse sitting up and have short legs, you may find that a low footstool, thick book, or coffee table crossbar raises your lap to support the baby and relax your lower back. Leaning back slightly or crossing one knee over the other may also work well when you nurse. As you become more practised, you'll find other creative ways to get comfortable. Try raising just one foot, so your baby's feet are lower than his head. A rocking chair is very useful for some nursing couples and not at all for others. A tip: if you decide to get a rocker, choose one that doesn't make lots of noise! For much more on "nursing props," see Chapter 4.

Soft Carrier? Almost Always!

One of the most helpful parenting tools is a cloth carrier, sling, or wrap, so you can "wear" your baby while you go about your day. Carriers come in all kinds of fabrics, colours, sizes, and patterns. There are many designs, from ones that tie in a crisscross shape to the basic kind, which is secured with one or two large rings. Look for one that fits you, meets safety standards, and is right for your baby's age and weight. And be patient – there's often a learning curve in wearing your baby!

Although having your hands free is great, babywearing benefits go far beyond a free hand. Baby carriers make nursing and skin-to-skin time easier, help soothe a crying baby, help you and your baby feel connected, and enable other caregivers to take care of the baby more easily.

Soft cloth carriers are not only baby carriers, they're also clean surfaces for nappy changing and blankets to cover a sleeping baby. Most people won't be able to tell when you nurse your baby in a sling. Some slings even have pockets for your phone and keys. La Leche League groups can be good places to see slings and other carriers in action.

A Plan for the First Few Weeks or Months

Just in case nobody has mentioned this to you yet – caring for a baby takes up a lot of time! You'll want to do what you can to streamline things or get help with all the other tasks you normally do each day, as Teresa learned:

> At my baby shower, one of my friends (who already had two children) gave me a slow cooker. It seemed like a weird present along with all the cute outfits, but it's been so useful! I can start dinner in the morning, while Daniel has his first nap, and it's all done and ready by evening – when all he wants to do is nurse.
>
> – Teresa, Ontario, Canada

Stocking your freezer is a good idea. You could ask for frozen or tinned prepared food instead of the typical new baby gifts. Online sign-up options for friends, family, and colleagues to bring meals or have meals delivered have also become popular in some communities.

Sometimes relatives or friends will pay for a cleaning service as a gift or visit and do housework and laundry if they live nearby. Partners on leave from work can also be a huge help. The more you can set up in advance, the better: it's tougher to get organised with a newborn in your arms.

See? You're already building your network and getting ready for your new addition – as well as building a strong foundation for breastfeeding.

My story begins with an enormous desire to bond with my son. . . . I knew the nutritional benefits of breastmilk, however, the deep desire to look into his eyes and caress his head while he was breastfeeding was the motivation. My husband and I, seven months pregnant, went to our first face-to-face LLL group talk. We were impressed by the closeness, understanding, and empathetic responses.
– *Sara Edith, Mexico City*

Want to know more?

You can find extra resources for this chapter
at the "Art of Breastfeeding" tab at
www.llli.org.

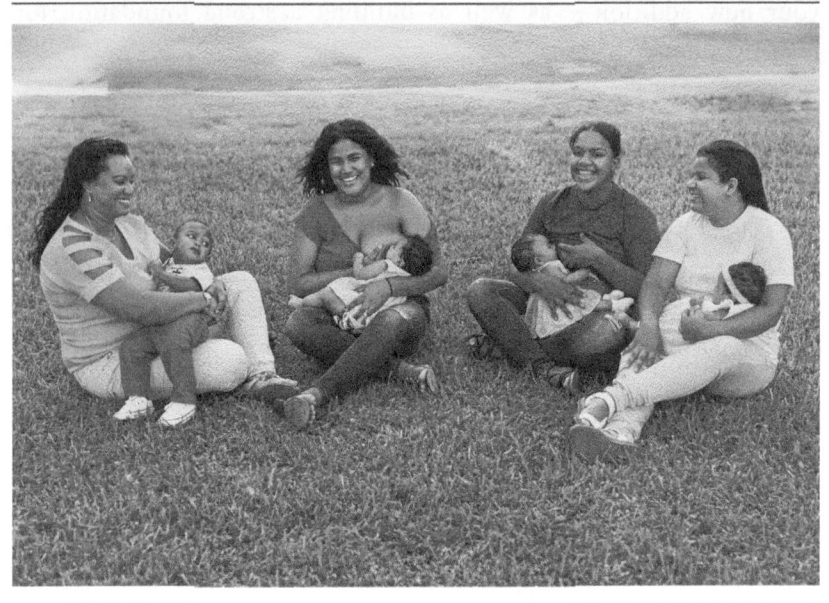

TWO

Connecting

We think of nursing as something that happens between two people: you and your baby. Yet having good support can make a huge difference:

> My mother was a blessing. She breastfed my siblings and me, and she was a wet nurse for a cousin. It was very common to see my mother, aunts, and older sister breastfeeding. My older sister is a blessing, too. She or my mother, and her dad when he can, take care of my daughter when I work. All my family were key to my breastfeeding and motherhood being so pleasant. Thanks to this support, I achieved my breastfeeding goals.
> – *Gisel, Mexico*

> I now know and believe that it takes a number of interconnected parts to establish a successful breastfeeding journey, and that it should not be the sole responsibility of us mothers.
> – *Kara, Australia*

> Breastfeeding is an art. During childhood, my day-to-day experience was being around women and their children, either on their breasts, backs, in carriers – always as one. Early in life, I learned the dedication required to support mothers so that they could breastfeed and raise their children, putting in daily effort to create an environment that is welcoming and healthy for families. We are here because of our mothers, grandmothers, and past generations. To honour them we need to be here for the current breastfeeding generation and for the ones to come!
> – *Heranush, rural New Zealand*

Are you wondering why we are talking about building a network of support when your baby may not even be born yet?

Here's why: having a support network is more important than you might think for meeting your feeding goals and smoothing the road to parenthood. It is a key part of the basic how-to.

What does a breastfeeding-supportive network look like? People who want to help you out might offer to feed the baby or take her overnight so you can sleep. But these offers can disrupt milk production (especially in the early months) and stress us out because we want our babies with us.

What you want are people who support your feeding goals, whatever those might be, and even if they change. You might decide to let your baby wean himself when you had planned to nurse only three months. Or you might decide to wean at one year, not two, as you originally thought.

> Our breastfeeding relationship started off well and it's been a wonderful part of parenting all my children. It's definitely a part-time job. Thankfully my husband is supportive. Breastfeeding is a physical job, but also emotional. I couldn't do it without family support.
> – *Vanessa, Florida, United States*

Supporting you with breastfeeding is doing all the other things, like cooking, cleaning, and laundry. It's company, encouragement, good listening, and suggestions for help if you run into problems.

> I don't think one parent can raise a child. I don't think two people can raise a child. You really need the whole village. And if you don't have it, you'd better make it.
> – *Toni Morrison, paraphrasing an African proverb*

Do I Need to Read This Chapter?

Maybe not! You might want to skip ahead if the following is true for you:

- You were brought up in a breastfeeding family.
- You live in a community where most babies are breastfed.
- You have spent a lot of time around nursing babies and children.
- You have knowledgeable, trusted people on hand to help.

We'd love all new parents to be in such a great position. But many of us are not so fortunate. So, what do we really need to help us feed our babies the way we want to?

More Than Information

For those who have access to the internet, there's a huge amount of information about breastfeeding. Yet all this information is no guarantee of easier breastfeeding – it may even leave you more confused.

We often hear new parents say, "Everyone tells us something different." Without prior knowledge, it can be hard to determine what's fact, opinion, or just plain wrong. We humans are social learners, learning best by watching others. Yet some of us have never seen anyone nursing close-up, or even at all. We need real-life role models, not just facts.

It's All About Relationships

Is learning to breastfeed a skill, like using a new gadget or app? There is learning involved, but nursing is not just a skill – it's a relationship. Your relationship with your baby is at the centre. This centre is part of a web of connections with

- your partner or key support person or people
- your family or others who brought you up
- your extended family and close friends
- your communities (cultural, faith, or other interests)
- your neighbourhood
- your healthcare providers
- your employer
- your wider society

If these connections support the way you want to feed your baby, you're in a great place to begin your parenting journey. Or you might feel like Ausilia, having her first baby in a new, unfamiliar home:

> My mother didn't support me exclusively breastfeeding. If it wasn't for a friend sending me the LLL book on day two of being a mum, my baby probably would have been bottle-fed. . . . I didn't have any friends or family in the same position as me, and all of my friends were at work, so it was quite a lonely time.
> – Ausilia, London, UK

Even if you come from a community with a long, proud breastfeeding history, you might not have access to that knowledge. Stephanie, an Indigenous parent, writes about how her community's breastfeeding heritage was stolen:

> Most of us Indigenous people from around the world would love to be able to say that we learned all about lactation from our mums and aunties. We would love to have the Traditional Knowledge or Stories about lactation, which we could use to motivate us to continue through the difficult first days or weeks. Most of us would also love to know our families, Nations, or Clans. But colonization took that away, too.
> – Stephanie, Six Nations of the Grand River, Ontario, Canada

Today, many new parents have a messy web of breastfeeding support for various reasons:

- Babies in their family weren't breastfed.
- Babies in their community aren't breastfed, or they are often fed other things (formula, other foods and drinks) along with being breastfed.
- They haven't spent much time around babies, breastfed or not.
- They don't know many people where they live.
- Their government or employer doesn't have policies for parental leave and breastfeeding.
- They might not know other families who look like them, share their feeding goals, or have stories like theirs.

If you have these gaps, it can be helpful to plan ahead to fill them. Every family is different, but all of us do best with a strong safety net of care and support.

What If It's Just Me and My Baby (Or Me, My Partner, and Our Baby)

Being isolated with your baby, even with a partner, isn't easy, but many parents have done it. Here are some ideas that might help you:

- **Professional support.** In some places, health organisations or agencies may provide a free or low-cost visiting home care attendant for a set time.
- **Postnatal doulas.** These trained caregivers provide practical and emotional support in your own home. In some places, doulas may be able to provide free or subsidised care.
- **Neighbourhood groups and faith communities** often provide support to new parents, such as meals. This is an excellent time to get to know friendly neighbours, if you don't already.
- **Parent groups.** Look for local support groups in your community. La Leche League might be one place to start!
- **Online groups.** Online support can be a great addition, although it can't fully replace in-person contact. You may find a local online group with options to meet in person.

Different Kinds of Families

There is no single ideal way for families to form and meet their children's needs for nurture, protection, and guidance. Humans are amazingly adaptable and creative. Most children live with at least one biological parent, many live with both, and a lot live with other members of their extended family as well as, or sometimes instead of, a parent. Some children are brought up in cooperative groups of related and unrelated adults. Others are adopted. All kinds of families are represented in La Leche League groups all over the world.

Different Arrangements for Feeding the Baby

Most babies are nursed by their birth mothers, but adoption, wet nursing (the baby being nursed by someone else), and shared nursing (the baby being nursed by more than one person) have also been practised throughout history. For more about these arrangements, see Chapter 18, Milk Sharing. In recent years, as scientific discoveries reveal more about the importance of human milk, we've seen a revival of some of these historical practices. Families are adapting traditional baby-feeding strategies for complex modern lives. There may be more variety than you think....

Some Indigenous Nations have stories of dads nursing their babies. Binary genders and strict gender roles were never ours originally.
– *Stephanie, Six Nations of the Grand River, Ontario, Canada*

We at LLL have experience with all these circumstances. Whatever your plan for feeding your baby, we're here to help. For more about this, see Chapter 17.

What's the Best Milk for Babies?

As shared nursing, wet nursing, and donor milk have become more common, the question is not simply "breastfeeding or formula?" Safe human milk is more suitable for almost all babies than formula.

If there is a choice about *whose* milk your baby gets, this is the order of preference:

1. **Your milk.** Your own milk is tailored to the exact age and stage of your baby and her specific needs as she grows. For more information about the special importance of colostrum (early milk), see chapters 3 and 17.
2. **The milk from someone who regularly nurses and cares for your baby.** This might be your partner, or a relative. During breastfeeding, the baby's saliva passes "information" to the breast about viruses she's been exposed to. This triggers the production of targeted antibodies, which are passed back to the baby through milk. That's why, when everyone else in the house gets ill, the nursing baby often gets a milder version of the illness, or is not ill at all. If the baby doesn't nurse directly, you can still get some of this protective effect as long as the person whose milk the baby gets spends time around the baby, coming into contact with the same germs.
3. **Human milk from another trusted source,** such as a registered milk bank, a wet nurse, or a milk donor. The baby won't get the

same protection from viruses as in the first two situations, but human milk still avoids many of the risks of formula. See Chapter 18, Milk Sharing.
4. **Formula.** For more about the differences between human milk and formula and between nursing directly and drinking expressed milk, see chapters 5 and 17. For more about bottles and other feeding tools, see chapters 5, 17, and 18.

Parenting (and Breastfeeding) as a Team

Most new mothers have partners. Many have others, such as grandparents, who share the baby's care. They might live with you or come and go. Whoever your support people are, working together to care for your baby may be the most important teamwork you ever do. When it works, it's hugely helpful for breastfeeding. Many describe their spouse, partner, or chosen co-parent as their most important breastfeeding supporter. Sometimes, though, co-parenting is more complicated. Adding a new child to a family can also bring extra stress as adults take on new responsibilities. Thinking ahead about how your parenting team will work is an investment in your family's future.

Keeping Yourself and Your Baby Safe

Close relationships are not always safe, for yourself or for your baby. The World Health Organization estimates that almost one in three women experiences violence from an intimate partner. The American College of Obstetricians and Gynecologists says that one in six abused women is first abused during pregnancy. If you are unsafe, you and your baby deserve help. Talk to your healthcare provider, a dedicated helpline, a domestic abuse organisation, or a trusted community leader.

For some couples, the first baby's arrival is the first time they haven't shared experiences as equals. Ivannia felt that her husband was missing out in the newborn period:

> I felt sorry for my husband because he felt lost in this new arithmetic of love. I wished he, too, had his support group of parents of breastfeeding

babies, because then maybe he would have understood the power of breastfeeding.

– *Ivannia, Costa Rica*

At first, babies tend to prefer their mother or primary caregiver. Their familiar smell, taste, sound, and feel are the new baby's safest place, especially when he is tired, hungry, uncomfortable, scared, or unhappy.

Fathers and Co-Parents (This Section Is for You)

You might be amazed at how much your baby will get from nursing. The breast is not just an alternative to a bottle. It's more like a Swiss Army knife: a multi-purpose tool that can calm, comfort, relax, and entertain your baby, soothe him to sleep and magically improve his mood. In the early days, some non-nursing parents wonder what they have to offer.

Rest assured; you are already important to your baby, and you'll become even more so as he grows. Children go through stages of intense interest in one parent, then the other. One day you will probably be his favourite person. In the meantime, there are already many things that you are best placed to do.

My husband has a unique relationship with his sons. . . . It is innate; he does not think about it. Each one has his own role; each one has his own strengths and resources; each one is unique, and so is each relationship. These differences are a richness for each of us. Breastfeeding doesn't take anything away from the dad; on the contrary, he discovers his own resources to build his own relationship with the baby, and he strengthens his confidence in his abilities as a dad.

– *Audrey, France*

Here are some ideas to support your partner while connecting deeply with your baby:

- **Calm the baby when she's upset but not hungry.** A baby who is "fed but frazzled" often settles more happily on a loved one who *doesn't* smell of milk!

- **"Wear" the baby.** Babywearing – carrying a baby in a sling or soft carrier – is great for babies' physical and mental development. Babies feel most secure when held close, and they love being on the move. As you hold the baby close, she'll probably be happier, and you'll learn your own ways to calm her.
- **Bathe the baby.** Being in the water is a great way to spend skin-to-skin time with your baby, especially if you shower or bathe *with* her!
- **Support the "nest."** Take on more household tasks or arrange for help while your partner adapts to their new role.
- **Encourage and affirm.** We all thrive on appreciation. If family members or others criticise or question parenting decisions, such as how your baby is fed, your partner needs to know they can rely on your support.
- **Call in reinforcements where needed.** You might already be an experienced parent of breastfed babies. Or you might love mastering a new skill and quickly become an accomplished breastfeeding helper! But if this is not you, don't panic. You're emotionally involved here, and you might not be best placed to assist with feeding issues. Help your partner find support, for example, by making, attending, and taking notes at appointments. About one in five women worldwide experiences depression in the year after giving birth. You are ideally placed to spot early signs of depression in your partner and help her find care. For more, see chapters 4, 5, and 18, Postnatal Mood Disorders.
- **Listen and talk.** This time just after your baby's birth is one of rapid learning and change – check in with each other often. What's working well, or not so well? Who needs what? What's urgent, and what can wait? When you're both tired, you might not always be your best selves. It can help to set some simple communication rules in advance, such as the following:
  o Let the other person talk until they've finished.
  o Assume good intent.
  o Offer advice only when asked.

One LLL member's agreement with her partner was that if they needed to discuss something difficult, they would hold hands while they talked. If you can stay connected while talking about the important stuff now, you will be excellent teachers for your child as she grows. If you find yourselves disagreeing strongly about things that matter, or if disagreements are distressing, it might be helpful to talk to a counsellor you both trust.

Strategic Helping

If you see your partner in pain or distress, it's natural to want to fix the situation quickly. Yet sometimes leaping in to help is *not* the most constructive response. For example, giving formula (or nursing the baby yourself – see the co-nursing section later in this chapter) early on can make it harder for a new mother to build her own milk supply. Here are some common suggestions that might or might not help, depending on your family's priorities.

- **Sharing feeding.** Although formula ads suggest otherwise, fathers and co-parents *don't* need to feed their babies to bond with them. It's not milk going into the baby that connects babies and parents; it's time spent touching, looking at, and enjoying each other. This happens without extra effort for the nursing mother, but partners can do it, too. Love doesn't always have to come with food. If you're thinking of giving a bottle because you're worried that nursing isn't going well, find breastfeeding help quickly. Most feeding problems are fixable, and the earlier you act, the easier it usually is to find a solution, or a workaround.

People insisted that Daddy wouldn't be able to bond because he can't feed the baby. A lot of nonsense, added extra pressure, mum guilt – but I stood my ground. He helped in many other ways, like taking care of the cooking.

– Lara, London, England

- **Taking the baby to give her a break.** Separations and missed feeds can complicate things for the new nursing mother. Breasts get full and uncomfortable. Supplementing or having someone else nurse the baby can reduce milk production. Nursing can be done lying down, while resting or dozing. For more about safe sleep, see Chapter 12. If you're worried that your partner is exhausted or overwhelmed, ask what *they* think would help. They might want some time alone; but if not, you can find other ways to give them the rest and support they need.

Co-Nursing

Co-nursing is when parents share the nursing of a baby – like Cyndel and her partner, Kendra:

Breastfeeding wasn't something new to me. I had breastfed Lennyx, our oldest. However, this time it wasn't me who was pregnant; my partner, Kendra, was pregnant. I was able to successfully relactate [start making milk again]. Though not even close to a full supply, I had enough milk to comfort Laveen when he was born. We developed a bit of a system. I knew that for Kendra's supply not to suffer, she would need to pump when I nursed him.

– Cyndel, Ontario, Canada

As Cyndel mentions, if you plan on sharing the nursing of your baby, it's important to understand how milk production works. If the birthing mother wants a full milk supply, she'll need to nurse as much as possible during the first month or so, while supply is still increasing (see Chapter 4).

And only the birthing mother makes colostrum – the immunity-boosting first milk (see Chapter 17). If you are relactating or inducing lactation (Chapter 17 explains how) to co-nurse your baby, you might focus on expressing during this crucial early period to build your own supply while your partner builds hers. Once your partner's milk supply is established, you can figure out the balance of nursing between you.

Other Than Parents

A dedicated support team of one is great, but a larger team is even better! Families benefit from the company, teaching, and caregiving of a community of trusted adults (and older children). Building your support team is a challenge if you live far away from extended family or move frequently. A bigger social circle can help in many ways.

> Our children's grandparents are lovely, but we don't live near them. I longed for the kind of care a nearby grandmother might have given our children – and me. So I adopted two "surrogate grannies." They were the main people who turned up at school events, helped out in emergencies, made me a meal, gave me a hug, and listened to my worries. I'm also delighted that my mum is a "surrogate granny" for a family in her own community. The different generations really need each other.
>
> – Clare, UK

Your Wider Community

Our ancestors brought up babies in communities, working alongside and helping one another. Mothers carried their nursing babies as they gathered food, did chores, and cared for older children. These older children learned to look after younger ones. Your baby doesn't know that he was born in the twenty-first century and not the Stone Age. You can see why one or two parents might feel outnumbered by one baby!

Some helpful things to know about a typical baby include the following:

- He is happier when he's being carried.
- He prefers being on the move to being still.
- He loves watching older children.
- He is often happier when his caregiver is in a friendly group rather than alone with the baby.

If you're outgoing, you might like a lot of company for yourself and your baby. If you enjoy solitude or dislike large gatherings, you might look for a small community. Tailor your network to your needs. Who will be in yours?

Filling in the Gaps: Patchworks of Support

Which of these statements best describes you?

- I have a strong sense of belonging, through family, culture, language, faith, local community. I know who I will be spending time with and can call on for help after my baby is born. They support breastfeeding.
- I have people who love and care for me, but they don't know much about breastfeeding, or they don't live nearby.
- My sense of belonging has been focused on work or study. I am not sure who I will spend time with or call on for help after my baby is born. I usually find information online.

Most new parents have support systems, but there might be gaps. A strong network is often made of many pieces joined together, like a patchwork quilt. The following sections describe some ways to fill gaps in your support quilt.

Virtual and Remote Support

When Diane's first baby was born in 1968, she was lucky to have a well-informed best friend:

> Without the help of my friend Sherry, and what she learned from La Leche League, I would never have been able to breastfeed. I still remember how desperate I was to breastfeed, and the wonderful feeling when I got the right information and help at just the right time.
>
> – Diane, California, United States

Early LLL Leaders helped new mothers by sending handwritten information through the post. We've moved on a lot since then! Some ways you can get help include:

- information searches online
- phone calls
- texts, emails, and messenger apps
- moderated chat groups

- video calls
- virtual group meetings

I attended a local Zoom support group, told them about my situation, cried, and an angel, Abbie, offered to lend me her pump. She came to my house, sat with me, and told me how to use it, all in the middle of the pandemic, through a face mask. I will never forget the support and solidarity I received from other breastfeeding mums.

– Mary, UK

Advantages of Virtual Support

- You're not limited by where you live or can travel to.
- You can access help 24/7.
- It might be easier to talk to people you don't know.
- You can connect with others in similar situations.

Getting the Most from Virtual Support

Make sure websites you use are trustworthy. Your best bet is a recommendation from someone you know and trust. Look for trusted credentials like LLL Leader or International Board Certified Lactation Consultant (IBCLC).

For some issues – perhaps your baby has a rare medical condition – national or international groups might be most helpful. Local parents are likely to be more helpful in finding local healthcare providers, activities, and places to meet other families.

Getting the Most from Your Healthcare Provider

As Tatjana found, getting the right information and support can transform your experience of having a baby:

In the eighth month of pregnancy with Stefan, I realised the light at the end of the tunnel – it was my doula! I thank her, to this day. Thanks to her commitment, and my great desire to succeed as a breastfeeding mother, Stefan is still nursing at fourteen months, in addition to three meals a day.

Doulas, breastfeeding counsellors/Leaders . . . there are so many wonderful, informative places – just look for them!

– *Tatjana, Serbia*

If you have any choice about your healthcare providers, you might want to look for these positive signs:

- **Baby-friendly designation.** This designation is awarded by the United Nations Children's Fund (UNICEF) to birth facilities that provide excellent basic feeding support (see Chapter 3).
- **Spaces free from commercial advertising.** The World Health Organization's International Code on the Marketing of Breast-Milk Substitutes is intended to prevent unethical formula marketing. It states that healthcare providers shouldn't display formula company advertising and shouldn't give out free samples. A healthcare office that offers free formula samples and advertising materials may not give unbiased care.
- **People you like and trust.** Look for those whose approach and experience are a good match for yours, as Natalie did:

I didn't imagine the challenges of a breastfeeding journey, or the difficult journey we would go through to become mothers via a fertility clinic (as an LGBTQIA+ two-mum family). The local postnatal lactation support team . . . in our small rural town . . . called shortly after we got home from the hospital to offer free support for breastfeeding. We were surrounded by a team of progressive female doctors and nurses. The quality of support we had in our small town of twenty thousand was pretty unreal, in a very good way.

– *Natalie, Canada*

For more about choosing a place to give birth, see Chapter 3.

How La Leche League Can Help

We're here to serve any family interested in nursing or providing human milk for their babies – whatever that looks like for you. All our services are free and provided by trained volunteers, who have all nursed or provided milk for their own babies. We'd be delighted to be part of your patchwork of support. There are many ways you can connect with us:

- If you already have a great support network, maybe you won't need anything from us except to dip in to this book from time to time! We publish other books, too, and much more breastfeeding information online, in many languages.
- In some areas, LLL offers antenatal classes for expectant parents to learn the basics of getting started with breastfeeding.
- LLL Leaders (breastfeeding counsellors) can support you by phone, messenger app, video call, etc., at any stage from pregnancy through the end of breastfeeding. Start at www.llli.org to see what's available in your area.
- If we don't yet have LLL in your area, you can still get help from our international social media, including virtual online meetings.

Karina was able to get support from LLL on a different continent when she gave birth far from home:

> I lived in Vietnam when I had my first baby. No one could really help me with breastfeeding until I contacted an LLL volunteer in Germany, my home country. The information from LLL made all the difference to me. Most of all, I loved the fact that the LLL solutions were free – they didn't suggest buying expensive supplies or equipment of any kind. I was so surprised, and I felt really taken seriously.
> – Karina, Germany

Our in-person support group meetings have been the cornerstone of LLL since the 1950s, and at the time of this writing they provide mutual support and a sense of belonging for families in more than eighty countries. We often describe an LLL meeting as a "buffet meal" – take any ideas you think will work for you and leave the rest behind.

What I was really grateful for was already having this support system [local LLL group] in place when I unexpectedly had a neonatal intensive care unit (NICU) stay with my second baby. Instead of trying to figure out my next steps during this difficult, stressful time, I was able to easily send a quick group message to all my Leader friends. In the middle of the night, as I sat in the dark hospital room pumping, they sent messages with support, encouragement, and helpful resources.
– Olivia, Canada

At La Leche League meetings, you can be encouraged and supported by:

- watching others as they nurse and care for their babies
- listening to their experiences and ideas
- asking questions
- borrowing books and other resources
- sharing how things are going for you in an accepting, nonjudgmental space
- figuring out what's normal baby behaviour and what might need attention
- problem-solving breastfeeding issues
- making friends with other families, who might be similar to you or very different
- learning from those who have more experience than you do and supporting those who have less

La Leche League friends can last a lifetime.

We're working hard to reach all parents who might benefit from our services, wherever they live, whatever their families look like, and however they prefer to get their breastfeeding support. We welcome feedback on how we can do better, and we welcome new volunteer LLL Leaders from all communities. We would love to meet you and your baby!

Want to know more?

You can find extra resources for this chapter
at the "Art of Breastfeeding" tab at
www.llli.org.

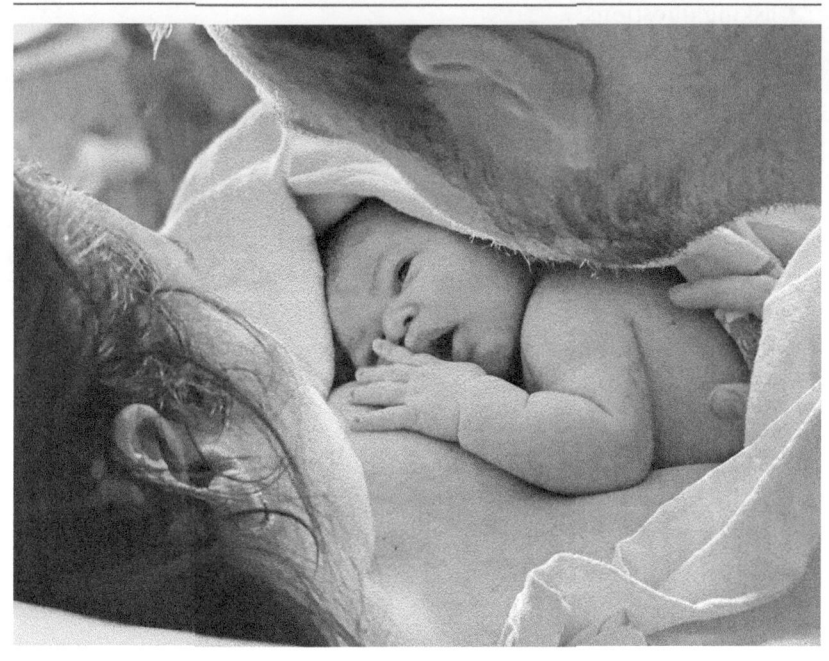

THREE

Birth!

> It was so incredible to me that a new being was created inside me. . . . I had given life. No one can imagine it until they live it, no matter how much you read stories about it. Every mother has her own story, each mother has a lot to tell. As a mother, I have thousands of stories to tell you.
> – Guajirita Alquizareña, from Cuba, living in the Netherlands

The Language of Birth

This chapter includes (and explains) a lot of birth-related words you won't hear every day. Birth has a whole language of its own! You may find it helpful to become familiar with the words your caregivers might use; the more you understand what's going on during your labour and birth, or what's being suggested to you, the more power you have to make the best choices you can.

Congratulations! You're going to have a baby (or babies!). This might be something you've waited and longed for, dreamed about.... Or perhaps it's a surprise, and you're not quite sure how you feel about that. Connecting with others who've already been through birth and the early days with a new baby can help you prepare for what's ahead.

How a baby is born has a big impact on how easy, or difficult, it can be to get breastfeeding started. Babies whose births were more complicated or difficult tend to take a bit longer to get going with breastfeeding – but they do get there. If you're going to be nursing a baby birthed by someone else, you might also find it helpful to understand how birth affects babies and what your baby expects as she arrives in the world.

For Clare, birth was an intensely joyful experience:

> I'd heard a lot of birth stories and was prepared for the worst. But my birth was easy (which doesn't mean it wasn't really hard work!). I wasn't scared during it, I had great support from the midwives, and I felt proud afterwards. And my baby was so beautiful! I was overjoyed to have her in my arms at last. Even though I was tired and a bit sore, I felt ecstatic for days afterwards, like I was walking on air. I couldn't stop smiling.
> – Clare, UK

Louise's second birth happened at home:

> I had my husband and official midwife present, but also a doula and two close friends. I felt safe, loved, and happy, and in between contractions we laughed a lot, and during contractions there were a lot of hands to take turns to squeeze. I got into the pool at the point where I felt so much pressure in my bottom, I was convinced that if my waters broke, my baby would come surfing out, and sure enough, there was a big "pop" and he was coming. In those final minutes I roared him out, wondering why this felt more intense than my first birth, but then as I pulled him out of the water, we realised why – he was a full kilogram heavier! We had our first feed snuggled on our sofa, eating the best toast ever. It was magic.
> – Louise, UK

Louise would be the first to acknowledge that she had a lot of factors working in her favour.

Many of us who are waiting to give birth have fewer resources and more complications. You may or may not have much choice about where you give birth, and who is with you when you do. There are many reasons why you might need, or prefer, your birth to look very different from Louise's. Whatever kind of birth brings them into the world, *all* babies are born expecting to breastfeed. But some need a little extra help and patience.

Preparing for Birth, Preparing to Breastfeed

Often when you're pregnant, especially if it's a first pregnancy, the birth looms so big in your mind that it's hard to think past it. Christina's experience is common:

> During my first pregnancy, I was very much preoccupied with the imminent delivery, but did not bother too much about what would happen afterwards.
> – *Christina, Germany*

Yet labour, birth, and the interventions you or your baby might experience can have a big impact on the beginning of breastfeeding, as Mandy remembers:

> First-time mum, so delighted to be pregnant but scared for the labour. Instructed to schedule the birth. Intervention after intervention, when will this end? Regret. Joy. Pain. Elation. A beautiful baby girl, who has her first feed with me. Cuddles. Delight. Then turmoil. Why can't I do it? Am I a good mother? Shame and regret and indecision. No matter what I tried: latching, relatching, asking others, borrowing pumps, struggling to understand what I actually needed to do to feed my baby properly.
>
> However, the second time round I was determined to have the information I needed. I had watched other mums breastfeed. I reached out for support, learned new things. I was ready this time to recognise it is hard but know where to reach out and take all the support I could get. I believe my birthing experience this time helped. Minimal intervention (even though it was heavily suggested) this time. I felt strong, empowered even. It hasn't been an easy journey. I understand that now, as a breastfeeding mother. I've let go of the guilt from not being able to feed my first baby as I had hoped. It's taken time and healing.
> – *Mandy, Northern Ireland*

Breastfeeding is likely to begin more smoothly if, before your baby arrives, you can do these things:

- *Inform* yourself about labour, birth, and the various interventions. You could read books, listen to podcasts, watch videos, and talk to friends who've already given birth.

- *Take* a childbirth class (in person or online) to prepare you for handling all kinds of labours and births. Most classes encourage you to attend with your partner or birth supporter.

Lola found her class had more impact than she expected:

I signed us up for a birthing and breastfeeding class alongside other couples entering the parenting role. Initially, my husband resisted attending because it was set for an entire weekend bootcamp. He didn't want to wake up early on a Saturday. Who does? We found the right place on the most comfortable sofa and were ready to learn alongside other new parents.

I still don't know exactly what did the trick for my husband during that intense weekend of learning. Was it the feeling of the place? Was it the ease of the instructor navigating complex topics? Was it the new knowledge he got that weekend? Or the lentil soup she made for us for lunch? That weekend was a life-changer. My husband became my biggest supporter and cheerleader during the birth and through the years of breastfeeding.

– Lola, Israel

Clare attended different kinds of classes with her second baby:

I went to classes that were based on movement (a kind of gentle yoga), and I found these even more helpful. We practised some possible positions for birth, like leaning forward over an exercise ball, and thought a lot about how it feels, rather than just getting information. I was absolutely rubbish at the yoga part – I'd never done it before, my balances were always wobbly, and I wasn't very flexible. But it really didn't matter.

I'm sure some of this is luck; I'm healthy, have a normal-sized pelvis, and had no pregnancy complications. But I do think that learning to relax into the process, letting my body do what it knew how to do, was hugely helpful. If you're not scared of birth, you can let go, open up, and let the baby out. If you're frightened or tense, everything closes up. I learned to stay upright and use visualisations, like letting the contractions break over me like waves. And some great little tricks, like relaxing your face – for some reason, if you can do that, it relaxes the other end of you as well! I went into birth feeling confident. My baby was born at home, and it was one of the most wonderful experiences of my life. I felt so powerful afterwards – it was amazing.

– Clare, UK

- *Find* a birth supporter you like and trust.

A La Leche League meeting can be a good place to start. Attending a meeting, or joining an online group, before your baby is born connects you immediately with other parents and parents-to-be. Then all you have to do is ask, "Do you know any good birth resources around here?"

Doulas and Birth Supporters

Research strongly suggests that one of the best ways to improve your labour and birth experience is to have the support of a trained doula (a person who provides practical and emotional support through labour and birth and/or after birth). Note that doulas are not medically trained. If having a doula isn't possible, then having a friend or family member with you, specifically to provide support, is also beneficial. This is in *addition* to your partner, if you have one. Giving you all the support you need is a tough call for your partner, because they may be doing this for the first time – like you! – and will be emotionally caught up in the experience.

As Clare found, a good doula will help as needed with older children, back massages, and muffins!

> I gave birth to my third child in my kitchen, in the middle of a batch of muffins. That's to say, the muffins went in the oven shortly before the baby arrived, and came out in time to feed the hungry midwives afterwards! I'd woken up that morning feeling restless, with an idea the baby might be arriving soon (though she wasn't due for nearly two weeks) and went into cooking overdrive. By the time the midwife arrived, around 9:30 A.M., I'd already made pasta sauce, bread, and chocolate cake. (Later, the midwife told me I was the only woman she'd ever seen wearing an apron at 7 cm dilated.) Staying upright and keeping moving probably helped get the baby out easily.
>
> I laboured in a birth pool in the middle of the kitchen, from which I issued cooking instructions. We had hired a doula, which turned out to be a great move – she helped my eldest child finish off the muffins when the contractions got too strong for me to carry on and massaged my lower back during each contraction, getting soaked in the process. (Apparently, with no sense of irony, I was shouting "Push *harder!*" at her every time.) The baby was born around 11:30, making it my most productive morning ever.
>
> – Clare, UK

If you give birth with the support of a trained doula, you're less likely to

- have an instrumental delivery (with forceps or vacuum extraction)
- use pain medication
- have a caesarean birth
- have a baby with a low five-minute Apgar score

INSTRUMENTAL DELIVERY: a health professional uses tools to help get the baby out.

FORCEPS: a metal tool that fits around the baby's head and is used to help the final stages of pushing, to move the baby down the birth canal to be born.

VACUUM EXTRACTION: a soft cup, with a handle and vacuum pump, applied to the baby's head to help the final stages of pushing, to move the baby down the birth canal to be born.

APGAR SCORE: the scale used when babies' health and well-being are assessed at birth and shortly afterwards.

Having a support person besides your partner during labour means you're more likely to feel satisfied with your birth experience. You're also more likely to start breastfeeding – even if the support person knows nothing at all about breastfeeding!

One of the most important tasks of a doula or birth supporter is to speak up on your behalf. Even if you're usually really good at communicating what you need, this may be more difficult when you're busy labouring, especially if you're in an unfamiliar place. A birth supporter can help advocate for your needs, especially if any of the following situations are true of you:

- You are going to be labouring (and parenting) alone.
- You have disabilities or communication challenges.
- You are part of a minority racial or ethnic group, especially in countries where there is a large gap in birth outcomes between majority and minority groups.
- You are LGBTQIA+, particularly if you are a transgender man giving birth.
- You have experienced trauma or abuse as a child, had a traumatic previous birth, or had another traumatic experience, such as a sexual assault, in your life.
- You have concerns that your voice may not be heard for any other reason.

> To this day, many Indigenous people, women and trans men in particular, fear taking ourselves or our babies to doctors and hospitals. Especially in the past two hundred years, we have been taught to sit down and not talk; to listen and obey. We have been unethically studied.
> — *Stephanie, Six Nations of the Grand River, Ontario, Canada*

If you're Deaf/deaf or hearing impaired and reliant on lip-reading, for example, your doula can remind staff to remove their masks or wear masks you can see through. A support person can help you understand what's going on and communicate your questions to staff if you don't speak the language fluently or find it hard to talk when you're overwhelmed. It's not helpful to be referred to as mum when you identify as dad, or to have to field questions about where the baby's father is when you're single or have a wife or female partner.

To find a qualified doula, check out doula websites for your area or ask around in your community for recommendations. Some doulas provide free or low-cost services for expectant parents who need them. If it's not possible to get the support of a formally trained doula, a friend or family member might fill that role.

Birth Decisions: Who and Where?

If you have any choice (and we know you might not!), you might be choosing between obstetricians, between a family doctor and a midwife, or between various midwifery practices. Your place-of-birth options may be home, birthing centre, or hospital. These decisions can make a difference in how easily breastfeeding happens, as Keiko found:

> I gave birth to my first and second babies at a large, public general hospital. I had a really tough time at the beginning, as mother and baby were kept apart in separate rooms, and I was supplementing the feeds by bottle-feeding expressed breastmilk. The story was completely different with my third and fourth babies, who were born after I had gained knowledge about breastfeeding from La Leche League. Parenting through breastfeeding was really enjoyable and felt easy, and I was shocked at how different things could be. I gave birth to my third child at a maternity clinic where mother

and baby were kept in the same room and bottles were not used. With my fourth child, I chose to give birth at home.

In Japan, the fraction of hospitals embracing the Baby-Friendly Hospital Initiative is unfortunately very low, at just a few percent, and the number of birthing centres is also very small. As was the case for me, most of those giving birth today have never seen a breastfeeding baby. Even if you felt you wanted to breastfeed, how easy would it be to say "I can do this!" about something that you've never seen done? I think it would be pretty hard. I wish for birthing facility policies to change in ways that will make breastfeeding more feasible.

– Keiko, Japan

The Baby-Friendly Hospital Initiative

In 1991, the World Health Organization and UNICEF sought to improve feeding support for all families by outlining Ten Steps to Successful Breastfeeding and urging all maternity facilities around the world to follow these steps and achieve Baby-Friendly accreditation. Over 10 percent of facilities in 168 countries have been certified. Is your facility one of them?

As Gabriela found, giving birth in a setting that's Baby-Friendly certified can make a real difference in your experience:

I had my first child at seventeen, and I would have loved to hear someone tell me that no matter your age, you are a mum now, and motherhood brings a huge gift: wisdom in just the right measure, that dictates from the heart what is best for your baby. I would have loved for them to share the Ten Steps to Successful Breastfeeding video with me and tell me that yes, I can! Get informed, Mum, you can do it!

– Gabriela, Ecuador

Choosing a Caregiver

Confused about who's who? Here are some basics to help you decide who to have care for you during your pregnancy and birth:

- **Midwives** most often work with uncomplicated pregnancies. In some places, they work under the supervision of doctors and in others they may involve a doctor if there are problems with the pregnancy or labour. Midwives provide emotional support as well as practical care for labour and birth. Most home births involve midwives; other midwives are hospital-based or work in birth centres.
- Depending on where you live, **family doctors** (called **general practice physicians** in some places) might attend births. Family doctors are less likely than obstetricians to intervene in the birth process, and they provide continuity of care for both you and your baby. Many give excellent care for uncomplicated pregnancies and births. In some areas they provide backup services for home births.
- **Obstetricians** are experts in the complications of pregnancy and birth, though they may have little experience with unmedicated birth. Midwives and family doctors will refer to an obstetrician if there are concerns. In some places you might see an obstetrician as your primary doctor for the pregnancy and birth even if there are no concerns.

If you or your baby have any known complications, you might be advised to give birth in a facility that provides a higher level of medical care. This happened for Laura:

> My daughter, Quinn, was diagnosed with a tumour on her lung at thirty-six weeks gestation on a routine ultrasound. Prior to this diagnosis, my doctors and I had planned for a normal vaginal birth. Between thirty-six and thirty-nine weeks gestation, we had met with two MFM doctors [maternal-foetal medicine specialists for high-risk pregnancies] and decided we would be travelling over three hundred miles to a world-renowned children's hospital to get care.
>
> – Laura, United States military

Many doctors (even those who work with newborn babies) don't have a lot of training about breastfeeding. But some are very supportive. Having a healthcare provider who understands the value of breastfeeding – and the importance of human milk – can be hugely helpful. Wendy, Theresa, and Gisel describe very different experiences:

My third pregnancy was very complicated.... I was in bed most of the time. After birth I tried to breastfeed, but my baby always suffered from severe pain in his stomach, and the paediatrician said it was because of my milk. I chose to give... formula. I long for that bond that is created between baby and mother when breastfeeding. I feel I should have insisted a little more for my baby, and I will always doubt if I did the right thing.
– Wendy, Mexico

At the hospital, a doctor told me no one could fully breastfeed twins. But it worked, and now I have been breastfeeding both of them for over two years.
– Theresa, Germany

My gynaecologist was a key piece; when I went to my post-op appointment, he asked me how I fed my baby, and my answer was breastfeeding. [He said,] "Congratulations – keep it up! Remember, there is nothing better than your milk to feed her."
– Gisel, Mexico

GYNAECOLOGIST: a doctor who specialises in women's reproductive health. Many gynaecologists are also obstetricians (they might use the abbreviation ob-gyn).

Choosing a Setting: Home, Birth Centre, Hospital?

It's been said that the first intervention in modern birth is leaving home. Research finds that home birth is just as safe as hospital birth for low-risk pregnancies, with lower rates of interventions and higher rates of breastfeeding. Midwives and doctors who attend home births are skilled in handling common problems. A hospital has more resources for overcoming more complex problems... but the hospital environment is what causes some of those problems in the first place.

Check out all the birth options available to you in your community. If possible, talk to parents who have had babies in more than one setting (usually easy to find at LLL meetings), and ask what differences they experienced in the birth, in breastfeeding, and in their relationships with their children. Find out what breastfeeding support will be available and when.

Changing Your Mind

Almost any birth decision can be changed at just about any time. You can change your planned place of birth or caregiver in your last month of pregnancy or even during labour. Trust your feelings. You don't owe people and places your loyalty; you owe yourself and your baby peace of mind. We know of mothers who'd planned to give birth at home but suddenly felt a strong urge to go to the hospital – and it turned out that was exactly where they needed to be. Parenting involves some very effective instincts; this may be the first one kicking in.

As Dawn found, births can sometimes hit unexpected snags. Good support makes a big difference, however your birth goes:

When my first son was born, he had quite a significant shoulder dystocia [the baby's head had been born but his shoulders got stuck]. This led to him requiring a full resuscitation, with an initial Apgar [score] of 0. The recommendation from the paediatrician was to send him to the NICU [neonatal intensive care unit, a special area of the hospital for newborn babies who need the most medical support] for hypothermia treatment, as he was having seizures. This meant he was placed on a cooling mat, which lowered his temperature into hypothermia for three days, another day to slowly increase it back to normal range, and then one day of observations before I could hold him or feed him for the first time. During this time, I was pumping every three hours and storing the pumped milk in the NICU freezer. I was very fortunate that my sister-in-law was a La Leche League Leader in a different province and was able to send me tips for pumping. I also was supported by a lovely NICU lactation consultant.

– *Dawn, British Columbia, Canada*

For more about NICU care, see Chapter 17.

Home
At home, you get to decide who will be with you for the birth. You may want just your partner and your midwife. You might like to have supportive family and friends around and feel safest and most protected within a fairly large group. And you may change your mind as labour progresses – it's okay to ask people to leave if you do.

Christina describes breastfeeding after having her second baby at home:

> The very first time breastfeeding our second daughter, right after giving birth at home, felt very different than I expected (and different than the first breastfeeding experience with my older daughter). It felt totally natural – like two matching puzzle pieces.
>
> – Christina, Germany

Clare's second baby was born at home, and for her one of the benefits was having her older daughter present for the birth:

> Our eldest wasn't quite three when our next baby was due to arrive, and we didn't have extended family around to help. This was one of the reasons we decided to have a home birth, so we could stay at home with her. It was about ten days before my due date, and a very hot day. In the afternoon, I took my daughter swimming at the local pool with some close friends. My heavy body felt almost weightless in the water. As we were getting dressed afterwards, I mentioned to my friends that I had a bit of a backache. They soon pointed out that it seemed to be coming every few minutes, and it really might be a good idea to go home *now*!
>
> Luckily it was a very short drive – the baby arrived less than four hours later. I laboured in a birth pool in our living room while our daughter ate her dinner. A midwife arrived, then a second one. At the moment when the baby was actually born, everyone (including our daughter) was crowded round the birthing pool to watch her come out. It was a wonderful day, filled with sunshine, water, and people I loved. By my usual bedtime, I was snuggled up in my own bed with my new baby. I hope that if my oldest daughter ever has children of her own, she will feel confident to give birth, because she knows it's a normal thing to do.
>
> – Clare, UK

There are no institutional routines to separate you and your baby after a birth at home, which helps in establishing breastfeeding. Sometimes, though, grandmothers, visitors, or even older children can end up "taking over" the baby. Right now your baby needs you most (and is safer from infection if she's not being passed around).

Birth Centres

Birth centres (sometimes called birth clinics) mean leaving home, but they are designed to recapture the course of normal birth after that first intervention. They can manage many types of complications while providing a homey atmosphere within a medical setting. The birth centre may be where you receive your antenatal care so you will become familiar with it. If not, ask for a antenatal tour, or at least a virtual one, to see where your baby will be born. Ask questions about whether options you're interested in – such as labouring in water – are available, and what help there is for getting breastfeeding underway.

Hospitals

Hospitals can also provide positive birth experiences and may be the safest places for higher-risk pregnancies and births. However, in a hospital one seemingly minor intervention can lead to another, and then another, turning what might have been a straightforward birth into something more complicated, as Sara Diana found:

> I was exactly forty weeks pregnant, and suddenly contractions started. It was my first pregnancy, but the moment the contractions started, I knew it was time. Several hours later, we headed to the hospital. The car trip itself was a nightmare – twenty minutes in the car, not being able to move as I wanted – it was really hard. When we arrived, we were assigned a private space to wait for the obstetrician. There, I started to feel stronger contractions, and even the feeling of pushing a little bit. I was doing well; I tried to disconnect from the world with each one and move freely. I forced myself to be in a "Zen" mood. And I believe I was getting it!
>
> The contractions were getting really strong. Then the obstetrician arrived and told me he had to do a vaginal exam. I didn't want it at all but didn't oppose it as it was my first birth, and I didn't know what to expect. With the vaginal exam, the nightmare came back at an even higher level. It was soooo painful! The doctor told me that my cervical dilation was only four centimeters and that it could take another few hours until it reached ten centimeters. And he asked me what I wanted to do. The shock and the pain prompted me to say, "I want an epidural – I can't bear this any longer!"
>
> With my second son I had a vaginal delivery without anaesthesia, and today I know that with my first, we were almost there – we only needed two or three hours more to have an easy vaginal delivery. If I had been able

to trust my instincts at that moment, I would have had my baby in my arms without further complications.

My first baby was born exhausted; he latched, but without energy. It was hard at the beginning; I had to fight hard to establish breastfeeding. I believe that because he was my first baby, I felt insecure, and one thing led to another: vaginal exam, epidural, contractions stopping, synthetic oxytocin, membranes being broken, caesarean section, breastfeeding problem.

– *Sara Diana, from Barcelona, living in Mexico*

CONTRACTIONS: the muscles of the uterus tightening and relaxing in powerful surges, moving the baby down the birth canal.
VAGINAL EXAM: a healthcare provider puts their fingers into the vagina to feel how open the cervix is.
CERVICAL DILATION: the cervix (the "neck" of the womb, the lowest part) opening during labour to let the baby out. Dilation is measured in centimeters. "Fully dilated" is about ten centimeters.
ANAESTHESIA: medication that blocks pain.
EPIDURAL: pain-relieving medication injected into the space around the spinal cord.
SYNTHETIC OXYTOCIN: an artificial form of the hormone oxytocin, given to restart contractions or make them stronger. Contractions stimulated by oxytocin tend to be stronger, longer, and closer together than normal contractions, and synthetic oxytocin doesn't have the same calming, pain-relieving effect on the brain.
MEMBRANES: also called the "amniotic sac" – the bag of fluid ("waters") that the baby is in. Membranes usually (though not always) break by themselves, before or during labour. Breaking them ("artificial rupture of membranes") can be done deliberately to begin or speed up labour.

Here are some ideas that can be helpful in reducing interventions, especially if you're giving birth away from home. You might not have all these choices available to you. In some countries you have an absolute right to refuse any medical procedure you don't want, while in others certain interventions may be non-negotiable in the facility you've chosen, or you may be told that to refuse a procedure would result in your medical insurance not covering your stay. Ask about your legal rights. Our aim is to equip you to make decisions within the constraints of your situation. Here are some ideas:

- **Protect your privacy.** Treat the room you're in as your (temporary) home. Keep the door at least partly closed and have your labour support person "approve" anyone who comes in, or at least ask them to introduce themselves and explain what they're doing. Bring your favourite music. Put up your own pictures. Wear your own clothes (with warm socks if the room is cool).
- **Stay on your feet.** For as long as you can. Walking helps your baby get in a good position for birth and keeps labour going. An exercise ball can be useful to sit or lean on. Wander the halls or go outdoors with your partner or supporter.
- **Cover the clock.** When labour really gets going, you won't care much about time anyway.
- **Question the need for routine vaginal examinations.** These examinations can increase the risk of infection and cause you stress. You'll know when you feel like pushing! But you can also ask to have a vaginal examination if knowing how much your cervix has dilated would help you decide whether to have a particular intervention.

How staff members interact with you can make a big difference in your experience:

> At almost six o'clock in the morning I felt a rumbling inside, and I realised that my waters had broken. But the doctor told me that I had to wait to see how things evolved. After my waters broke, my contractions began to intensify, and when they examined me at eight in the morning, I was six centimeters dilated. At that moment I really believed that with each contraction and pushing, I could not go on. I am very grateful to the doctor who touched me; she spoke to me by name, and that helped me to be able to continue.
>
> – *Guajirita Alquizareña, from Cuba, living in the Netherlands*

- The **bathroom** can be a good place to labour. Try sitting backward on the toilet, resting your head on your arms. We're used to relaxing and opening up on a toilet. Your partner or support person can massage your lower back in this position, too.
- **Get yourself into warm water.** A shower can help you relax. Soaking up to your neck in a bath can be an amazing comfort, and both can be great for pain relief. Some hospitals and birth centres have birth pools specially designed for labour. It's safe for babies

to be born underwater if there are no complications – they don't start to breathe until they come out into the air. Some families borrow, rent, or buy a birth pool to use at home.
- **Remember that the staff are there to support you,** so let them know what you need – like extra pillows, a darkened room, or closed door.
- **Ask the medical staff not to offer you medication** or an epidural. If you want pain relief, you can ask. Plan with your birth supporter to suggest other comfort measures.
- **Gravity can help** if you find a comfortable upright or side-lying position for pushing, where your sacrum (the large triangular bone at the base of your spine) is free to move, allowing your baby plenty of space for birth. Gravity will work against you if you lie flat on your back (you'll have to push the baby uphill and the sacrum will get in the way). You can also give birth squatting, standing, or kneeling with support. You might want to practise some of these positions with a doula or supporter beforehand.

After Your Baby Is Born: Keeping It Simple

After birth, keep your baby with you, on your body, bare skin against bare skin, at least until after he has that first nursing, which could continue off and on for several hours.

Anita had great support to do this immediately after her birth:

> The nurses were very good and positive, and they gave me lots of advice, even though they knew I had four other children. I knew more with Mohamed, and he fit right on the breast. He was a hungry little man and just started right away while we were still in the little room where he was born.
>
> – Anita, Sierra Leone

There's abundant research to support the importance of skin-to-skin contact immediately after birth and during the hours that follow. It helps with breastfeeding and with keeping your baby warm, calm, and protected from infection – which in turn will minimise a host of other problems. Sometimes, though, hospital routines can get in the way, as they did for Shoko when her baby was presented to her fully dressed:

When I was reunited with my newborn baby after an operation to have my retained placenta removed, he was snugly wrapped up in two layers of clothing plus a hat, and in my exhausted state I just accepted this clothed-baby situation as the status quo.... After all, why wouldn't a baby be clothed just as we are (with the addition of a hat)? There was no question that the baby wouldn't be in the transparent box next to my bed whenever I wasn't feeding, being kept warm by his clothes, blankets, and special hot-water bottles for babies (the last being so typical in the Netherlands that they are listed as something you are expected to have at home in preparation for your baby's arrival). All of this being presented as standard meant that it simply didn't occur to me to question any of it.

– *Shoko, the Netherlands*

Even after the first few hours, your baby will be happiest and healthiest in your arms, next to your body, or on another adult's body, 24/7. Skin-to-skin contact after birth helps protect you from excessive bleeding, too. And it can feel wonderful!

Another of the moments that caused me the most happiness and amazement was when they put my son to the breast for the first time; almost with his eyes closed, he knew how to find the nipple, latched on quickly, and sucked very hard. That filled me with peace and love; everything around me ceased to exist, and only he and I were enjoying our first time together.

– *Guajirita Alquizareña, from Cuba, living in the Netherlands*

Almost any measurements or procedures, except for weighing and surgery, can be done while your baby lies on you, even if the hospital staff are not used to doing things that way. The sooner you're home, the sooner you can do things your way. On the other hand, if you're needing help getting comfortably positioned for feeding, and you're getting good help where you are, you might prefer to stay a little longer. Again, follow your instincts, and don't be afraid to ask for what you need. Most caregivers want to help!

How Birth Interventions Can Affect Breastfeeding

The various medical interventions during labour and birth can make breastfeeding more challenging at first – as Cindy found:

> I gave birth to a little boy named Elios, with a deep desire to breastfeed after having seen my mother breastfeed my little brother for two years. Unfortunately, after many pitfalls (induction, long birth, incubator, jaundice…) it took us a long time before our milky adventure finally became enjoyable! After the rain, there is always good weather; we are now at two years and three months of breastfeeding!
> – Cindy, France

Our goal in sharing this information is *not* to make you feel bad if you choose, or end up having, an epidural or a caesarean birth, or anything else. An intervention can be the best possible choice when the potential risks are weighed against the potential benefits. And everyone has to weigh those up for their own situation. What we hope to do is prepare you to make more informed decisions, and to have the information you need to be able to deal with any challenges.

Induction

When labour doesn't start as expected, or if there are complications, or sometimes simply for convenience, your doctor or midwife may recommend **induction of labour** (labour is started off artificially, by a health professional).

B.J. found herself in this situation:

> I ended up ill with pre-eclampsia with our first daughter and needed to be induced. The speedy birth led to me requiring surgery afterwards, so I was whisked away. My wife held our daughter and fended off midwives who were eager to give the baby formula right away. My wife, Fi, knew that I wanted to try breastfeeding and she understood that if we allowed bottles from the start, this would interfere with my wishes. Fi brought the baby to me as soon as I got to the recovery room, and our breastfeeding relationship started in earnest.
> – B.J., England

How can induction affect breastfeeding?

- Induction of any type tends to **increase the need for pain medication** because contractions often start out quite strong and you don't have time to build up to them.

- If the amniotic sac is broken to help get labour going (**artificial rupture of membranes**), the **risk of infection** increases.
- **The baby's heart rate is more likely to show signs of stress,** increasing the chance of you needing an emergency caesarean.
- Depending on when the induction is done, **your baby may be born a bit early,** so getting breastfeeding going may take some extra effort.
- If you have **IV** synthetic oxytocin (intravenous medication given directly into a vein), the added fluids can cause **more breast engorgement** (*extra fluid, in this case, in the breasts*) a few days after the baby is born, causing discomfort and making it harder for the baby to latch on and get milk. Some engorgement is normal, but IV fluids have been shown to increase it. For what to do if you get engorged, see Chapter 18, Engorgement.
- **Added fluids also increase your baby's weight** at birth. Then, when the baby wees away that extra fluid during the first few days, it looks as though she's lost too much weight. Supplementation with formula may be recommended, even if it's not really needed. Some researchers have suggested calculating the baby's weight loss based on their weight at twenty-four hours, rather than at birth, to give a more accurate picture.

Epidural Pain Relief

Epidural anaesthetic in labour is very popular in some communities. Sixty percent of those giving birth in the United States currently have an epidural, compared with 30 percent in the UK, where most births are attended by midwives. And epidurals are popular for good reason: they can completely block the pain of labour while leaving you awake and aware, so that you experience the moment your baby is born. But – you probably knew this was coming – epidurals can negatively affect breastfeeding in these ways:

- When you have an epidural, there is a risk that **your blood pressure will drop.** To prevent that, you need intravenous fluids. As mentioned in the previous section, this can cause breast engorgement and artificially inflate your baby's birth weight.
- Research has shown that **babies are more likely to be in less desirable positions for birth** after an epidural because you're not able to move around. Difficult positions for birth increase the

need for vacuum extractions, forceps, and C-sections. These in turn can affect breastfeeding.
- **The medication given in the epidural reaches your baby** (through the placenta) and might affect his ability to find the breast, latch, and suck effectively, especially after higher doses of anaesthetic. (Research findings in this area are mixed, however; some studies find no difference.)

Cutting the Umbilical Cord Immediately

Full-term babies are normally born with a good amount of iron stored up if the **umbilical cord** (the tube that connects the unborn baby to her mother, providing oxygen and food) is cut after it stops pulsating. What does this have to do with breastfeeding? Doctors sometimes recommend supplementing breastfeeding with formula because it has a lot of iron. But if your baby was born at full term and the cord wasn't cut prematurely, her iron stores will usually be sufficient until she starts eating family foods. For more about iron, see Chapter 8.

Caesarean Birth

In some countries, a majority of babies are now born by C-section. Wherever you live, a C-section is a possibility that you need to consider and plan for. Caesarean birth can be a lovely experience, as it was for Gisel:

> We started our successful breastfeeding the same day my tenderness was born. Her name is Angela, and her arrival in this world was by scheduled caesarean section. She was born at 9:00 A.M., but her first feeding was an hour later, because there was a small problem and we had to make sure that my daughter's health had not been affected. That's why at first they only showed her to me, I kissed her, and they took her to the paediatrician. When they had finished checking her and me, the nurse put her on my chest. Finally, I latched her to my chest as if the nine months in my belly had been training. One of the times that she let go, a drop of superyellow milk ran down her cheek and I said, "Of course, as long as it comes out, it doesn't matter that it was a caesarean section."
>
> – Gisel, Mexico

The effects of medications and IV fluids given during a C-section and the difficulty in finding comfortable positions for breastfeeding when your abdomen is tender from surgery, can make breastfeeding more difficult. And it's challenging to recover from major surgery and look after a new baby at the same time. This doesn't mean that you can't breastfeed after a C-section – many, many of us have! – but if you can safely avoid one, it's worth considering.

The evidence is stacking up that caesarean birth may have potential long-term health effects, too. Babies born by C-section have higher rates of obesity, allergy, eczema, asthma, diabetes, and other autoimmune conditions. Some researchers think the difference in the babies' gut microbiomes may play a role.

All of us have microbes (bacteria, etc.) living in our digestive systems. They help with digestion, prevent illness, and they provide other health benefits. During a vaginal birth, babies pick up their mothers' microbes, and these form the basis of the baby's healthy gut microbiome. Babies born by C-section, though, grow a gut microbiome different from that of babies born vaginally. Research suggests that swabbing the baby's mouth, nose, and skin with the mother's microbes as soon as the baby is born (sometimes called "vaginal seeding") may help her grow a gut microbiome more like that of a baby born vaginally.

If you know ahead of your baby's birth that you will have a C-section, you can ask your healthcare providers about the latest research in this area and what they recommend.

How Can You Get Breastfeeding Off to the Best Possible Start?
Here are some tips to help:

- **Skin-to-skin contact** is the nearest thing anyone has found to magic for helping nursing get on track, as Shoko found:

    The skin-to-skin time that my baby and I had was one of the most significant factors in our breastfeeding journey kicking off to such a smooth start, despite him being born at thirty-six weeks (hence being "premature" and needing to be birthed in hospital, despite my plans for a home birth). It was one of the most glorious feelings, my baby lying against me and not being able to tell where my body ended and his started.
    – *Shoko, the Netherlands*

- If your baby is to be taken to a hospital nursery, or if your hands aren't free, you might want to have him **touched to your cheek first. Nuzzle him, smell him;** maybe have someone take photos or video of this moment to keep with you. One mother of caesarean-born twins found that she fell in love with the first, who had been touched to her cheek immediately, faster than the second, whom she saw but didn't touch.
- **Nurse your baby in the operating room** if possible, while the surgery is being finished. Your baby can be laid on your chest above the drape; your helper can hold him and help position him near your breast. This is a memorable moment for both of you, no matter what your baby does. If he nurses, it's a wonderful extra. His smell and touch can go a long way towards emotional healing from the surgery.

After the Birth

Like Natalie, you may have had a very long journey to get to this moment:

> Long before conceiving our son, I had always imagined breastfeeding my child/children. I didn't imagine the difficult journey we would go through to become mothers via a fertility clinic. After two years of injecting my body with many hormones, numerous IUIs [intrauterine inseminations], driving through snow squalls for hours in the dark of many early winter mornings, countless blood tests, internal ultrasounds, and an emotional rollercoaster – finally IVF [in vitro fertilisation] worked and we got pregnant on our second embryo transfer with our son! After twenty-four hours of labouring and two and a half hours of pushing, our beautiful, healthy eight-pound, four-ounce bundle of pure joy was placed immediately on my chest, and he latched like I'd always dreamed of.
>
> – Natalie, Canada

No matter what interventions you've had, there are lots of things you can do after the birth to connect with your baby and begin breastfeeding. And if you're going to be nursing a baby birthed by someone else, these tips can help you, too.

Drying Your Newborn

The simple act of drying our babies probably contributes to our feelings of love. When mammal mothers are deprived of the chance to sniff and dry their still-wet babies, their bonds with the babies are weakened.

Skin-to-Skin (Again!)

The best hospital warmer can't warm a baby as quickly or as well as full-body skin contact with his mother – his *bare* chest and stomach against her *bare* chest and stomach. (There's no need to remove your shirt completely if you don't want to, just open it up.) In fact, if you have twins, the temperature on each breast rises and falls to warm or cool them independently! It's no surprise that stress hormones are much higher in babies who are kept away from their mothers in these critical first hours. Skin-to-skin contact is what your baby expects. And it's a powerful way to get to know your baby, as Mary describes:

> I had done some reading, and straight after the birth I was ordering the midwives not to wash her [my baby's] hands and to let my daughter find the breast herself. I couldn't believe the energy and strength of this tiny being as she charged her way towards my breast for the first time. I panicked and asked the midwives, "What do I do? How does it work? Is there any milk there?!" One came over and squeezed my breast, and four points of thick yellow colostrum poked out. Our first feed together was euphoric. Holding her, I recognised her pointy bottom from the weeks and months I had felt her wriggling inside me. I remember saying to my husband, "That's what we kept thinking was her knee poking out!" The midwives commented that she was hungry, as she stayed latched for a long time. Then she slept for hours.
>
> – Mary, UK

After a Caesarean Birth
Skin-to-skin contact after birth helps you and your baby get on track – whatever kind of birth you've had. Linett got good support from her medical team to start skin-to-skin contact and nurse straight after her C-section:

> It all started with a C-section, which I didn't plan on, but that's another story! After my baby was delivered into my arms to complete the "Golden Hour," my baby was transferred to the breast, and the paediatrician helped me to feed my baby.
>
> – Linett, Mexico

Babies have powerful instincts to nurse, even after a complicated entry into the world, like Audrey's baby:

> My son was an emergency C-section baby; he was "transverse breech" – his head was stuck in one pelvic bone while his butt was in the other. They had to do a T-incision to remove him because they couldn't get him out. But he latched quickly with no troubles.
>
> – Audrey, United States

Skin-to-skin holding helped Susana start to heal from a difficult birth:

> When my baby and I met for the first time, after an unnecessary, medicated, and long process which concluded with a C-section, I offered my breast and she immediately accepted. That was the first moment of joy, when I could finally breathe and rest, and I'll never forget her face, asleep in my arms. That was three years ago, and I still see that little face in the first hours; every time she falls asleep while breastfeeding, I recall the feeling. That became the safe place of my life, the very best instant of my whole existence, and it will remain treasured.
>
> – Susana, Havana, Cuba

- **In the recovery room, you can ask for help with breastfeeding.** Your baby can nurse in any of a number of positions: lying across your chest towards your opposite shoulder or below your opposite breast, cuddled in your armpit, even lying alongside your face with his feet towards the headboard. Any position that gives your baby access to your breast without being near your incision can work. After surgery, while the incision is still numb, may be the simplest time for you and your helper to find a breastfeeding position that will work well for the next couple of days.
- Like Fatmata, you might opt to **have family or friends with you 24/7**, or as close to that as you can manage, so you can have your

baby with you even though you're immobile or affected by medications:

> I had a C-section and was very weak and tired. My mother's auntie was with me in the hospital.
>
> – *Fatmata, Freetown, Sierra Leone*

If you're not able to be with your baby because you need medical care or rest, the next best place for your baby is skin-to-skin with her other parent, or another support person. Audrey describes the impact of early skin-to-skin contact between her baby and his father:

> My husband's relationship with our son began during the pregnancy, but especially from the birth, after the caesarean section, when I told my son, "I love you, you're going to go with Daddy," and he was with his father during those first four hours of life without his mother.
>
> – *Audrey, France*

What If I'm Higher Risk?

If you've been told that your pregnancy is high-risk, like Ali was, your birth plans (and dreams) may go out of the window.

> At thirty weeks pregnant I was diagnosed with a pregnancy-related liver condition and told to prepare to have my baby very soon. One of the first things I did when hearing the news was contact a local lactation consultant. She helped me write out a nursing plan for a premature baby. She painted a picture of what we might be up against: a very sleepy baby who may not want to nurse. We ended up being able to make it all the way to thirty-seven weeks, and once baby came, to our surprise he was big, healthy, and seemingly full-term.
>
> My lactation consultant had very firm suggestions about doing skin-to-skin immediately after birth and to stay like that for as long as possible. We were able to do this. For the entire twenty-four hours we were at the hospital after his birth, he stayed in my arms. During this past year I've had zero supply issues, zero latching issues, zero weight concerns for baby, zero worry about our breastfeeding journey. Sure, you can call it luck. . . . Maybe there's a bit of that, but I think our success is rooted in the support of my

lactation consultant. I felt I had the right education, support, and tools to succeed.

— *Ali, California, United States*

Most babies can breastfeed even after the most severe birth complications. The more complicated the birth, though, the more time and patience it's likely to take to get started. So line up your resources, and know that there's plenty of help out here. La Leche League groups can offer solidarity and support – many of us have had a more difficult start, too, and have found ways through (see Chapter 17).

Moving Forward After a Difficult Birth

If you feel that what happened during birth is getting in the way of your relationship with your baby, you're not alone. Many babies won't latch right away after a difficult birth, and some mothers aren't sure they even want them to. This makes a lot of sense biologically – neither of you received the sequence of motions and hormones that makes for an easy start. You and your baby need to connect in a fundamental way. The good news is that, as Lizzeth found, human babies and mothers are amazingly adaptable – we can get back on track after all kinds of births and early challenges. We just need enough time, patience, and support. Liz tells her story:

> When my baby girl was born in the thirty-eighth week – because she began to slow down her movements and I had a caesarean section – she was born very small. Although by that week she was no longer considered premature, she was still small. In the hospital they helped me a lot with breastfeeding, but even so, it crossed my mind that she was not eating enough. When I got home, I checked if I had a bad latch. I got cracks in a nipple. Then Monica, my lactation consultant, came, and she helped me a lot. This, and the fact that my baby was gaining weight, motivated me more.
>
> — *Lizzeth, Mexico, baby born in the United States*

Here are some ideas to help you connect with your baby:

- **Keep your baby with you 24/7,** even if you don't feel like you want to be with her yet. The familiarity that develops with being together will help your bodies to recognise each other on a primal

level. Moment by moment, hour by hour, you'll find more about her to like.
- **Have your baby's bare skin against your bare skin as much as possible.** Smell her, feel her, caress her, savour her; again, even if you don't feel like it. What connects you and your baby is not magic but hormones. We understand a lot now about how these hormones work: the more you hold your baby, the stronger they'll flow.
- **Take a warm bath together.** You might like to add candlelight and mood music, to enhance the falling-in-love vibe! Stroke and massage your baby as you enjoy the soothing water. Admire her skin, nuzzle her, kiss her toes. Let her nurse while you soak if she can and wants to. You might want a helper on hand to lift her (and help you) in and out of the tub, especially if you're not yet very mobile after birth. If not, have a thick towel on the floor beside the tub where you can place the baby while you get in and out.
- **Hold your baby and watch his face while friends or family members give you a relaxing massage** – foot, scalp, shoulder, back, anywhere that feels good. Give yourself over to the sensation and open yourself up to the enjoyment. This releases hormones that help you connect.
- **Make some decisions about your baby** – what he'll wear, how to hold him, how to comfort him. Taking responsibility for him helps you feel more nurturing towards him.
- If your baby isn't nursing yet, **know that it's probably just temporary.** Babies are born expecting to breastfeed – it's a basic survival behaviour. Their feeding instincts are really strong, and last for months. Keep up your milk production, and keep offering, but there's no benefit in trying to force it. For more on how to get your milk production going while you wait for your baby to be ready to nurse, see chapters 4 and 5. For more about encouraging your baby to nurse when he's ready, see Chapter 17.

Post-Traumatic Stress Disorder (PTSD)

For some parents, the birth experience is so difficult that they experience **PTSD** (also called "birth trauma" when it occurs after birth), an anxiety disorder caused by a very frightening, shocking, or distressing event. Post-traumatic stress disorder is not necessarily related to the pain of the birth, although that can be a factor; it can also be the result of emotional trauma, such as fearing that your baby might die, or that things were done to you against your will, as Sandra describes:

> The only preparation I had during pregnancy for childbirth and breastfeeding was a book that my sister had given me, and the truth is that I didn't give adequate importance to these issues. I thought that childbirth and breastfeeding being something natural, my body would know how to do it – what a mistake. I didn't count on all the medical interventions and obstetric violence that we were going to experience. My labour, like that of many women, ended in a probably unnecessary caesarean section because once I had started labour, my movement was limited, and there was no dilation. During the caesarean section my arms were tied, I had no skin-to-skin contact, they took my son to a nursery, and I didn't see him until a few hours later, even though we were both in good health. I asked to see him more than five times, and I did not.
>
> – Sandra, Mexico

Post-traumatic stress disorder can also be experienced by partners or other people who witness a traumatic birth. And for some of us, birth is complicated by past traumas, such as sexual violence or abuse. Traumatic memories can be so huge and scary that they overwhelm our usual ways of coping with bad experiences. These memories can pop up when you least expect and can haunt your dreams. A particular smell, noise, or sensation can trigger intense "flashbacks" that make you feel you're back there, experiencing it all over again. You might feel jumpy and on edge and find yourself unable to relax. Maybe you feel like something awful will happen to your baby if you take your eyes off her.

Kara describes how good care, and nursing her baby, helped her start to recover:

> In the after effects of my birth trauma, despite being set back physically by my severe injuries and intensive surgeries in the first few days, establishing breastfeeding became the glimmer of hope. It became the thing that I gripped onto when everything around me was out of my control. Thanks to my incredibly supportive partner, who assisted with hand expressing, caring for our baby, and providing unconditional encouragement both emotionally and physically. It was also critical that we had access to quality lactation support in the early weeks after birth. Without having all these supports, education, and community combined, I don't know if I would still be

experiencing the most connected breastfeeding relationship I have with my now two-year-old daughter. And for this I am forever grateful.

— *Kara, Australia*

If your birth (or any other traumatic memory) is still interfering with your daily life and making you miserable even several weeks later, please reach out for help. You're certainly not alone. Support is available, including effective treatments for PTSD, and life can get better. Nursing or providing milk for your baby can be part of the process of healing. Sandra, who experienced the traumatic caesarean birth described in the previous section, writes:

> I loved my breastfeeding, from start to finish. Breastfeeding came to move everything in me; I was born as a mother and reinvented myself as a woman. My advice: breastfeed your child, but also breastfeed his soul, fill him with love and life and may all the good of you be sown in him; breastfeed his heart.
>
> — *Sandra, Mexico*

Owning Your Birth

Whatever happens, this is *your* birth. No one else gets to tell you how to feel about it. As Aurelia writes, the conflict between how you think you *should* be feeling and how you actually feel can be intense:

> There was grief that my own body wasn't capable. Because after many hours of labour followed by four and a half hours of pushing, I went in for an emergency C-section. And there was grief that because of this, I couldn't hold my baby right away. And instead I spent an agonizing couple of hours in solitude, because I wanted her dad to go with her. But I had to wait for the anaesthesia to wear off before I could see her again and hold her the first time.
>
> I felt like I'd been tricked. That I'd been promised some wonderful, magical moment, but somehow failed at earning the right to have it. I was legitimately traumatised by this, and I was devastated that my body had let me down, even as I simultaneously experienced inexplicable joy because my body had in fact provided for me, by creating this miracle in the form of my daughter.
>
> This was the birth of a beautiful, healthy, perfect-in-every-way baby! This is the time to celebrate life! How could I possibly be feeling pangs of

grief in this moment? There must not be permission for it because we never, ever talk about it. And logistically speaking, there really isn't time to feel grief; there's a baby to be cared for around the clock, for goodness' sake! And there isn't space to feel grief because there is so much joy and love. And the people around us are so happy, and we are, too! And we feel ashamed that there might be some negative emotion rising up, so we push it down and try and ignore it away.

At least this is what I did. I had all this grief, and I didn't have time or room to feel it. And even if I did, there was no sense of permission to talk much about it, but it was there, living in my body.

– *Aurelia, Texas, United States*

When you're ready, it can help to tell your story to a caring friend (one who won't say, "But at least you got a healthy baby") or write it down or create a piece of art, collage, selection of photos, or video. Your story will become precious to you for exactly what it is – the beginning of your life with your child. It may even become precious to your child, as it did for Kristin:

For my birthday, a few years back, my mother scanned several pages of her handwritten diary for me and put them into a thick manila envelope, which had the words "The Story of Your Birth, to be read with a cup of hot tea" written on the front. As I read through them, steaming mug in hand, I became absorbed into every thought she had, and every action she took. Hour by hour, minute by minute, she described her fears, her excitement, her frustration, her conviction, her pain – and, finally, her joy and relief when I made it into the world. It bonded me even closer to her. I am so thankful that she gave her time and energy to putting her memories down into words mere hours after bringing me into this world. I will cherish this gift for the rest of my life, and one day pass it along to my own children.

– *Kristin, United States*

No matter how the birth goes, most babies can go on to nurse. And even if they can't, you still have a unique connection with your baby. Providing your own milk by some other means, as Emma did, is a different way you can nurture your baby, if nursing is not possible. For more about alternate routes, see Chapter 17.

My daughter, Amelie, and I share such a close bond. I didn't think it would be possible without breastfeeding, but it really is! Amelie is fed with a PEG (stomach tube). Two days into our neonatal intensive care unit experience, we were taken into a room and told about her kidney problems: her kidneys hadn't formed properly – there was no cure – she would need a transplant when she was big enough. I was also told that this meant her potassium levels were dangerously high, so I'd need to replace most, if not all, of her breastmilk with a special low-potassium milk. At some point I will donate a kidney to her.

If I have another baby, I will pump milk for her again, to help when she is immunosuppressed. To anyone who cannot feed – for whatever reason – I feel you – but always remember that you can and will still bond with your baby. I had to leave my lovely LLL group because it became too painful to hear about breastfeeding. But I will always be grateful for the experience of feeding my babies as much as I could.

– Emma, London, UK

In the following chapters, we'll show you the basics of keeping your milk supply high, your baby well fed, and your breasts a happy place while you and your baby recover from whatever kind of birth you have. There are good days ahead.

Want to know more?

You can find extra resources for this chapter at the "Art of Breastfeeding" tab at www.llli.org.

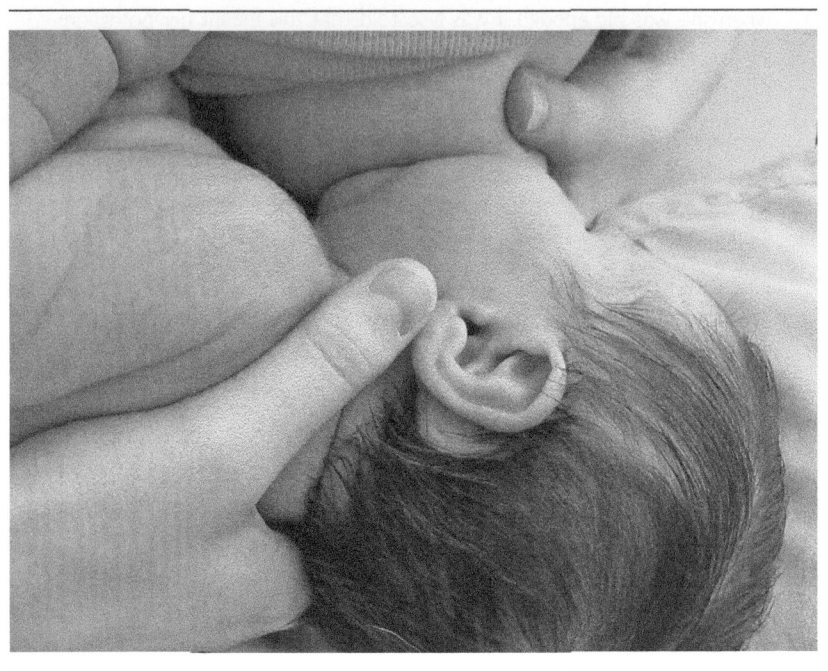

FOUR

Latching and Attaching

> When my baby was born, he immediately latched on to the boob and I was fascinated. It seemed crazy to me that he knew that he should go there and that he should suckle. The instinct with which they are born! I don't quite understand instincts, but they seem to work; we seem to be programmed that way.
> – Guajirita Alquizareña, from Cuba, living in the Netherlands

You and your baby have instincts and abilities not just for birth but for breastfeeding as well. Yes, it may seem a little awkward at first – but although this is *your* first time, it's a process that has worked *billions* of times before.

From Womb to World

Babies are born prepared to crawl to the breast and attach. You'll probably want to help – that's instinctive, too.

Ideally, your baby will be in your arms moments after she's born. Swedish researcher Ann Marie Widström calls the first hour or so after birth the "golden hour," describing nine instinctive stages babies move through to transition to the big outside world. This is why the first hour is so important and helps your baby start nursing well.

Your birth helper can help you hold your baby safely in a comfortable, semi-reclined position. Your baby can lie on top of you, her front on your front, with a blanket over the two of you for warmth. There! Gravity pastes her body against yours, while your hands are free to stroke her. That's really all you need to do at first – find a comfortable way to cuddle together so that you're supported – head, neck, shoulders, body – by whatever you're leaning back against. Your baby might search for your breast immediately, or not. If the birth was a rough one, she may just cry at first. As one helper says, "She needs to tell her story." And you can tell her yours. Soothe, stroke, snuggle, and talk to her. If it's been a complicated birth, or your baby was born prematurely, she may not show feeding behaviours right away. It's okay. You both have *plenty* of time. Keep her close, skin-to-skin as much as you can – you will see her feeding reflexes emerge when she's ready.

You can find lots more about getting breastfeeding back on track after a slow start in The Three Keeps later in this chapter, and in chapters 5, 6, and 17.

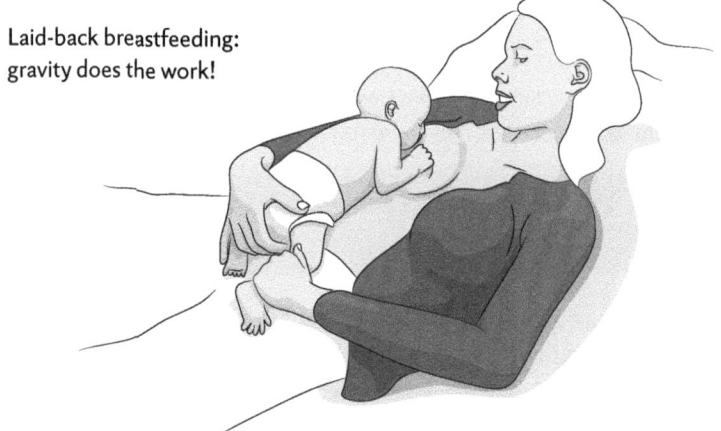

Laid-back breastfeeding: gravity does the work!

Starting Positions

"How should I hold my baby when I nurse him?" is a common question. In past years, you might have been told to "sit up straight and hold your baby like *this*." In the last couple of decades, breastfeeding supporters have worked out that things often go much better if you just trust your baby, and your body. This is not really a new idea. It's a rediscovery of what our ancestors must have known – that babies are competent feeders.

Stephanie, an Indigenous parent and lactation consultant, puts it beautifully:

> We believe that Creator, in the last months of pregnancy, teaches our infants how to nurse all by themselves. Infants don't have primitive reflexes.

They have knowledge. Seeing babies as sentient from birth allows us to parent them from their perspective.
— *Stephanie, Six Nations of the Grand River, Ontario, Canada*

Nursing a new baby is like dancing with a new partner. How are you meant to do that? You *could* be given a list of instructions, or photos to show you the "correct" positions. Having danced with a previous partner helps – to some extent! But you will find your own way together. Lola found that instinct was a more reliable guide than videos:

I anticipated problems since it was my first time, but thankfully, I didn't overthink the technique. I even followed videos on how to latch correctly, videos that gave me validation that I was doing it just right. As if there is one way to do it!
— *Lola, Israel*

Leaning back and nursing baby-on-top works well most of the time. With her belly against yours, and her hands and feet on your body, all your baby's feeding reflexes are engaged. On her back or side, she's pretty helpless, but tummy-down, she's strong and competent. Get ready to be impressed!

This kind of nursing is sometimes called

- laid-back breastfeeding
- natural breastfeeding
- Biological Nurturing (popularised by British midwife Suzanne Colson, PhD)

The emphasis of this approach is on comfort and instinct. There *is* no long list of instructions – just a few tips!

- Gravity sticks your baby against you so you don't have to worry about supporting his weight with your hands or arms.
- You decide on your position and your baby's position, how to hold or move your breast, and how to move your baby.
- Your body opens up so that your baby can lie on you in any position. If you're laid-back, the arrangement becomes whatever is most comfortable and stable for you and your baby. You can adjust the angle for the sizes of your body and your baby.

- Gravity brings your baby *towards* your breast as he bobs around, instead of pulling his head *away from* it.
- Your baby's whole body touches yours, encouraging instinctive responses in both of you.
- Your baby isn't as likely to flail his arms and get in his own way. He uses his hands (and feet) with purpose to move himself around.
- You have a hand free to stroke your baby or pick up that drink you're suddenly thirsty for.

It's okay if this approach doesn't work for you. There are many possible ways to nurse your baby – read on for more!

Laid-Back – *Not* Lying Flat

Lying completely flat, face down on your body when you are also flat on your back, may increase babies' risk of sudden unexpected postnatal collapse (SUPC), a very rare but serious event: the loss of consciousness and breathing in a seemingly healthy, full-term newborn, usually in the first week of life. Risk is increased if

- you smoke
- you had a complicated birth (shoulder dystocia, vacuum extraction, or forceps)
- your baby needed to be resuscitated after birth

In the early days after birth, you and your baby are safer if you have someone with you to make sure you're both okay.

Here are some things to remember when you're reclining with your baby at any time in the newborn period:

- Lie at an angle, with your head higher than your legs.
- If you're using medication that makes you drowsy, or you're extremely exhausted, have another adult stay with you.
- Pay attention to your baby. Using a smartphone while lying down with a newborn has been linked with sudden unexpected postnatal collapse. If you really need to use your phone (for example, if you're autistic, using it for self-regulation), have someone else with you to watch your baby.

Sitting Up, Baby Leading

If you (or your baby) prefer to nurse sitting up, try starting with your chest bare and no bra. You can wear an opened shirt, robe, or hospital gown tied at the front, not the back. These steps may help:

- Undress your baby down to her nappy.
- Lean back a little bit (not quite as much as with laid-back breastfeeding) and get comfortable.
- Hold your baby vertically against your chest, facing you, with her head under your chin, your hands behind her shoulders and bottom, and follow her lead.

As your baby rests on your chest, he'll begin bobbing his head and working his way down towards one breast or the other. Be prepared – he might make a sudden lunge! Keep his body against yours, and help him in any way that feels right. When his cheek or nose is near your nipple, he'll probably move his head, open wide, and take your breast.

Like laid-back nursing, this approach lets your baby "make the trip to the kitchen" on his own, as other mammal newborns do.

Baby supported behind back and shoulders, head resting on your arm

Sitting Up, Shortcut

You can also choose a breast for your baby and hold her so her body angles across yours. Her hip rests on or near your thigh, with her whole front against your front, "tummy to mummy."

- Snuggle your baby in close by holding her behind her back and shoulders. Her head can rest on your wrist or forearm.
- If you hold her so that your nipple falls in the space between her upper lip and nose, she can tip her head back slightly to take it into her mouth.

- If she fusses, calm her by holding her upright for a minute or two, talking to her, patting gently, then try again.
- If she doesn't latch, express a few drops of colostrum and rub it around your nipple and areola. The smell of your milk can help her find her way.

What Babies Need to Breastfeed

The approaches described in the previous section all let the baby lead the way. Some babies need a bit more help at first. So now we'll show you some more parent-guided approaches. Let's look first at what babies need.

Babies Need to Be Calm

If your baby is upset, take time to soothe him. Try the following:

- Bring him up higher on your chest, stroke him, bounce him a little, talk to him. You'll gradually learn what calms *your* baby.
- Respond to early cues for wanting to eat – sucking on his hand, smacking his lips, turning his head towards you. He'll have more patience if he's not too hungry.
- If he's hungry and upset, calm him with a little expressed milk. You could use a dropper, spoon, cup, or bottle (see Chapter 18, Supplementing).
- Babies rely on their hands to explore their new world and to find the breast. When they pat the breast just after birth, they put the amniotic scent on the breast. Baby mittens can get in the way. If you're concerned about your baby scratching himself (or you!), you can gently smooth his nails with a nail file. Some parents find it easier to nibble soft baby nails gently with their teeth.
- Others can also help calm the baby: they can hold the baby upright, swaying gently or walking.

For more ideas for calming an upset baby, see Chapter 6.

Babies Need Good Support

Whether you're reclining or sitting up, your baby will be better able to nurse if she's well supported. If you're lying back, gravity does this for you. If you're sitting up, hold her behind her back and shoulders and remember "her front to my front." Her bottom and shoulders need to be tucked in close to you. This helps keep her stable while she moves her head to search. Babies who don't feel stable may wave their arms around, which can make latching more difficult. Some babies prefer the support of a firm pillow when they're lying on your lap.

Babies expect to use their stepping reflex (pushing with their feet) to move towards the breast. If you're sitting up and your baby is lying sideways, she might appreciate something (a pillow, your hand, or a chair arm) to brace her feet against. Or you may find that touching her feet just distracts her. Every feed helps you get to know each other better.

Babies' Lower Jaws Need Room

Your baby's *lower* jaw needs to be deeply placed on your breast. His upper jaw doesn't move much with nursing. Try this: rest your index finger under your nose like a mustache – on your upper jaw – and make exaggerated chewing motions. Your finger doesn't move, does it? Your baby is the same: his lower jaw is his moving jaw, and it needs plenty of room. If your fingers are in the way of his lower jaw, he won't be able to latch well. You can shape your breast or lift it, if you want to, but do it from a respectful distance, with your fingers well away from where his chin and lower jaw need to be.

If you're wearing nursing clothing with openings, you might have to move the fabric. Better still, wear clothes you can open up completely or go topless for now. While you're learning, clothes can get in the way.

Babies Need a Big Mouthful

Milk is mostly in the alveoli in your breasts. The baby who just chews on a nipple won't get much, and it'll hurt!

Samantha noticed that when nursing was sore for her, her baby wasn't as settled, either:

> Her latch was a bit off and my nipples got really sore and blistered before I knew it. She was also quite fussy and wanted to be permanently attached.
> – *Samantha, from the UK, living in Bali, Indonesia*

It's called breastfeeding (not nipple-feeding) for good reason. When your baby has a good big mouthful of breast *beyond* your nipple, *that's* when it's comfortable. And *that's* where the milk is. So, when it *feels* good, it *is* good.

Babies Need the Breast to Fit

It might be helpful to slightly compress your breast, like you would a sandwich. You want to shape the breast parallel to your baby's mouth. When you eat a big sandwich (burger, burrito, or kebab – almost anything you need two hands to eat!), you keep your thumbs back, so there's room for a bite. In the same way, if you hold your breast, keep your lower-jaw fingers *w-a-y* out of your baby's way.

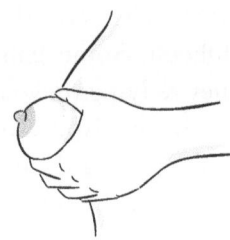

The breast sandwich

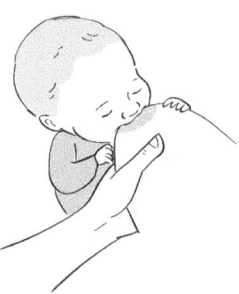

If you have smaller breasts, you might not need to hold or compress them.

Babies Need to Choose Their Own Timing

Instructions for nursing sometimes say, "Latch your baby when her mouth is open really wide." Mammal mothers rarely need to take that much control over a feed, and their babies don't expect it. Unless there's a specific need, your baby will probably do best if *she* picks the moment. Your job is to have your baby well supported, within easy reach of the breast.

Babies Need to Be Able to Tilt Their Heads Back

To nurse, your baby needs to approach the breast chin-first, then stay in close chin contact with the breast, nose lifted free or nearly free from the breast. Tipping his head back a bit helps with swallowing, too (try swallowing with your chin tucked towards your chest – you'll soon see why!).

You don't need to *make* your baby tip his head back – put him in the right place and he'll know what to do. Line him up nose-to-nipple (not lips-to-nipple) before he opens his mouth. As he opens his mouth and latches onto the breast, he'll tip his head back.

You might be tempted to push on the back of his head, or a nurse

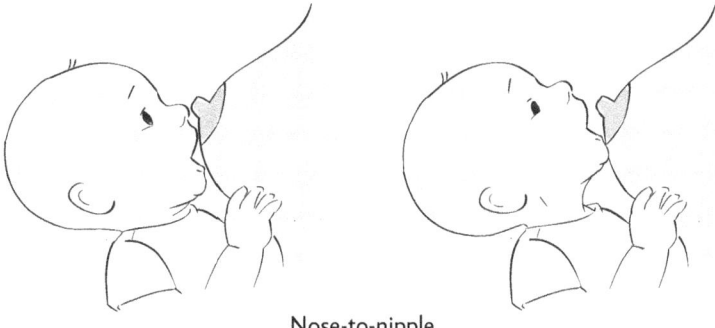

Nose-to-nipple

or birth attendant might try to do that (you can ask them not to). Pushing on the baby's head doesn't help! It can even put babies off nursing, especially if they're more sensitive or have a sore head from birth. Pushing on his head also pushes the baby's chin towards his chest, making it hard for him to get a good mouthful if he does latch on. If you're tempted to push his head forward, keep your fingers off the back of his head. If you're sitting up, you can support your baby's head on your same-side forearm – or use your thumb and fingers in a C shape to support the bony parts behind your baby's ears.

Babies Need to Breathe

In most cases, babies get plenty of air if their heads are gently tilted back a little. Even if her nose is lightly touching, your baby can still breathe just fine. If she can't, she will let go. But what if her nose is buried? Tip her head back a bit more, maybe by hugging her back in closer. You can also press gently on your breast with your hand or finger to give her some breathing room. Or press your hand flat just above your breast, to tilt it upward.

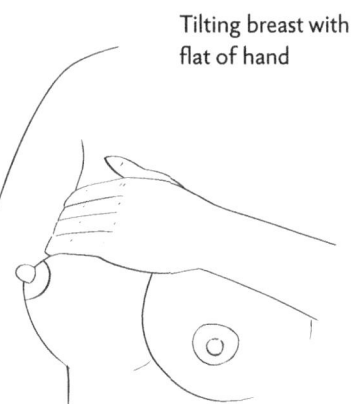

Tilting breast with flat of hand

Babies sometimes lean their heads to one side when nursing in laid-back positions. This head position might look uncomfortable for the baby, but as long as it's comfortable for *you*, you can leave her to it – after all, she chose to do it!

Do I Have to Lift or Hold My Breast Throughout the Feed?

Depends! See how it goes *without* holding or lifting your breast. Some babies need to have the breast stabilised for them as they latch, or shifted slightly to make breathing easier. Give your baby a minute or two to settle into rhythmic sucking. *Then* you can remove your hand from your breast, keeping the baby close. If she lets go, put your hand back where it was. Eventually, she will probably remain attached without your help, giving you a hand free to grab a snack yourself.

What About Those Holds and Positions?

Over the years, breastfeeding helpers have tried to find ways to help babies get a good latch, especially babies who may be sleepy or have post-birth complications. One approach has been to hold the baby in certain ways. When all is going well, specific holds and positions don't really matter, because you and your baby figure out your own system. But if you're having trouble, it can help to have a "recipe" to follow until you know what works for you. So, let's talk a bit about each hold.

The **cradle hold,** or some variation of it, is what many of us use when the baby is a bit bigger and we're pretty good at nursing, but you can try it at any stage. It's the classic position you might see in old paintings of nursing mothers. Try these tips:

- Hold your baby with the arm on the same side as the breast you're nursing on, his tummy against your body and his head on your forearm. Your hand can support his lower back or bottom.
- You might want a pillow to help support his weight. You can also bring your other arm underneath him for support once he's latched.
- Position him so your nipple is near his nose. If he doesn't open his mouth or move to latch on, use your other hand to support the breast (or compress it) and brush the nipple against the baby's top lip, just below his nose. Or brush the nipple against his cheek at the corner of his mouth. Once he opens his mouth wide to latch, you can tuck his bottom in closer to help him tip his head back.

The **across-the-chest hold,** or **cross-cradle hold,** works especially well with small babies and is often taught in hospitals. Here are tips for this hold:

- Hold the baby with your arm that's opposite the breast she is going to take. Your hand supports the base of her skull and neck (not the back of her head). You may be able to support a small baby on your forearm.
- A pillow across your lap might help if your baby is bigger.
- You can use your other hand to shape the breast if you want to.
- As she opens her mouth and takes the breast, gently hug her in by her upper back to help her tilt her head back a bit.

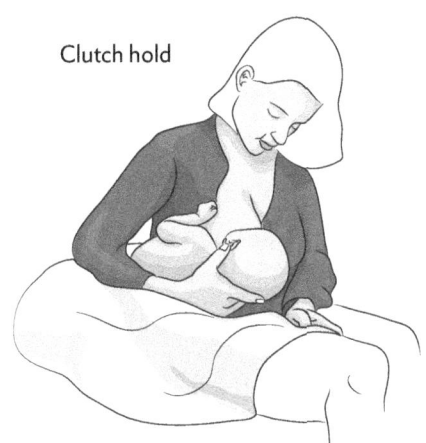

Clutch hold

The **underarm** or **clutch hold** (also called the **"football"** or **"rugby hold"**) may help if you've had a C-section, because the baby's weight is kept away from your incision. It's a bit awkward once your baby is bigger, and you may need pillows or blankets to help support his weight, so most people switch to other positions after the first couple of weeks. But it can be a useful "starter" position. This is how to do it:

- Position your baby on his back, with your hand behind his shoulders, neck, and the base of his head and his body lying on your forearm.
- Tuck him along the side of your body with his head at your breast and his feet towards the back of whatever you're sitting on.
- You can use pillows, cushions, folded blankets, or something similar to help support his weight so your arm won't get too tired.
- Keep him close to your side with his chin facing the bottom of your breast. Touch near his nose with your nipple, so he will open wide and latch. Support his shoulders as he does, so that his head can tip back a bit.
- You can use your other hand to support your breast if needed.
- If your breasts are small, you may need to move the baby into a semi-sitting position so that he can get close to the nipple.

- If your baby pushes off the back of your seat/headboard with his feet, either sit further forward or try a different position!

My Baby's Hands Keep Getting in the Way!

Sometimes your baby starts waving her hands around and pushing back against the breast. Or just as you think she is going to latch, she starts sucking her fingers, moving her head away from the breast.

Babies naturally use their hands to help them find the breast and the nipple, so swaddling or restricting their hands can frustrate them.

What to do? Patience can help – let her do what she needs to do with her hands, talk to her gently, and she'll probably move to latch on her own when she's ready. If she's upset, take a minute or two to lift her up to your shoulder and calm her, then try again. You may want to try a different position where she is more in control of the process, such as laid-back breastfeeding.

Side-lying makes feeding at night much easier and can help a baby who has difficulty latching. You might like this position if you have large breasts. Since you don't hold the baby, your hands are free to shape or move your breast.

It may take a few tries to learn side-lying, but often it becomes the most comfortable and relaxing position of all. Practise in the daytime before you try to do it in the dark! Here are some ideas to help:

- Set up your bed safely (see Chapter 12).
- Lie on your side, facing your baby. Your knees will be bent and your body will be curled around your baby's. (You can read more about this "cuddle curl" in Chapter 12.)
- A pillow under your head and behind your back gives you support. One between your knees is helpful if you have any pelvic pain. If you have a long or curved nursing pillow, it could go behind your back *and* between your knees.
- Place your baby on his side facing you, and move him so that your nipple is level with his nose.
- If you have larger, softer breasts that tend to flatten, a folded towel or cloth under your breast (but well away from your baby's face) can raise it to the right height.

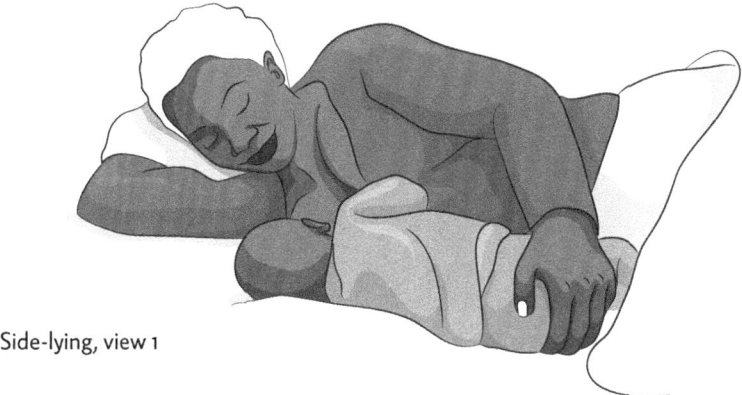

Side-lying, view 1

- If you have small breasts that your baby can't easily reach, try putting him on a folded blanket or towel (avoid soft pillows) to give *him* a lift.
- Touch the nipple near your baby's nose. It might help to shape your breast like a sandwich so that he can latch more easily. Remember to keep your fingers well back from the nipple.
- As he latches, gently press on his back to bring him closer and help keep his head tipped back.
- Once your baby is comfortably attached, you can tuck a rolled-up small towel or blanket behind his back to hold him there.
- If you have fairly large breasts, you might be able to give your baby the second (upper) breast just by leaning over.

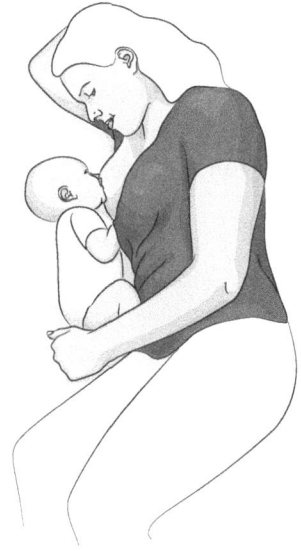

Side-lying, view 2

- To change sides, sit up and lift your baby to the other side, then turn over to face him. If you have help, your helper can move the baby while you get comfortable lying on your other side. Later on, after you have recovered from your birth, you can hold the baby close against your chest and roll over together. For more about sleep and sleep safety, see Chapter 12.

Nursing on the Move

Sometimes babies latch better if you **stand up.** You can sway or bounce gently to help calm your baby, keeping her head near your nipple. Try holding her vertically. As always, support your baby, let her lead the way, and see what happens. Once your baby is latched, you may be able to sit down again.

It's also possible to nurse on the move in a sling or carrier – a more advanced skill! Right now, mastering one basic position might be enough. Eventually, you'll make all kinds of positions look easy – as Shoko describes:

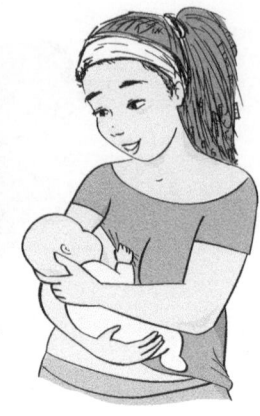

Nursing standing up

Breastfeeding positions know (almost!) no limits – I've done breastfeeding with my babies (and myself!) at a multitude of different angles and with various methods/levels of support (single-handed hold whilst standing or walking around and carrying something in the other hand, anyone?).

– *Shoko, the Netherlands*

La Leche League groups can be good places to pick up tips on where to get slings, and give you an opportunity to watch babies nursing in all kinds of positions.

Adaptations

Nursing After Episiotomy or Caesarean Birth

If you've had an **episiotomy** (cut that widens the birth canal opening) or a C-section, or you're in any other pain or discomfort, there are many ways to get more comfortable when nursing:

- **Episiotomy:** Side-lying nursing takes all the pressure off your bottom. Laid-back positions can also work; experiment to see if there's an angle that feels okay. If you need to sit up, ice packs wrapped in a towel can help ease discomfort. It's also possible to get specially shaped cushions to sit on. Or you could nurse standing up.

- **Caesarean:** Side-lying can work well; use a small pillow or folded blanket or towel to protect your wound. Or you may be more comfortable sitting upright with a pillow or two behind your back. You could use a clutch or a cradle hold with a pillow across your incision.

Make sure you've got the pain relief you need (see Chapter 18, Medications). For more information on post-birth recovery, see Chapter 5 and talk to your healthcare provider.

Body Adaptations

If you're living with a condition like carpal tunnel syndrome or arthritis, or with limb deficiencies, you are probably used to adapting your activities for your own body – as Mariana was:

> I don't have my left arm; I had an accident when I was three years old. Since that age, I learned to do all things with only one hand, and breastfeeding was no exception. If I was at home, I could find a pillow to hold my baby's head, if [away], I would use my handbag for support and breastfeed my baby anywhere. I did that with such a natural approach I think many people didn't realise what could have been a difficulty.
>
> – *Mariana, Guatemala*

You can help your baby latch using your forearms. A partner or support person can help you and your baby find comfortable positions. For more information about adaptations for different bodies, see Chapter 17. We're here to help.

Breast Size and Shape

There are many ways to adapt all these positions for the shape and size of your breasts:

- If you have very large or soft breasts, you may find your baby latches best in a laid-back position while you use the "breast sandwich" technique described under "What Babies Need to Breastfeed."
- Or if you have obesity or overweight, you may find that side-lying is a good way to start. Once you get yourself positioned, you don't

have to support your breast as you help your baby latch. Some have found that using a sling (not the baby carrier type, but a sling like you'd use for a broken arm) under the breast can help lift it for easier nursing in a sitting-up position.
- Most nipples don't point straight forward – they point at least a bit downward, and out to the side. If your nipples point towards the floor, a rolled-up cloth placed between your breast and rib cage may help while you and your baby are learning. It slightly lifts your breast, making it easier to see what's going on at the "business end."
- If your breasts are small and you are long-waisted, it's quite a distance from your lap to your breast. If you want to use a cradle hold, support your arm with as many pillows as you need to bring the baby to the right height. Try laid-back breastfeeding, or sit upright with your baby facing you, straddling your leg on the side you want to feed on.

Whatever your shape and size, nursing can work just fine for you. If you'd prefer not to nurse in front of other people, let your breastfeeding supporter know. Many LLL Leaders and other breastfeeding supporters are able to help you with holding and latching your baby by phone or video call if you prefer to get your support from home.

He's Latched On, But It *Hurts*!

The feeling of your baby nursing may surprise you. That's a strong little mouth, and it may tug your nipple more than you thought it would, as Clare found:

> It felt weird at first – like a vacuum cleaner was attached to my nipple! Once I got used to it, and we worked out how to get a nice deep latch, the experience was really nice.
>
> – Clare, UK

If it feels pinchy or painful, try moving his body or yours around a bit. A small adjustment can make things more comfortable.

If you've taken pain relief medication – or if you're filled with "happy hormones" after a straightforward birth! – you might not feel pain even if your nipples are getting sore. It's a good idea to look at your nipple when your baby unlatches. It will probably look longer because your baby stretches it into the back of his mouth as he nurses.

It's a sign that something needs attention if you see

- your nipple looking squashed, misshapen, or compressed (like the letter *V*)
- any damage to the skin (chafing, blisters, bleeding, cracks)

Anita found some relief for sore nipples with her older children – but even though her youngest baby nursed a lot, she wasn't sore:

> With my other children, if I got sore nipples or my breasts were sore, I'd rub palm oil on and that helped. Baby Mohamed hardly gave me a break, but even though I was tired, I didn't get sore this time.
> – *Anita, Sierra Leone*

Soreness is common but not inevitable.

You can find more information on sore nipples in chapters 5, 8, and 18. Again, don't forget the pain relief if you need it.

Tongue-Tie

Occasionally, however hard you both try, a baby just *can't* get a big mouthful and nurse well because her tongue can't move properly. Annalee got plenty of support and worked hard on latch, but nothing helped until her daughter had a **tongue-tie division** (often called a "tongue-tie release," a minor surgical procedure to correct tissue that restricts tongue movement). Tongue-tie needs to be diagnosed and treated by a specialist. Your local breastfeeding supporters may know of services in your area.

> My daughter's first latch was great, the second felt intense, and the third was when I started to think "This doesn't feel right," and from then onwards for the next six weeks I experienced intense, toe-curling, burning pain every time my daughter breastfed. My daughter's "minor" tongue-tie came up a few times. . . . At the six-week mark [the healthcare provider] revised the tie, and immediately the pain disappeared. It was that easy!
> – *Annalee, Canada*

Latch difficulties don't always resolve quite this fast after the procedure, as Shoko found. As her story also shows, tongue-ties can run in families:

> Some challenges when my eldest was a newborn may have had something to do with his tongue-tie, which wasn't diagnosed and treated until he was three and a half weeks old, when I was at rock bottom and knocking on depression's door with severe mastitis and sleep deprivation. It took a couple more weeks before I noticed any change in his latch, and all the while my health issues continued.
>
> Given this experience, my husband insisted that we have our next baby checked for a tongue-tie early. Thankfully, both the diagnosis and the treatment happened quickly, and this time I noticed an immediate improvement in my baby's latch, with his growth picking up pace afterwards.
> – Shoko, the Netherlands

It may take a week or two after a tongue-tie division to start seeing a change – but when a baby's tongue movement is restricted, treatment can make a big difference.

Good breastfeeding has little to do with how good it *looks* and everything to do with how well it *feels* and *works*. It's going just fine as long as he's able to get the milk he needs without getting too tired *and* you both feel comfortable. If either part of that description isn't working – if you're feeling pain or if the baby isn't getting milk well – then something needs adjusting. It's often possible to make adjustments while your baby is nursing. If these don't work and you need to unlatch, you can prevent pain by gently breaking the latch, not pulling your baby off while he's sucking. Put a finger in the corner of his mouth, right between his gums, to break the suction. Then slip your nipple from his mouth and start again. Try not to do this too many times, though, because it can be frustrating for both of you. Instead, get some help finding a more comfortable approach. Here are some ideas you might try:

Tilting Your Nipple

Hold your breast with your thumb on top and your fingers on the bottom. Place your thumb well back from the base of the nipple. Make sure your fingers won't bump your baby's chin. Press in with your thumb. This will tilt your nipple up. Bring your baby to your breast so that his chin is touching. When he opens his mouth to latch, release your nipple at the last second by removing your thumb. This allows your nipple to fall deep into your baby's mouth.

You may have heard this trick called a **flipple,** because you're flipping your nipple to an upward angle. Remember to keep your baby snug against your body and let him control his head himself.

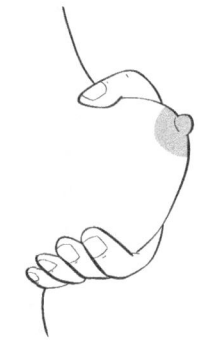

Tilting your nipple can help your baby take a bigger mouthful of the breast

Narrowing the Sandwich

You probably compress a sandwich so you can get it into your mouth. Narrowing the "breast sandwich" to make it easier for your baby to get a deep mouthful will do the same thing. You can combine this with the nipple tilt. Remember to keep your lower-jaw fingers well away from the nipple.

Pillows

If your body supports your baby, there's no need for pillows to support her. Pillows can put extra space between her body and yours, and they can get in the way of easy nursing, as Luisa found:

> The midwife showed me how to attach my son so he could nurse, and I was delighted that it worked immediately. What didn't work for us was the nursing pillow. A lot of people told me what a great thing that was, but I just couldn't find a way to make it work. That showed me that we had to find our own way, and that our own way was perfectly fine.
> – Luisa, Switzerland

If using a pillow means you have to lift your breast to your baby, you probably don't need the pillow! But you might find pillows useful, especially in the early weeks after birth, when you spend so much time nursing. Here are some pillow tips:

- Normal bed pillows are fine – there's no need to buy expensive breastfeeding pillows.

- The exception is when you have twins or other multiples – special twin nursing pillows can be useful for nursing two at once or keeping one close by while you nurse another. For more info, connect with other parents of multiples and see Chapter 17.
- You may do better with a flat-surfaced pillow. Babies tend to roll off the curves of rounded ones.
- If you have a long curved nursing pillow, you could experiment with putting it around the side of your body on the side you're nursing on rather than in front. This way the pillow can support your back and arm, and the baby is less likely to roll into the gap between the pillow and your body. Babies usually nurse better with their heads higher than their bottoms.
- One or more pillows behind your back can be comfortable when sitting, lying, or reclining.
- If you need just a *little* support under an elbow or wrist, small cushions, folded baby blankets, and towels can work.
- While your baby is nursing, ask yourself, *Where am I using my muscles?* Your partner or supporter can help you prop that area so you can relax.

Nursing Props

If you're nursing sitting up and have short legs, a low footstool (or thick book, brick, yoga block, or table) can raise your lap to support your arm and baby. Cross your legs, or try raising just one foot, so your baby's feet are lower than his head. You may also be comfortable sitting on the floor.

When you first start nursing outside your home, take a pillow or other props if you need to. As you become more practised, you'll find other ways to get comfortable. A bag, sling, folded coat or baby blanket, pushchair wheel, or chair rung can become a temporary nursing prop.

None of This Is Working! My Baby Isn't Latching!

Some babies just aren't quite ready to nurse yet. Your baby may need more time if

- she was born prematurely (even a week or two), or small-for-dates
- your birth was complicated

- you had labour medications
- she has any extra complications, like low blood sugar or jaundice (see Chapter 18)

It's upsetting and frustrating when you want nothing more than for your baby to nurse happily. You might feel pressure from others to "make it happen *now*." But difficulty nursing is a temporary setback that many families have overcome. A baby who *won't* nurse, *can't* nurse. She *wants* to nurse. She's not lazy or stubborn. She just needs some help and time. The key is to be patient, and to have good help. Babies are hardwired to breastfeed. A healthy baby will get there. In the meantime, there are three main things you can do to protect your milk supply and your baby's health:

The Three Keeps

Look after these Three Keeps, and you'll be ready and able when your baby is.

1. *Keep* Your Milk Flowing

Your milk supply will start to increase automatically in the first couple of days, whether you remove milk or not. After that, *the amount of milk you remove tells your breasts how much to make long-term.* If your baby isn't nursing yet, start expressing your milk so you'll have plenty when your baby is able to nurse. This is the most important task for you to do at this stage. Babies have weeks or months to learn how to nurse. Milk production, though, increases the most in the first two weeks and peaks in about a month. For more about milk production, see Chapter 6.

In the first few days, colostrum is thick and often easier to remove by hand expressing (see Chapter 15) than by pumping, though it's fine to try a pump (and may be advisable if your baby is premature). Massage and breast compressions also help.

- Start expressing colostrum in the first few hours after birth. Ask for help from your caregiver.
- Then, express your milk at least eight to twelve times every twenty-four hours (see Chapter 6).

- If your baby isn't nursing by the second to fourth day after birth, when your milk increases, you can continue to hand express as well as use a hospital-grade breast pump. For more on pumps and pumping, see Chapter 15.

For more tips on increasing your milk, see Chapter 18, Low Milk Supply.

2. *Keep* Your Baby Fed

You'll want to give your baby as much of the milk you express as possible. At first you may get only drops. This is normal – a little colostrum goes a long way!

You might find it easiest to hand express into a spoon and tip whatever you get into your baby's mouth. You can put the spoon down on a flat surface to express into or hold it with one hand. If you get enough colostrum, you can collect it from the spoon with a dropper or syringe to give to the baby.

If you're hand expressing into a pump funnel or pumping, you can wipe precious drops off the funnel part with your finger (and let your baby suck them off) and collect the colostrum from the pump's bottle with a dropper or syringe.

For more about feeding tools, see Chapter 18, Supplementing. If your baby needs more than you can express, see Chapter 18, Low Milk Supply and Milk Sharing.

3. *Keep* Your Baby Close

Your baby's bare skin against yours helps encourage his feeding reflexes. And being close to you, he won't burn valuable calories trying to stay warm. Your heart and breathing will pace and steady him. And he'll have lunch close by, ready and waiting. These ideas may help:

- Let him doze on your breast, and have your breast nearby when you feed him. Try holding him skin-to-skin with his cheek against the breast during a feed (by dropper, spoon, cup, or bottle), ending with him content and asleep, pillowed on your breast. Your chest is the most satisfying place in the world, even if it may not seem like a food source just yet.
- The first step towards nursing may be that your baby will mouth

your nipple but not suckle. Express a few drops on your nipple to encourage him to lick and suck.
- A nipple shield (a thin piece of silicone shaped like a nipple/areola, placed over your own nipple) can be very helpful when your baby can't stay attached on his own (see Chapter 18, Nipple Shields).

These feeding times can be relaxed, happy, low-pressure. Play at nursing when you both feel like it, instead of working at it because it's mealtime. Time, trust in the process, and a breastfeeding helper are your best allies.

Peggy's experience echoes those of thousands of other families whose babies got there in their own good time:

> My baby would not latch initially. He actually pushed me away and cried every time I put a boob in his face. We saw a lactation consultant, tried everything that people suggested, including using a breast shield, but the baby still would not drink from the boob. I almost gave up, but we tried every few days. Around two months, the baby just started taking the boob – like duh! Or as if he'd been doing it all along. Just wanted to share with other women to not give up, because their baby may just decide one day that this is how they will eat now.
>
> – Peggy, United States

For more ideas for enticing a baby to the breast, see Chapter 17.

Find and *Keep* a Breastfeeding Helper

We'd like to add one more Keep. Find and keep in touch with a kind, experienced helper who understands your unique breastfeeding situation, someone who supports your choices and whose approach is a good fit for you. This can make all the difference! Shanna struggled for a long time before finding a home in her local LLL group:

> When my first daughter was born, I had difficulty getting a comfortable latch. It wasn't until I went to my first La Leche League meeting, when she was five months old, that I finally learned how to breastfeed comfortably. I remember walking into that meeting and being greeted by the friendliest women I had ever encountered. The Leaders were especially warm and welcoming.
>
> – Shanna, Ithaca, New York, United States

Some breastfeeding difficulties may exceed a Leader's skills, but Leaders usually know other local and specialist resources for families. You can also check www.ilca.org for regional International Board Certified Lactation Consultants. Cities may have more resources, but technology has brought virtual breastfeeding support to many rural families. Support and solidarity from other parents can sometimes be the most help of all.

There's a reason your baby isn't breastfeeding, and helpers will keep looking as long as you want them to … or until, suddenly, "magic" occurs, and your baby starts nursing! We've seen babies who suddenly "got it" at two weeks, four weeks, six weeks, three months, six months, and later. When LLL Leaders work with families, we usually don't worry that the baby will never latch. We worry that the parents won't be able to persevere until it happens. Breastfeeding usually works… eventually. In the meantime, there are ways to keep your milk supply strong, as Andrea found:

> He was in an incubator for a week. Every morning I woke up and climbed the stairs slowly to lock myself in a room where there were other mothers waiting for news of our babies. All of us with our breasts out expressing breast milk to give to our babies. Days went by and I could not touch or hold my baby in my arms; I could only see him through a glass window. This wonderful day a nurse came out and said, "Aguila Martinez's baby." I could not believe it; I turned around and saw the most beautiful child in the world. I took my child in my arms for the first time, and with tears in my eyes, I listened to the nurse and uncovered my breast to feed him. How wonderful – my little baby had no difficulty taking my breast and began to suck without any problem.
>
> – Andrea, Mexico

Babies are built to breastfeed. Early babies, small babies, ill babies – they're all designed to feed at the breast.

A few babies *can't* nurse directly – yet human milk is even more important for a baby with complex medical needs. For more about alternate routes, see Chapter 17.

Practice Makes Perfect (or Good Enough)

It takes time for you and your baby to catch on to this new skill. Fortunately, you'll be getting *a lot* of opportunities to practise.

Eventually, you'll be able to nurse on this chair and that sofa, in a parked car and in the park, lying on your side in bed or sitting cross-legged on the floor, even getting up to answer the door. Maybe you'll settle on a style wildly different from anything we mention – something tailored to your breast size, waist length, favourite postures, and baby's preferences. Your baby will be a pro. And you will be, too.

> Latching never hurt – my baby knew exactly how to feed and I guided him so naturally. Breastfeeding came so easily for us together and I cried with joy, watching him feed. Somehow, everything I had been through seemed to fade away as I nourished my little one and held him tight. Finally, it felt like everything was just right.
> – Lauren, New Mexico, United States

Want to know more?

You can find extra resources for this chapter at the "Art of Breastfeeding" tab at www.llli.org.

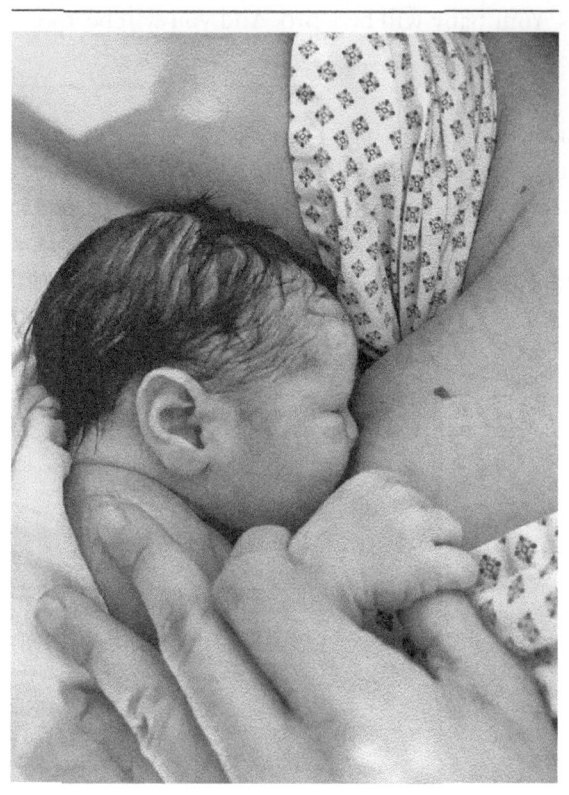

FIVE

The First Few Days: Hello, Baby…

> Melissa had begun breastfeeding just minutes after her birth, but the nurse told me she'd probably sleep quite a bit for the next few days. Hah! That wasn't Melissa's plan. She'd nurse for twenty minutes, doze in my arms for fifteen minutes, then nurse again. I spent most of those early days in bed with her, just gazing at my beautiful daughter.
> – Julie, Canada

Here you are – you and your new baby (or babies!). Your emotions are all over the place, and your body hardly feels like yours. Holding your baby might be even better than you'd imagined… yet your whole world has tilted, and you know there's lots to learn.

As you and your baby learn together, your priorities might change, like Noémie's did:

> Breastfeeding wasn't necessarily at the heart of my visualisation of the new mum experience. However, I was open to trying it, at least for the first few days of my son's life, knowing the benefits it could bring. From the first time I tried it, I was moved by the experience. It was finally the close relationship that convinced me to continue this magnificent milky adventure.
> – Noémie, Québec, Canada

Each new baby starts from a unique place. Your nursing experience may be very different from others around you – and from what you expected. Wherever you find yourself right now, we're here to help you find a path that works for you.

Things to Keep in Mind

Lots of things are going on during these first few days. Breastfeeding is only one of them. At the same time, there can be pressure to get that nursing part working well quickly. But it's not *now or never*. Even if things aren't going well at first, there is plenty of time to get it all sorted out.

Also, breastfeeding isn't *all or nothing*. Yes, there are very good reasons to breastfeed exclusively. But if that isn't working, partial breastfeeding (temporarily, or on an ongoing basis) is valuable. Or if nursing at the breast isn't going well, you can provide your milk in other ways for as long as you choose.

And remember, *it gets better*. Your baby will grow stronger and more capable, your changing body will settle down, and things that seemed awkward or tricky will start to feel natural and easy. As Guajirita describes, life smooths out:

> The first few days were difficult, but now that they are over, I can look back on them in a different way and remember them as something wonderful. I had a lot of milk, I spent all my time with the baby on the boob, I learned to dress him, to hold him, to give him the boob, to bathe him, everything that I was so scared of because I didn't know how to do it.
> – *Guajirita Alquizareña, from Cuba, living in the Netherlands*

So, if your baby still isn't latching, or your milk supply is still low, or your nipples hurt *so much*, we promise you – *it isn't over*. It will get better, and getting the right kind of support can help you along the way. You're not alone.

Nobody Told Me!

Despite childbirth classes and experienced friends, some little things about those early postnatal days aren't usually mentioned. Or like Claudia, you might be told things that you later discover simply aren't true:

> When my baby was born, I was the victim of a lot of misinformation, such as: breasts should hurt at the beginning of breastfeeding; the long list of foods I should not eat; when there is colic I should not breastfeed the baby; I could not breastfeed with a fever; I should change her from one breast to

the other every ten minutes, and not offer the breast again for three hours; my baby should be in the crib and not on me, etc. It was a hard beginning, but thanks to a group of mums, I joined the La Leche League Cuba WhatsApp group. From then on, everything was much easier, and I understood each stage that my little girl was going through.

– *Claudia, Havana, Cuba*

So here are a few things it might be helpful to know in the early days after birth. (If you didn't birth your baby yourself, parts of this list may still help to fill in some detail on what your baby expects.)

- **Colostrum** is the very concentrated milk produced from late pregnancy through the first few days after birth, packed with immune factors that protect your baby's gut and kick-start his own immune system. The small amount gives your baby the chance to practise feeding. Colostrum can be white, bluish, yellow, orange, or clear.
- Your baby's first couple of poos will be sticky and black – that's **meconium,** the waste that filled your baby's intestines before he was born.
- You'll have **lochia,** a bloody discharge similar to a menstrual period that can last up to six weeks. Early on, the flow can be very heavy. Standing up can cause quite a gush. You might want to use "overnight" pads with underwear you don't care too much about, and keep a pad or dark-coloured towel on the bed. Contact a healthcare provider right away if you pass any clots bigger than a golf ball.
- You may also have a gush of blood each time you nurse your baby, as your **uterus contracts** in response to the hormones released by your baby's suckling. The contractions or afterpains can be strong enough to hurt, especially with second or later babies. You might want some pain relief on hand – even if you didn't use any during labour. Weeing before you nurse can help; so can a hot water bottle or heating pad.
- You may be extra **hungry** after the birth. You've just had a real workout, and you deserve some real food. If you've had a tough birth or other complications, though, you may not feel hungry. Your milk production won't be affected by how much (or what) you eat – but you'll feel better and recover faster if you're well nourished.

- **Your baby doesn't fit the books** (not surprising, since babies can't read). And every baby has a unique, inborn temperament, so even if this baby is not your first, you're likely to have some surprises.
- **You can't sleep.** Part of it may be the mental turmoil of becoming a parent. Then there's the shift in hormones. Being a new mother raises your radar – you sleep more lightly and wake more easily – especially if your baby isn't with you. As Allison found, if you keep your baby close, you'll probably sleep better:

> When I brought my little one home from the hospital, I fully intended her to sleep in a crib while I slept in a bed in the same room. But I simply couldn't fall asleep! I wasn't having what I would have considered anxiety, or worried if she was breathing – I simply couldn't relax enough to fall asleep without being able to see and touch her.
>
> – Allison, North Carolina, United States

Your wakefulness will probably settle down in a few days. If it doesn't, you might need extra support with your mood (see Chapter 6). For more about sleep, see Chapter 12.
- You might **feel overwhelmed by visitors.** If you're in hospital and desperate for peace and quiet, let the staff be your gatekeepers. Ask them to stop visitors and suggest they come to see you when you get home. If you're home, you can post visiting hours (short ones!) on the door and stay in your dressing gown.
- You leak from everywhere. We've already mentioned lochia. Some mothers also find they have **bladder issues** that are usually temporary. That means weeing a little if you cough, sneeze, or laugh. Talk to your healthcare provider if this doesn't improve over the next few weeks. Pelvic floor exercises can help.
- If it **stings when you wee,** drink plenty of water. Pour warm water over any stitches or sore parts while you wee and rinse the area afterwards. Your healthcare provider may have more ideas, such as cold compresses, numbing spray, or witch hazel pads, for reducing discomfort.
- As your milk increases rapidly, you might **leak milk,** especially when you hear your baby (or another baby!) cry. You might want to wear breast pads and sleep on a towel. As this mother found, the early days after birth can be a pretty damp time:

> This delivery left me with a grade III tear.... Even so, breastfeeding was wonderful; we had milk gushing, the three of us woke up bathed in milk, the house smelled of milk, and our connection was magical.
> – Caro Santi Sebas, Medellín, Colombia

- You may **sweat** at first, too, especially at night. Keep extra nightclothes handy. You're probably figuring out by now that new parenthood involves a *lot* of laundry! Your body is going through hormonal changes and needs to get rid of extra fluid, including any IV fluids from labour.
- Once she starts getting a lot of milk, your baby will begin filling **nappies,** so there are also *her* fluids to deal with. During these first few days, babies usually poo every single day, with the colour changing every day. See Minding Your Wees and Poos later in this chapter.
- And your eyes... well, they seem to **tear up** over anything! More than one new mother has had to have someone else call for breastfeeding help because she keeps breaking down on the phone, especially around the third or fourth day after birth. Don't worry if you call and burst into tears – we'll wait patiently until you feel ready to talk.
- Although most parts of you leak easily after birth, bowel movements might be difficult. **Constipation** is common, and it can feel scary to exert any effort – especially if you've had stitches or a tear. Drink plenty of water and eat food rich in fibre. Stool softeners and laxatives are compatible with breastfeeding, but contact your healthcare provider if you don't poo within a couple of days.
- You may have swollen eyes, fingers, breasts... everything. **Swelling** is usually due to normal hormonal changes, although IV fluids make it worse. You can help get rid of swelling by drinking plenty of water, wearing loose clothing, elevating your legs, and doing gentle exercise. A massage may also help. For swollen breasts, see Chapter 18, Engorgement.
- Maybe you're recovering from a caesarean birth, episiotomy, or tear – or have some other kind of discomfort, like Denise:

> I had a really lovely, pain relief-free water birth. However, at the very last push, I unfortunately fractured my tailbone. This made sitting down very difficult and painful. My husband would bring the baby to me to feed, or we

would safely co-sleep. It has taken a long time to recover, but I found positions that didn't hurt as much, like lying on my side or dangle feeding, and having a donut cushion when I did need to sit. Family and friends to talk to were so important, as it could feel isolating and frustrating. As well as going for short walks and physio to help recovery.
— Denise, UK

Make sure you've got as much **pain relief** as you need — there are many options you can use while breastfeeding (see Chapter 18, Medications). Check with your healthcare provider if you're not sure what's safe.

Baby Blues

The first weeks after birth can be a perfect storm. Physical changes, discomfort, emotional highs and lows, and sheer exhaustion can combine to make us weepy, irritable, or downright despairing for a day or two. This is the time for supportive people to step up, providing food, reassurance, and loving care. Some of us, like Liz, got nowhere near enough:

My now husband started a new job the day I came out of the hospital, and so I sat at home alone, constantly feeding with hardly even a chance to eat.
— Liz, UK

Others, like Clare, were much better cared for:

Even though we don't have family nearby, our friends were great. I especially remember the experienced mum of three who dropped off a meal and fresh fruit. And my thoughtful mother-in-law gave me special luxury toiletries for myself, not just gifts for the baby. I felt loved.
— Clare, UK

For ideas on how to build your support network before (and after) your baby arrives, see Chapter 2.

While some tears and emotional days are common, if you're feeling anxious or low for days at a time, be sure to let your healthcare provider know. These feelings could be the beginnings of postnatal depression (see Chapter 18, Postnatal Mood Disorders). Getting help quickly can help get you back to enjoying your baby.

Conflicting Feelings

You may be stunned by how much you love your baby. Or you may be stunned that you don't. As Aurelia writes, there can be a big gap between how we think we *ought* to feel and what we actually *do* feel:

> There was grief, even though I felt joy and unconditional gratitude for the gift of my child. And even though I felt the presence of God's very grace as a result of this gift, there was also deep sadness. And it was really, really confusing and no one told me that was gonna happen, that grief might be a part of all the feels I was feeling. But it was there.
> – Aurelia, Texas, United States

It takes time for many of us to feel connected to our children, especially after a tough start. Fortunately, babies come equipped with many ways to help us fall in love with them over weeks, months, and years.

Being a mother is a twenty-four-hour-a-day responsibility, and it can be hard. You might feel shell-shocked at first by the challenge of taking care of a new baby. Where are the breaks you used to get at work? This is why a network is so helpful: you need people who will take care of *you*, so you can nurture your baby. It's okay if you feel sad or angry at times. This huge transition involves some real short-term losses along with the gains – especially in communities where your new role is not highly valued or well supported. And some of us just find change harder than others.

When you become a parent, change becomes the "new normal," as Rosie describes:

> I have found that having a baby just means constant change. No phase lasts very long, no matter how endless it may feel while you're in it. . . . It's a constant process of figuring out where we both are in this dynamic, of finding myself in the relationship, and of allowing the balance to fall where it needs to at any given stage.
> – Rosie, England

Whatever you're feeling right now, you're not alone. Many of us have been there, and we know that it will be okay. You can find ideas on how to regain a sense of control later in this chapter.

The Night Shift

These first few nights can be tough, especially if you're exhausted after a long labour or surgery. Take as many naps as you can! If you can't sleep during the day, resting and putting your feet up is still beneficial. Think about nighttime lighting – you want enough light to see without turning on bright lights. Blue light, from a phone or TV screen, is more likely to disrupt your sleep than dim nightlights.

One mother unwrapped an energy bar and set it on her bedside table so she wouldn't have to unwrap it at 3:00 A.M. A drink beside your bed is also a good idea. Your nights will settle down eventually. Online support groups can be ideal if you need company during the night – there is always someone else awake with their baby!

Secrets to a Good Beginning in the Early Days

1. Skin-to-Skin

Skin-to-skin contact with your baby is the closest thing to magic we have in getting breastfeeding going (see Chapter 3). Being together skin-to-skin continues to be a wonderful way to connect with your baby – not just in the first few hours.

If you're providing expressed milk or formula for your baby rather than nursing directly, skin-to-skin provides your baby with some of the touch he'd get from nursing. Your baby might enjoy being fed (by cup, bottle, etc.) while she's snuggled skin-to-skin. Success in feeding doesn't always look the same. Emma's new baby couldn't nurse – but Emma was determined to provide her with the protection of her own milk:

> My daughter was born with bilateral cystic dysplastic kidneys. She also had collapsed lungs. I was a very experienced breastfeeder and was still feeding my two-year-old son. I got to work on pumping straightaway – it was easy as I already had a supply, which had massively increased since giving birth. I knew she was getting the good stuff from the get-go, even though via an NG [nose-to-stomach] feeding tube.
>
> – Emma, London, UK

2. Removing Milk Tells Your Body to Make More Milk

In the first twenty-four hours, an average feed is 5 to 10 ml (1 to 2 teaspoons). Volume increases quickly, roughly doubling daily in the first few days. By two, three, or four days (occasionally, a little later), many of us experience obvious signs of increased milk production: tender breasts that feel warm, heavy, full, and temporarily uncomfortable. You might start leaking milk and feel your milk rushing down as you nurse. This change is sometimes called "milk coming in" (though this isn't accurate, because you were already making milk, even before your baby was born). The technical terms are *secretory activation, lactogenesis II,* or *onset of copious milk production,* but it will happen whether or not you know that!

An increase in milk production is likely to happen a little later under these circumstances:

- This is your first baby.
- You have diabetes or other metabolic issues.
- You had a really difficult birth.

But however long it might take, for almost all of us, it *will* happen!

When my milk finally came in, I wept with joy. I have a vivid memory of proudly pumping two ounces and taking a selfie with my little bottle of transitional milk. So proud of my body for once!
– Lauren, New Mexico, United States

The increase in milk production is initially caused by the placenta leaving your body. Even if you decide not to breastfeed, your breasts will increase milk production during the first few days. After that, **it's milk removal that tells your breasts to make more.** If you don't remove any milk at all, your milk will dry up over the next couple of weeks. Nursing early and often these first few days encourages your milk to increase rapidly, giving you the best possible chance of making all that your baby will need. This is especially important if you are at risk of low milk production – because, say, you have a history of breast surgery or had low milk supply with your previous babies. Getting good feeding help right at the start can make a big difference.

Most newborns need to feed at least eight to twelve times in twenty-four hours. Many will feed more. Feeding fewer times than this is linked to lower milk production later. Ideally, it's your baby's effective feeding that removes the milk. If your baby isn't yet nursing efficiently, or at all, you will need to hand express your milk or use a breast pump. Having to do this doesn't mean breastfeeding "isn't working" – this is how you keep your milk production up, so that when your baby's nursing improves, you'll have plenty of milk. See Chapter 15 for more about expressing.

3. Get Help Early

At first it can be hard to know what's normal and what you might need some help with. Maybe it *really* hurts when your baby nurses, but your friends all said they had pain, too, and you wonder if you just need to tough it out. (You don't; see Chapter 4 and Chapter 18, Sore Nipples.) Maybe your baby cries when you put her down after nursing, and you're worried she might still be hungry. (Maybe, or maybe she just wants to be held.) Perhaps your baby is sleepy and sucks a few times before dozing off and you aren't sure if that's a problem. (It might be.)

Ask for help! As Diane says,

> It really is amazing that just getting the information you need, at your most vulnerable, can make the difference of being able to breastfeed or not.
> – Diane, California, United States

Breastfeeding issues tend to be more easily fixed the earlier you deal with them. If you had difficulties with a previous child, or physical issues that make feeding more challenging for you or your baby, early help is even more important. If you're not sure whether things are going okay, or think they might not be, we encourage you to reach out for help right away.

It's easy to assume that everyone everywhere has internet access. Remote areas can have limited access or none, though, and no local LLL Leader. If that is the case for you, you might reach out to someone locally who has nursed her baby, a non-profit community group, or the local health department. You might also check to see if any nearby organisation (such as a post office, library, or health clinic) can give you internet access.

Breastfeeding Begins: The First Few Days

We often hear three questions at this stage: how long, which side, how often?

How long? Your baby can nurse as long as he wants. How long a baby nurses doesn't tell us how much milk he got. Suprising, maybe – especially if you're using an app that records feed lengths – but it's true! An unmedicated baby may nurse for an hour or more at a time in the first few days. A medicated, sleepy baby may need extra encouragement to keep going. You can find key information in this section about how to tell whether your baby is getting enough milk.

Are these long feedings going to be hard on your nipples? Fortunately, nipples don't wear out with overuse (we've tested this!). A deeply attached baby can nurse as long as he likes without damaging you.

Which side? In these first few days, you may find that your nipple or your arm or your itchy nose wants to switch sides before your baby has stopped sucking. That's fine! Change sides – or don't change sides – for any reason you like. As long as it's comfortable, you can keep up your switching all day and only good will come of it. Do make use of both sides over the course of the day. Your baby probably doesn't care which side you start with; you just need to offer the other breast whenever he wants a change, and to keep yourself comfortable. As your milk increases, you will be responding to how full each breast is as well. Some babies always take two sides during a feeding, some only ever take one, and most do a bit of both. It's the same for adults – you might not always want dessert, but it's nice to be asked!

How often? If your baby is an active and eager nurser, nurse him as often as he wants. Unmedicated babies who stay with their mothers often nurse more than twelve times in twenty-four hours. They're putting in their order for abundant milk.

If your baby isn't waking enough on her own, you may need to encourage more frequent feeds. This is more likely if she was born early, was small-for-dates, is ill or jaundiced, or had a difficult birth. Starting about six hours after birth, aim for *at least* eight feeds in twenty-four hours. The feeds don't need to be evenly spaced – your baby just needs enough of them whenever she's sufficiently awake. Targets are more useful than schedules. Keep her skin-to-skin and she's more likely to "wake up and smell the milk." Offer the breast at the first signs that she's stirring, before she goes back to sleep. Once she's growing well, you'll be able to relax and follow her lead.

You don't need to feel trapped on the bed or sofa with your baby. If you want to go to the bathroom or get a snack, slip a finger in the corner of your baby's mouth to break the suction, slide her off, and do what you need to do. Your baby may want to nurse again when you come back.

Bottom line: feeding patterns don't tell you much. If your baby is full-term, healthy, growing as expected, and pooing and weeing normally, you can trust her to manage her own eating. If she's not, work closely with your healthcare provider and a breastfeeding supporter. As long as your milk is flowing and your baby is well fed, you have time to work on any feeding issues (see Chapter 4, The Three Keeps).

My Breasts Are *So Full*!

Breast engorgement (swelling caused by extra fluids) is common around two to four days after birth. Not everyone gets engorged. But engorgement can happen fast and come as quite a shock, as Natalie remembers:

> My milk came in abundance, and I was severely engorged from milk and fluids.... I was so engorged that my son couldn't latch, and we were both in tears. That is when my husband reminded me, "Hey, didn't you go to that breastfeeding thing [La Leche League]; you need to call them!"
> – *Natalie, Ontario, Canada*

Engorgement usually settles down in a day or two, but while it lasts, you can find out what to do about it in Chapter 18, Engorgement. As Kat describes, an older nursling can also help!

> Tandem feeding was brilliant because, whenever I felt engorged, the toddler was happy to be the comfortable breast pump.
> – *Kat, United States, babies born in the UK*

Some new mothers have a short-term, low fever with breast engorgement. If your fever rises or you feel ill, contact your healthcare provider right away.

Nights and Naps

If your baby was born in a hospital, you may encounter one of these three likely nighttime scenarios:

1. **Babies go to a "central nursery"** – a room with babies in cribs and nurses watching over the whole group. This practice is not recommended by authorities such as the World Health Organization and has been phased out in many places, including the UK. Your baby (even one with health concerns) does better when he can stay close to you 24/7. When your baby is separated from you, his heart rate is less stable, the risk of infection is higher, and breastfeeding is less likely to get off to a good start.

Enable mothers and their infants to remain together and to practise rooming-in twenty-four hours a day.
– Ten Steps to Successful Breastfeeding,
World Health Organization and UNICEF

---

2. **Rooming-in** means sharing the same room with your baby. When your baby stays with you, you can have him on your chest, in your arms, or at your side as much as you like during the day. However, many hospitals don't want a mother to have her baby in her bed at night for safety reasons: hospital beds may be high and narrow, and parents who have just given birth are more likely to be medicated and immobile.
3. **Bedding-in** is used in some places. You and your baby share the same bed both day and night, nursing as you choose, beginning to synchronise your sleep patterns, getting to know each other, and bringing in an abundant milk supply.

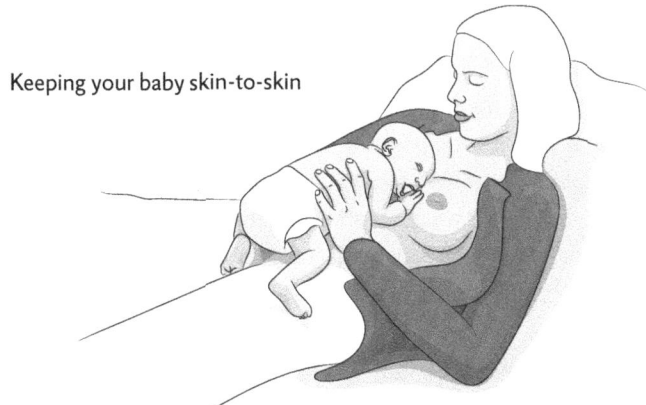

Keeping your baby skin-to-skin

Sharing Sleep Safely in a Hospital

If you're using pain or other consciousness-altering medications, or if you smoke, your baby is safer in someone else's arms, or in a bedside crib or sidecar bed, when you feel drowsy or plan to sleep. It's also riskier for a premature or ill baby to share your bed. Otherwise, sharing sleep safely in hospital mostly depends on the bed.

- Some hospitals now have double beds, enabling you and your baby (and partner) to sleep safely together.
- You may be able to use an extra hospital sheet to make a safe space in bed for your baby. "A flat sheet can be laid sideways across your bed so that more of it hangs off one side than the other. You and your baby lie on the sheet with the free end running up over the rail and back under the two of you again. Put some slack in it so it lies flat on the bed and put your baby between your own body and the now-solid rail" (from LLL's book *Sweet Sleep*).
- Try discussing sleeping arrangements with the hospital staff on the night shift. Shoko managed to communicate well with her nurse, even though the nurse was dubious at first:

Fast-forward to my second child, and we've had a completely different start to our breastfeeding journey. We had skin-to-skin contact for almost the entire time I was in the hospital (about thirty-six hours after his birth), including during my night stay, with the nurse finally accepting that nothing she said would deter me from insisting that I would have my baby with (on!) me during the night in my bed, and after coming home. We did laugh about all of this together the next day, before I was discharged – we parted with smiles.
– *Shoko, the Netherlands*

If co-sleeping in your birth facility is not an option, you will soon be home. There, you can use whatever arrangement you and your baby like best. For more about normal baby sleep and sleep safety, see Chapter 12.

Newborn babies wake often to nurse. They have tiny stomachs and lots of growing to do, fast! We know this newborn period is tiring, though, especially if you don't have much support.

New parents are sometimes led to believe that if they can just get more milk into their babies, the babies will sleep longer. But babies wake for many reasons other than hunger, and they nurse for many reasons other than milk. Giving them extra milk will not necessarily give you more sleep, but it can lead to overfeeding.

Some newborns do need more milk than they can get at the breast. To figure out whether your baby might need more milk and, if so, the options for giving it, see Minding Your Wees and Poos and Weight Watchers later in this chapter.

Just a Little Formula?

If you run into early breastfeeding issues, formula might be offered, or suggested. While we recognise that formula is sometimes needed, we, along with the World Health Organization, UNICEF, and public health experts, condemn the underhand marketing tactics used by profit-driven companies who sell it – but that's another story. Where breastfeeding isn't possible or desired and donor human milk isn't available, formula is the only safe substitute. We're here to support you with breastfeeding, whether or not you're also using formula.

> Do not provide breastfed newborns any food or fluids other than breastmilk, unless medically indicated.
> – Ten Steps to Successful Breastfeeding,
> *World Health Organization and UNICEF*

While formula can be essential in some situations, formula used *when not medically necessary and without guidance* can make breastfeeding less likely and full milk production more difficult, as Hitomi describes:

> I did not receive adequate support when I gave birth the first time. For the first six days after giving birth, my baby and I were in separate rooms and my baby was given formula (with no explanations and without my consent) before direct breastfeeding sessions. There was no support for the positioning and latching of my baby for breastfeeding. I just had to keep bearing the constant nipple pain I had, and because the time allowed for direct breastfeeding was short, my baby's intake of formula kept increasing.

> When I think back to this time, getting to exclusive breastfeeding from this starting point was the most painful process I experienced in my sixteen years of parenting.
>
> – Hitomi, Japan

Formula also introduces extra risks to the baby. Montoya was well informed, and determined to avoid unnecessary formula for her baby:

> I was almost certain that with my condition and age, one child could possibly be it for me. I vowed to do everything that I could to give him a great start, and breastfeeding was number one on my list. Prior to giving birth I read and watched almost everything about and related to breastfeeding, mainly because I had no one close to me who had been on the journey long enough to provide adequate advice. Right away we had issues with breastfeeding, he barely latched; therefore, being in a non–Baby-Friendly hospital, I had to stand my ground about *no* formula. *Period.* I actually fed Kanaan with a spoon for about a week after our return from the hospital. Once he latched, our breastfeeding journey was right on track.
>
> – Montoya, Mississippi, United States

Parents don't make decisions about feeding in a vacuum. Mary's story shows how unethical marketing, misinformation, and cultural expectations combine to put babies at risk:

> On the cans in the market, they said it [formula] was good for babies ... and I thought I could stop nursing, save my breasts, and Samuel would be fine. Other women said I could just feed him formula mixed with milk [powdered milk intended for older children and adults – not suitable for babies], and he would gain weight. ... I heard from several of my friends who'd got pregnant and had babies. They said breastfeeding would spoil my breasts and men wouldn't want me anymore. They told me all sorts of things. What did I know? They had experience and knew more than me ... or so I thought. I'm definitely going to nurse this [next] baby. I want this baby to be healthy, and I know not to stop breastfeeding for a man. Samuel had some health problems when he was a baby. I know more now and am not going to listen to my friends.
>
> – Mary, Freetown, Sierra Leone

Studies show that babies are often given formula in hospitals for reasons other than medical indication – maybe staff are overstretched or don't have the skills to support breastfeeding. Healthcare professionals may have received training or "educational materials" from formula companies and been influenced to see formula-feeding as normal. Parents (targeted by formula advertising during pregnancy) may ask for formula, and it might be given without full information about the potential risks.

If anyone suggests that your baby needs formula, it's worth asking a few important questions before you decide:

- Why is it necessary?
- How urgent is it?
- If it is not an emergency, is there someone who can help me with breastfeeding or expressing milk?
- Is donated human milk available?

If formula is medically necessary for your baby, or your baby has already had formula in hospital, there's good news. Recent research suggests that if formula is used carefully and sparingly, your chances of going on to breastfeed your baby are still good. Work closely with your healthcare provider and breastfeeding supporter, and check out Chapter 18, Supplementing.

Traditional Supplementation Methods

Wet Nursing

The thought of another woman feeding your baby has a yuck factor for many modern parents. But is it really weirder than feeding a baby a manufactured, ultraprocessed product made from the milk of another species? It's interesting to think about where our ideas of normal come from. Marketing may play a bigger part than we realise.

Wet nursing is the traditional way to feed a baby whose mother can't meet all the baby's needs – and it's still practised in many places:

> Aria would fall asleep from the effort without having eaten, or she would eat but she struggled a lot to know what to do. In desperation, I asked a

cousin who was breastfeeding her own baby at the time to help me and feed Aria. When my cousin breastfed Aria, she ate ecstatically.

– Linett, Mexico

My mother was feeding her own eleven-month-old baby, and for a while she nursed my baby. I watched, and after a few days, when I felt stronger, I took the baby and could nurse her. My mother said I should feed the baby the first milk so the baby would get vitamins.

– Fatmata, Freetown, Sierra Leone

At the beginning I thought my little one had a problem because she did not attach to my breast, but when I asked my sister to offer her the breast, my little one latched on so easily, and then my mind changed – I knew we would make it – and so it was. With my third child I had a postnatal complication, but fortunately there was my sister, who breastfed my newborn. . . . When I got home, I found a newborn in peace.

– Alma, Mexico City

Informal milk sharing (using milk expressed by someone else) is a growing trend. Modern breast pumps make this a realistic option for many families. For more about how to share milk as safely as possible, see Chapter 18, Milk Sharing.

Born at Home

If your baby was born at home, you don't have to deal with hospital rules. Yay! But once your midwives and other caregivers leave, you might be a little nervous: this tiny new human is now *your* responsibility! We're here to say: you've got this. Stay in bed as much as you can to rest and relax with your baby. Stay in your nightwear so nobody will expect you to get up. You can set up whatever sleeping arrangement works for you (see Chapter 12). If possible, let your partner or supporters manage visitors, keep you well fed, and take care of older children, so you can spend time getting to know the newest member of the family.

Minding Your Wees and Poos

Not being able to see "what goes in" to the baby can seem like a problem if you're in a community where formula-feeding is the norm. Fortunately, babies come equipped with several built-in indicators to tell us whether they're doing okay. (Something to think about: even if you *could* see how much milk was going in, how would you know it was the "right" amount? Some babies take more than twice as much as others!) We explore this topic further in Chapter 13. **What's in your baby's nappy** gives more useful information than how often or long she slept or nursed, or how many breasts she took each time.

The following table tells you what to expect in the early days. If your baby does something different, check with your healthcare provider.

Nappy Output in the First Week

When	💧 What to look for (pee)	▲ What to look for (poo)
Day 1 after birth	💧 One slightly damp nappy.	▲ One sticky black (meconium) poo.
Day 2	💧💧 Nappies are getting heavier (more pee). You might see orange-red "brick dust" (urate crystals) in the nappy.	▲▲ Same as or more than day 1. Poo may start changing to dark brown.
Day 3	💧💧💧 Same as day 2. *(The weight of the nappy tells you more than the test strip some nappies have, which changes colours if it's wet. Babies sometimes wee but miss the strip.)*	▲▲▲ Poo is changing colour, from brown to dark green.
Day 4	💧💧💧💧 If you're still seeing urate crystals in the nappy, check with your healthcare provider—your baby may need more milk.	▲▲▲ Poo should have changed from brown to dark green to yellow by the end of this day.
Day 5	💧💧💧💧💧 At least five soaked nappies a day. Urine should be clear or pale and smell mild. *(Try putting 3 tablespoons of water on a dry nappy to get a sense of how heavy they should feel!)*	▲▲▲ At least three yellow poos, each one at least 25 to 30 mm, or 1 inch to 1.5 inches in diameter. This is what to expect every day for at least the first month.

 Contact your healthcare provider straight away if
- your baby doesn't poo for twenty-four hours
- you see "brick dust" (urate crystals) in the nappy after the third day
- your baby's poo hasn't turned yellow by the fifth day

A word of caution: *don't* be fooled by anyone who says, "It's fine for a breastfed baby not to poo" (occasionally, we even hear about doctors who've said this). Or, like Mary, you might be told that your baby's lack of poo is due to constipation, when it's really due to needing more milk:

> We were told how many dirty nappies to expect and contacted the midwife we'd been assigned when we were still on meconium nappies on day three. She said the baby must be constipated, and to give her orange juice and water in a bottle. I knew this didn't sound right.
> – Mary, UK

Babies might poo less *after* the first month, but in these early days, not pooing every day is a warning sign for not getting enough milk or having some other health issue.

Once your baby has a solid track record of growth, you can stop looking at the details.

Weight Watchers

Many medical caregivers advise that babies shouldn't lose any more than 7 percent of their body weight before they start gaining, and they absolutely shouldn't lose any more than 10 percent. They should be back at birth weight by ten to fourteen days. Be aware of this potential issue: **weight inflation.** If you had a lot of IV fluids during labour, your baby got some of those fluids, too. With those extra fluids on board, your baby's weight at birth will seem higher than it really is. Once he begins to get rid of those extra fluids (by weeing them out), it will look like he's lost lots of weight – but some of that weight is really just those fluids. Some research has suggested that weight loss be calculated based on the baby's weight at twenty-four hours after birth. With this guideline, fewer babies seem to be losing too much weight.

Also, watch your baby's behaviour, as well as the scale. Here are some things to look out for:

- If your baby has lost a bit of weight but is eager and organised when she eats, swallowing well, and pooing more often, then she's probably doing fine. Watch to make sure her good progress continues; it probably will.

- On the other hand, if your baby has lost little weight but is sleepy, not nursing well, and not pooing, then she probably needs some help digging herself out of a temporary hole. You may need to take charge of her meals by feeding her more often or expressing some extra milk. Expressing does two things: gets more food into her so that she starts pooing, and protects your supply. Check with an LLL Leader, other breastfeeding helper, or your doctor if your baby's still not pooing as expected within a day or two.

Surviving with Your First Baby

You're headed home from the hospital, or your helpers are headed home, and you're suddenly, with no previous parenting experience, caring for a new baby! You may wonder how this can even be *legal* without a license.

Camilla felt very unprepared:

> I never thought to use a bottle because in my mind my dream was to breastfeed her, but no one tells you what you have to do and how hard it can be. There are many courses online about how to change nappies or about the first bath, but there isn't enough information about breastfeeding. I thought it was something absolutely natural. In hospital, the midwife showed me how to do a good latch, and then good luck at home.
>
> – *Camilla, from Italy, living in the UK*

Keep in mind that parenting has worked throughout history. As María discovered, you have the instincts you need – and nursing your baby can help you find them:

> I was very young when I started mothering – my baby was born when I was eighteen. I didn't purchase bottles because the most logical thing to do was to breastfeed my baby. While holding my baby in my arms, I enjoyed seeing him grow and being healthy. Inside myself a great feeling of satisfaction started growing every time that I held him or nursed him.
>
> I never imagined that breastfeeding could impact my life, the changes that it entailed, and, above all, the priorities that I established through it. I always thought that breastfeeding would occur in the most natural way and without complications. For me, the road was not easy. However, it was breastfeeding that helped me to search within myself for the answers,

listen to my inner voice, and in this way, we managed to overcome all adversity and turn that adversity into a connection – a connection so strong that a new woman was born in me, with strengths that I never imagined having.

– María, Guatemala

Your baby won't break if you hold her "wrong," or if the bathwater is a bit too cool, or if she coughs or sneezes or startles. Since she can't clear her throat yet, you may hear some weird sounds coming from her at times. But your baby is an excellent teacher, and your instincts and common sense are excellent students. You'll get all the truly important lessons.

Your Baby's Second Night

Don't be surprised if your baby is *much* more unsettled on Night Two than she was on Night One. That first night, she was probably sleeping off her birth. Now she's awake enough to realise that it's dark, and quiet, and still . . . all things that help adults to sleep but feel *really* scary for new babies. She may need to tell you that it's all a big shock and doesn't feel right *at all*! Keep her close, skin-to-skin as much as you can, and offer the breast often. If you've worked out your sling or carrier, that's probably also worth a try. A partner or supporter can take turns holding and carrying her while you get some rest. Plan to do as little as possible tomorrow – she'll probably be much calmer once the morning comes, and you can catch up on sleep. It will get easier.

Babies Who've Had a Difficult Start

Some babies, like Praveena's, had extra complications:

Arjun suffered meconium aspiration and required oxygen for the first few days of his life. The amazing NICU nurses and lactation consultants stressed the importance of hand expression and pumping immediately so that I could build up my supply until Arjun was able to nurse after he was weaned off oxygen. I was finally able to nurse Arjun when he was around a month old, which made the hassle of constant pumping less daunting.

– Praveena, Texas, United States

Other common early issues are hypothermia (getting too cold), hypoglycaemia (low blood sugar), and jaundice (a build-up of yellow pigment in the baby's blood, which comes from the breakdown of extra red blood cells). For more information on all these conditions, see Chapter 18.

These issues are more likely if your baby was born early (or very late), or small-for-dates, or is ill. The tailor-made protection provided by your own milk is even more important for a premature baby or a baby with medical complications. It might take a little more time to get nursing running smoothly. But as long as you keep your milk flowing, and your baby well fed, you have plenty of time to work on it.

My daughter was born via a planned C-section and had surgery to remove a lobe of her lung immediately following birth. She spent five days intubated, and another seven days learning how to feed from the bottle. From the second she was born, I had supportive nurses and lactation consultants guiding me through my pumping journey. They were so kind and encouraging. My milk took about three days to come in. As a new mum, I was anxious it wouldn't come, but they kept saying it *will* come in, keep pumping. They had signs around the NICU promoting breastmilk for neonatal patients, stating how crucial breastmilk is to their recovery and overall health.

We got home after twelve days in the hospital, and that night, she latched for a full feed. She latched and never wanted to stop. She realised I was a milk source, and I feel in my heart that the comfort of being close with me while feeding after everything she had been through just took all of her worries away. She was finally where she was meant to be, in the arms of her mama, and that's where she stayed for months and months. I wouldn't trade our breastfeeding journey for anything. The hard work was worth it every time she felt comforted by my breast (which was the majority of her first year!).
– Laura, United States military

Concerns You May Have in the First Few Days

Here are some of the early-days issues that LLL Leaders most commonly get asked about. No question is silly, any more than it's silly to ask the French word for bread when you're trying to eat in France.

You really are learning a new language. You'll be fluent soon, if you get your questions answered! If your questions aren't addressed here, you may find answers in Chapter 18, on LLL websites, or by contacting a local breastfeeding supporter.

Should We Wake the Baby for Feeds?

Like other mammal babies, healthy human babies sleep when they need to sleep and wake when they need to wake. We have instincts for all kinds of situations, but waking a healthy baby isn't one of them. Our instincts are geared towards soothing and encouraging sleep. If you had no medications, if your baby stays in close contact with you, if he eats well when he eats, is gaining weight, yet is sleeping longer than three hours at a stretch... that's probably just who he is. Keep an eye on his weight and enjoy watching that long TV series or reading that book the other new parents don't have time for!

Waking a Sleepy Baby Who Needs to Eat

Sleep guidelines are different for babies who are born prematurely or small-for-dates, or who are jaundiced, ill, or not growing as expected. Their appetite might not be working properly yet, or they may not have enough energy to nurse as much as they need to. Here are some ideas to help you learn your baby's cues:

- **There are wake-able times and non-wake-able times.** If you lift up your baby's arm, then drop it, and you feel some tension in it as it falls; if you see eye movement under those tiny lids; if her mouth is making little sucking movements; or if any part of her is making movements, waking will be easier.
- **Keep your baby skin-to-skin as much as possible.** Skin-to-skin contact keeps your baby calm and warm, saving her energy for eating. With your baby snuggled on your chest, you'll notice the very first signs of movement.

Encouraging a Sleepy Baby to Nurse

- Dim any bright lights. It's easier for your baby to keep her eyes open if she doesn't have to squint.

- Undress her.
- Stroke her and say her name. Rub her feet. Maybe gently wipe her face with a damp cloth.
- No luck? Lay her on her back, no wrappings, so she can't feel you at all. That's unsettling enough to wake many babies.
- Gently roll her from side to side, from all the way on her left side to all the way on her right side, and back and forth. Almost all babies will open their eyes to see who's rocking their world.
- Hold her along your forearms, head in your hands, feet at your elbows, and lift her so that she's more vertical, then lower your arms so that she's horizontal, up and down, up and down, talking to her gently as you do so.
- As a last resort, put a little milk on her lips and in her mouth – just a bit, waiting for her to swallow before adding more. Occasionally, a baby will sleep through a whole meal or two this way. She might also latch and nurse in her sleep, especially if she's in a laid-back breast-feeding position (see Chapter 4). That's fine. Your real goal, after all, isn't to wake up the baby so much as it is to help her eat.

Should We Swaddle Him?

SWADDLING: wrapping a baby in a blanket or sheet restricting his movements with the intention of calming the baby or encouraging sleep.

If your baby has been taken from you and comes back swaddled – wrapped up like a burrito – unwrap him and snuggle him against you with a blanket over both of you. Some babies are calmed by swaddling; it may have its uses. But not for most healthy babies. A baby who *can't* be held (say, in an incubator) might benefit from swaddling as a substitute for what they're missing right now – the comfort of being held. There's no need, though, to swaddle a healthy brand-new baby who could be blissed out on your body, his body soaking up warmth and love from yours. Skin-to-skin contact after birth is one of the World Health Organization's Ten Steps to Successful Breastfeeding.

Swaddling has been practised in many cultures at different times, but it is important to be aware of the potential risks, including overheating, (perhaps) respiratory infections, and an increased risk for SIDS (sudden infant death syndrome). For more on swaddling, see Chapter 12. If you do swaddle your baby, dress her lightly, and make sure her legs can turn up and out at the hips. Leave your baby's hands out of the swaddle, as many babies use their hands to calm themselves.

What Can I Do for Nipple Pain?

Ouch! While it's often said that "breastfeeding is not supposed to hurt," research and experience tell us that some level of tenderness, soreness, or pain is a common early feeding issue, as it was for Diane:

> My breastfeeding wasn't going very well, to say the least. I had no idea how important positioning was, so with my baby on his back and his head turned towards the breast, I was just raw.... I called my best friend, Sherry, to come over and help me, because I was ready to quit breastfeeding. I will never forget her coming in, looking at my sore nipples, and calmly saying, "Let's start over." And we did.
>
> – Diane, California, United States

Fortunately, in most cases the causes of nipple pain are quickly sorted out, maybe with some help from a friend or breastfeeding supporter. In the meantime, you don't need to just grin and bear it if you're sore and miserable; there are a lot of safe options for pain relief while you're nursing. The biology of breastfeeding is flexible, adaptable, and sturdy. Babies are no lazier about feeding than they are about breathing. Getting help earlier rather than later will probably help you – body and mind – feel better faster. For more information, see Chapter 18, Sore Nipples.

> I'd been in pain during every feed for days and my nipples were quite severely damaged, but I wasn't going to give up now I'd started. I remember crying on my husband's shoulder that maybe we should just switch to formula. Fortunately, he was my strength when I had lost mine. I'll never forget him asking me "What do you want to happen?" I replied, "I want to feed her, but not if it's harming her." He said, "Well, if that's what you've decided, we'll make it happen." I'm still feeding my daughter, who is now two.
>
> – Mary, UK

Plan B

It's your call whether you can tolerate nursing if you're really sore. You always have the option of expressing your milk to keep your baby fed and your milk flowing while you heal. Doing this could be for the occasional feeding or for a couple of days or more. Nursing is hardwired into your baby – he won't forget how if you need to take a complete break for a while. Line up breastfeeding support for when you're ready to try again. As long as your milk supply is protected, you have *plenty* of time to work towards comfortable nursing.

How Can I Tell If He's Really Eating?

Nappies tell you a lot, of course, and by three days or so, you'll probably start to notice swallowing. Good swallowing of ample milk will usually sound like this: whisper the sound "keh...keh...keh" at about one "keh" per second. Some babies spend some time gulping (and there's no mistaking that). Some may make the "keh" sound with every few sucks. But that whispered "keh" is usually a swallow.

During the first few days, you may not hear a steady, rhythmic swallowing sound; the amount of colostrum that a baby takes can vary a lot. Listen for the "keh" sound for practice – you'll hear it now and then – and you may notice that your baby's lower jaw drops a little, maybe with a hesitation or pause when it drops. That drop – *pause* – close motion is also a swallow. Not every noise a nursing baby makes is a swallow, and some babies who nurse well are nearly silent. But watching and listening for swallows can be encouraging – they tell you that colostrum and milk really are going from breast to baby. This is working! Some parents find it helpful to video a feed – you may be able to see and hear more clearly in playback.

Maybe your baby won't swallow when he first latches. First, he may make some quick, fluttery little sucks that mean he's organising everything in his mouth and settling into a place where he can massage your breast and trigger a milk release. Call this *preparing* to nurse. Then he'll probably start some slower sucks, especially if he's getting nice mouthfuls of milk.

A word of caution: even really experienced breastfeeding

supporters can't tell for sure how much milk a baby is getting just by watching her feed. Nappies and weight are the most reliable indicators of whether a baby is eating enough. A baby who is mostly doing light, fluttery sucks that are all the same length, and little or no swallowing, is probably not pooing as expected. She might keep losing weight or grow very slowly. If this is your situation, you'll want to find help fast. Breast compressions can help the baby get more milk while she nurses. Compressions are like hand expressing into her mouth when her sucking slows down. When the baby stops sucking and swallowing, you could also express some milk and offer it to her later. As her energy picks up, and your milk production increases, her active nursing will last longer, until eventually she can do all the work for herself (see Chapter 18, Low Milk Supply and Supplementing).

They Say Everything's Fine, But I'm Petrified

Many of us have felt this way despite reassurances from our healthcare teams, especially when we had our first babies and hadn't been around newborns before. Caring for a newborn can feel like moving to a new country – or planet! Or maybe, like Amanda, your last breastfeeding experience was far from what you hoped for:

> Three years later I had my second child. I never felt more motivated in my life to be successful with something. I was determined to make breastfeeding work. I was still deeply affected by how things went with my first baby, Molly, and I needed for hers to not be my only breastfeeding story.
> – Amanda, Ohio, United States

You will get through this. These tips have helped other families navigate the early days:

- **Put the baby first.** He won't be a newborn for long. He needs to nurse and be held. Those needs are intense and continuous for a few weeks. Most other things will wait. If you're worrying about other things, make a list and focus on the most urgent ones (you might want to add "sleep" in there!). Delegate as much as you can.
- **Don't worry about organising.** It's fine to put everything in piles or toss things in baskets. Keep your baby supplies where you're likely to be eating, sleeping, and nursing. Go with the flow of this

moment rather than trying to establish some perfect pattern from the start. Things change quickly!
- **Make several possible places to nurse, sleep, or eat.** Kirsten had nursed Willem just fine in her flat, stiff hospital bed but somehow couldn't get it to work anywhere else. She put a pad of blankets on the living room floor and used that while she and her baby slowly learned other nursing positions. Whatever works – go for it, as long as it's safe. You might stash water bottles and snacks in each location.
- **Conserve your energy.** You have healing to do. That means rest, time with the baby, and something to eat and drink. Your baby needs you most. If possible, get help with older children and chores. Lie down, or at least sit down, as often as you can. Staying in your nightwear reminds everyone that it's not "business as usual."
- If you have a partner or key support person, **work as a team,** with the baby as the focus. Keep communication open (but when you're both exhausted is not the best time for important conversations). Don't compete about who's the most tired. A hug or compliment can go a long way. This is a big adjustment for you both – expect some bumps along the road. It's okay to make mistakes. Your child will make many in the years to come, and you will respond gently, because you know that she's a beginner. So are you.

Nursing After Loss

If you've lost a pregnancy or child before this one, had a difficult time with your previous baby, or are struggling with birth trauma, the anxiety you're feeling might be spillover from that earlier experience. Intense joy, grief, and fear all at the same time can be bewildering and overwhelming. This is Verity's story:

I have breastfed all my three children with relative ease. The most challenging time for me was breastfeeding again when my second baby, Ruby, was born. My first baby, Marianne, died of spinal muscular atrophy (SMA). She was diagnosed with the condition at five weeks old. She had a nasogastric tube, and I expressed breastmilk for her until her death eight weeks later. I became pregnant again two months after Marianne died. . . . When Ruby arrived, she was completely different from Marianne, which was a blessing. The way she breastfed was different, too. Marianne had always needed a lot of support to feed, taken a really long time, and looked so exhausted. As a new mum I thought this was normal, but looking back, it was part of her medical condition.

It was a few days into our feeding journey that I started to find things overwhelming. Looking down at Ruby, and seeing Marianne there, I felt like my mind was playing tricks on me. It was lovely to be breastfeeding again, but I felt guilty that I had had another child; like I was betraying Marianne somehow. Then, when thinking about her so intently, I felt as though I wasn't considering Ruby as an individual. When Ruby cluster-fed, it felt more intense than when Marianne had been at the same stage. I had to keep reminding myself that Ruby was a healthy baby and Marianne had been ill all her life, so the previous experience I was basing everything on was false, because I had not had a normal baby yet.

With all the postpartum and breastfeeding hormones swirling around with the grief, it was hard to see the truth of our breastfeeding problems. If Ruby had trouble latching, I immediately thought she was ill or dying. I was terrified she would stop feeding, like Marianne did, and that it would be a sign of terrible things ahead. But thankfully LLL was there. I contacted [an LLL Leader], who reassured me that all the problems Ruby was having with fussiness and latching were normal. She helped me get back to basics and suggested more skin-to-skin and just going to bed with the baby for the day. She also suggested that I write my feelings down. . . . So I started writing to Marianne while I was feeding Ruby; that way I felt like Marianne was there in a positive way, but I was focusing on Ruby as well. Breastfeeding after loss is very hard, but never being able to do it again would be much harder.

– Verity, Oxfordshire, UK

Talking, journalling, and creating artwork can be ways to work through feelings of grief, anxiety, or fear. If they're invading your daily life, making it difficult for you to enjoy your new baby, reach out for support.

What Can I Do to Help My Partner Breastfeed? (Partners and Supporters, This Section Is for You)

Here are ways you can support your partner:

- **Keep the food coming.** Think of no-fix, easy-to-eat, one-handed foods – and keep the water bottles or drink glasses full. Nursing a newborn is kind of like running a marathon – it makes you much hungrier and thirstier than usual! Make sure the food and drinks are within easy grabbing range. There are few more frustrating experiences than being stuck under a baby with a snack just out of reach. Everyone feels better, and recovers faster, when they're well fed.
- **Set up a sleeping arrangement that works for all of you.** You may need to try a few setups to find the best one, and it could involve separate sleeping spaces for a while. This won't be forever. For more on sleep, see Chapter 12.
- **Act as gatekeeper.** Manage visitor flow and be ready to shoo guests out the door if you can see your partner is tired or overwhelmed. Or refer them to the job list on the fridge to get a little work out of them before they go!
- **Listen.** Your partner might want ideas and help to fix issues, or they might just want to tell you how they're feeling. Try to just listen with empathy, unless they specifically ask for ideas. Roller-coaster emotions and tears are common in these early days – for both of you! If they're met with kindness and encouragement, things will probably soon settle down. If you're not sure what would be helpful – ask. It might be different from day to day.
- **Call for breastfeeding help as needed.** Ordinarily, LLL Leaders and other breastfeeding helpers want the nursing mother to call. But when we hear her voice in the background giving you information to repeat to us, we know exactly what's going on. We've been there ourselves. Another good option is to put the phone on speaker, so we can talk to both of you together.

Floating the Right Way Up

One new mother described the first few days after birth "like being thrown out of a ship at sea." Totally disorienting, all the usual landmarks gone, not even sure which way is up. A few weeks later, this same mother was at an LLL meeting chatting knowledgeably about her baby's preferences, nursing on an unfamiliar sofa while drinking tea and eating cake with one hand. She had become part of the community of mothers. She was finding her way. If you're feeling lost right now, your baby and your instincts are your best guides – and there's *lots* of support out here. Welcome.

Want to know more?

You can find extra resources for this chapter at the "Art of Breastfeeding" tab at www.llli.org.

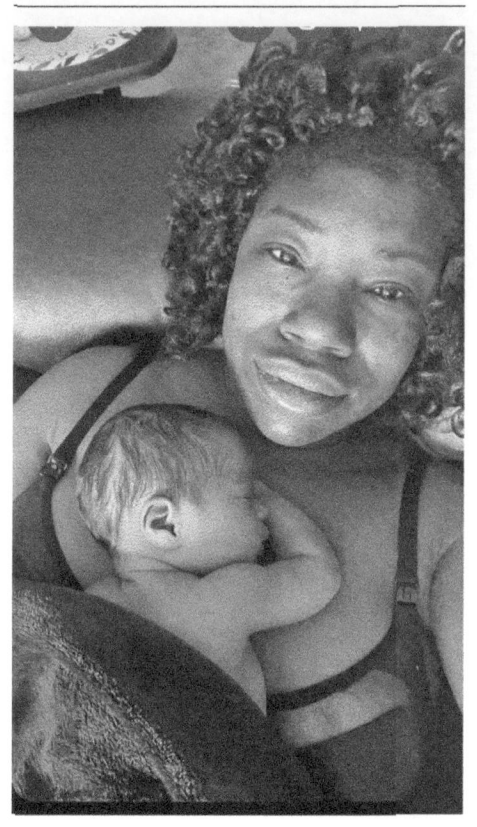

SIX

Four to Fourteen Days: Milk!

> The early days with my first baby were the most intense of my life. I was so happy to have her in my arms at last. I also felt like someone had thrown me out of the airlock into space! All the things that used to shape my time had disappeared or gone blurry. My body felt soft, slow, and weirdly empty, except my breasts, which were in overdrive. When I walked, it felt like my insides might fall out. The world felt unsafe. I loved this baby more than anything, but I didn't know her yet. I didn't know if I was going to be a good enough mother. It took a little while before I was able to trust my baby and my body, and find rhythm in our days.
>
> – Clare, UK

You've made it through those first days. Your emotions might still feel like a roller-coaster ride. How has one baby turned the world upside down? You can expect moments full of joy and amazement as you look at your baby. Even asleep, her expression changes moment by moment. Awake, she looks at you with wise and knowing eyes. What is she thinking? Many of us wonder, at first, if we can cope with the responsibility of caring for this tiny human. But your baby trusts you completely.

There's a reason this book is called *The Art of Breastfeeding*. It's an *art*, not something with instructions. You can learn from other people – and books! – but you and your baby will find what works for the two of you.

In the early weeks after birth, these are the key things to focus on:

- input (what goes into your baby)
- output (what comes out!)
- rest and recovery

More Milk

By now, the amount of milk your body is making should have significantly increased. You can expect it to continue increasing – not as dramatically! – over the next few weeks.

Your breasts may feel heavy, warm, and sore as the milk volume increases. This will pass.

Trevor, a transgender dad, had had chest masculinisation surgery when he was younger, and his baby needed supplements of extra milk after a couple of days. By day five, he noticed something:

> My chest tissue was changing. Fast. My skin started to feel tight. Then hot, and even hotter.
> – *Trevor, Manitoba, Canada*

You can still be making plenty of milk even without the swelling, though, as Clare remembers:

> I barely noticed the changes I was warned to expect around the fourth day, such as uncomfortable breasts. My baby was feeding well – maybe she was just taking it as fast as I was making it! The main thing I noticed was that her poo turned yellow.
> – *Clare, UK*

Nursing Now: First Two Weeks

Many new parents wonder how to tell whether their baby is nursing well. Luckily, you don't need to know how much milk your baby has taken to know if he's getting enough!

The amount of milk your baby drinks will be different at each feed, and that's normal. It may also be different from the amount taken by another baby of the same size.

Your Milk Ejection Reflex (Milk Release)

Some of us start to *feel* our milk release a few days or weeks into breastfeeding. It can be quite uncomfortable at first. It may help to use breathing techniques (such as the ones you might have learned for labour) or distract yourself. The sensation often eases off or stops after a few weeks, as Lieke found:

I always feel my milk ejection reflex at the beginning of a feed. At first it was really unpleasant, a tingling, sharp sense in my nipples. After several seconds it faded away and then I could continue feeding in a relaxed manner. After a few weeks, the first seconds did not hurt anymore either, though I always felt the milk ejection reflex as a tingling sense. And thirst; I always have a strong "thirst reflex" just before my milk ejection reflex comes.
– Lieke, the Netherlands

You can't always tell when your milk has released. You might have several releases (milk ejections) in a feed or pumping session, but it's common to feel only the first one or two – or none at all. If you watch your baby, you might see him start to suck more deeply when a new rush of milk releases.

Rosie's experience as her milk released was more emotional than physical:

In the beginning I found breastfeeding soporific. The letdown made me wretched. My limbs would become physically too heavy for me to lift, and my entire body would burn and ache. My mood would also drop. I felt like nothing was good in the world, and I dreaded every feed. I think that I have some form of dysphoric milk ejection reflex, which significantly marred the early newborn days for me. Happily, the symptoms did subside. Now I don't get the full-body aches or heaviness and I barely even notice the mood drop most of the time.
– Rosie, Oxfordshire, UK

If you have very strong negative feelings when your milk releases, see Chapter 18, Dysphoric Milk Ejection Reflex (D-MER) and reach out to a breastfeeding helper.

Here's what to look for to know nursing is going well:

- **Nursing is comfortable.** Pain is a signal that something needs attention, not an inevitable part of breastfeeding (see Chapter 18, Sore Nipples). Your breasts feel softer by the end of most nursings.
- **Your baby nurses at least eight times in twenty-four hours.** More than that is fine. Nursings can last from a few minutes to forty minutes per breast. If your baby often nurses longer than this, work with a breastfeeding helper to check whether your baby is nursing efficiently.
- **Your baby settles into deep sucking.** Babies begin feeding with little fluttery, fast sucks. As the milk flows (usually within a minute), those quick sucks change to longer, slower sucks, with a whispered "keh" sound, or a hitch or pause in the jaw motion as she swallows. You'll probably notice a swallow with every few sucks. After a while, she rests, neither sucking nor letting go. Just like you, your baby likes to "put her fork down" now and then! She takes a break, catches her breath, and waits for the next milk release. As her meal progresses and the flow slows down, there are more sucks before each swallow.
- **Your baby ends the feed satisfied.** After periods of slow, steady sucking and some pauses, her eyes usually close. She may relax so much that she starts to lose the breast and does a couple of sucks to draw it in again. After a bit, she falls asleep, totally relaxed. Your nipple slides from her mouth; or if you slide a finger gently into the corner of her mouth to release her grip, she doesn't rouse enough to complain. Or she finishes her meal awake, calm, and alert.
- **Your baby is gaining enough weight.** Look for a return to birth weight by two weeks. Average gain after that is a little more than 30 grams (1 ounce) a day, but your baby may gain somewhat more or less.

What *doesn't* matter is

- how many minutes on each breast
- how many breasts per feed
- the time between feeds
- the same feeding pattern each day

Finish the First Breast First

There's no need to interrupt the feed to switch breasts. You can let your baby nurse from the first breast until he lets go or falls asleep. Sometimes he'll take your other breast if you offer, and sometimes he won't. Just like adults, babies don't want all their meals the same size.

Which Side First?

Should you use something (a wristband, an app) to remind you which side you nursed on last? Many experienced nursing mothers simply prod each breast to check which feels fuller, and offer the fuller one first. Most babies don't mind which breast you start with. If you forget, and nurse on the same side a few times in a row, the other breast will remind you!

Your Baby's Output – More on Poos and Wees

When milk goes in, nappies get filled up and weight goes up. It's helpful to keep an eye on wees and poos in the beginning. The number of wet and pooey nappies should increase day by day through the first week. Rule of thumb: from the fifth day through the first month or so, most babies who gain weight well have *at least* three poos a day that are at least 25 to 30 mm (1 to 1.5 in.) in diameter. More, of course, is fine. If you see fewer, check with your healthcare provider. Don't be fooled if someone says, "Breastfed babies often stool only once every few days, so it's normal that your newborn is having so few stools." That may be true of an eight-week-old, yet it's *almost never* true of a ten-day-old.

Here are some things to expect about your baby's poo:

- Most exclusively breastfed poos are **mustard-coloured** (bright yellow or yellowish brown) after the fourth or fifth day. If your baby's poos don't turn yellow by the fifth day, let your healthcare provider know. The texture may be smooth, or lumpy like small-curd cottage cheese. Green poos later on can result from letting an ordinary yellowish poo sit for a while, from *way* too much milk (this baby will be gassy and uncomfortable, too), from taking iron

supplements, from eating lots of dark green leafy vegetables, or from foods with green food colouring.
- Breastfed poos tend to **smell** like buttermilk, bread, even cheddar cheese or popcorn – yeasty or sharp, but not unpleasant. Occasionally, an exclusively breastfed baby has poos that smell bad. This may signal an illness.

Bottom line: colour, consistency, and smell don't matter *at all* in a thriving, happy baby, but they can help in figuring out the problem if the baby isn't happy or thriving.

Counting wet nappies? It's possible for a baby to fool you with nappies that seem sort of wet without having many stools or much weight gain. If a baby has plenty of *pooey* nappies, she's usually taking ample milk and has plenty of wet nappies. A month or more from now, she may switch to less frequent (but larger) stools, but by then you'll have all sorts of ways to know she's doing fine.

Rarely, babies may not poo or wee enough because of medical conditions. If you notice that your baby's poos are fewer than expected, or seem dry and hard, or if you notice dark reddish crystals in your baby's nappy, contact your baby's healthcare provider right away. You should also contact a healthcare provider if you see that your baby's mouth and lips are dry, if the fontanel (soft spot) on the top of your baby's head is sunken, or if your baby's skin looks loose or wrinkled.

Bottom line: as long as your baby is pooing, weeing, growing, healthy, and happy, it doesn't matter at all what his feeding pattern is. Thriving babies have a huge range of feeding patterns.

What If Something Isn't Going Well?

Brenda's baby had a slow start, but with help she was able to get breastfeeding on track:

> My baby slept deeply after the birth and didn't wake up to eat for two days. On the third day he cried a lot, seemed to be very hungry but didn't want to eat. He didn't sleep because he wanted to eat, but he didn't eat because he wanted to sleep. I cried a lot. I had a phone consultation with a consultant. She explained that I should not go so

long between feedings, that for a couple of days I should express some milk, give it to him with a dropper, and when the baby reacted, bring him closer to the breast. It became easy. We successfully established breastfeeding thanks to a little patience, information, and taking the time to get to know the baby.

– Brenda, Mexico

Signs That Your Baby Might Need More Milk

Your baby might need more milk if you see

- pink "brick dust" (urate crystals) in the nappy after the third day
- poo that has not turned yellow by the fifth day
- fewer than three yellow poos every twenty-four hours from the fifth day on
- that your baby is becoming sleepier overall and more difficult to wake
- that your baby is tense and unhappy after feeding

If you have concerns, talk to a healthcare provider to check your baby's weight and general health. A breastfeeding helper can help you figure out some strategies. Most people whose milk is slow to increase can make enough milk – you're just having a slow start, and you will catch up soon. Expressing your milk helps to tell your breasts that more milk is needed. Hand expression works well for many, but a pump (ideally a hospital-grade one if that's available) can be helpful.

For more about expressing, see Chapter 15. For more about feeding expressed milk to your baby, see Chapter 18, Supplementing.

Breast Compressions: Stimulating a Milk Release

A baby who is sleepy or not very efficient at feeding might need a little help to get more milk at the breast. One way to help is compressing the breast **while he's nursing** (you can also do this while pumping). Here's how to do it:

- Wait for your baby to pause in sucking.
- Depending on your position and preference, press your breast against your chest or cup it between your thumb and fingers (away

from the nipple) and squeeze gently – it shouldn't hurt.
- Your baby will probably start swallowing again.
- When the swallowing stops, release your hold to allow more milk to flow into the area you were compressing, then compress again.
- Shift your hand to compress different areas.

It's like hand expressing right into the baby's mouth (or pump). Compressions can be useful in these situations:

- **If your baby is frustrated that your milk isn't coming fast enough,** this can help push out more milk.
- **If your baby stops actively sucking,** this can stimulate him to start again.
- **If you're increasing your milk supply,** this can help ensure that your baby gets more of your milk.
- **If you're pumping,** this may increase the flow and give you more milk.
- **If you're in a hurry,** this may shorten a nursing. Worth a try, anyway!

Your Milk Output: How Milk Production Works

Just as you don't need to know what goes on under the bonnet to drive a car, you don't need to understand how milk production works to feed a baby. But when you're trying to figure out problems, it can be helpful to understand some of the basic science.

The first few days after birth, your breasts continue making colostrum, as they did in pregnancy (though the volume increases every day). The big change is triggered by the delivery or removal of your placenta. This allows the release of breastfeeding hormones – though you won't see the results for a couple of days or so.

Placenta Problems?

If any of the placenta is retained (remains in your uterus), it interferes with the milk-making process. If you have very heavy bleeding, or lighter bleeding that lasts for more than six weeks, or if you pass big blood clots after the first week, and your milk production is low, it's worth checking with your healthcare provider to see if you have retained placental fragments. Having these removed may increase milk production.

Now a new process kicks in: milk keeps being made only if milk keeps being removed from your breasts. The more milk is removed, the more milk is made. If your milk is not removed at all, milk production slows and stops within two weeks or so.

It's ideal if the milk is removed by the baby, but hand expressing and pumping also work. The more milk removed during these early days, the higher your long-term milk supply will be. The process starts fresh for each baby.

Around four weeks after a full-term birth, milk production usually reaches its peak level. So these early days and weeks after birth are the ideal time to work on increasing milk production if you need to.

Concern about not having enough milk is one of the main reasons parents turn to formula, and sometimes even stop nursing altogether.

Many of us who worry about having enough milk are making plenty:

- **Maybe nothing's wrong.** You just didn't expect your baby to need to eat this often.
- **Maybe it's the way you look at it.** For every parent who says, "I think something's wrong. If I'm not holding her or nursing her, she's crying," there's another who says, "I figured it out! All I have to do is hold him and nurse him and he's right as rain."
- **Maybe someone is scaring you.** Having someone say, "Are you *sure* she's getting enough? I think she shouldn't be eating *again*," is enough to worry anyone! Try to surround yourself with people who've enjoyed breastfeeding and know how it works. La Leche League meetings are one place to find them.

Sometimes, there really is a problem, and figuring it out quickly can help you turn things around:

- **Maybe your baby isn't taking your breast as well as she might.** You might be holding the baby too far away, too high, too low – all things that keep her from getting milk easily. Sore nipples are a major tip-off that things can be improved (see Chapter 4). If feeding is painful for you, it's probably not working as well as it could for your baby, either. Lots of sucking without much swallowing is another sign. If you don't quickly get more comfortable and your baby doesn't seem more satisfied, find a breastfeeding helper.
- **Maybe your baby can't suck effectively** because she has a physical problem such as a tongue-tie (see Chapter 4 and chapter 18, Tongue-Tie).
- **Maybe you're following a parenting programme or schedule** that doesn't fit you and your baby. Try going with your baby's cues and you'll probably see a happier baby and more pooey nappies within a day or two. Sometimes it can take a bit longer to turn a milk supply around if it's dipped too low.
- **Maybe you have a fussy or unhappy baby.** Some babies have periods of crying that are hard to figure out or soothe. These may not have anything to do with nursing. They might be just her intense and sensitive temperament. Focus on pooey nappies and weight gain to reassure yourself. You can find some ideas on soothing sensitive babies in When Your Baby Is Unsettled later in this chapter and more information in Chapter 18, Crying and Colic.

Still concerned? Keep reading! And talk to a breastfeeding helper as soon as you can. You and your baby deserve quick help.

Low Milk Production

Not being able to make enough milk is something that many of us worry about. In some communities it's taken for granted that babies need extra milk, fluids, or foods. According to the World Health Organization and other authorities, though, most mothers who have given birth are able to make enough milk for at least one baby. Additional fluids and foods are unnecessary and pose health risks. There are good health reasons for babies to receive only their mother's milk, where possible.

> Breastmilk is the ideal food for infants. It is safe, clean and contains antibodies which help protect against many common childhood illnesses. Breastmilk provides all the energy and nutrients that the infant needs for the first months of life.
> – *World Health Organization*

While most of us can make plenty of milk for our babies, some of us genuinely can't – as Sandra discovered:

> After breastfeeding for three years I was diagnosed with "mammary hypoplasia." This means that your mammary glands are not 100 percent developed and do not produce a full milk supply. You may require donated milk or formula to feed your baby. I met other mothers with breast hypoplasia; we were all unaware of our condition. Many of them were unable to exclusively breastfeed and grieved for it. Mothers with hypoplasia have found that timely diagnosis allows us to learn about other feeding techniques, allows us to know our body and its limits, but also helps us find that body-to-body contact with our children strengthens our bond.
> – *Sandra, Mexico*

Research showing that human milk and nursing are really important for babies is encouraging more families to try breastfeeding – including those facing extra challenges, such as

- premature or ill babies
- disabilities or health conditions
- previous breast surgery
- babies who arrived through adoption or surrogacy
- co-mothers in same-sex relationships
- trans parents
- and many more

Some parents in these situations have fully breastfed. You never know how much milk you can make until you try!

If you have any of these challenges, consider connecting with a breastfeeding supporter before your baby is born or as soon as possible afterwards. They can help you make the most of your milk-making potential and check whether your baby is getting enough milk. If your baby needs extra milk, they can help you find a way of feeding your baby that works well for your family.

Angi's breastfeeding experiences were also complicated by insufficient glandular tissue (IGT, also known as hypoplasia – underdeveloped breasts; see Chapter 18, Breast Tissue Insufficiency). She found a different way to provide human milk for her baby:

> I never thought I would be standing at the kitchen sink at 11:45 P.M. thawing out another woman's breastmilk for my son. IGT is real, and rare. I didn't know I had it when I had my daughter. I just resorted to breastfeeding her some and formula-feeding the rest, to eventually just formula supplementing.
>
> I wanted my second pregnancy to be different. So I set up an appointment with a lactation consultant at thirty-four weeks gestation. After a hopeful conversation, I got into a gown to be examined. That's when her hope turned into doubt. But we both remained hopeful! Fast-forward five weeks later, I'm calling to set up an appointment with her, to do a weighted feeding [weighing before and after feeding] with my son.
>
> During the exam, I found out that he was only getting about a teaspoon or two from me. My heart broke. Not enough tissue to produce the adequate amount of breastmilk my child needs.
>
> I told my husband that one of our friends, Kalicia, who has a three-month-old, said she could donate breastmilk to Cole. He said to reach out to her. So I did, and since then I have been driving an hour and a half one way to get her milk to provide for my son.
>
> So, I never thought I would be standing at the kitchen sink at 11:45 P.M. thawing out another woman's breastmilk for my son, but I am so thankful that for now, the door is open for me to feed Cole that way. And thankful for willing friends to provide not only for their flesh and blood but for loving my son like their own, to do this for him, and for me!
>
> – Angi, United States

For more about using donor milk, see Chapter 18, Milk Sharing. For more about the causes of low milk production, see Chapter 18, Low Milk Supply.

If you're not able to make all the milk your baby needs, it can feel really disappointing. But, as Lauren writes, breastfeeding, with extra milk if necessary, can help you gain confidence in your body's ability to nurture your baby:

> Breastfeeding my baby became the catalyst for trusting my body again for the first time in years. After three long years of infertility and a lifetime of random health diagnoses, all of which I felt "too young" for – I had slowly stopped believing my body knew how to do anything right.
> – Lauren, New Mexico, United States

Nursing is about much more than just milk. Whatever amount of milk it turns out you can make, you can nurture your baby at the breast or chest. We can support you to find a balance of feeding that works well for your family. For more about living with low milk production, see Chapter 17.

Too Much Milk?

Many mothers overproduce at first, and it can take a month or more to settle down to the amount of milk your baby needs. If you have lots of milk, your baby may grow more quickly. Sometimes, babies *look* like they're struggling with too much milk, but it's because they have feeding issues that make it difficult for them to manage normal amounts.

Be cautious about reducing milk production unless your baby is growing very well (see Chapter 18, Oversupply).

Meeting Your Own Needs, Too

Food

Life with a new baby often seems to revolve around the baby's feeds. Breastfeeding takes lots of time, and at first you often need both hands to manage a feed. But what about *your* feeds? When will there be time for lunch?

Many of us are surprised by how hungry and thirsty we feel in the early weeks after birth. You probably won't feel like this the whole time you're breastfeeding – your appetite and thirst will settle down. All most of us need to do is eat when we're hungry and drink when we're thirsty. If you find that you're so focused on your baby at first that you forget to eat or drink, you could try setting an alarm to remind you. These are signs to watch for:

- If your wee is dark-coloured and smells strong, you need to drink more.
- If your energy is low or you feel dizzy, you might need to eat.

Keeping Yourself Fed

Here are some tips from the LLL community to help keep yourself nourished:

- Keep a water bottle in each place you usually nurse.
- Stock up on foods you can eat with one hand.
- Have a snack ready to eat during night feeds.
- If someone asks if you need anything, request a homemade meal, easy-to-cook groceries, or take-out food. Some new parents ask every visitor to bring a meal.
- Ask your partner to make something for your lunch before leaving for work.
- Eat or prepare food before your baby's most unsettled time (see When Your Baby Is Unsettled later in this chapter).

When I woke up to feed newborn Neve during the night, I'd find that Jon had left a plate of cut-up fruit on my bedside table. I can't tell you how much I appreciated that.

– Emily, from Canada, living in the UK

Rest

Looking after a new baby is tiring, especially if you don't have lots of practical support. And you're also recovering from pregnancy and birth (or surgery if you've had a C-section).

Young babies need to wake often for milk and a sense of safety, both day and night. They get scared if they think they are alone. The gap between this reality and "seven to eight hours of unbroken sleep" might seem huge right now. With time and experience, you will learn how to get the rest you need while meeting your baby's needs. The keys to getting enough rest and sleep are making sleep a priority, being flexible, and drawing on support when you need it.

Daytime Downtime

You've probably heard people say, "Sleep when the baby sleeps." You might be thinking, *With so much to do? The kitchen is a mess, I haven't taken a shower, and visitors are coming!* Right now, rest *is* more important. Maybe you can't always sleep. But you *can* rest. If you like to achieve goals, try putting "rest" at the top of your to-do list.

Find places in your home where you can comfortably practise laid-back mothering, leaning back at a relaxed angle, supported by pillows as needed, your baby snoozing on your chest (with your shirt open when you can). If she wakes up to eat, she can take care of most of the job herself. Relax in that position whenever you can, whether she's eating or sleeping. Rest, with or without sleep, speeds healing and helps keep you from feeling overwhelmed. Your baby's frequent nursing pattern can encourage resting, as Rosie learned:

> I had not expected how much of my time breastfeeding a newborn would take, or how much I would struggle with that. My baby would feed for an hour at a time and it felt like such a chore. I told my husband daily how much I hated it. The hormone cocktail of those early letdowns made my entire body physically ache with exhaustion (even my teeth hurt!) and I would sit and watch the clock, waiting for the glorious moment where my baby would vigorously unlatch herself with a loud "pop!" and fall asleep. And then all of a sudden she got a lot more efficient at feeding, and a lot more interested in the world and my hours of sitting vanished.
>
> I've often wondered in the months since what exactly it was that I resented so much about all that sitting and cuddling and feeding. I think a lot of the problem was just how non-negotiable it felt. My body and my time were not mine, but my child's, and it was hard to have my days and nights dictated to me by this little person who depended on me totally. Looking back, I wish I could have made those early weeks of breastfeeding my own and found ways of putting my feet up and enjoying myself. Now that I have a nine-month-old, the idea of an uninterrupted hour on the sofa in front of the TV sounds like bliss!
>
> – *Rosie, Oxfordshire, UK*

Nighttime Downtime

New parents may feel torn between how they believe (or are told) they *should* handle sleep and what babies need. Separating mothers and babies at night is a recent idea. Our ancestors, and many parents around the world even today, would find it very strange. Mothers and babies have slept together since the beginning of human history. For more about safe co-sleeping, see Chapter 12.

Even keeping your baby close doesn't guarantee a good night's sleep at first. She was probably used to partying at night before she was born (remember those kicks that woke you up at 2:00 A.M.?). Many babies are still very wakeful at night in the early weeks. But she'll gradually learn the difference between day and night. By six or seven weeks, most babies seem to understand, at least a bit better, that nighttime is for sleeping (although of course they still need to wake for feeds). You can help your baby by

- taking her out into the daylight, especially in the mornings
- keeping the lights off, or low, when it's dark outside
- trying to avoid blue light – the kind you get from most computer and phone screens – at night (it disturbs the hormones needed for sleep)

One nighttime job to work on during the day: learning to nurse lying down. For some hints on side-lying, see Chapter 4. For much more about sleep, see Chapter 12.

Your Body and Emotions

As one mother at an LLL meeting put it, "After birth it's all highs and lows. There's not much in between!"

If your birth was straightforward and you have plenty of support, you might feel happy and excited. But even when things are going smoothly, feelings can be intense. If your journey has been far from smooth, or you don't have much support, you might feel like you're in the middle of a storm.

> Cyndel was nursing the son her partner gave birth to and found the reactions of other people made it challenging:

> Not long after Laveen was born, I suffered some pretty serious depression and anxiety surrounding the way others viewed me as his mama. I had never before had to struggle with caring about how people saw our family from the outside, but for some reason, I found myself there. The bond we created having our little quiet moments really helped me overcome some of that.
>
> – Cyndel, Ontario, Canada

Baby Blues

During the first two weeks after birth you may get hit with the "baby blues" – a day or so of *What have I got myself into? Where has my life gone? I've lost myself. Now I'm just my baby's mum.* Now is when a loving partner, family member, or close friend can be extremely helpful. Not necessarily by solving problems or having answers, but by being there with a shoulder for you to cry on, a listening ear, or gentle hands that you can trust your baby to for a bit.

Baby blues may make you tearful, uncertain, forgetful, restless, or irritable. You may have nightmares, or even negative feelings towards the baby. Breastfeeding helps ease these feelings. They usually leave – and good riddance! – within a week. If you're unsure whether you have baby blues or more serious depression, see Chapter 18, Postnatal Mood Disorders, and reach out for help. You're not alone.

Important to Know

Rarely, postnatal depression can turn into postnatal psychosis (PPP). This is more likely if you have had mental health concerns in the past or have a close relative who has had PPP. Symptoms include sudden, extreme changes of mood; severe anxiety; loss of appetite; insomnia; confusion; and delusions or hallucinations. Postnatal psychosis can also include thoughts of harming yourself or your baby. It's risky for you and your baby, and it's a medical emergency. If you're having any of these symptoms, you need medical help immediately. If you're a partner or family member reading this, and see that the new mother has these symptoms, get her medical help right away.

After a More Difficult Start

Many of us start parenthood with more challenges. Maybe your baby was born early or has health concerns. Maybe the birth was very different from what you hoped for, or you're in pain.

How your birth went "on paper" only tells part of the story. A birth that the doctor thought was straightforward might have been really scary for you, while a planned caesarean, with a partner holding your hand, can be a lovely experience (though still major surgery). Talking, writing, or making art about your birth might help you make sense of it. If you are bothered by gaps in your memories or understanding, it may help to go through your medical notes with a doctor or midwife. With a little time, painful memories often lose their power. If you continue to be troubled by dreams or flashbacks, or you just can't stop thinking unhappily about your birth, it might be helpful to talk to your healthcare provider, or a counsellor or therapist.

Anxiety

New parents often feel anxious. A certain amount of anxiety is helpful – it makes you pay attention to your baby. You notice how your baby responds to what you do, and gradually learn his normal behaviours. If he is ever not okay, you will quickly notice. Too much anxiety, though, can get in the way of tuning in to your baby. If your pregnancy or birth was complicated, or your baby has been ill, your anxiety dial might be turned up to high. Being on high alert all the time is exhausting and robs you of relaxation and enjoyment.

If you're anxious, it can be very helpful to talk to someone you trust. Anxious thoughts don't mean you are going to harm your baby; your mind is working overtime to keep him safe. You deserve help. It may take time to reset the sentinel part of your brain. There is no shame in getting support with doing this – lots of us have been there. For more about anxiety and related disorders (like obsessive-compulsive disorder), see Chapter 18, Postnatal Mood Disorders.

When Your Baby Is Unsettled

Tests and Procedures

In many places, babies have blood tests in the first few days to check for various illnesses. Some babies may have additional procedures, such as circumcision or ear piercing. Nursing is excellent pain relief. It can be helpful to nurse your baby beforehand, so she's peaceful and relaxed. Or you might even be able to nurse while the procedure's happening. After a more major procedure, your baby might need to recover by sleeping for a few hours. When she wakes up, expect plenty of nursing for comfort, especially if she's still a little sore.

If you aren't able to nurse through the procedure, you can comfort your baby at the breast right afterwards. If your baby is not nursing directly yet (for example, if she was born prematurely), the taste and smell of your milk is still comforting. You could try dripping some milk into her mouth with a syringe, offering a finger or dummy dipped in your milk, or placing a used breast pad next to her nose. Gentle touch, and the sound of your voice, also reassure and soothe your upset baby.

Evenings (and Nights)

My baby feeds all evening, and my breasts feel empty – have I run out of milk?

Every time I try to put my baby down to sleep, he cries! What am I doing wrong?

Why does my baby cry at the breast even though he still seems hungry?

Sound familiar? Most new parents are surprised by how much they need to calm and soothe their babies at the end of the day. It's one of the most common reasons they contact LLL Leaders!

For the first week or so, most babies are either eating or asleep. During the second week, many babies seem to "wake up," often quite suddenly. Now they have more needs than just milk and sleep. There may be times when they don't know what they need so they ask for help – loudly!

A lot of babies are frazzled by the evening. They've spent the whole day taking in the sounds and sights – new activities for them – and they're *up to HERE* with it all. The comfort they know is nursing, so they often nurse on and off all evening long.

Here are some time-honoured suggestions for getting through an evening with an unsettled baby:

- **Carry your baby during the day.** This helps calm him before the evening fussy time hits.

- **Take a nap together in the afternoon.** This will make you less frazzled, even if he is fussy!
- **Offer to nurse about an hour before he usually gets upset.** Soothing your baby before he becomes worked up may make for a more peaceful evening. At worst, it will give you both a little rest.

You might notice (especially if you're expressing your milk) that milk flow seems slower in the evenings. You haven't run out of milk! The emptier your breasts, the higher the fat content. Slower flow at this time of day may even be a "design feature" – it means your baby can do lots of sucking for comfort without getting overwhelmed with milk. If this change in flow frustrates your baby, you could try breast compressions (see Breast Compressions: Stimulating a Milk Release, earlier in this chapter) to put a bit more "oomph" behind your milk release.

Your baby may not want more milk, though, and might get upset when you offer the breast yet again. This is not because your breasts have suddenly malfunctioned. Your fussy baby just doesn't want any more milk right now. He may be settled more easily by a person who *doesn't* smell of milk!

Fussy Babies: Partners and Supporters, This Section Is for You

Calming a baby isn't magic; it's something anyone can learn with practice. You might not have done this before – but neither has your baby. These tips have worked for other families:

- **Carry the baby in a sling or soft carrier.** Most babies who are frazzled but not hungry love the close contact, especially if you get moving right away. If the baby is not used to using a sling yet, try it first when she's calm. You could practise with a cuddly toy first!
- **Walk, sway, rock, or dance.** See what music the baby likes (she might surprise you!).
- **Head outdoors.** A change of scenery can calm everyone – try standing under a tree so the baby can see the pattern of light through the branches.

- **Go where other people are.** Babies feel safer when the person caring for them is surrounded by a friendly group. You could also turn on the TV, radio, or a podcast so she can hear other people talking.

The Magic Baby Hold

Also called "the colic hold," this way of holding your baby has helped calm almost every well fed but fussy baby we've met. Hold your baby's back against your chest so the two of you are facing forward. Bring your left arm over your baby's left shoulder and hold his right thigh. He'll have one arm on either side of your arm, and you'll have a solid grip on his leg. You can hold him so that he faces the floor, hug him against you so that he faces out, or even rest your left hand, still holding his thigh, on your hip. Your shoulders are relaxed, and you have a hand free. You can try either side if you like, but using your left arm also puts your baby on his left side, which some babies find especially soothing.

Now add the "baby bounce." You can start with swaying, but it may be that your baby needs at least a sway with a hitch in it. You won't be able to see his face with this hold, but you'll feel your baby's body's tension. If you see the back of his head start to wrinkle or feel his body start to tense, turn just a bit. Now he has completely new scenery in front of him. Most of the time, the baby bounce and the new scenery as needed will help. Nothing really helps a baby who needs to nurse, though, except more nursing.

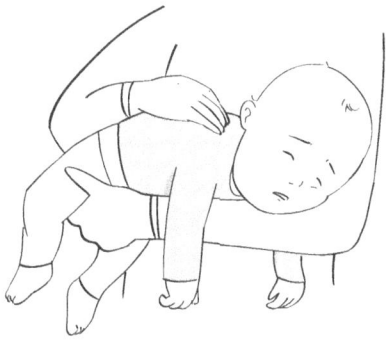

Magic Baby Hold, sometimes called "tiger in the tree" hold

Swinging

A strong, fairly fast swing from head to toe can interrupt crying and help your baby get organised again. Hold the back of your baby's head and shoulders in one hand and her bottom in the other. Position her upright, facing you. Swing her up and down in front of you, along a wide arc, as high as your face and as low as your hip. Hold your baby securely, and watch her face to see if this movement is helping (some babies don't like this). Try whispering "Shhh, shhh" in her ear while moving her.

We hope one of these options helps you calm your upset baby... or you might find your own way that works even better.

Pre-soothing

Why wait for the wail? Keeping your baby close and getting him on the move *before* the crying starts means less crying overall. Don't hesitate to interrupt what you're doing to offer comfort – a quick response will mean your baby will be settled again more easily. Think Baby First rather than about tasks like nappy changes and baths. If your baby says it isn't working, *stop* to nurse and console, then try again. You'll both be happier. It won't be long before baths and nappy changes are playtime. In the meantime, there's no need to make them added stresses. In the first couple of weeks, most of your baby's fussy times are just adjusting to life on earth. Life will improve as you and your baby settle in a bit more.

If you have a **hard-to-comfort baby** for reasons you just can't figure out, check out more information about crying, colic, reflux, and other common causes of baby distress (see Chapter 18). If your baby sounds like he's in pain, or cries for long periods and isn't calmed by any of these ideas, contact your healthcare provider.

First Two Weeks: FAQs

These are some of the first two-week issues often raised at LLL meetings. If your questions aren't addressed here, you'll probably find them answered in Chapter 18 or on LLL websites. And you're always welcome to contact an LLL Leader.

How Often Do Babies Eat?

Healthy babies who are growing well have hugely different feeding patterns. Some feed only five or six times in twenty-four hours (very rare!). Others feed fourteen times or more. Eight to twelve times is typical in the early weeks. How often your baby needs to eat depends a lot on how much milk your breasts can hold in one go (your "storage capacity") and his stomach capacity. You can't see it, but your baby can figure it out and find a feeding pattern that works for him.

Your baby might also want to eat more or less often depending on the following:

- **How he's feeling.** Babies nurse because they're hungry and also to calm down, warm up, enjoy some company, go to sleep, and feel better if they're uncomfortable or tense. And sometimes they want to nurse more, or less, and we never know why. Maybe your baby's been exposed to a virus, or is about to grow faster. Maybe being cuddled by his cousins was very exciting. Trust him!
- **The time of day.** Many young babies nurse most in the evening and at night.
- **The weather.** Expect more feeding when it's hot. (You're probably drinking more, too.)

Feeding schedules might work for the few babies who happen to fit them but not for most. If you think your baby might want to nurse, and you're willing, go for it. Even if it's the eighteenth time that day. Plenty of nursing in these early days will help ensure plenty of milk in the future. Nursing won't always feel as intense as it does now. In the blink of an eye, your baby will be running around, and if you want to cuddle him, you'll have to catch him first!

What If My Baby Is Very Sleepy and Doesn't Ask to Eat?

Your baby may need extra encouragement to eat if

- she was born early (even just a couple of weeks)
- she had a difficult birth
- she was small-for-dates or large-for-dates
- she has jaundice or is ill
- she lost a lot of weight in the first few days

If you're concerned your baby is not nursing enough, try these tips:

- **Keep her close,** skin-to-skin as much as possible (undressed down to her nappy). Feeling and smelling the breast reminds her she needs to eat. Baby carriers are good for skin-to-skin while doing other things.
- **Watch for small movements,** signs that she's waking up. Offer the breast before she fully wakes or goes back to sleep. For early signs of your baby needing to nurse, see Will My Baby Feed Better If I Hold Off Until She's *Really* Hungry? later in this chapter.
- **Aim to nurse at least eight times in twenty-four hours.** It's usually easier to count feeds than to watch the clock.
- **Offer some expressed milk or formula first.** Doing this can give a very tired baby enough energy to nurse (see Chapter 18, Supplementing).

If you're worried that your baby might not be getting enough milk (see Signs That Your Baby Might Need More Milk earlier in this chapter), contact your healthcare provider and get breastfeeding help quickly. As long as she is fed and you keep your milk flowing (by expressing if necessary), you and your baby have time to work on breastfeeding. For more on premature and early-term babies, see Chapter 17.

How Long Should a Feed Be?

It depends! Some babies who are growing fine feed for only a few minutes on each breast. Others nurse for as long as forty minutes on each breast. How long they nurse doesn't tell us how much milk they are getting. Babies know best about how long they need to nurse.

On the other hand, you can interrupt your baby's feeding if you need to! If you have to hit pause on a feed – to help an older child, answer the door, go to the bathroom, grab a drink – that's fine. You have needs, too. Just offer to nurse again when you can.

The Very Slow Feeder
Some slow feeders just like to savour their food and are doing fine. They gain weight well and are happy after nursing. Maybe they will grow up to be chefs, or restaurant critics. However, if your baby's weight gain is not as expected, the long feeds might be a sign that he's not nursing effectively. Some of these babies sleep really well at night not from

contentment but to save on energy. If this describes your baby, see Chapter 18, Weight Gain Worries.

The Superfast Feeder
A few babies can routinely zip through a whole feed in five or six minutes in the early weeks and be satisfied for some hours. But they get their milk so fast and end up so full that they may not have a chance to linger over dessert, snacking and napping in their mothers' arms in typical newborn fashion. If your baby is a superfast feeder, make sure you give him extra time to be carried and snuggled.

If you think your baby always gets too much, too fast, see Chapter 18, Oversupply.

One Breast or Two?
Other mammal mothers don't worry about minutes or changing sides. They nurse as long as they want to and change positions when they feel uncomfortable, or when the baby lets go but still seems hungry.

A few babies only ever take one breast per feed, and some always take two. Most babies sometimes take one, and sometimes two (or more). Babies don't always want their meals the same size. If you're eating out, you might not always want dessert – but it's nice to be asked!

If you're working on increasing your milk production or your baby's intake, you will want to use each breast (nursing or pumping) as many times as you can. Switch sides whenever the flow of milk, or the baby, slows or stops. This may be several times in one session. If you have way too much milk, using only one breast per feed may help.

Do I Need to Empty the Breast?

Babies don't usually change sides because the breast is empty. On average, babies take only about two-thirds of the available milk. They change sides because they want a change of speed, flow, taste, or maybe just position. Full-term, well babies can choose how many "courses" to have, and how much of each.

How Long Does My Baby Have to Nurse to Get to the Hindmilk?

Foremilk is the thin, low-fat milk that comes at the beginning of the feed, and *hindmilk* is the creamy, high-fat milk that finishes the feed. Well... truth is your breasts *make* only one kind of milk. The reason it *seems* different is that cream rises. If you nurse really often, it all stays swirled together. Wait a little longer between feeds, and some of the fat in your milk can creep back up the ducts, leaving a lower-fat milk behind. Think about mixing water and oil and letting it sit for some minutes; the oil will rise. More or less the same thing happens in your breasts. If you nurse your baby again fairly quickly, the fat content will still be higher. Otherwise, at the next nursing the fat gets squeezed down again, gradually mixing back in. It's all nutritious, and the fat variations give your baby some variety. This isn't an issue, except for babies who find themselves with too much collected "soup" to work through to get to "dessert."

Even that's not a problem most of the time; *all* your milk is good milk. If your baby is growing very well but seems unhappy and has green or frothy nappies, see Chapter 18, Oversupply. Otherwise, know that the system is built to have variations, and yes, *all* your milk is good milk.

Trust the Fists

When a baby is hungry, she tends to clench her fists tightly and bring them towards her face. If she falls asleep hungry, her fists usually stay clenched. But when she gets milk she relaxes, starting with her face. Then her shoulders relax, and finally those fists unclench. Eventually they're as limp as the rest of her. Think of her hands as her built-in fuel gauge!

Will My Baby Feed Better If I Hold Off Until She's *Really* Hungry?

This is sometimes suggested, but it tends to make life harder for both of you. A baby starts asking to nurse with these small nursing cues:

- his eyelids fluttering open
- his hands coming towards his face
- his mouth movements

If he doesn't get a response, he makes the signals bigger:

- rooting (turning his head or moving his whole body) towards your chest
- whimpering

If you offer to nurse as soon as you see the early cues, or when he starts rooting, he'll probably take your breast gently and easily. If you don't, as his hunger builds, his body and mouth tense. He starts to cry. By then, he can be too stressed to eat, and harder to calm. The nursing will take longer. The American Academy of Pediatrics says, "Crying is a *late* indicator of hunger." So by the time your baby is crying, he has probably been *politely* asking to nurse for a while.

If you often delay feeds, especially in these very early days, you may end up with less milk overall, and your baby may not grow well.

Some babies seem to go from fast asleep to "I'm starving!" in about two seconds flat (we think of them as turbo-charged babies). If your baby is like this, keep him close and offer the breast as soon as he starts to stir, before he's fully awake. If you've missed the moment and he's beside himself, you might try calming him in these ways:

- swinging him (see Swinging earlier in this chapter)
- letting him suck on your finger
- offering some expressed milk

His patience will probably grow as he gets more experienced at feeding.

Are There Special Milk-Making Foods or Drinks?

Yes and no. Many cultures have their own herbs, foods, or recipes that have been used for centuries to support milk production. But there's nothing in particular needed to make enough nutritious milk. Your milk is made from your blood. If you haven't been worrying about the quality of your blood lately, there's no need to worry about the quality of your milk! To learn more, see Chapter 18, Diet and Weight (Yours).

Across the world, nursing mothers eat every kind of food and can make milk just fine:

- You don't need to **drink** anything in particular. It doesn't take milk to make milk. Dairy cows drink water!
- If your baby is **fussy,** don't automatically blame it on your diet – more likely reasons for your baby's fussiness are discussed in When Your Baby Is Unsettled earlier in this chapter. Some cultures whose diets include spicy foods have a special, milder diet for nursing mothers. But after about the first month, *most* babies are not bothered by *any* foods in their mothers' diets. Your favourite foods will flavour your milk somewhat, and your baby will learn the family menu through breastfeeding.
- If there is a **food problem,** the most likely culprits are cow's milk and dairy products. Some babies are fine as long as their mothers don't eat large quantities of these foods at one time; others will react to even a small amount. If your family has a history of severe allergies and anaphylactic reactions, you are wise to be cautious. Talk to a breastfeeding supporter or your healthcare provider if you're concerned your baby might be reacting to something you're eating.
- **Go easy on caffeine** for the first month or so. Watch your baby for jitteriness once you add caffeinated beverages, and go light enough that you can nap easily when you get the chance.

Is It Normal for Breastfed Babies to Have This Much Gas?

All mammals have intestinal gas every day. We adults are (usually) just more discreet about it. The baby who's gassy and who isn't bothered by it is fine. But sometimes gas makes a baby truly uncomfortable. And even a baby who isn't bothered by gas most of the time might have a meltdown if he feels a bubble in his tummy when he was already frazzled. To help move those gas bubbles around painful corners, you could try these suggestions:

- nurse
- use the Magic Baby Hold described earlier in this chapter

- carry the baby upright against your shoulder or chest (a sling is great for this)

A gassy and uncomfortable baby who is also growing very quickly might be getting milk faster than he can cope with (see Chapter 18, Oversupply).

How Do I Burp My Baby?

Cultures that carry their babies a lot usually don't understand the notion of burping them. The baby who is carried upright most of the time will naturally burp when he needs to. Burping a baby is more often needed when bottle-feeding because more air is swallowed. Wind can also be an issue if you lay your baby down immediately after nursing. Lying flat tends to trap air in the baby's stomach (how do *you* feel when you lie down after a big meal?). Some babies seem to squirm a bit at the beginning of the feed, especially if the milk comes out fast and they are noisily gulping. They may need a quick burp early on in the feed so the air doesn't get trapped under all that milk.

If your baby needs to burp, you could try these tips:

- hold him against your shoulder (covered by a cloth to catch the likely spit-up) and rub or pat his back gently
- sit him up in your lap, bend him forward, and then straighten him up again while you gently pat his back
- search online for videos on "wonky winding," a nifty way of shifting your baby around to help the bubbles come up.

What Can I Do About Spitting Up?

Many babies don't seem to be bothered by spitting up. And the amount of milk they spit up usually looks like a lot more than it really is. Spitting up can happen as a result of larger meals at longer intervals, so try nursing more often. Your baby may keep smaller volumes down better. Carrying your baby upright, especially after nursing, also helps.

If your baby is spitting up so much that it is hard for her to feed, she is not growing well, or she is really miserable, contact your healthcare provider (see Chapter 18, Reflux). If your baby has additional symptoms, such as green poo, eczema, or nappy rash, or is wheezing, talk to your healthcare provider.

How About Dummies?

The amount of time new babies want to spend at the breast sometimes shocks new parents. Maybe your baby doesn't need more milk, but he wants to be calmed or go to sleep – and the breast works almost every time. Would a dummy help? Here are some things to consider when making this decision:

- Some parents swear by dummies, whether to calm a bottle-fed baby between bottles or to reduce the time spent at the breast.
- Breastfeeding researchers tell us that when mothers want to breastfeed, using a dummy sparingly in the early months doesn't mean an end to breastfeeding.
- Some studies say dummy use at bedtime helps protect babies against sudden infant death syndrome (SIDS). It's not clear why this is so. Other researchers suggest that if the baby usually uses a dummy, not using one on a given night might increase the risk of SIDS.
- Using a dummy can affect the development of the mouth and teeth, raising a child's palate and crowding his teeth, as well as narrowing his nasal passages and leading to an increased risk of sleep apnoea. Orthodontists and dentists tend to warn against the long-term use of dummies, though they note that it is usually easier to stop a child from sucking on a dummy than to keep him from sucking his own fingers or thumb.
- Speech and language therapists tell us that overuse of dummies during the daytime may slow down language development.
- Research suggests that dummy use may be linked to increased ear infections in babies and toddlers.

A dummy is a substitute for the breast. When nursing babies want to suck, it's the breast they're looking for, and nursing can meet many needs besides food, as Laura found:

> She wanted to nurse practically 24/7. It was her comfort and escape from any and all discomfort. I was so happy to have it as a tool rather than having

to rely on other comfort items as she refused to attach herself to lovies, dummies, blankies, bottles, etc.

– Laura, United States military

Nursing meets those sucking needs with skin contact, good jaw development, and a full tummy thrown in.

There are times when a baby really can't nurse, though, such as

- in a car seat
- in an incubator
- when separated from the nursing parent
- before surgery, when she can't have milk for several hours

Some families might consider using a dummy in these situations, especially if their baby is really distressed. If you are thinking about using a dummy at home, you can keep the risks to a minimum if it's only used to settle the baby to sleep.

How Soon Can I Get My Baby on a Schedule?

At first, feeding the baby looms larger than anything else. You might think that if you could schedule the feeds, life would get back to "normal" faster.

Ah, but feeding will soon be a really *minor* event – one of the easiest, quickest, most casual and flexible parts of your day. You'll be able to fit it in among other things. Going to the supermarket? Top the baby off with a quick nursing before you go and you can shop longer without stopping. Babies rarely refuse these little extras when you offer. Paying the bills? Talking on the phone? Watching TV? You can do any of these and more while you nurse the baby. Sometimes you won't even notice you're doing it until you see a surprised face when you answer the door, baby still attached!

If you schedule feedings, you might end up trying to fit more complicated events around your baby's meals. It can be hard to leave the house, for example, because you feel you have to stick to your feeding schedule. Most babies simply can't wait the lengths of time many schedules suggest, or they can't follow a schedule and gain weight *and* keep your milk supply in good shape. Setting up a schedule risks an underfed baby and early weaning – and a more complicated life.

Nursing, once you and your baby have had some practice, is just not that big a deal. If you've got a sling you can nurse in, you can nurse on the go.

Most families find that feeding finds its own rhythm by about six to eight weeks, and life starts to feel a bit more predictable. Some babies, though, are just never very "regular," and it's easiest to just go along with them.

If you're the kind of person who needs a plan to feel in control, you could

- get up each morning around the same time
- have your meals at about the same times
- take the baby out for a walk every morning
- go to bed each night around the same time
- set up a weekly calendar of outings and social meet-ups

It may be more useful to track what your baby actually does, rather than what you think she should be doing. Baby-tracking apps can be a distraction, taking the focus off the baby. But some parents find apps reassuring as they help them learn their baby's unique rhythms.

Your baby's feeds can fit flexibly around the things you plan to do – this is *much* easier than trying to fit both your life and your baby's around feeds at set times.

My Baby Isn't Nursing at All Yet, or Not Very Well

When Natalie had a tough start with nursing, support from her wife made all the difference:

> During that first month, 24/7 around the clock I breastfed on demand, then pumped while my wife supplemented our baby with syringes and bottles for every single feed. Those first few weeks were a whole team effort; it was not a one-person job, and I am grateful for all the support I had. It would have been impossible otherwise.
>
> – Natalie, Canada

A tough start doesn't mean it is too late. Many babies take some time to be ready to start nursing or to nurse well, especially if

- your baby was born prematurely
- your baby has health concerns
- your baby has been separated from you because one or both of you needed medical treatment
- your baby had a difficult birth
- your baby had upsetting experiences at the breast that have put them off trying
- your baby was birthed by someone else

If your baby isn't nursing yet, don't panic. Babies are hardwired to breastfeed. Most babies will keep trying for at least two or three *months* after birth, even if they're meeting a breast for the first time! We've seen many babies start nursing much later than this, too. Here are some ideas that may help your baby start nursing:

- Focus on cuddling your baby skin-to-skin and just hanging out together. He might surprise you one day, finding the breast and latching on all by himself.
- Try offering the breast when he's fed and calm, rather than hungry and upset.
- If you're trying hard and it's feeling stressful, take a break from nursing and try again in a few days.

For more ideas for enticing a baby to the breast (and stories about babies who started nursing long after birth), see Chapter 17.

Focus on expressing your milk; it's a great investment in your future breastfeeding relationship. If your goal is to provide all the milk your baby needs, your target for now is to express at least that much. You've got plenty of time for nursing to fall into place. For more on how to keep your milk supply strong until your baby is ready to nurse, see Chapter 4, The Three Keeps.

Is It Possible to Spoil a Baby?

Maybe! You could buy your baby lots of expensive things she doesn't need. But spoiling with cuddling and attention? Not possible.

The word *spoiling* suggests giving your baby more than is good for her. It isn't possible to hold a newborn baby more than is good for her. She was born expecting to be held close most of the time. You're not making her dependent — she already is. And in just a few months' time, she will crawl, walk, and then run away from you. Even if you hold her all the time now.

Meeting your baby's needs now gives her a totally reliable base for exploring the world. In these early months, her wants are the same as her needs. We can meet either one without worrying about spoiling. When she is a year old, sometimes her wants and needs will be different. She might want to pull the cat's tail, but she needs to be kept safe (and so does the cat). It will be up to you to help her sort out these things — to help her learn patience, tolerance, kindness. But for now? All she needs to learn is love.

Perhaps you feel similar to how Teresa felt:

> I remember nursing my baby boy and thinking, "This is the most beautiful baby in the world." I would go to the store with him in a baby carrier and think, "All the other mothers must be so jealous that I have this perfect baby." I felt sorry for them, really. My mum told me that she felt the same way when I was a baby — and when my younger sisters arrived, too: an almost overwhelming feeling of love. It was like an extra connection to my mum to have the same feelings.
>
> — *Teresa, Ontario, Canada*

Want to know more?

You can find extra resources for this chapter at the "Art of Breastfeeding" tab at www.llli.org.

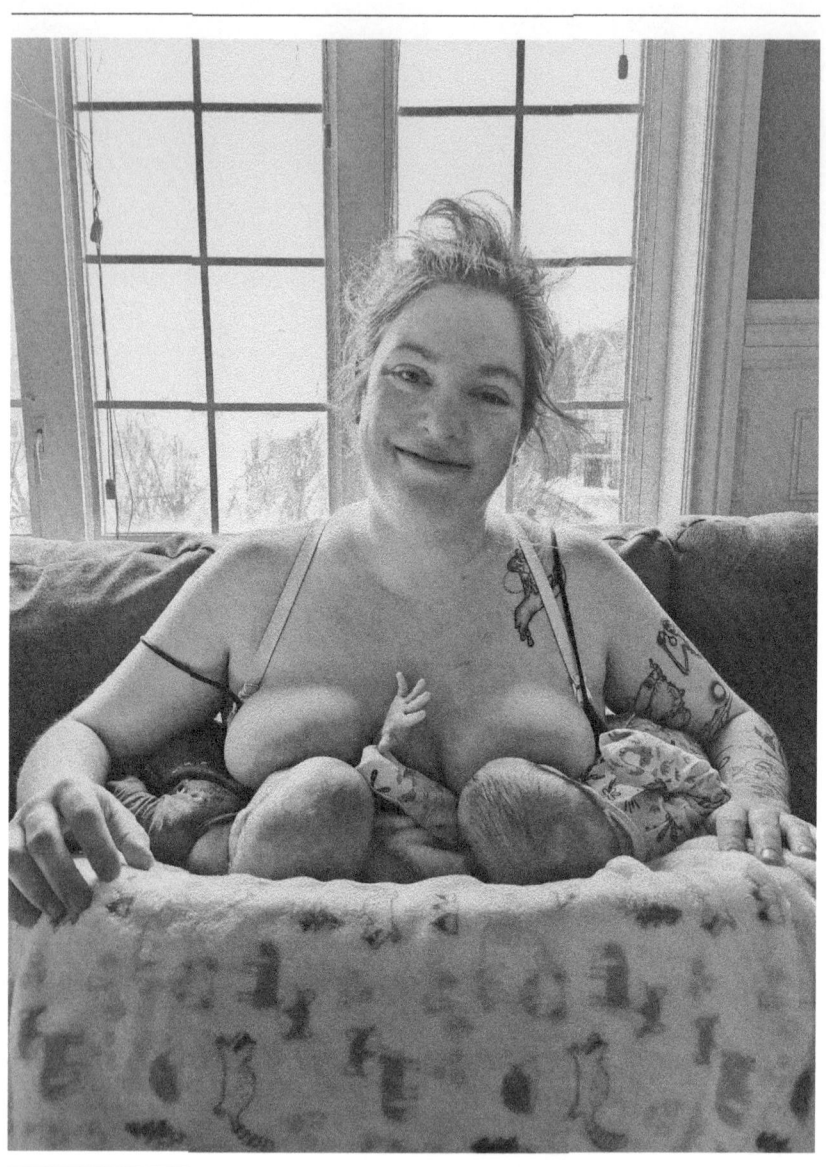

SEVEN

Two to Six Weeks: Finding Your Way

> No one really told me what exactly to do next. One day I didn't have a baby and the next day I did, and I can remember looking at her and thinking, "What do I do?" Like, I don't know how to take care of a baby. Thankfully, one thing people did tell me is that I would just know what to do. That this instinct would just kick in. And they were right.
> – Aurelia, Texas, United States

Well, look at you! You've made it through the first few weeks. Your baby is getting a little bigger and stronger, and the two of you are getting to know each other. You've started to figure him out – you know how he likes to be held, and the early signs that he wants to nurse. He's getting to know you (and your breasts!), too, and figuring out how to feed effectively. Your body is healing, and your falling-in-love relationship with your new baby is beginning to grow.

On the other hand, you might not be feeling completely on top of things. Your days probably aren't smooth and comfortable yet. That's not surprising; you're still a relative beginner – although when you meet a newer parent, or someone who's still pregnant, you already have a ton of experience to share.

Learning to nurse a baby, and building a milk supply, is like learning anything new: the hardest work is right at the start. But *babies settle down*. A newborn baby has no experience and no perspective. Everything surprises her. Cold air on bare skin? Needs to poo? She can react like it's the end of the world. You try your best to help, but it's pretty much trial and error.

By six weeks or so your baby will be more used to being here, and you'll be much more used to her. When she's unhappy, you'll know what has worked before. It all gets easier.

And it will get easier faster if you have enough support. Many communities once supported new mothers with "lying-in," a time when relatives would care for the new mother so she could recover, rest, and nurse the new baby. (A newer version is the "babymoon" – a honeymoon-type month or so of help with housework and meals.) Your community may provide this time of support for your family.

Our milk is sacred to us. Nursing parents are tended to in the first month, or more, so they can tend to their babies. Rest. Good food. Traditional Medicines.

– *Stephanie, Six Nations of the Grand River, Ontario, Canada*

Nowadays, unfortunately, many of us are not given this time to learn and recuperate. In some countries, there is no maternity leave. We very much hope that will change.

Even if you've had a baby before, each time may be different, leaving you feeling like a beginner all over again – as Roxana and Theresa found:

When my second son was born I thought things would be a little easier because I had already been a mum; however, the first few days without the support of LLL I thought I would die trying. I felt overwhelmed. Now I am breastfeeding my second child, and I am healing small wounds in my body, mind, and soul.

– *Roxana, Havana, Cuba*

After my older daughter, I thought that I now knew everything perfectly for the next sibling. And then I had twins. . . .

– *Theresa, Germany*

It takes time to get to know this new little person (or people!) and find your new normal. A new baby is a new relationship – not a gadget that comes with a set of instructions. It isn't possible, or necessary, to do everything perfectly. This is a time of learning, trying things out, and muddling through. Apart from safety basics, there is no "right" way to care for and feed your baby – only what works for now. Be as gentle with yourself as you are with your baby. It will get easier.

Nursing Beginnings – Two to Six Weeks

Healthy, full-term babies at this age may still be disorganised with latching. Samantha found it took some time before nursing Ruhi (her third baby) was easy:

> I hadn't anticipated any breastfeeding problems, but it actually took us a good few weeks to get into it.
>
> – *Samantha, from the UK, living in Bali, Indonesia*

As you become more practised, you'll start to notice that both of you are more in sync – even if you lead, your baby follows almost perfectly, making everything smoother and simpler.

If your baby was premature, or had any complications, breastfeeding may also take more time. As long as you protect your milk production and focus on The Three Keeps (see Chapter 4), you have *plenty* of time to work everything out.

A baby this age is usually focused on eating, but you'll also see quick smiles on his face when he's feeling good after or during nursing. These early eyes-closed smiles mean he's happy and content – they're not caused by gas. By six weeks, you may even begin to see love smiles, with eyes open and looking right at you.

Pain is always a signal to pay attention to, no matter how good "the latch" looks. If your nipples are still bothering you (or have started hurting when they didn't before), reach out for help.

Mariatu got support from experienced mothers in her community:

> It was tough. I was going to stop, till my auntie showed me more. I watched [my auntie and my neighbour, who were also nursing] and was around them, so I put Ibrahim the same way. I guess he learned, and so did I.
>
> – *Mariatu, Freetown, Sierra Leone*

Rafaela contacted LLL:

> The first few weeks were really painful; I often cried while breastfeeding. I am so grateful to [the LLL Leader] – without you, I would have given up.
> – *Rafaela, Austria*

If you haven't yet tried laid-back breastfeeding approaches (see Chapter 4), you might like to give them a go. They often help to make nursing more comfortable and relaxing. You can find more information in Chapter 18, Sore Nipples.

I Still Don't Know When to Nurse My Baby

At a party, the hosts don't usually ask if you're hungry before passing the snack tray. They offer frequently, and *you* decide whether to eat or pass. Or the food may be available as a buffet, where you can help yourself. You are your baby's host with the snack tray or buffet! Offer to nurse whenever your baby seems interested or unsettled. She will let you know if nursing is not what she wants right now. Here are some ideas that may help.

Whim Nursing

Nursing can be your baby's whim, or it can be your whim. You can offer to nurse for no other reason than that it feels as if it's been a while. Or you miss your baby, want to finish reading that article, are about to run an errand, or just... feel like it!

Nursing can be your baby's whim, too. Maybe he's just had a scary dream. Or maybe he has a bubble of gas and nursing will help his intestines pass the gas. But it doesn't really matter what the reason is. If it makes you or him happy, that's good enough.

Why Does My Baby Need to Nurse Twice as Often as My Friend's?

> For me it came down to one simple thing – feed the baby when she wants to be fed. My daughter always wanted to be fed, so I fed her.
> – *Janedy, Taiwan*

Some babies can't get milk as efficiently as others or tire before they're really full. They may gain weight well as long as they can eat frequently. Some breasts simply can't store a lot of milk, so the baby needs to feed often to get enough. Some sensitive babies nurse often to help them cope with the many little things that cause them stress throughout the day. Frequent nursing not only fills babies' tummies but keeps your milk supply in great shape.

Andrea's doctor helped her learn to trust her baby and her body:

> There was a time when I was very anxious about not knowing how much milk my baby was getting and whether she was satisfied, because sometimes she would let go of the nipple and start crying. I consulted my paediatrician, and she told me not to "think" when feeding the baby, but to let the body do what it is designed to do.
>
> – Andrea, Bogotá, Colombia

As long as your baby is gaining enough weight, the number of feeds is unimportant. If your baby *isn't* gaining well even though nursing often, contact your healthcare provider, and find breastfeeding support quickly.

Why Is My Baby Nursing Much *Less* Than My Friend's?

If your baby is growing just fine, then nursing less isn't concerning. Maybe your breasts hold more milk than your friend's, so your baby can take more milk in one go. Maybe your baby has a stronger suck or a different metabolism.

Julie's baby, who was later diagnosed with sensory processing disorder, seemed to resist nursing – but she managed to get plenty of milk:

> I offered her the breast frequently, but she only latched on when she wanted to, usually every three to four hours. She would pop off after a couple of minutes and scream; I would try to calm her down, and eventually she would latch again for a minute or two and repeat the pattern until she refused to latch completely. I worried about Alice's intake, how she could survive on such short, infrequent feedings with so much spit-up. However, she gained incredibly well. Because of her high muscle tone and strong, coordinated suck, she was able to transfer a large volume of milk very quickly. I really tried to listen to what Alice was trying to tell me about her needs. I noticed when Alice was fussing for hunger and offered the breast. When she unlatched and fussed, I let her lead the

movement and noticed she wanted to switch sides, so I let her. When she unlatched after a couple of minutes, she would lean back to the first side. It was unusual for a newborn, but we finally had nursing sessions without screaming.

— Julie, Ontario, Canada

Babies with sensory processing issues are a lot more, or less, sensitive to life than most babies. They may

- feel very tense (high tone) or floppy (low tone)
- get extremely upset by nappy and clothing changes, noise, lights, and crowds
- dislike things that calm most babies, such as being touched, carried, or snuggled
- have ongoing feeding issues, such as gagging or tiring easily at the breast

If you're concerned about your baby, talk to your healthcare provider.

Most babies need at least eight feeds in twenty-four hours (it doesn't matter *when* they have them). If a baby's weight gain is low, and he's not asking to feed this often, you can encourage him. Keeping him close, skin-to-skin as much as possible, will calm your baby and save his energy for feeding. If he can feel and smell the "buffet" nearby, he's more likely to remember he needs to eat. If he still isn't gaining weight as expected, or you suspect there's a bigger problem, contact your healthcare provider and work with a breastfeeding supporter. It's important that your baby gets enough to eat while you figure out what's going on. For more on keeping your milk supply high, see Chapter 4, The Three Keeps, and Chapter 18, Weight Gain Worries, Supplementing.

Should I Watch the Clock?

The clock is a pretty recent invention. Most babies in human history have been nursed without one. Many still are, as Fatmata describes:

There are lots of new babies in the area, and we talk, we cook, we visit each other. Other mothers have shared how they care for their babies, and I learned to feed my girl whenever she wants. We don't have a schedule.
– *Fatmata, Freetown, Sierra Leone*

In the past, in some places, mothers were advised to feed on a schedule – every two, three, or four hours. This practice often led to breastfeeding problems, especially low milk production, so the recommendation changed: feed the baby whenever she shows signs of wanting to nurse – her feeding cues.

Support mothers to recognise and respond to their infants' cues for feeding.
– Ten Steps to Successful Breastfeeding,
World Health Organization and UNICEF

Trouble is, the idea of the schedule still lingers for many parents. The phrase "Feed the baby on cue…about every two (or three, or four) hours" is still heard in some places. Some people believe this regularity gives you control of how much your baby eats. But it doesn't. For more on how you can *really* tell whether your baby is getting enough milk, see A Thriving Baby later in this chapter.

Some mothers say they're feeding on cue – when they feel it's been long enough. They may bounce the baby, change a nappy, try a dummy – anything other than nursing. The baby may be fussing, even crying, but mum or dad says, "It's only been an hour, how can she possibly want to nurse *again*?"

Haven't you ever suddenly craved ice cream, or a cup of coffee, a few minutes after dinner? *Babies don't have to be hungry to nurse.* If you offer, and nursing *isn't* what your baby wants, he'll tell you. Or he may respond with relief, as if to say, "Well, *finally*! Weren't you *listening*?" If he's been crying for a while, he may be too upset to nurse right away, so calm him first then offer again.

Offering the breast when he cries won't spoil your baby. His body is geared to constant holding and frequent feeding (exactly as it was in your womb). Your milk is geared to frequent feeds as well. Deliberately holding a baby off can lower your milk production, slowing the baby's growth. A baby can't gain weight well if they don't take in plenty of milk, and following your baby's cues helps him do just that.

It's also normal for a baby to "cluster-feed" at times, meaning he takes several short feedings during an hour or two. He may be "tanking up" in preparation for a longer sleep, as well as calming his brain, frazzled by a day of learning and excitement. The concept of a feed as a Big Event — something that needs preparation — is probably an import from bottle-feeding. In communities where breastfeeding has always been the norm, babies are more likely to stay close to their mothers, nursing on and off around the clock. No one counts or times feedings. Anita learned to nurse as she went about her usual work:

> I wasn't able to manage the house, cook, and tend to the family while continually breastfeeding. One of the nurses advised me to wear a lappa [a piece of material often worn to carry babies on backs], and she showed me how to tie it so Mohamed was in front. I didn't wear a blouse, and the baby was against my chest. Whenever he was hungry, he'd move around and find my nipple and drink.
>
> – Anita, Sierra Leone

The Pleasingly Plump Breastfed Baby

Some parents worry about their baby growing too fast. This baby's growth astonished even his doctors:

> The baby drank lots and lots of milk. He got all chubby; so much so that the doctor didn't believe that I was just breastfeeding him and I didn't believe it either, but there were no little dwarfs in the room that were sneaking in to fatten him up for me!
>
> – Guajirita Alquizareña, from Cuba, living in the Netherlands

Overfeeding is a valid concern — childhood obesity has reached epidemic levels in much of the world. A roly-poly, exclusively breastfed baby, though, is not a cause for concern. Samantha's baby also grew fast:

> My supply was fairly prolific and there were litres of it. Amalya weighed 11 kg at nine months old so we knew it was highly nutritious, too! And so, for six months, I donated lots of milk to my local NICU!
>
> – Samantha, from the UK, living in Bali, Indonesia

As your baby becomes mobile, this healthy fat will be used for fuel. Breastfed babies tend to grow fast in the early months but slim down by a year. Formula-fed babies often grow more slowly than breastfed babies at first, but their growth rate doesn't slow down in the same way – a pattern linked to overweight later on.

It's easy to overfeed a baby by bottle if you're not careful, but pretty much impossible if they're just nursing at the breast. If you're feeding your baby expressed milk or formula by bottle, see Chapter 18, Weight Gain Worries, on how to reduce the risk of overfeeding.

Nursing satisfies many more appetites than just a hunger for food. If we focus only on feeding cues, we miss out on the many other needs that nursing meets for our babies. This is why many health professionals now prefer to talk about *responsive feeding*.

Responsive breastfeeding involves a mother responding to her baby's cues, as well as her own desire to feed her baby. Crucially, feeding responsively recognises that feeds are not just for nutrition, but also for love, comfort, and reassurance between baby and mother.

– *The Baby Friendly Initiative, UNICEF UK*

It can be very freeing to throw out the whole idea of schedules and offer to nurse whenever your baby is unsettled, even if you nursed just ten minutes ago. Or whenever *you* happen to feel like nursing. Maybe, as Gisel describes, your breasts are getting a little too full:

My everyday life was and is to take care of my daughter, feed her and contemplate her. I produced a lot of milk, my breasts were very full, but my daughter always emptied them. When I put her on one breast, the other side would leak; I used disposable pads to avoid getting wet. I did not collect it, because I was always with her – I did not think it was necessary. During the day, when she slept for hours at a time, mountains would form on my breasts and become hard; when my daughter woke up, they would disappear in a matter of minutes.

– *Gisel, Mexico*

As nursing becomes harmonious, responding fluidly to *either* of you feeling like doing it, you may find that whim nursing quickly begins to include conversational nursing.

Conversational Nursing

Nursing is a key part of your baby's first human relationship. It's part of how she communicates with you, and how you communicate with her. Those deep gazes that the two of you share at times are communication, too. Nursing represents your longest conversations – and you can hold them whenever you and your baby like.

You've probably already found that sometimes you kiss your baby for no reason. Did you look at the clock before you did? What would you think if you were told to kiss your baby only once or twice a day? In the early 1900s, some books *did* advise mothers to handle their babies as little as possible, and refrain from showing affection. There were some very unhappy mothers and babies as a result. More recent research has shown the dangers of this advice: touch is *vital* for babies, promoting brain development and learning. It turns out that the "social brains" of babies who are starved of interaction end up smaller. The "love hormone," oxytocin, which flows during close contact, including nursing, has been described as "fertiliser for the brain." Your baby deserves all the loving contact you can give.

Whim nursings and conversational nursings – all these no-clear-reason nursings – put those healthy creases on your baby's arms, make you and your baby feel secure and happy, get your lifelong relationship off to a good start, give your milk supply a solid base, and make parenting easier.

Isn't He Just Using Me as a Dummy?

Exactly! Nursing feeds your baby, pacifies him, puts him to sleep, comforts, reassures, and relaxes him. Isn't it amazing that you can do so much for him? If you offer your breast only as food, you'll cut out some of the calories he gets, you could end up with supply problems, and you'll lose the pleasure of – literally – going with the flow.

Tied to the Baby? Feelings About Your New Role

When you're finding your way with breastfeeding, a mixture of feelings is very common, as Lynn describes:

> Sometimes it was a little bit challenging to know my body was solely responsible for feeding my baby girl, but at the same time it felt amazing and unbelievable.
>
> – Lynn, Turnhout, Belgium

Being *needed* so much can be uncomfortable for some of us, perhaps especially if our own baby-needs weren't generously met – or if we're feeling anxious about putting a career on hold. Clare writes about how she recognised her anger, even though she was enjoying her new baby:

> A few weeks after my first baby arrived, I realised that I was furious – furious with my husband, whose life had changed so little while mine had changed so much. It wasn't even that I disliked my new role – I was loving it. But it was the first time I'd experienced economic disadvantage and loss of status because of my sex, and I had to come to terms with that, before I could get on with enjoying my baby. Once I'd seen it, I could make a positive choice to let it go.
>
> – Clare, UK

If you're feeling pressured, or trapped, don't just stuff those feelings down; it's better to talk about them. Resentment can come between us and our babies, and other people we're close to. An LLL meeting can be a good place for these honest conversations about the losses as well as the gains of your new role.

Other Questions You May Be Having Between Two and Six Weeks

These are common concerns parents ask LLL Leaders about at this stage of rapid learning – for you and your partner, if you have one – as Christina describes:

> After our baby girl was born, we struggled through the first difficult weeks of breastfeeding, and eventually I was able to close some knowledge gaps.

> At last, we as a family (yes, including my husband!) became real breastfeeding "pros."
>
> – Christina, Germany

If your questions aren't answered here, you'll probably find them answered in Chapter 18 or on LLL websites. Always feel free to contact your local breastfeeding helper. Sometimes a supportive voice or smile in real life means a lot. Websites and books can only take you so far. You deserve real people, too!

Help! My Breasts Are Soft!

Remember how in the early days your breasts felt full and firm if your baby went a bit longer between feeds? By six weeks, many of us find we rarely feel full anymore, except if the baby goes a lot longer than usual between nursings.

The change can be sudden; it might feel like your breasts have deflated overnight. Don't panic – as long as your baby is still producing plenty of wet and pooey nappies, and gaining well, your milk hasn't vanished. Luisa's experience is common:

> Sometimes I thought that I didn't have enough milk because my breasts felt empty. But our son gained weight in a way that assured me that what I gave him was enough.
>
> – Luisa, Switzerland

Some of what you felt before was tissue swelling, not milk (see Chapter 18, Engorgement). By now, excess fluids and excess milk have sorted themselves out. Supply and demand have balanced, and your breasts have settled down. After the early weeks, it's normal for a lactating breast to feel... well, normal!

You may stop leaking milk as much as you did in the first days, too. As the weeks go by, milk begins to flow only at your baby's request (although sometimes a baby's cry, or even thinking about her, can still lead to a little leaking).

Thinking back on leaking in the early days of nursing, Clare recalled this memorable moment:

> I was in the supermarket with my baby. An older woman came up to me and said, "I'm so sorry to bother you, but I think your milk is leaking." I clutched

my chest. Then realised she meant that the four-pint container of cows' milk in my trolley was leaving a trail along the floor!

– Clare, UK

Some of us find that we leak for much longer – maybe even for as long as we breastfeed. That's normal, too (if a bit of a nuisance).

Or maybe you're thinking, *My baby is gaining well, but my breasts have always been soft,* or *I've never leaked!* That might be because you have a lot of storage capacity or because your baby nurses often enough to keep them from overfilling. Whether or not you feel full, or leak milk, the same guideline applies: a happy, thriving baby who's growing well is proof that your milk supply is fine.

A Thriving Baby

Many of us worry about making enough milk, especially with first babies. Most of us don't have to. Here are some signs of a thriving baby at this age:

- She is **gaining weight appropriately**. It's a good idea to have your baby's weight checked regularly by a healthcare provider, at least until you're confident that feeding is going well. Babies with health or feeding challenges usually need to be more closely monitored.
- She has **at least three yellow poos and five or more clear to pale yellow, mild-smelling, and heavy, wet nappies each day** during the first month or so. After this, some babies will start pooing less often, but they should still be producing plenty of wet nappies, and of course, growing well.
- She **has no trouble latching** and easily **stays attached**.
- She **usually has her eyes open** and looks interested for the first part of the nursing.
- She **has slow, deep sucks** for part of every nursing, beginning soon after the feed starts.
- She **is content** for at least a few minutes after nursing.
- She can almost always be **consoled by nursing again**.
- She sometimes has **calm, alert times** between feeds.
- She **is visibly filling out**: plumper thighs, fuller cheeks, and deepening creases on her wrists. Her skin looks smooth, not loose or baggy.

- **She is growing in length and head circumference.** Your baby's clothes will look shorter and her hats smaller!

If any of these signs aren't happening for your baby, check with your healthcare provider and find a breastfeeding helper. In some countries, you can use baby-weighing scales in pharmacies. Weighing your baby at home is not usually necessary.

How Much Milk Is He Getting?

The amount of milk a baby requires varies hugely among babies and from feed to feed. By about four weeks old, babies take an average of 750 to 800 ml (25 to 27 ounces) of milk a day. But this is just an average – some babies take 550 ml (19 ounces), while others drink as much as 1,300 ml (46 ounces).

The daily intake of a breastfed baby remains remarkably constant through the first six months of life. By the end of the first week, if all's going smoothly, you're producing about three-quarters of that amount. By two weeks, you're nearing your long-running peak.

But do precise figures matter? Not if things are going well. The amount of milk your baby takes varies from nursing to nursing, day to day. Your supply bounces up a little or down a little to accommodate his needs. Is it hot? He might want a bit more to quench his thirst. Is he really hungry? He'll take both sides and maybe go back to the first again. He knows his own appetite. As long as he's gaining well, you can forget the numbers, watch your baby, and let him tell you what he needs and when he needs it.

If your baby is *not* growing well on just nursing, contact your healthcare provider and find breastfeeding support. And check out Chapter 18, Weight Gain Worries and Low Milk Supply.

She's Suddenly Started Nursing a Lot! Am I Losing My Supply?

As long as your baby's nappy output stays high and she's growing well, you can be confident that your milk production is working well. It's common for babies to go through periods of intensive feeding and increased fussiness, sometimes called "growth spurts." Babies do grow in fits and starts, so more nursings might be about putting in a temporary order for more milk. But it's just as likely that these "frequency days" are about what's going on in your baby's brain, not her stomach. Parents often notice that times of more nursings happen just before their baby does something new: becomes more interested in the outside world, rolls over, sits up, and so on. As long as you follow her lead, after two or three days your baby will probably go back to her usual feeding pattern.

When do these frequency days happen? Around ten days, three weeks, six weeks, three months, and six months... but they can happen just about any time. And here's a secret: if you're nursing your baby whenever either of you likes, you may never even notice them.

I'm Still Worried About My Milk Supply

We use the term *milk supply* throughout this book because it's what most people say and we couldn't come up with another word, but there really isn't any such thing. To say that you have a milk supply is to imply that the amount of milk you produce is pretty rigidly set. It isn't. Take milk out and more milk will be made. There's an upper limit, of course, which is a bit different for each person. (And we are seeing more parents who, for various reasons, need to use donor milk or formula to supplement the amount of milk they can produce. For further discussion of milk production issues, see chapters 6 and 18.) If you're concerned about your milk supply, the sooner you deal with it, the more likely you are to be able to increase it.

Eline's babies were all slow to gain weight at first. Really good support transformed her experience with her third baby:

> I come from a family in which my younger brother was fed for a long time, so I could see myself breastfeeding my baby not just for the first few weeks but for months or years. When my first child was born, I supplemented with artificial feeding after a week. Baby was not gaining enough weight, was restless, not pooing enough. I fed her for five months, but with more and more artificial feeding. I didn't think I had enough milk.
>
> My second daughter was a big baby. Again, I started breastfeeding and wanted to do it exclusively. I had read up better, but again, in the second week I gave a bottle due to restlessness and not gaining weight. This again provided confirmation that my children did not get enough at my breast.
>
> During my third pregnancy, I became even better informed. My big son didn't gain enough weight the first week. I kept trusting my body and nature; the support of my husband helped a lot. I got all the space I needed

to lie down a lot and be skin-to-skin with my baby. The clinic also gave me extra weigh-ins and confidence that some babies take longer than protocol to gain weight. I also had a lactation consultant come in. She taught me that the baby could latch on to the breast naturally. After 3.5 weeks, my son was at birth weight and started to grow well. Knowledge and support from those around you and daring to deviate from protocol and expectations are so important in breastfeeding.

— Eline, the Netherlands

One potential issue at this stage is hormonal contraception, which is sometimes started soon after birth, or around six weeks. Methods containing oestrogen (such as the "combined pill") are known to suppress milk production and aren't usually recommended during the early months of breastfeeding. What is less well known is that progesterone-only methods (including the "mini pill," hormonal IUDs, and implants) can also sometimes reduce milk production. For more about contraception, see Chapter 9.

I Feel Like I Have Too *Much* Milk!

Your body has a lot of "backup systems" for living — two lungs, two eyes... and two breasts. Many women who've had one breast removed can make plenty of milk for their baby with the remaining breast, and some have nursed twins and even triplets.

By the end of these first six weeks, most of us find our breasts are making just what our babies need. But some of us have breasts that just don't want to quit — and may need a little persuasion to cut back. For tips on how to do this, see Chapter 18, Oversupply. The usual measures worked well for Denise:

> I had oversupply of milk and a very strong letdown. Within thirty minutes to an hour I would be engorged. If Baby slept two hours straight I would get very uncomfortable and I ended up getting mastitis [breast inflammation — see Chapter 18 for more information] three times. At my most frustrated point I reached out to LLL, and a lady called Kathryn was like an angel. Right away she listened to me and identified quickly what the issue was. She gave me tips on the positions to use to reduce the strong letdown, and also how to regulate the oversupply. For instance, lying back and having Baby feed lying on top or feed on one breast for two rounds, then the other. Also, that I could express a little bit in

between feeds to ease off the engorged feeling, but not so much that I would trigger fresh supply.

— Denise, UK

Over-production of milk (hyperlactation) is rarely much more extreme. Praveena tells her unusual story:

I knew something was off immediately when the nurse handed me a medicine cup at two hours postnatal for me to hand express into, and it ended up overflowing with colostrum in under a minute. She brought me a breast pump, and I proceeded to pump four ounces of colostrum in ten minutes.

Little did I know this was the very first warning of oversupply that would plague the next ten months. I got my first clogged duct at five days postnatal. I was unable to work the clog out and ended up with high fever and body aches due to mastitis two days later. I suffered excruciating pain and a debilitating feeling of sickness, but the clog and mastitis finally resolved after about four days on antibiotics and constant massaging and pumping.

My newborn son could not handle my fast milk flow and would choke when I tried to nurse him, so I ended up exclusively pumping for the first four to five weeks. During that time, my supply continued to increase rapidly. By six weeks postnatal, I was pumping about ninety ounces a day. My amazing lactation consultant guided me through this, helped me deal with the constant clogged ducts, and helped me avoid mastitis numerous times.

She had me try every trick under the sun to bring down my supply, but unfortunately, it just would not budge. With her help, I was finally able to nurse Arjun when he was around a month old. I was able to nurse Arjun for ten months, and he drank my pumped milk for another year. After an especially terrible bout of mastitis that had me hospitalised, I decided I could not continue breastfeeding anymore. I could not cut down on my supply by naturally weaning as I ended up with clogs or mastitis, so I took a medication to stop my breast milk supply. After giving birth to my second child, I had even worse oversupply, but thankfully I knew the drill this time and was able to avoid mastitis for the most part.

I still don't know the cause of my oversupply. I had some blood work done, but everything was within normal limits. While it might sound like a blessing to some, dealing with oversupply was by far the most difficult part of motherhood for me. I am so thankful to have had the guidance of my lactation consultant, my obstetrician, my physical therapist, and so many others who helped me through my journey.

— Praveena, Texas, United States

Those of us with oversupply can grow so accustomed to overfull, dripping breasts and choking babies that we think we're losing our supply when it stops happening (see the section A Thriving Baby earlier in this chapter). Make changes gradually, and keep an eye on your baby's weight while you're working on bringing your milk production under control.

My Baby's Less and Less Willing to Nurse at All

A breastfeeding supporter can help you figure out what's going on. Here are a few possible reasons:

- **The milk is coming too fast.** Your baby might gag, cough, and splutter when your milk releases, and come off the breast, leaving your milk squirting. He might manage better in nursing positions (laid-back, side-lying) where he can easily move himself out of the way. Have a cloth handy to catch squirting milk while he waits for the rush to slow down. Avoid expressing any more milk than you absolutely have to. Expressing increases the amount of milk you make. If your baby is obviously struggling with the amount and speed of milk, *and* he's growing really fast, by six weeks you could think about taking measures to control your milk supply (see Chapter 18, Oversupply).
- **The milk is coming too slowly.** Very slow flow is most likely when overall milk production is low. Work with a breastfeeding helper to see if you can increase your supply. You can also compress your breast with your hand while nursing to encourage milk to release, and switch to the other side when your baby starts getting frustrated. If these tips don't help, a nursing supplementer (see photo at the start of Chapter 17) can be used to speed up and even out milk flow at the breast. This device works by delivering expressed milk or formula via a thin tube placed next to your nipple (see Chapter 18, Supplementing).

  A few of us have normal milk production but **delayed milk release.** This can happen because of a thyroid condition or extreme stress. Warmth, relaxation, visualisation, massage, and laughter can all encourage a shy milk ejection reflex (see Chapter 15, Tips for Pumping).

  Babies who are used to fast, effortless feeding from a bottle may come to prefer the bottle, especially if something, such as low milk production, is making nursing difficult for them. Paced bottle-feeding can help, along with working on any nursing issues. Some families choose to switch to a nursing supplementer or cup instead of a bottle (see Chapter 18, Supplementing). Limiting or stopping dummy use can also encourage a reluctant nurser to do more of his sucking at the breast.

- **Your baby is ill or uncomfortable.** A stuffy nose can complicate nursing (see Chapter 18, Colds and Minor Illnesses). White patches in your baby's mouth – on the gums, inside the cheeks, and on the roof of the mouth, not just the tongue – may be signs of candida (a kind of yeast) infection, often called "thrush." This infection can make it uncomfortable for the baby *and* for you to nurse. Thrush can be passed back and forth between you and your baby, so both of you will need to be treated (see Chapter 18, Yeast (Thrush/Candida Infections)).

Check with your healthcare provider if your baby isn't nursing as well as usual and doesn't seem quite right to you. A sudden refusal to nurse in a young baby who was nursing well is most often a sign of illness.

My Baby Still Hasn't Even Started Nursing

There are lots of reasons babies take a while to start nursing. Sometimes, like Sien and her baby, you just need a little time and help:

> When Noor was born, it was my intention to breastfeed for a year. In the hospital we didn't receive a lot of help or info on how to get started. So when we went home it became clear it didn't go so well, and she wasn't drinking. The midwife gave us a bit more info, and after three weeks of hard work, we finally were on a roll.
>
> – Sien, Belgium

Asia took longer to get to full breastfeeding but felt it was worth the effort:

> We left the hospital bottle-feeding, as any attempt of breastfeeding would end up with the baby asleep within a few seconds. I hoped to try again in the privacy of my own home. Having left the hospital, I was faced with a difficult personal situation. Living in an extended family arrangement, I did

not have the privacy I needed. Instinctively I felt that I could succeed in getting the baby to latch properly if I was given time alone with her.

On day five or so my milk came in, and it disappeared faster than it came in. I cried every day due to my inability to breastfeed, but the loss of milk made me feel worse, probably on the borderline of depression. Following LLL advice, which I found on their website, and with the help of my mum, I gathered the strength to act. I kept my baby girl skin-to-skin as much as I could. The next day a miracle happened. I was given the privacy I needed, and my baby just suddenly latched! After that, it took a long time to establish exclusive breastfeeding – it didn't happen until around four months old. But it was definitely worth it.

– Asia, UK

Premature babies need plenty of time before they can nurse well. In the meantime, your milk is the best possible food and medicine for them. Verena worked hard to provide milk for her premature twins – and other babies!

After two weeks in the hospital, our twins were born at thirty-three weeks plus two days by emergency C-section. The C-section was traumatic for me, and I only heard my children cry briefly. I saw them sixteen hours later. With both of my children being cared for in the ICU, there was only one thing for me to do: get as much colostrum as I could. I started pumping four hours after the C-section, and it carried me through the difficult first few days and the exhausting next four weeks that my children spent in the hospital.

Within two weeks I pumped myself up to 2.2 litres of breastmilk a day, brought my milk to my children, and donated over 20 litres of milk to the human milk bank. In the clinic, my children were fed by feeding tube and then bottle-fed. After my twins were home, I was able to feed both of them exclusively at the breast relatively quickly.

– Verena, Vienna, Austria

Babies born a little early (say, three weeks) are often treated like full-term babies because they are usually healthy and can go home quickly. But at first they often feed more like earlier preemies: sleepy and low in energy. They're eager to nurse but might need support from expressed milk until they're ready to nurse for themselves. Take your time and keep a close eye on your baby's growth while you make a gradual transition from expressing to nursing. Expect it to take at least until your baby would have been forty weeks, plus a bit longer

– babies born early have more to cope with in the outside world than they would have if they'd been born later. You can find much more about feeding premature and early-term babies in Chapter 17.

Babies weighing less than about 2,500 grams (5.5 pounds) at birth, whether or not they were born early, may also act like premature babies. They usually need extra time and support until they can do all the work of feeding – like Jo's baby:

> My second-born was born underweight, which we didn't expect. He latched on right away, so the midwife was sure he'd gain weight quickly. However, when we took him home, I noticed that he slept a lot, and when he fed, his suck was weak, and he didn't stay on the breast for very long.
> – Jo, Kigali, Rwanda

Ideally, you'll have a breastfeeding helper used to working with premature and small babies. La Leche League can also offer solidarity and encouragement from other families who've been there.

If your baby has complex medical needs, your feeding plan will need to be tailored to her condition and medical care. Except in very rare situations, your own milk is even more valuable for your ill baby, and any time she can spend at, or near, the breast will help calm and comfort her. See Chapter 17 and LLL websites for resources on feeding babies with complex medical needs.

Or maybe your baby is full-term and healthy, but something else is making feeding difficult. The most common reason for early feeding difficulties is taking a while to get the hang of deep, effective attachment at the breast (see Chapter 4). Some of us have additional challenges, like very large, soft breasts, milk production issues, a premature baby, or tongue-tie. A breastfeeding helper can help you find solutions or workarounds to these challenges.

If nursing is very far from where you hoped it might be, these early weeks might feel like they're dragging on forever. But babies are hardwired to breastfeed and will keep trying for at least two or three months after a (full-term) birth – often much longer (see The Three Keeps in Chapter 4). As long as you're protecting your milk production and your baby enjoys being at or near the breast, there's plenty of time for things to fall into place.

If you or your baby have extra complications, see Chapter 17. There is almost always a way to nurse your baby or provide your milk. We're here to help.

Exclusive Pumping

We're seeing many more mothers who, from choice or necessity, are expressing instead of nursing. This is a massive labour of love and a recognition of the importance of human milk, especially for babies with extra challenges – like Rae's son Gideon:

> When Gideon was ten days old, we got a positive diagnosis for Prader-Willi syndrome (PWS). In babies, PWS is characterised by extreme hypotonia (floppiness) and failure to thrive. Most PWS babies never breastfeed, and many never manage bottle-feeds, relying instead on NG tubes [a tube goes through the baby's nose into his stomach]. As none of my babies have had formula, I really didn't want that for Gideon – he had enough to deal with as it was. Providing him with milk was the one thing I could do, so it gave me something to concentrate on.
>
> I continued to try and put Gideon to the breast – he simply did not know what to do. He didn't root, he didn't latch. I found the experience frustrating and soul-destroying. By eight weeks, I'd met another mum with a daughter with PWS, who helped teach me how to bottle-feed Gideon. This meant his NG tube was removed. I spoke to PWS professionals across the world looking for an "answer" – the magic technique that would enable Gideon to feed at the breast.
>
> Gideon just doesn't have the strength to breastfeed effectively, nor does he have the correct suck/swallow/breathe coordination. There is no magic answer. Instead, I try and focus on my successes: Gideon was exclusively breastfed for six months; he has never had formula, and at thirteen months I am still giving him breastmilk.
>
> – Rae, Great Britain

The EP (exclusive pumping) online community has unmatched know-how on all aspects of expressing, storing milk, and using expressed milk. If you find yourself EPing, for now, or longer-term, a warm welcome awaits you in EP social media groups, and of course, in LLL. For more about EPing, see Chapter 17.

My Baby's Unhappy but Doesn't Want to Nurse Right Now

This is one of the most common reasons for new parents to contact LLL Leaders. After the first sleeping-or-nursing weeks, babies start to wake up – often quite suddenly! – and the list of things they might want at any given moment gets longer. Nursing will satisfy most of the items on that list: food, comfort, company, soothing, warmth, pain relief, and more. But sometimes babies need something different. The first few times this happens, you might wonder whether your breasts have malfunctioned. As long as your baby's growing well and nursing is mostly going smoothly, it's most likely that your baby is just fed-but-frazzled right now.

Try some other things, like changing her nappy. Some babies hate a wet nappy, while some don't care at all. Shoko found that her babies became unsettled when they needed to wee or poo:

> When a baby simply won't latch on (and latching isn't usually a problem), chances are that baby needs to wee or poo, whether this is happening at the start of a feeding session or during one. A baby can become very agitated if he is encouraged to be kept on when needing "to go." Knowing this has helped me on countless occasions with my second baby (I didn't know this when my firstborn was a newborn) to not feel the frustration one might feel for baby popping on and off and not maintaining a latch – he will be able to, just as soon as his other pressing need "to go" has been met.
> – Shoko, the Netherlands

Your baby might need a change of position, view, or motion. Lieke found that taking her baby outside worked well:

> If the baby is restless, I always first try offering my breast. Then my other breast. If this doesn't help, I try burping her. I check her nappy. Sometimes I offer the breast again. And if that doesn't help, I go for a walk with the baby in a carrier. One block around the neighbourhood is usually enough to let her fall asleep. Sometimes I go for a walk three times on a single evening.
> – Lieke, the Netherlands

It's hard to calm a frazzled baby if you're frazzled yourself. A fresh pair of arms (that belong to someone the baby knows well, who *isn't* producing milk!) might be just what your baby needs. If she really doesn't want to nurse now, being near your breasts can be confusing for her – and you. Her instincts will probably take her there anyway, but she may just say a loud "no, thank you!" Audrey found that baby Leo slept well with her partner:

> Leo took a lot of naps with his daddy, who had started telecommuting after he was born. Leo was sleeping on top of his father doing 3D animation in videogames.
>
> – Audrey, France

When she's calmer, maybe after a "reboot" nap, offer your baby the chance to nurse again. Nursing solves a multitude of baby problems besides just hunger. At some point, nursing will probably be your baby's answer, even if it wasn't his original question.

Not understanding normal baby behaviour – especially fussiness and crying – is a major cause of early, unintended weaning. Companies that want to sell you formula will tell you their products make babies happier and more settled – and not mention their known risks.

If your baby is often unhappy and you can't figure out why, see Chapter 18, Crying and Colic, talk to your healthcare provider, and find breastfeeding help. Nursing problems almost always have nursing (or expressed milk) solutions. But the problem may not be related to feeding at all.

What Are Some Causes of Crying Besides Hunger?

The most common reason for babies to cry is that they're on their own. We're a "carrying" species – our babies expect to be kept close. Being nearby isn't enough for a newborn. He can't see far, so if he can't *feel* you, he doesn't know you're there. For our ancestors, being left alone was a threat to a baby's survival; so babies are programmed to protest if they think they *might* be alone. And the nervous system of a baby is unfinished at birth. He relies on caretaking adults to help him manage his feelings, calming and comforting him when it all gets to be too much.

The more babies are held, the less they tend to cry. Across the world, parents and others instinctively pick up, hold, and soothe babies by talking and singing to them. This is ancient knowledge, as Stephanie, an Indigenous parent and lactation consultant, writes:

> We know that babies need skin-to-skin as emotional centring with their parents. When they need to be held more, we know the baby needs us. They aren't regressing. Babies know what they want and like, and what they don't want and don't like. We honour this by learning from their knowledge.

We see the baby's needs and desires from their perspectives. That's how we attach to each other.
– Stephanie, Six Nations of the Grand River, Ontario, Canada

Experienced baby-holding adults know that upset-but-not-hungry babies are happier on the move. They instinctively sway in a gentle dance, or rock the pram. Clare found clever solutions:

A combination of a sling and an exercise ball meant I could keep up with my emails – gently bouncing at my desk, baby snuggled close. With my third baby, I learned to nurse in the sling as well – multitasking at its best!
– Clare, UK

While your baby may want *you* and no one else if he's upset, fortunate babies have people who can take turns holding them. A sling or soft carrier enables you (or someone else who loves your baby) to meet his need for closeness while getting other things done. And no – you won't spoil your baby by keeping him close. You'll be developing his brain, and his trust. Relaxed, well-loved babies have the best chance of growing into confident, happy children and adults who know how to make loving relationships. In a few months' time, your baby will be ready to start moving away from you – whether you're ready or not!

These are some other reasons for crying:

- A baby might be uncomfortable, overexcited, or tired.
- Occasionally, a baby reacts to a food you're eating. Talk to your healthcare provider if you think this might be a problem for your baby.

Sometimes, crying is a mystery. This understanding changed Luisa's experience:

In my thoughts, my breastfeeding relationship with our son would go smoothly. But it didn't. Which doesn't mean it was bad, I just had to learn that something doesn't have to go smoothly to be wonderful. For example, one day our son screamed at my breasts the whole time. That day I cried a lot, too. I then asked a lactation consultant for help, and with her help I could accept that some days are hard, but better days will come.
– Luisa, Switzerland

For some less common causes of crying and more tips for comforting your baby, see Chapter 18, Crying and Colic. If you have a truly unhappy baby – especially if she's unhappy most of the time, not just an hour or two here and there – consult with your baby's healthcare provider. Caring for a crying baby can be very distressing for adults, especially if you've had many experiences of not being comforted yourself. Ask for as much help as you need. La Leche League groups are good places to meet families with babies of all kinds.

Adapting to the Baby You've Got

Ask any parent of more than one child: each baby comes with their own personality. While you'll be watching it unfold over years to come, some aspects of your baby's **temperament** start to show up in these early weeks.

Temperament refers to the way someone naturally behaves, feels, and reacts. It's believed to have a biological basis, as the various characteristics start to be seen from soon after birth and tend to be fairly stable during a person's whole life. Psychologists have suggested lots of different ways to look at temperament, but no matter which model is used, all agree that it influences your life in many ways. For babies, some characteristics that can be useful to think about include:

- how physically active they are
- how sensitive they are to what's going on around them, and to their own bodily sensations
- how intense their reactions tend to be
- how regular they are; whether they tend to eat, sleep, and poo at roughly the same times each day, or not
- whether they are happiest in company, or on their own with just family
- how easily they make transitions, such as between being asleep and being awake

---

Some babies wake up calm and cheerful, and fall asleep easily, staying asleep even if the dog barks right by the crib. They soon fall into regular patterns of eating, sleeping, and pooing. When they get a little older, they smile charmingly at strangers, who comment on what easy, delightful babies they are. If you have a baby like this, enjoy them – but try not to give advice to anyone else!

Other babies need lots of help to wind down for sleep and to ease the shift back to being awake. They wake up if a dog barks a block away. Minor physical discomforts – getting undressed, pooing, burping, a clothes label that itches – can really upset them. They're highly sensitive, high energy, and high maintenance. As one tired father put it, "She just doesn't seem to like being a baby. I figure she'll find life less frustrating when she can walk and talk."

And your baby is likely to be a unique combination. Julie found that the strategies she'd learned with her first baby didn't work for Alice, who later turned out to have sensory processing disorder:

> My second baby, Alice, came into the world in a rush. From the beginning, she was strong, loud, full of energy, had a good deep latch but would pop off after a couple of minutes, screaming. She pushed away when we tried to hold, rock, or soothe her. She protested with her whole body, arching her back and pushing with her arms. We wanted to engage in attachment parenting with Alice, but she didn't. We tried to co-sleep and carry her in a sling, but she screamed and struggled. When we put her down in her bed or on a blanket on the floor, she quieted or fell into a deep sleep.
>
> – Julie, Ontario, Canada

Whatever kind of baby you have, life will go better for both of you if you adapt accordingly. Very placid babies might need to be reminded to eat. It can be easy to ignore them, but they need plenty of company and brain stimulation, too. Your highly sensitive baby won't hesitate to tell you – loudly! – if he's not getting what he needs. Keep him close and experiment to see whether he does better with calm and quiet or plenty of activity. Surround yourself with supportive people who remind you what a great job you're doing. Try not to be intimidated by parents of easy babies (maybe they'll get one like yours the next time).

I'm Just Not Enjoying Any of This

Some babies, and some breastfeeding situations, take more work than others. Two to six weeks is also the time when postnatal depression or anxiety can make its appearance. You're in the middle of a massive life transition, with hormones all over the place. Even the happiest pregnancy, easiest birth, and greatest joy about becoming a mother can still result in moments where you burst into tears unexpectedly.

Moments of sadness that come and go are sometimes called the baby blues, and they're a normal reaction to the changes you're going through. Usually, this time of ups and downs passes. If feelings of anxiety, unhappiness, or depression continue for more than a few days, talk to a person you trust or a healthcare provider, or contact a postnatal depression support group. Most medications for anxiety and depression are compatible with breastfeeding. For more information, see Chapter 18, Postnatal Mood Disorders. Some people get very strong feelings of aversion or agitation when nursing. This can be really distressing. It's more common as babies become toddlers and preschoolers, or if you become pregnant while nursing, but it can happen earlier, too. You can find more info in Chapter 10, I Feel Terrible When I Nurse! If you feel awful every time your milk releases, see Chapter 18, Dysphoric Milk Ejection Reflex.

Those who already live with mental health issues, like Annabé, need especially good care in the months after birth:

> When I met LLL, I was going through one of the most wonderful times, my second pregnancy, but the circumstances of my life and my mental health condition made that whole stage one of the worst times of my life. I only saw and felt darkness, pain, and a lot of loneliness. I started attending LLL meetings with my second baby. I had no problems with breastfeeding. Finding a space to share about breastfeeding and parenting topics and having my experience and motherhood valued was a completely new and fresh feeling. LLL allowed me to learn that I can see beyond the dark, I can put any battle on hold, and for as long as it takes I can simply let myself be carried by the intention to offer, to give, to be there. I learned that I can be, feel, and live beyond my disorders.
>
> – Annabé, Latin America

The arrival of a new baby is a time of extra stress, for sure – and it can also be an opportunity for change. Whatever your challenges, LLL Leaders can help you find strategies and workarounds, or help you choose another way to feed your baby.

How Do I Nurse When I'm Out and About?

Learning to nurse beyond your home is part of the art of breastfeeding. Many countries have legal protection for the right of babies to nurse wherever they need to. The law is only part of it, though – you will quickly get a sense of whether nursing in public is "the done thing" in the places you live or visit. Helen, who is from the UK, noticed that nursing was much more publicly visible in Ecuador:

> In Ecuador, women will very openly uncover their breasts in public to feed their babies. When a flash of nipple appeared, everyone politely looked away. There was never a suggestion that the mothers should cover themselves or remove themselves to a toilet cubicle to feed. Without embarrassment, nipples are uncovered in restaurants, churches, playgrounds, you name it! The country has no need to produce "Breastfeeding Welcomed" stickers, as pretty much every place welcomes it.
> – Helen, UK

Depending on your community's support for breastfeeding, and how you feel about your body, you may be very comfortable nursing wherever you go – like Luisa:

> I breastfeed in public and think that this has to be normalised (quite a shame actually, it should be normal anyway). In the beginning, I just fed our son wherever I was (of course trying to create a space with minimal distraction for him). Then I found out that several shops/cafés, etc. offer a special room for breastfeeding, which was a big help.
> – Luisa, Switzerland

In some places, it's awkward or unacceptable to nurse where others can see you. And some of us have been taught to feel ashamed of our bodies. Other people probably will not get more than a brief glimpse of skin and may not even notice that you're nursing. (It's amazing how much more nursing we see once we're aware of it!)

The more often breastfeeding is noticed, the more it will be accepted. Many of us nurse away from home because we suddenly don't have a choice – hungry baby, public setting. Through giving birth and feeding our babies, many of us have come to value our bodies for what they can do, not what they look like.

These ideas may help you feel more at ease with nursing in public:

- Practise at home – in front of a mirror if you want to see what others see.
- Wear clothes you can nurse in comfortably. They don't have to be specially designed for nursing, although having special nursing clothes might help if you feel anxious.
- Try the two-layer approach: a stretchy tank top that pulls down, plus a top layer you pull up. Your baby's body hides almost all the bare skin.
- You could wear a tank top underneath your top, with circles cut out for nursing. Your outer shirt covers the circles, and the tank top covers anything that your outer shirt doesn't.
- A cardigan, jumper, jacket, or loose button-up shirt can cover anything your baby's body doesn't.
- While nursing on one side, pressing your forearm against the other breast may help to prevent leaking. If you do leak, adjust your clothing so any wet spot won't be right over your nipple. Dark-coloured prints help to hide wet spots.
- If you usually use pillows or other feeding props at home, you might feel safer taking them out with you at first. See Chapter 4 for out-and-about nursing props and positions.
- Practise nursing sitting cross-legged on the floor.
- The most awkward moment when nursing in public may be when your baby actually latches. You can turn your body away from other people during the latching process, then turn back once she's nursing.
- Meet other people's eyes with a friendly, open expression, or avoid eye contact. Most people will automatically match your behaviour.
- A blanket or specially designed shawl or cover-up may help – though it may attract more attention than just nursing. Babies usually prefer to see your face while they nurse.
- Start by nursing somewhere that feels like a home away from home, like at a family member's or friend's place – and expand outward from there.
- Ask around (La Leche League meetings are one place you could start) about the popular baby feeding spots in your neighbourhood. You might even make some new friends while you nurse.

Do I Need to Introduce a Bottle? Will It Help?

If you're able to spend six months or more with your baby, you might not need to use bottles at all – she can go straight on to a cup. Babies who are already eating plenty of family foods when you go back to work will often manage fine with just food and water while you're away. Companies that sell feeding equipment would like us to see bottles (and pumps) as normal parts of nursing, but it's worth remembering that most human babies never used them. Chapter 14 has lots of tips on separations from your baby.

If you want to use a bottle because you're going back to work, consider waiting until your milk supply has settled down (around a month) and nursing is going smoothly. There's no magic window of opportunity for introducing bottles. Of course, there are other reasons for expressing before this time, if nursing *isn't* going smoothly (see Chapter 4, The Three Keeps).

Some families choose to store some milk in the freezer for emergencies – for example, if you have a medical condition and might need to go to the hospital on short notice. Verity-rose decided to do this after a stressful experience with her second baby:

> With my third baby I decided to harvest colostrum. My second baby had been in the Neonatal Intensive Care, and I had to swiftly learn how to hand express, as he was too poorly to feed directly and needed milk via NG [nasogastric] tube. I decided that this time I would collect some pre-birth as it would mean, should I need it, I didn't need to worry. Thankfully I never needed it, but knowing the syringes were in the freezer gave me peace of mind.
>
> – Verity-rose, UK

Even if your baby won't take a bottle, there are lots of other options for feeding him milk (see Chapter 14).

Having someone else give a bottle to "bond with the baby" misses a key point about breastfeeding. Breastfeeding doesn't just fill a stomach – it's a relationship. Partners, other family members, and friends can hold, carry, calm, change, and bathe your baby. Of course you can share feeding, if this is what you all choose. But it's not the transfer of milk that connects nursing mothers and their babies – it's all the time spent holding, touching, and gazing at them. Non-nursing parents (and others) can do this beautifully, without getting involved in feeding. Love doesn't always have to come with food. Even in families with two mothers who are both nursing the baby, there can be times when "only the birth mum will do." The baby's relationship with each person is unique.

Chris reflects on his role as a father of babies with very different feeding stories:

> As a new father, I didn't give feeding much thought. I figured it was best to let my wife handle it – after all, she's the one with the boobs. At first, I was disappointed when my firstborn wasn't initially breastfed. I didn't understand why this process could be so difficult. While I initially felt like giving my child a bottle was a shortcut to bonding, it soon became apparent that there was more to it than that. I resented the bottles and the realization that my child wasn't getting the best start possible. I imagined bonding through playing, educating, and watching films together.
>
> After a few months, my wife relactated (which is astounding). However, not having the milk could be frustrating at times. If my child was hurt or needed soothing, the milk was the first thing that came to mind. I had to find other ways to soothe them, such as rocking, cuddling, or distracting them.
>
> With my fourth child, I had become accustomed to my wife being the primary soother. However, my youngest comes to me for cuddles and soothing, even though I don't lactate. I'm even the one who helps her to sleep. I've come to realise that the milk isn't a barrier to being an active parent.
>
> – Chris, UK

For more about relactation, see Chapter 17.

Using bottles doesn't save time or give you more sleep. Ask any mother who's *had* to express for a baby who wasn't nursing yet – expressing usually takes longer than nursing. And research has shown that exclusively breastfeeding mothers get the most sleep of all mothers – especially if they sleep with their babies. For more on sleep, see Chapter 12. If you're feeling dangerously tired, there's an "emergency sleep plan" in LLL's book *Sweet Sleep*.

If you do use a bottle from time to time, it's well worth the extra effort to use your own milk in it if you can. Using expressed milk protects your milk production and your baby's health. Where this isn't possible, any amount of your milk that your baby gets benefits him in ways nothing else can. For more about formula, see Chapter 5.

People Are Saying I Need to Get Away from My Baby

New parents hear a lot that they need to get away from their baby. But you might or might not feel like going. It's your call. This is the falling-in-love stage with your baby, and many of us find that it just doesn't feel right to be too far apart, as Clare found:

> When my baby was a couple of weeks old, I thought I "should" take a break from being with her, so I decided to walk round the block. As I reached the end of the street, losing sight of the house, I started to feel a pull backwards, as if my baby and I were joined by elastic. I was only away about ten minutes, but that stretched feeling was so uncomfortable that I didn't do it again for months!
>
> – Clare, UK

On the other hand, some of us find we feel "touched out" at times. This might be a matter of personality, though lack of support may also be a factor. In some places new parents have help all the time to take a turn holding the baby. Some of us aren't so lucky. If you feel alone, or have health challenges and need more rest, it's okay to ask for help from people you trust.

Most adults (and many teens) love holding babies. If you're short of help, maybe there's a grandmother nearby who's missing her grandchildren, or a young adult far from home who'd be delighted to be "adopted" by your family. Or if your budget allows, you could consider hiring some help, such as a postnatal doula. This can be a good time to make new connections. For more on building your support network, see Chapter 2. For more on handling separations from your baby, see Chapter 14.

Depending on your personality, you might be happy hunkered down at home, or you might be going stir-crazy. Babies at this age are very portable. You can go out walking, to lunch, the movies, or any activity you like with your baby. A baby sleeping in a sling is almost invisible. If your baby cries, most other people will be less bothered than you are. A baby who is unsettled at home might be more relaxed on the move. Bring him with you, and you might all have a better time.

What About Sex?

Will you ever have sex again? Sure. Many parents already have at this point. Others haven't yet, and that's common, too. Discomfort from birth, vaginal dryness, and tiredness can reduce the inclination for a while. Others find an exhilarating increase in their libido, responsiveness, and orgasm intensity. It helps to have a sense of humour about leaking milk (or a towel underneath you). And maybe some lubrication. Talk to your healthcare provider if discomfort persists. Pregnancy, birth, and nursing can be a great opportunity to shed some inhibitions and gain a new appreciation for what your body can do. There is a very, *very* wide range of normal experiences. And remember: the way things are now is *not* the way they'll be forever. For more about reestablishing intimacy with your partner, see chapters 8 and 12.

Being Home So Much Can Be Lonely!

Being home with a baby doesn't have to mean spending all your time actually *at* home (unless you want to). And it doesn't have to mean being alone.

Clare found unexpected benefits when her friend needed company:

> My friend had her first baby a few months after mine. She developed postnatal anxiety and didn't want to be alone. Her husband called and asked if she could spend time with me. She'd come over most weekday mornings, or I'd go to her, and we'd hang out together for the day. We attended LLL meetings and baby groups, went for walks, made and ate lunch, did housework, maybe gave the babies a bath. It's much easier for two adults to take care of two or more babies than for one person to take care of a baby alone. What started as an emergency became a friendship.
>
> – Clare, UK

Historically, women taking care of babies and children spent time together working, sharing chores, news, knowledge, and friendship. Research suggests that women often don't have a fight-or-flight response to stress. When we're under stress, we release oxytocin, which makes us want to take care of our children and seek the company of others. Oxytocin, tending children, seeking friends? La Leche League welcomes you.

Raquel found that LLL meetings gave her more than just feeding support:

> My daughter Lucía is undoubtedly the best thing that has happened to me and, at the same time, the hardest experience I have ever had. For me, breastfeeding support groups were much more than breastfeeding support. There, many of us mums found a shoulder to cry on when we felt the world

was falling on top of us, and the best advice not only for breastfeeding but for all kinds of doubts about postnatal recovery and baby care.
– Raquel, Madrid, Spain

At LLL meetings, you can meet people who have been through the same things you are experiencing. You will see how experienced mothers nurse, carry, and hold their babies. You may see how they deal with older children and juggle multiple competing needs. New parenthood is different from any other club. We all flounder at least a little, and we all have at least a little something to give. As one attendee said after their first meeting, "I was going from here to the paediatrician's office to get some of these questions answered. Now I think I'll just go home and enjoy my baby."

While virtual meetings can work really well, there's nothing like being with people in real life. If you don't have an LLL group in your area, you could look for a childbirth class reunion, baby activity class, or parenting group, or consider asking one or more friendly-looking families if they'd like to form a playgroup with you. They're probably looking for company just as much as you are. If they're already in a group, they'll probably be happy to have you join!

Your baby will probably enjoy the company, too. Babies are born expecting a lively community around them, with adults and children of different ages. Some babies get bored at home. You may find yourself saying about your fuss-free or peacefully sleeping baby, "But she's not like this at home!" You may have found the community you both need. Babies who react to noisy groups with tears may feel secure in a baby carrier or sling, while you get the company you need.

Learning to Trust Yourself

Every ordinary mammal mother comes equipped to raise her ordinary baby. Special circumstances may call for some specialised knowledge, but even then, the bedrock of that specialised knowledge is instinct. We're unsettled by the sound of a baby crying, so we pick up the baby and comfort him. Pure instinct!

You're now starting the most complicated job of your life, without an instruction manual. Actually, your instruction guide is right in front of you, incredibly cute, with big wide eyes. Your baby knows how to complain if she's in need, and you have an internal urge to respond when she complains. The two of you will work out the details as you grow together. Cyndel reflects on how she has developed with each of her children:

> Each child I have nursed has helped me overcome something through that breastfeeding relationship. As I help them to grow physically, they have helped me to grow and change and heal alongside them. I am so thankful to each of my children for the person they have made and continue to make me become.
>
> – Cyndel, Ontario, Canada

The arrival of a child may stretch us in ways we never anticipated. Melissa's son Andy has cerebral palsy:

> Two things make all the difference in breastfeeding – support and determination. The same things make all the difference in parenting, and especially in parenting a child with special needs. Andy's birth completely changed the course of my life in so many ways. I cannot imagine where I would be today if I had not breastfed Andy. I am grateful for all that our breastfeeding journey taught us.
>
> – Melissa, Tel Aviv, Israel

You might be thinking, "I don't know what my instincts are. This feels like alien territory." Or the whole topic of motherhood (or fatherhood) may just leave you feeling really sad. If this is you, you're not alone. You may be an "unmothered mother," or an "unnurtured parent."

Some of us are motherless, having lost our mothers to death or abandonment. Nicole felt her mother's absence deeply:

> My mother passed away when my first baby was only three months old. I dearly missed sharing all the exciting milestones as my daughter grew older. I was breastfeeding and was not aware of the LLL group in my city. Another woman I knew, Rebecca, had four breastfed, grown-up kids. She gave me plenty of moral support. Later I became a member of our local LLL group and enjoyed all the benefits of a monthly chat with like-minded mothers – but I always wished I could have my own mother's help.
>
> – Nicole, South Africa

Some of us have a living and involved mother but have not had the "good enough" mothering we needed. Where our inner mothering template should be, we have painful memories, confusion, or just a blank – as Aurelia writes:

> There was grief surrounding my abandonment issues of my mother leaving when I was a kid – as I looked down at my little baby and wondered in a new way how any mother could ever choose to go. There was grief because I felt so totally unprepared and unworthy of being a mother myself.
> – Aurelia, Texas, United States

The good news is that we can learn and heal. Becoming a parent is a huge opportunity for change. La Leche League meetings are one place to nurture and grow our instincts through exposure to positive models, as Anna discovered:

> I did not go to LLL with my first child. I thought it was only for parents who had breastfeeding problems, and breastfeeding was uneventful for us. During my second pregnancy, a good friend asked me to mentor her expectant stepdaughter. She had concerns that the young woman might be abusive or neglectful to the baby, as she was unkind and critical to her stepson. I thought of a wonderful, loving, nurturing mother we knew who was an LLL Leader. I took this young woman to an LLL meeting and was surprised to find that I had found a home. I had found mothers for myself, when I had not even realised how badly I needed them. So I went to LLL for someone else, but stayed for myself, and for my family.
> – Anna, Texas, United States

Having a baby gives us the chance to connect with others in new ways. Many of us have learned about nurture for the first time as we learned to do it for our children. With time, patience, and loving support, we can learn to nurture ourselves, too.

Want to know more?

You can find extra resources for this chapter
at the "Art of Breastfeeding" tab at
www.llli.org.

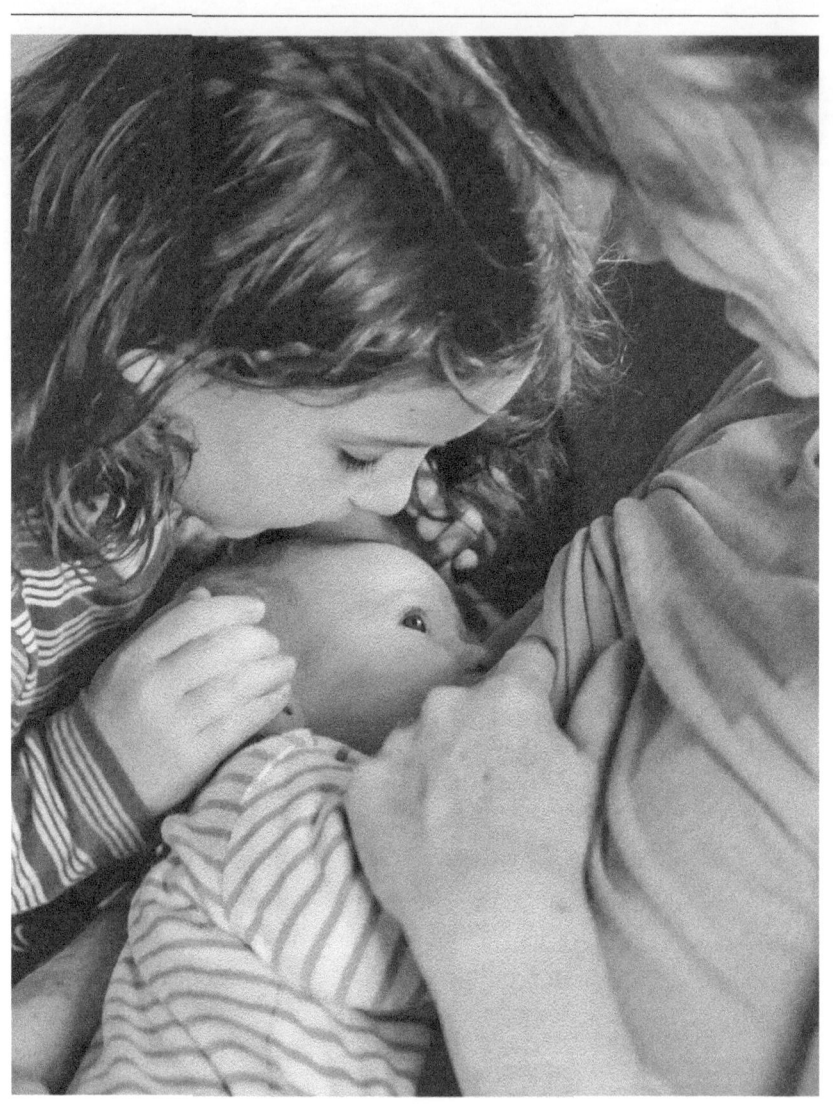

EIGHT

Six Weeks to Four Months: Hitting Your Stride

> I'm four months postnatal and I've exclusively breastfed my baby thus far. My milk supply is excellent, and nursing continues to be a joy. As I lay my sweet baby Julien down to sleep, full of milk – I pat myself on the back for the work we've done together. As I've sat and nursed my baby through my maternity leave, I'm reminded in my reflections that despite the complications, the trauma, and the difficulty, my body did do exactly what I had hoped – eventually. My healthy, fat, sweet, perfect little boy is in my arms and I'm keeping him alive, just me, just us, just right, despite the bumpy road along the way.
>
> – Lauren, New Mexico, United States

Congratulations! You've reached a milestone recognised across many cultures: the first forty days after birth. You're no longer a beginner. Now you have a ton of knowledge to share. And you're probably more confident about your milk production, like Lauren, or have worked out how to work with what you've got, like Raquel:

> The milk production I was getting was not ideal, so I started to supplement with formula until I started complementary feeding. I always breastfed on demand, because despite the pain and the difficulties, she found comfort in suckling. It may seem contradictory, but it was not. It was difficult for her to breastfeed, but at the same time she found that refuge of love and peace that breastfeeding is.
>
> – Raquel, Madrid, Spain

You've learned to recognise some of your baby's cues: to nurse, change sides, play, sleep. You don't have to *think* so hard about everything. You just respond to your baby, and it works. As you trust your instincts, and your baby, you can really find your stride.

Barbara writes about how this process was for her:

> I finally realised that if I would just abandon myself to my baby, and relieve myself of expectations (usually other people's) of how she "should" behave, then everything would be so much easier and so much more enjoyable. This took a few months, but it changed my life!
> – *Barbara, North America*

Claire, an LLL Leader, puts it this way:

> Imagine that you and your baby are alone on a desert island. Imagine what you would do to care for your baby, and then do it.
> – *Claire, Texas, United States*

Nursing Now – Six Weeks to Four Months

By now, you've probably been through some "frequency days" (sometimes called "growth spurts" or "leaps"), those fussy times when your baby needs more nursing and soothing than usual. When this first happened to Lynett, she thought there might be a problem with her milk production, until her doctor reassured her:

> Soon the first growth spurt started, and she started to fight with the breast, wriggling and complaining a lot, and again I thought, *I don't have enough milk.* I talked to my paediatrician and she told me that this attitude was normal since the baby needed to suckle more so that more milk would come out, and she would soon pass that stage. And that's how it was for more than a week, but the good thing is that it passed.
> – *Lynett, Mexico*

Maybe your baby does need to eat more because he's in a fast-growing phase. Or maybe it's not about milk at all. It could be a sign of brain growth and development. Babies react to what's going on in their outside world, too. Any change in their usual environment really upsets some babies, while others love anything new and get bored and cranky if you stay home too much!

If you take those frequency days out of the equation, your baby is probably crying less now, overall. He's more used to being in the world and is no longer surprised by everything. He's much more aware of what's going on around him. When he smiles at you – which he's probably doing more often now – his whole face lights up. When he's really happy, his whole body "smiles." Lola noticed her son was thriving and his reflexes aided him:

> [He breastfed] with delight, gusto, and passion. The audible gulps, body movements, head nodding, and playful hands indicated satisfaction.
> – Lola, Israel

Now that you're settling into it, you might also feel a deep satisfaction (at least sometimes!). As Shanna puts it:

> I wish I could convey the simple, immense pleasure of nursing my three children. Nursing was a primal, deeply essential connection for us, a full-bodied hug. Nursing my children was our love language.
> – Shanna, Ithaca, New York, United States

By four months your baby may be giggling. And talking! It's not words, but it's definitely speech – controlled sounds that she tries to produce evenly, taking turns with you as you chat. You might find yourself pausing your shared conversation until she's finished nursing, since she can't talk with her mouth full. And sometimes your baby, nursing busily, catches your eye, smiles, and starts to leak milk around the smile. Then she comes off, just to smile at you. Did you think she only loved you for your milk? Absolutely not.

The Fourth Month: Big Changes

By about three months, many of us feel like we're finally getting the hang of this. You and your baby are in sync. Then all of a sudden – things change again.

Somewhere around three or four months, parents often call an LLL Leader saying, "I can hardly get my baby to nurse *at all*!" (If your baby was born prematurely, this may occur a little later.)

What's going on? These are some of the possibilities:

- **Your baby is starting to develop outside interests,** interests besides nursing. He can hear and see better now, and he's got more control over his movements. He can raise his head, or put his hands in his mouth. The world is opening up to him: from only being able to see about as far as your face from your lap, he can now see across a room. There are so many interesting things to discover! He wants to spend as little time as possible eating so he can spend as much time as possible exploring. And trying to get the attention of everyone he sees.
- And **he's an expert at getting milk.** Though you're worried he's barely nursing, your baby manages to take a whole feed in just a few minutes. If you had milk supply issues early on, have experienced an eating disorder, or are generally feeling concerned about your nursing relationship, these changes might seem alarming at first. If you try to nurse your baby when he's more interested in something else, or continue nursing when he's done, it probably won't work. You really *can't* make a child eat. It's your job to make food – in this case, the breast – available. It's *his* job to decide when and how much to eat. (This is likely to come up again once your baby is a toddler! See Chapter 13.)

At this stage, just like when your baby was younger, he's doing just fine, as long as the following are true:

- He's growing as expected.
- He has plenty of energy.
- He's developing normally.
- He seems happy with the amount of milk he's getting.

After the first month or two, most babies tend to take fewer and shorter nursings each day. They may also start having longer gaps between some feeds – but they *don't* get less milk overall. They're just getting more efficient.

If you're worried your baby really might not be getting enough milk, check in with your healthcare provider and contact an LLL Leader or other breastfeeding supporter.

Nursing a very distractible baby can be frustrating. Babies may stop nursing every time they hear a new sound or catch a movement out of the corner of their eye. And they don't always remember to let go of your nipple when they turn around to see what's going on! Teresa found a way to prevent this from happening to her:

> At three and four months old, baby Lisa was always getting distracted by her rambunctious two-year-old brother when I tried to nurse her. I put a hook and eye at the top of my bedroom door and added a box of quiet but interesting toys in my closet. Then I could lock the door, lie down on the bed to nurse Lisa, and my little boy would happily play with the "special" toys on the carpet.
> – *Teresa, Ontario, Canada*

Here are some tried-and-true approaches for keeping a baby's interest in nursing:

- Nurse in a quiet, dark room, or in a sling while walking.
- Offer something fun to do while nursing (sometimes called "counter-distraction").
- Change nursing positions. Maybe several times in a few minutes!

You can find more tips in Chapter 9. Some babies – just like some adults – have a tendency to forget to eat when they're busy and benefit from gentle reminders. But even if you do nothing, chances are this will be a short-lived (if annoying) phase. Once some of her curiosity is satisfied, your baby will become a more focused nursling again. Meanwhile, nighttime feedings may be especially important, because she can concentrate better when nothing else is going on.

Is My Baby Regressing? Changing Sleep Patterns

No matter how your baby was sleeping before, it's very common for babies to wake more often around four months of age. If your baby had already started sleeping for a longer stretch at night, having those periods of uninterrupted sleep stolen from you may be more of a shock! Your baby isn't regressing, and it's *not* that you've done anything wrong. The trend during the first year is for babies to sleep for longer stretches at night. But progress towards a whole night's undisturbed sleep tends not to go in a totally straight line. Expect some ups and downs along the way.

While your baby temporarily needs you more at night, it's okay to go with the flow. Nursing will help him get back to sleep faster and ensure a good milk supply, especially if he's too busy to nurse much during the day. Sleeping for shorter periods and waking more frequently will also keep him from spending too much time in deep sleep states, reducing his risk of sudden infant death syndrome (SIDS). The risk of SIDS is highest between about two and four months – could this be one reason babies this age *need* to wake more often?

For now, take a daytime nap with your baby when you can, or go to bed a bit earlier. You might find it reassuring to connect with other parents of four-month-olds – many of their babies will be doing just the same thing. Though we can't tell you exactly how long this wakeful stage might last, it's probably just a temporary blip. For more about sleep, see Chapter 12.

Questions You May Have Between Six Weeks and Four Months

My Baby Hasn't Pooed in a Week! Is He Constipated?

For the first few weeks, every pooey nappy is a sign that your baby is getting enough milk. Around six weeks or so, though, some babies stop pooing as often. Some start pooing once a day, and some wait several days. The change can come abruptly, and can really throw you if you'd stopped thinking about your baby's nappy output.

What's going on with the ones who poo only once a week but continue to gain weight and seem active and healthy? We don't really know! When these babies do finally poo, it's still very soft, not the hard stools you'd see in a constipated baby. And in time, these babies often go back to a more typical pooing pattern.

What Is Constipation?

Constipation is not defined by how often a baby poos or whether she seems to strain when she poos; it's about her having hard, dry stools that really hurt her to pass.

> Straining but then passing soft yellow poo is probably just a sign that she's still learning to coordinate the muscles required for pooing. There's even a word for it: *dyschezia,* also known as "grunting baby syndrome"! There's nothing you need to do except keep your baby as calm as you can and wait for her to outgrow it.
>
> Let your baby's healthcare provider know if your baby's stools are hard and dry or if they cause any bleeding when she passes them.

What we do know is that a longer than usual time without pooing is *not* a reason to add formula, juice, corn syrup, or other foods to the baby's diet.

Of course, if it's been several days or longer before your baby finally poos, the results can be really messy – a blowout instead of skid marks. After a week, expect a mudslide. Sometimes these deliveries are made over the course of a day. The parents of very predictable babies may not even bother with a changing bag for much of the week ... but they plan to stay home on Poo Day.

Some babies start to feel uncomfortable and cranky as they work up to having a big poo. Nursing may help; it stimulates the baby's digestive system to "move things along." But sometimes the uncomfortable baby refuses the breast, maybe because it just makes her tummy hurt even more. You can try holding her in an upright or squatting position to see if that helps, or try bicycling her legs, or gently massaging her belly. You might also want to try sitting her in a warm, shallow bath. Be prepared – you'll need to wash out the tub if this works!

Is My Baby Teething?

Most babies begin teething sometime after four months, but some babies do get teeth early (a few are even born with them). For the most part, teeth are irrelevant to breastfeeding; although as Ali says, you might hear otherwise:

> I am very lucky to live in an area where there is lots of support for new mothers. I hear too many stories and too many reasons why people were not able to breastfeed, or had to cut their breastfeeding journey short. Reasons like "baby did not like to nurse" or "they got teeth so early."
>
> – *Ali, California, United States*

You may have to wiggle your baby into a more comfortable nursing position at times when the teeth first come through. And some babies try to bite down while nursing during those particularly sore times when the teeth are trying to surface. For now, even if your baby isn't ready for teeth, he may be *getting ready* for teeth.

Actual teething may involve fist gnawing, a lot of drooling, crankiness, and doing weird things with his jaw to soothe his gums during nursing. Helping relieve the discomfort often relieves any temporary nursing issues, too.

In some countries, health agencies don't recommend numbing ointments for babies. And numbness may make nursing feel funny to your baby and even to you. You could try a breastmilk ice lolly or a teething toy instead. "Teethers" allow your still-awkward little one to hold on to them anywhere and get something satisfying into his mouth.

For more about when teeth are most likely to appear, see Chapter 9. For more about cavities and night nursing, see Chapter 12.

Will Exercising Affect My Milk?

Exercising is basic to mammals – because their lives depend on it. Mice, desperate to stay alive, have always run from cats... and then nursed their babies. Cats, desperate to eat, have always run after mice... and then nursed their babies. Breastfeeding wouldn't work very well if babies suffered every time their mothers ran to catch dinner or ran to avoid *being* dinner! Not surprisingly, most studies have found no significant difference in the volume or composition of milk after exercise.

But would it really *matter* if your baby weren't thrilled with the taste of your post-exercise milk? It may well be that your baby also isn't thrilled with the taste of, say, cinnamon or broccoli in your milk. No problem. If a baby takes less than usual at one nursing, she'll just take more than usual at the next.

There are, of course, plenty of benefits to exercising and staying fit while you're breastfeeding. Working out can improve your mood, reduce your stress levels, give you more energy, strengthen and tone muscles, and help you sleep better at night. So go ahead and exercise! Here are some suggestions:

- Breastfeed your baby right before you work out so your breasts are less full during the exercise and your baby doesn't interrupt it.

- Wear a supportive bra (or two!) to help you feel comfortable.
- Wear breast pads if leaking is still an issue.
- Take a quick shower or towel-dry before you nurse if your baby doesn't like nursing when you're sweaty.

What if you're training to the point that you might, in your childless days, have stopped having periods? That means you're exercising so intensely that your body wouldn't even try to raise a baby, and your milk production may be affected. On the other hand, one of the reasons we gain weight during pregnancy is to sustain a child during possible famine (see Chapter 18, Diet and Weight), so there is probably no problem if you want to train hard. Social media abounds with stories of athletes breastfeeding or expressing their milk while competing, so you're in good company!

Milder exercise is absolutely fine. Walking with your baby in a sling or stroller can be a good way to start. Finding a walking partner makes a walk a social event. Fitness centres often have postnatal programmes where you can bring your baby along. Some even work the baby into the routine. For more exercise tips, see Chapter 14.

Should I Be Doing Anything to Lose Weight?

Well-nourished women often tend to lose around 0.8 kg (1.75 pounds) per month during the first six months of nursing. Most of the rest of us maintain our weight. Some of us, like Lynn, find that our bodies prefer to hold on to a little extra "insurance" all the way through breastfeeding:

> Unfortunately, I didn't go back to my prepregnancy weight, while some women who breastfeed do this rather effortlessly.
> – Lynn, Turnhout, Belgium

If this is the case for you, you might find that you naturally lose some weight after weaning. For more about diet and weight, including some important safety information to be aware of if you're considering any kind of calorie restriction, see Chapter 18.

Are There Environmental Pollutants in My Milk?

Environmental pollutants have been a trending topic for years. Every year we know more about them. And yes, there are environmental contaminants in human milk. They're *everywhere:* in the food we eat, the air we breathe, the ground we walk on, and in many products in our homes.

So should you stop breastfeeding? Of course not! Formula contains *far* more environmental contaminants than your milk does. Formula-feeding is a complicated process with many steps, and each potentially adds contaminants:

- the diet and environment of the cows whose milk formula is made from
- the manufacturing processes that produce formula
- the packaging formula comes in
- the water used to mix formula
- the plastics formula is served in

Regardless of the level of pollutants, your milk is almost always *by far* the safest, healthiest food for your baby. And human milk helps offset the effects of pollutants by boosting your baby's brain development and immune system.

If you have a job that puts you in contact with very high levels of pollutants, talk to your employer about ways to reduce your exposure. Some firefighters, for example, are reassigned to non-active duties while they're breastfeeding. La Leche League Leaders can provide information to help.

If There Are Antibodies in My Milk, Is That the Same as My Baby Being Vaccinated?

Breastfeeding builds your baby's immune system and helps protect him against bacteria, viruses, and parasites. Your milk will give him antibodies to fight illnesses you have had and those you have been vaccinated against. But the amounts of antibodies transmitted in your milk are much less than the levels usually created by vaccination.

Breastfed babies will actually achieve higher immunity levels with their vaccinations than formula-fed babies will. Talk to your healthcare provider to make informed decisions about vaccinations for your baby.

Should I Be Giving My Baby Vitamin D?

Vitamin D helps us absorb and use calcium properly and keeps our immune systems strong. We can manufacture vitamin D in our skin by exposure to sunlight. It's also available in some foods (like cod-liver oil). But getting enough sun on our skin has become tougher for a number of reasons:

- Fewer of us work outdoors.
- More of us live in urban areas with tall buildings and air pollution, which block the sun.
- As a result of awareness about skin cancer, people tend to use sunscreen generously when they're outdoors.
- Above certain latitudes, you can't get enough vitamin D from sunlight in the winter.
- People with darker skin need more exposure to the sun to acquire enough vitamin D.
- Some women cover their skin for religious or cultural reasons.

As a result, many pregnant and breastfeeding women are deficient in vitamin D, and this deficiency can affect their babies (as well as their own health). Rickets is a condition in children who receive too little vitamin D, resulting in softening of the bones and bowed legs. Fortunately, this condition is very rare. But low vitamin D may put us at higher risk of other long-term problems, such as diabetes and cancer, too.

While it isn't possible to get too much vitamin D from sunlight, it *is* possible to get too much through supplements and enriched foods. Excess vitamin D can cause a buildup of calcium in your blood, which can eventually lead to bone pain or kidney problems.

If you're concerned, you can have your and your baby's vitamin D levels checked by a simple blood test. Discuss the results with your baby's healthcare provider to decide whether you or your baby need vitamin D supplementation. In case your baby needs higher vitamin D levels, here are some ways you can help her:

- **Expose her to more sunshine** – but in a way that minimises the chance of sunburn. This is the best way to increase your baby's vitamin D level. If you carry your baby in a car seat, there's no need to throw a blanket over the whole thing unless it's a really cold winter day. Research suggests that five to thirty minutes of sun exposure, particularly between 10:00 A.M. and 4:00 P.M., either daily or at least twice a week to the face, arms, hands, and legs without sunscreen may be enough. This will depend very much on your location and skin colour, so talk to your healthcare provider about your individual situation.

- In some countries, routine vitamin D supplementation is recommended for all breastfed babies and for you during pregnancy and breastfeeding. Again, talk to your healthcare provider if you have questions.
- If you are uncomfortable with supplementation of vitamins other than D (since your milk alone provides optimal amounts of those nutrients), you may be able to get a **vitamin D–only preparation** for your baby rather than multivitamins.

Does My Baby Need Other Vitamins and Minerals?

Other than access to sunlight for vitamin D, a breastfed baby's life hasn't changed that much over the millennia, and his food supply hasn't either. Your milk contains what your baby needs.

If you follow a vegan diet (plant-based, no animal products), then you probably already know that you need to supplement your diet with adequate vitamin B12. If your vitamin B12 levels are good, your baby will receive enough through your milk.

You might be told that your baby needs extra iron, but that's because formula-fed babies need extra iron. There isn't a lot of iron in your milk, but there is exactly the amount there is supposed to be. The iron in your milk is much more completely absorbed by your baby than the kind of iron found in formula, baby cereal, or iron supplements. Also, your milk contains a protein called "lactoferrin," which binds to extra iron that your baby doesn't use, keeping it from feeding harmful intestinal bacteria. Iron supplements can overwhelm the lactoferrin so that the bacteria thrive, often resulting in diarrhoea and even microscopic bleeding.

Formula is a different story. The kind of iron in formula isn't readily absorbed by babies, so more has to be added to compensate. The extra iron can cause microscopic intestinal bleeding that ends up reducing babies' overall iron levels.

But your baby may indeed need iron supplementation if the following is true:

- Her **cord was cut before it stopped pulsating.** In this case her iron stores may not last until she starts eating family foods (see Chapter 3).
- She was **premature,** because she may not have been born with the same nutrient stores as a full-term baby, so the general guidelines may not apply to her.
- She **starts on solids prematurely** – before she would begin eating them on her own – so her iron stores may drop. Some fruits and vegetables can bind with the iron in your milk before the baby has a chance to absorb it.

If iron supplements are suggested for your baby, it may help to know that you can't increase the levels *in your milk* by taking iron supplements yourself or by eating more iron-rich foods. You can always ask for a blood test for your baby to confirm the need for more iron before starting her on iron supplements.

Help! My Hair Is Falling Out!

Many of us, like Shoko, notice that our hair begins falling out around three months after birth:

> When my second child was about ten weeks old, the amount of hair coming off my head went from nearly nothing to seemingly tons. I was reminded the same thing had happened around two to three months after my eldest was born. I had already read an article about hair loss in breastfeeding mothers being quite common (and also that it would stop at some point!), so I knew to expect it and it wasn't a complete surprise or shock when it started happening.
>
> – *Shoko, the Netherlands*

This period of hair loss is a normal and temporary stage, and it's not caused (or made worse) by breastfeeding. During pregnancy your hair doesn't fall out as much as usual and may grow thicker – and now all that extra hair reaches the end of its natural lifespan and starts falling out. If you feel the amount of hair you're shedding is extreme, talk to your healthcare provider. Excessive hair loss can rarely be a sign of problems that can be treated.

What About Travelling with My Baby?

Travelling really makes you appreciate the ease of nursing! And if your baby is accustomed to sleeping with you, he'll feel at home wherever you go.

Milk to Go

If you're expressing your milk, as well as or instead of nursing directly, travel needs more planning, but it is still possible.

Travel can be more challenging if you're using supplemental donor milk or formula. If you're using formula, you may find that ready-to-feed is safer and more convenient for travel, even though it is more expensive than powdered. Ready-to-feed will also eliminate concerns about different water supplies.

For more about travelling and human milk storage guidelines, see Chapter 15. If you need information about specific resources at your destination – for example, if you have disabilities or medical needs – LLL Leaders may be able to help.

Car Travel

Travelling by car with a nursing baby doesn't take much advance preparation – no formula or bottles to pack, and pooey nappies aren't too stinky. But when your baby wants to nurse? A bit more challenging.

It's safest to pull over to feed the baby, even if you're not driving. But don't assume you'll have to take the baby out of the seat. The stop may be shorter and the baby happier if you lean over to nurse the baby right where she is. All that taking out and putting back can rouse a baby who's fallen blissfully asleep in your arms. Some *really* flexible mothers have been able to nurse from both breasts without taking the baby out or moving to the other side of the car seat. Or you may both appreciate the stretching and in-arms time a stop allows. If you're supplementing (and are not the driver!) you can feed on the move – but you may still appreciate a stop to cuddle your baby and stretch.

Staying in the backseat if you're not driving lets you interact with your baby, sing, and pass over toys. And some parents find their babies will take a dummy while in the car. But let's face it: trips that used to take two hours can now easily take three or four. This is life with a baby for now. One day, hard to believe, your baby may be driving the car!

Plane Travel
One of the advantages of travelling with a breastfeeding baby is the ease of "nursing up and nursing down" to avoid those blocked ears that make many children cry when the plane takes off or lands. If nursing during takeoff and landing isn't possible, for example, because your baby is in a car seat (recommended by some airlines), you might see if he will suck on your finger or a dummy.

If you're using an at-breast supplementer, as some adoptive and non-birthing parents do, it may be helpful to have the supplementer already looped around your neck and ready to go. Parents with disabilities may pre-board to get comfortable before others board the plane. Let your flight attendant know of any assistance you may need with your baby.

Nursing is also helpful during the rest of the flight, as Imogen found:

> We travelled to India to visit my in-laws. Breastfeeding was an amazing way of comforting both my girls while on the long flights from the UK to India.
> – *Imogen, UK*

And one more thing: transfers and waiting at airports may be much easier with a sling. If you have a sling, you won't have to take a baby stroller – though strollers can be useful for transporting your changing bag and a carry-on suitcase. Your sling can also help you nurse discreetly in the waiting area – or as you walk around, as Mimi describes:

> Whenever I went out with Riri, the sling was always with us. It seemed to me that Riri felt safe by being able to feel attached to me, and wherever we went (whether by train, by plane, or on foot), she would never make a fuss. The sling was very convenient and could also cover the breast, so I could quickly offer her a nipple whenever she would start rubbing her mouth against the breast. No one ever noticed that I was walking around breastfeeding!
> – *Mimi, Osaka, Japan*

A sling can also double as a surface to put your baby on while you deal with passports and boarding passes, and it can even serve as a changing mat.

Other Means of Transportation
Imogen found herself nursing in all kinds of vehicles during her travels:

> While we were in India, I breastfed my younger daughter in some unusual places – sitting in the backseat of cars (car seats are not a legal requirement yet in India, so my baby sat on my lap while in a car), on overnight trains, and in autos (open-sided, small taxis that are very common in Indian cities and can seat up to three grown-ups on the seat behind the driver).
> – Imogen, UK

Where the use of seatbelts or infant seats is mandatory, like on some long-distance buses, nursing-on-the-move is trickier. You might need to make a stop or carry expressed milk. But as soon as you stop or get off, you'll be able to nurse. Where seatbelts aren't needed – like on the train or underground – nursing is straightforward. If you're worried about the reactions of other passengers, a sling can make nursing more discreet. Though as one mother put it, "If I ever feel embarrassed about breastfeeding on the bus or train, I remind myself that it's much kinder to the other passengers than making them listen to my baby crying!"

On Arrival
Once you get to your destination, you may want to avoid passing your baby around at first. Even a very young baby can be frightened by a group of loud, excited strangers all clamouring to take her away from you. Wait until she settles in a bit, and set whatever ground rules you're comfortable with. You may be going to visit your sister, but this is *your* baby!

Should My Baby Be on a Schedule by Now?

The mothers of long ago had tasks to do and no safe place to keep the baby except carried or at their side. Parents today have busy lives, too, and fortunately, babies are still born with the expectation that they'll fit naps and feeds around whatever else is going on.

Although at first life with a new baby seems chaotic, at some point in these early months you'll probably find that your day has taken on a pretty reliable rhythm. That rhythm makes life feel more predictable, though for most babies it won't be something you can set your watch by (and a few babies don't follow any kind of regular pattern at all).

There will still be days when your baby eats all day, and days when he sleeps all day. Add in "frequency days," running-around-doing-errands days, and teething days, and it may seem like every day is an exception to the rule! Or maybe you've already gone back to work or school, so you and your baby are already adapting to someone else's timetable. But whatever your situation, you're increasingly able to read your baby, weaving both your needs into the pattern of your days and nights. And he's becoming more able to fall in with your plans, entertaining himself with new sights and sounds or napping as you go about your day.

An actual schedule may only make things more complicated, and spacing out nursings to suit a clock can jeopardise your milk supply. While you can nudge your baby towards predictability, there will still be a certain amount of unpredictability. The good news is that unpredictability is a close relative of adaptability; the baby who won't nap at the expected time today is the same baby who'll obligingly sleep through a frantic last-minute errand tomorrow. As one mother said, "We have a routine, but we don't have a schedule. A schedule would mean he naps at three. A routine means we usually have a bath after supper."

If you're the kind of person who really needs a clear structure to help you feel in control or manage your anxiety, you can find some ideas in Chapter 6, How Soon Can I Get My Baby on a Schedule? There are lots of aspects of life that you *can* take control of while allowing the flexibility that babies, and breastfeeding, need. You can read more about anxiety in Need a Backup Plan? later in this chapter.

What About Sleep Training?

At this age, many babies still get a hefty portion of their calories at night. Unless she's chosen it on her own, sleeping through the night can slow your baby's rate of growth, and it risks early weaning. Your baby will sleep for longer stretches when she's ready. But we know how important sleep is right now, which is why Chapter 12 is all about how you and your baby can get more of it.

I'm Going Back to Work (or Study) Soon

By now you've settled into your new normal. You might be starting to think about returning to work or study. If you don't have maternity leave where you live, you might be there already.

Some parents decide ahead of time that one of them will stay home with the baby. Although people often assume the stay-at-home parent will be the birthing parent, your partner might have more parental leave; or you might be the higher earner and your family can't manage without your income. If you're parenting solo, staying home may not be an option. It's also possible that you made a decision before your baby arrived but changed your mind now that he's actually here. Whatever your situation, there may come a time when you need, or want, to be separated from your baby while you work.

There's no way around it: leaving a young baby for long periods of time is difficult for both of you. Biology expects you to be together most of the time while your baby is small. When you are not, you have to think about who will take care of him, how to express milk, how many times, how to store it, and a lot more. All while still recovering from the birth and being woken throughout the night by a hungry baby. Absolutely not fair, and it's something that too many parents have to cope with, often within a few weeks of giving birth. The longer you're able to delay separation from your baby, the easier it tends to be.

For starters, you could try to just take the baby to bed with you an hour earlier than you would normally turn in. That extra hour of being horizontal in a dark room, even if you don't sleep through all of it, can mean you're better rested the next day. For many more ideas on sleep and a thorough discussion of going back to work, see chapters 12 and 14.

I *Still* Have Too Much Milk!

By about six weeks, you probably have a good sense of whether you're dealing with a true oversupply of milk. It might be time to start calming down your overenthusiastic milk production, if your baby is growing really fast and either of the following is true:

- Your baby often coughs, splutters, and gets upset when your milk releases.
- She often has green, bubbly stools and gut pain.

If you haven't yet tried it, a simple first step to deal with this problem is using only one breast at each nursing, commonly known as block feeding. For a longer discussion of this topic, see Chapter 18, Oversupply. Or you could donate your extra milk for vulnerable babies, as Dawn did:

> After feeding was started at the breast, my son gained one pound in twenty-four hours. With some help from my local LLL meeting and my midwives, I was able to figure out that I have a very fast letdown. I learned to use laid-back and side-lying [positions] to try and help slow the flow. And eventually some block feeding to try and reduce my supply a bit. After a bit, I decided to start pumping and donating to the local human milk bank. I was able to donate just over 100 litres in eighteen months.
> – Dawn, British Columbia, Canada

To read more about donating milk, see Chapter 18, Milk Sharing.

Maybe everything's going fine except for leaking. Nuisance that it is, leaking does reduce your risk of blocked ducts from extra milk. You may need to wear breast pads and keep an extra pad on the bed for a little while longer. If you're wearing any kind of milk collection device, or using a squeezy silicone milk collector, that could be what's encouraging the extra flow. You could stop using them and see if it helps.

Is It a Problem That My Baby Is So Easygoing?

Having a happy, easygoing baby certainly can make the first weeks and months a lot easier. Sometimes, these quieter babies start out gaining well when you're paying close attention. But later, when you're back to getting chores done, you miss subtle feeding cues, and they're too polite to complain when a meal is missed. This is especially true in childcare settings, where the most assertive babies get most of the attention. Even though the easygoing baby doesn't insist on constant holding, she'll benefit from being held, carried, and nursed frequently just as much as any baby.

I'm Still Dealing with a Fussy Baby

You don't even want to *hear* about those calm, contented babies because yours certainly isn't one! He's thriving, and happy some of the time, but is easily upset by things like itchy clothes, having to wait more than thirty seconds to be fed, being held in a way he doesn't like, and a long list of other dislikes. Sometimes he's just inconsolable.

If your baby gets fussy easily, it can be worth checking for things like allergies, food sensitivities, and oversupply (see Chapter 18 and LLL websites), but it may just be his personality. For more about baby temperament, see Chapter 7.

Julie benefited from extra help with her baby, who later turned out to have sensory processing disorder (see Chapter 7, Why Is My Baby Nursing Much *Less* Than My Friend's?):

> Alice didn't like to be touched, held, or carried unless we had big, swinging movements. She was happier on a blanket on the floor, and slept best when laid in a dark, quiet room. She napped at the same time every day, and she would not fall asleep anywhere other than her quiet space. When she was about three months old, the Baby Talk group had a guest speaker who demonstrated infant massage. Massage helped Alice's digestion and reduced the spitting up as well. Her strong, tight muscles visibly relaxed. Infant massage was the first time I was able to touch my daughter's skin without her struggling to pull away.
> – *Julie, Ontario, Canada*

What worked with your previous baby – or works for your friends' babies – may not work for this one. Heranush describes it beautifully:

> With time I have understood that breastfeeding is a dance that needs to be learned with each child.
> – *Heranush, rural New Zealand*

Olivia's second child was very different from her first:

> With my first son, breastfeeding seemed like his top priority in life. It could soothe him to sleep. It could comfort him after a bump. He didn't let me far from his sight, day or night! My second was different. He did enjoy nursing, but it was short and to the point. He was more interested in the world around him. If there were sounds around him, he couldn't focus. If he was hurt, he would need to calm down before he would latch on. I was surprised how different it was the second time around. It was the same mum, same upbringing, but different personalities.
> – *Olivia, Canada*

Maybe you've got an intense baby who needs input! Input! Input! She's bright and curious and wants to discover the world. Or maybe your baby finds the world beyond your arms overwhelming. She just wants to stay close to you. Look for other parents of intense or high-need babies to share notes with. Keep a sense of humour and try not to compare. And keep your baby close – your presence, touch, and of course, your breasts will often go a long way towards calming her, as Alexa found:

> My daughter breastfed frequently, on demand, everywhere. She was a very alert and energetic baby and toddler, and I carried her at my chest often. Looking back, sensory processing issues (sensory seeking, audio/visual processing) were probably there right from the start, but she was so happy and contented, and nursing was an immediate calming balm I could offer to her at any time and in any place.
> – Alexa, New York, United States

For more about sensory processing issues, see Chapter 7, Why Is My Baby Nursing Much *Less* Than My Friend's?

Need a Backup Plan?

The hormones of parenting and breastfeeding make us want to soothe and comfort our babies when they cry. But what if you try *everything* and the baby is still crying, and you're exhausted and at your limit? As this mother describes, parenting can bring out the worst in us as well as the best:

> I feel that having a child is something wonderful and that it brings many new ways of being happy. It is an extreme experience, extreme in positive feelings, also extreme in challenges, and it dusts off a lot of your negative things that you need to fix.
> – Guajirita Alquizareña, from Cuba, living in the Netherlands

Now's the time for a backup plan. Raising a child was never meant to be something you do all by yourself; parents have always needed communities of support around them. If you are starting to feel overwhelmed, maybe you can do one of the following:

- Call a trusted person to come over and take the baby for a walk.
- Call someone just to talk to them, even if they can't come and help in person.
- Bring the baby with you to a neighbour's house for a visit.
- Contact an LLL Leader for some comforting words.
- Do something for yourself – have a warm bath (with or without your baby), enjoy a special snack or soothing warm drink, put some music on and dance (maybe even with the baby). One mother kept a stash of chocolate for use on these tough days.

If you're feeling desperate, you might need to do the following:

- Put your baby down in a safe place and step away.
- Breathe deeply.
- Take a few minutes to notice how you're feeling.

It's natural to be upset when your baby is crying and can't be consoled. And your stressed-out feelings are a sign that you need more support than you are getting. Take some time to calm yourself down, maybe reach out to some potential support people. When you're ready, go back, pick up your baby, and smell the top of his head – that amazing smell that only he has.

If you still feel like you want to run away, or like you could harm your baby, you need some help right away. If you're spending a lot of time *worrying* about hurting your baby, even though you would do anything to protect him, see Chapter 18, Postnatal Mood Disorders. These upsetting thoughts are probably a sign that you're suffering from anxiety. You're not a bad parent for feeling like this, and there is good help available.

I'm Still Really Anxious

Some of us have lived with anxiety for years before we have a baby. For others, anxiety seems to arrive *with* the baby. If you've had a difficult start to life with your baby – especially if you've been frightened for your own or your baby's safety – it can feel like an alarm is constantly sounding in your mind. It takes a while for your "threat level" to dial down to anything like normal. For more about anxiety, see Chapter 7, I'm Just Not Enjoying Any of This.

If anxiety is robbing you of any pleasure in your baby, or

overwhelming your ability to manage day by day, please reach out for help. We've written Chapter 18, Postnatal Mood Disorders, with you in mind. You're not alone.

I'm Going Through the Motions, but I Don't Love This Baby Yet

Some of us fall in love with our babies as soon as we first realise we're pregnant or when we see the first ultrasound. Others are smitten as soon as their babies are in their arms. For some of us, love takes longer to grow. It's not uncommon to feel a sense of emotional distance after a traumatic or complicated birth, or if you and your baby have been separated. Or maybe you're feeling disconnected because your experience, or your baby, is very different from what you expected.

If you sense that love for your baby is not growing, give yourself more time. If that feeling of detachment persists, though, it can help a lot to find someone who understands – a counsellor or friend, maybe a support group related to birth, breastfeeding, or early parenting. This is the kind of conversation we have at LLL meetings all the time. There's no shame in feeling this way. Lots of us have been there, and we know that as you keep doing the things that nurture your baby, the feelings will follow. For more about this, see Chapter 5, Conflicting Feelings, and Chapter 3, Moving Forward After a Difficult Birth.

Intrusive memories, flashbacks, or physical birth injuries that have not healed can be very distressing, and they can affect your enjoyment of your baby. For more about birth-related trauma, see Chapter 3, Post-Traumatic Stress Disorder.

What About Sex?

Some of you are thinking, *So what? I've been having sex for weeks now,* and others are thinking, *Sex? Why would I even think about sex?*

The timeline for reestablishing any form of sex after birth varies greatly. It might be affected by

- how easy or difficult your birth was
- your recovery from birth
- how breastfeeding is going
- your baby's personality and needs
- your relationship with your partner
- norms in your community

There are at least as many other issues as there are couples.

Where Anita lives, there are taboos about sex during breastfeeding:

> I was breastfeeding, and in my culture we believe "kombras" (nursing women) shouldn't lie with our husbands while the baby is nursing.

She decided to do it differently with her next baby, after getting new information:

> With this baby, I followed the nurses' advice and will breastfeed for as long as I can. I now know lovemaking can go along with nursing.
> – Anita, Sierra Leone

You may find that your new body and role are real aphrodisiacs for you or your partner. Or maybe the urge to have any kind of sex life has completely disappeared for a while. If you find yourself in the second situation, you can reassure yourself (and your partner) that this part of life isn't over.

In the meantime, you – and your partner when you feel ready – can get to know and enjoy your changed body. If your culture's ideal of female beauty is a slender teenager's body, you might be eager to "get your body back" to how it was before. You might feel embarrassed or even ashamed about how you look now. It may be hard to imagine how anyone could see your body as attractive. We've got good news: bodies that have given birth and are making milk are beautiful and sexy. They are powerful. They can give – and receive – pleasure, as well as life and nurture.

Affection keeps your relationship strong and holds the door open for intimacy. Although you might be getting more than enough touch from your baby, your partner might be getting much less than before. A big hug (and a compliment) can go a long way in a relationship. Or how about holding hands, a shoulder or foot rub, or a gentle pat or squeeze?

You may find at first that anything more than this is beyond your means. But over time, things change. Clare found a good use for a traditional aphrodisiac:

> To be honest, I could happily have managed without sex for a good few months after the birth, as I had the constant "warm fuzzy" of a baby to

hold. But the physical intimacy meant a lot to my partner, and with patience and humour, we gradually got there. A breakthrough was when I decided that to get in the mood, chocolate would need to be provided. It's still being provided, years later!

– Clare, UK

Sex doesn't have to be all-or-nothing. Any kind of intimate, pleasurable touch is a good start. This can be a chance to rediscover sex. What you enjoy may have changed. Your breasts may be more sensitive, especially in the first few months – but they may also feel sexier. And, of course, they now contain milk. If you want to keep milk out of your lovemaking, nurse the baby or express on both sides beforehand. But milk can also be fun, if you want it to be. Where there is orgasm, there may be milk. In fact, that very same hormone (and the milk it can trigger these days) might also be released by having a great meal, seeing old friends, or cuddling a pet. When good times happen, sometimes milk happens! You can massage with it, or joke about it.

You may need extra vaginal lubrication, because breastfeeding hormones can cause dryness. Try an over-the-counter lubricant instead of one containing oestrogen, to avoid any possible effect on milk production.

And where is your baby while all this is going on? Some babies nap soundly and are easily moved where you want them. You can even start your romantic moment with a drive that puts the baby to sleep and leave her in the car seat nearby. If your bed is big enough, you can just move her to one side while you two enjoy each other. Or place her in a co-sleeper, or crib. Remember, *the baby doesn't care what's going on*. Separate bedrooms (and beds) are a modern luxury. You might be uncomfortable with an audience, but a baby's only concern is that her needs for food and comfort are met, and during these early months she may stay asleep best if you're not far away. And if she wakes up when you least expect – or want – her to, your hand on her back may be all she needs.

What if you're still just not interested in sex? After spending all day being intimate with the baby, you might not have anything left over. The time that you're devoting to your baby is an investment in your family's future well-being. Understanding and patience (with yourself, and your partner if you have one) can make a big difference.

Sometimes, a very decreased interest in sex can be a symptom of depression – and not just in you. Partners can also experience depression in the year after birth. Reach out for help; effective treatments are available (see Chapter 18, Postnatal Mood Disorders).

Your love life is just one more area where things have changed for now. The words to remember are *for now*. Life *will* gradually become less intense, and the sex life you previously enjoyed can gradually resume – maybe even be better!

Relationships Under Stress

However committed your relationship, and however much you've looked forward to becoming parents, don't be surprised if you feel distanced from your partner at times. You're both dealing with a huge amount of change – but it affects each of you differently. One of you might be missing work, while the other feels extra financial responsibility. One of you feels touched out, while the other is lonely. Time you used to spend together is swallowed up by the basic tasks of getting through the day (and night) with a new baby.

Communication is key. It's easy to assume that your partner should know how you feel. But they may not – unless you tell them! You may think you know how your partner thinks and feels, too, but it's worth checking before you act on your assumptions. One mother who worried that her partner didn't find her attractive anymore discovered that he had been traumatised by watching their baby's delivery by forceps. He was terrified of having sex, in case he hurt her. An honest conversation quickly got them back on track.

Three mantras to stress-proof your relationship after birth are **keep talking, listen well,** and **be kind.** These ideas might also help:

- **Don't wait until relationship cracks turn into chasms. And don't wait for there to be "time to talk."** You'll need to *make* time.
- **Try going for a walk or drive with your baby** just after she's been fed. The movement will probably lull her to sleep, leaving the two of you to talk.
- **Young babies tend to be calmest in the morning.** There's no rule that says important conversations have to happen after dark.
- **Set some ground rules,** like not calling names. Some things, once said, are difficult to recover from. Focus on the issue in hand, not your partner's character or past offences. Some find it helps to hold

hands during the discussion. Constructive discussions rarely happen when people are angry. Arrange to talk again when you're both feeling calmer – and make sure you follow through.
- **Get help if you need it.** Talk to a counsellor if you're still struggling.

Can I Get Pregnant?

If you're having sex, as in male-female intercourse, then yes, you can get pregnant! If you want to avoid another pregnancy, the lactational amenorrhea method, LAM for short, is a natural contraceptive method based on the way the hormones of breastfeeding can stop ovulation and menstruation. This method can be very effective in preventing pregnancy for the first six months after birth. The World Health Organization found a pregnancy rate of about 1 per 100 women per year with consistent and correct use of LAM. But note: it's reliable only if *all* the following criteria are met to prevent ovulation:

- Your baby is less than six months old.
- Your periods haven't resumed (before six weeks after birth, bleeding, spotting, or vaginal discharge with some blood is not a period).
- Your baby is breastfeeding exclusively, without regularly receiving any other food or drink, including water, and no regular use of dummies or bottles, or you remove the milk from your breasts (by nursing or expressing) at least every four hours during the day and five hours at night.

There's biological logic behind LAM. The baby who's getting all his food, day and night, from his mother, isn't ready to share her. His mother's body isn't ready to take on a second intense job.

Your body may assume it's safe to get pregnant again if the following is true:

- Your baby is fed with formula, which causes your hormone levels to drop faster to their pre-pregnant levels.
- Your baby is encouraged to sleep through the night without nursing, like an older baby, or he uses a dummy and spends less time at the breast, like a baby who's weaning.

If you have to be away from your baby but want to keep up the LAM protection against pregnancy, you'll need to express milk as often as your baby would nurse at home. Of course, in some jobs this may not be possible – in which case, LAM is not a good birth control option for you.

If you want to use another kind of birth control, it may be a good idea to steer clear of all hormonal methods – pills, contraceptive implants, hormone-impregnated intrauterine devices (IUDs) – for at least the first six months because of their potential effect on milk supply.

Hormonal contraceptives include

- birth control pills containing both oestrogen and progesterone (often called the Pill or combination pill)
- birth control pills containing only progesterone (often called the mini pill)
- progesterone implants, such as Implanon
- progesterone injections, such as Depo-Provera
- IUDs that emit hormones (oestrogen and/or progesterone), such as Mirena

If you want to use hormonal contraceptives, consult with your healthcare provider and remind them that you're breastfeeding. It's well known that oestrogen-containing hormonal contraceptives lower milk production; they're unlikely to be prescribed for you.

Progesterone-only methods are usually fine, but a small number of mothers also report decreased milk production when using them. IUDs (intrauterine devices) and implants can be removed if necessary – but there's nothing you can do to reverse the effects of hormonal contraceptive injections, which are designed to last for months. Starting the mini pill is a popular option for those who want to use a hormonal method, because you can easily stop taking it if you think your milk production has been reduced.

For more about protection from pregnancy *after* six months, see Chapter 9.

I Haven't Been Away from My Baby Since He Was Born. Is That Okay?

Over the past few weeks or months of hard work and little sleep, this little one has become such an important part of your life that you miss him when you're not with him. It's attachment. It's the spell a baby weaves to keep you from leaving him behind (a wildly unsafe situation from the baby's perspective). Those solid instincts have worked in favour of mothers and babies for millennia.

If you don't *want* to leave him, and you have the resources to choose, staying with your baby a while longer is a choice you're unlikely to regret. As the saying goes, "On their deathbeds, most people don't wish they'd spent more time at work."

But everyone is different, and you may find that you want or need to be away from your baby for a while. Some of us really need solitude to recharge and feel like ourselves. Your great-grandmother probably had lots of people around who could hold the baby when she needed a break, but that might not be an option for you. Conflicted feelings are part of the complexity of modern life with a baby, as Olivia describes:

> I've had to learn how to sit with the dualities of breastfeeding – feeling two different things at once. I am exhausted from the night wakings, but love being needed. I would love a date night out, but don't feel comfortable leaving him with someone yet. I love being the sole source of life for this little one, but would also love an hour to go get my hair done. I'm grateful for the support of my partner, but in the nights I feel angry he gets to sleep through. I'm so grateful my body is sustaining my little child, but I also long for the days my body was for myself. I feel so proud of myself breastfeeding successfully, but my heart aches for my friend who is struggling with it. I can feel it both, and I can feel it all.
>
> – Olivia, Canada

If you can, start with short separations – an hour or two. Nurse right before leaving. Your baby may just sleep until you're back. You might want to leave some expressed milk with the person looking after her, for peace of mind. Check in as often as you like and, if possible, plan so you can come home early if she needs you. For more on handling all kinds of separations, see Chapter 14. La Leche League Leaders are always happy to help you figure out the logistics.

We've said it before, but it's worth repeating: you're not on your own. Samantha's first few months with her baby turned out to be tougher than she expected. Alongside support from family, she found a "home" in LLL:

I was living in a new city, she was born in the depths of winter, my husband went back to work when I was five days postnatal, and my baby and I really struggled to get to grips with breastfeeding. We didn't really hit our stride until she was around four months old. Had it not been for our mums and the community and support I found through LLL, I think that my mental health would have suffered significantly more during those early postnatal months.

– *Samantha, from the UK, living in Bali, Indonesia*

Just as we did for Samantha, we would love to provide a safe haven for you, too.

Is it easy to be exclusively breastfeeding? It is not easy to be available 24/7 for every feeding. I can't say it was easy or simple. And I never imagined it would be. But to see his little face . . . that while he's eating, he's looking at me and laughing, it just melts me. To see that connection that is forming day by day, to see how he is growing . . . it is priceless. And I thank LLL because I have really learned and felt supported in this process.

– *Lizzeth, Mexico*

Want to know more?

You can find extra resources for this chapter at the "Art of Breastfeeding" tab at www.llli.org.

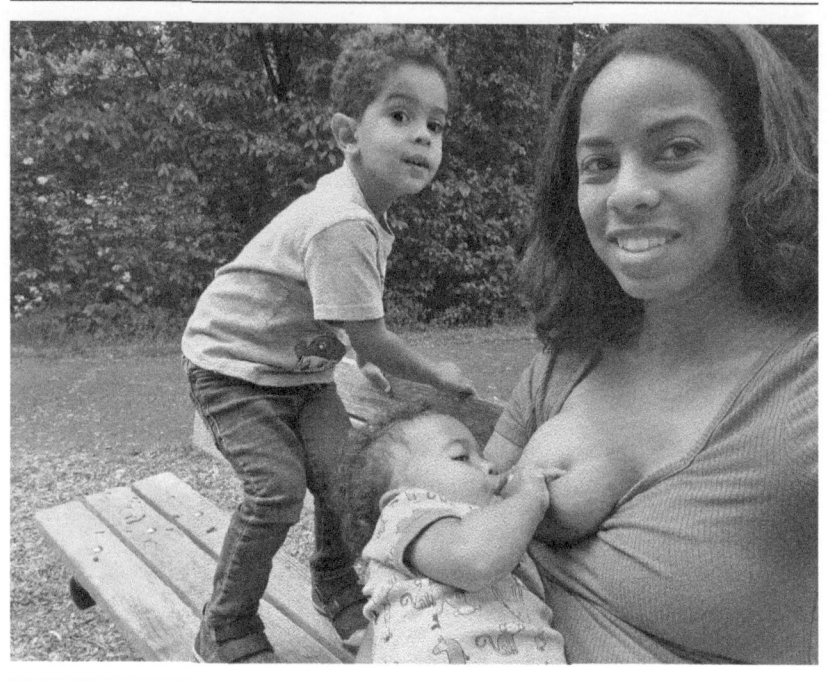

NINE

Four to Nine Months: In the Zone

> I didn't appreciate at the time the ease of breastfeeding an older baby – how comfortable and practised we both were by this point in our breastfeeding journey, to be able to feed anywhere and everywhere, without a second thought. My favourite times were out on country walks with my husband. We needed nothing, my son and I; we just found ourselves a spot on the grass. We were self-sufficient. We were out there in public. I wish I'd fed him more in public, to be honest, I wish I'd helped normalise feeding an older baby. The power of hindsight, eh? I do wish, looking back, that I'd allowed myself to relax and enjoy this stage of breastfeeding more than I did at the time. Enjoy it wholeheartedly, treat it more like a reward for getting this far.
>
> – Kate, England

It's only been a few months since your baby has arrived, but when you take a moment to look back, you can see just how far you've come. Your early breastfeeding goals might have changed, since you've solved or found workarounds for any problems you had then, and nursing is now just a normal part of your day. You're in the zone.

At this age, your baby might be on the move. Julie's baby was an early crawler – and a fast nurser:

> By the time Alice was about five months old she was crawling well all over the place. She was now less fussy: she was too busy exploring and playing and using her muscles. She would crawl over to me to nurse, and five minutes later would be done and ready to play again.
>
> – Julie, Ontario, Canada

Your baby's personality is coming into focus. She may be outgoing and friendly, her main aim in life being to escape out of the door and see what the neighbours are doing. Or she may be more reserved, preferring to watch the world from the safety of your lap or sling. Sometimes a baby's temperament is an easy fit for her parents, and sometimes not. If your baby gets overwhelmed by crowds and you're very sociable, you might need to stay home more often than you'd really like. Your shy friend, on the other hand, might need to go out a lot more than usual, to keep her active, outgoing baby from getting bored! Understanding the baby you have makes life easier for both of you. For more about temperament, see Chapter 7, Adapting to the Baby You've Got.

Nursing Now: Four to Nine Months

Nursing has probably become second nature to you now, but like everything with babies, it keeps on changing. Luisa changed how she held her baby:

> At first, I fed our son only in the cradle position. But as he got bigger and heavier, I tried different positions – for example, sitting him on my knee so he could drink upright.
>
> *– Luisa, Switzerland*

Your baby probably needs a lot less help with nursing than in the beginning. Nursing "gymnastics" often start as he tries out different positions and invents new ones!

Speeding Up

Your baby is more efficient now: getting the same amount of milk in less time. Some babies this age can take a whole meal in five minutes. If you had a slow feeder to begin with, or issues with slow growth or low milk production, this change might feel a bit alarming. As long as your baby continues to grow well, seems satisfied after nursing, and has plenty of energy, you can be sure she's getting all she needs.

Hanging Out

Now it's obvious that nursing isn't only a meal – it's a conversation. Your baby might come off the breast just to smile at you, milk dripping down his chin. Louise remembers one of her baby's favourite nursing jokes:

> How do you respond to your seven-month-old as they repeatedly blow raspberries on your nipples before pulling off to giggle at you? It's both intensely tickly and irritating, and adorable.
> – Louise, UK

In the early months, nursing can be an opportunity to get other things done, like catching up on your messages. Your four- to nine-month-old baby, though, sometimes craves having you put down your phone or book. He might even get a little fussy at the breast if he feels he's being ignored.

The Yo-Yo Baby

Babies who have been lovingly cared for have usually developed deep attachments by this age. Your baby gazes at you adoringly. You're the bright star at the centre of her solar system, and all she wants is to be with you. Whenever you go out of sight, she's heartbroken. Around seven to nine months is a common age for separation anxiety to begin – your baby, having worked out that you're a separate person, is very upset when you leave.

Then there might be other phases, when her natural curiosity about the world sends her off exploring: "Too busy to nurse – got to check out that noise" or "There's the cat...see you later!" Expect more nursing at times when she's all about connection and less when she's all about exploration.

Tips for Nursing Distractible Babies

Being easily distracted isn't a sign that your baby is ready to wean – it's just a developmental stage. If he's nursing less than you'd like – if you're feeling disconnected, or your breasts are uncomfortable – see if you can make nursing a little more interesting for him. Here are some ideas to try:

- **Change position.** If your baby's proud of his new abilities to sit or stand, could he nurse in one of those positions? While a newborn can't comfortably turn his head to feed, an older baby can sit sideways

on your lap, turning his head to the nipple. To nurse your baby while he's standing up, try sitting on a step stool or on the lowest stair.
- **Nurse on the move.** You can nurse with your baby in a sling while walking, or while bouncing gently on an exercise ball or swivelling in a desk chair.
- Look for quiet times to nurse, like **naptime, bedtime, and nighttime.**
- Try **nursing in a quiet, dark room** during the day. Some families have a daily afternoon "rest time" – older children do quiet activities; you lie down with the baby.
- **Chat or sing** while he nurses.
- Let him **use his hands** (see the next section).
- **Model focus for your baby.** Give him your full attention.

Little Fingers

Your baby is becoming skilled with her hands now, and she loves to practise using them – including while nursing. Favourite activities at this stage include

- massaging, patting, or kneading your breast (babies, like kittens, figure out that this can trigger another milk release). Some babies pinch, which you will want to discourage sooner rather than later
- playing with your hair
- poking your nose or teeth (many of us wonder if we're nursing a future dentist)
- fiddling with your clothes, your other nipple, or a mole or skin tag (ouch!)

Nursing Manners

Fidgeting can quickly become part of a baby's nursing ritual, especially when he's tired or going to sleep. You might not mind, or you might find it very annoying.

B.J., who lives with chronic pain, needed to balance her own needs with her babies':

> Since childhood, I have suffered from migraines, and I was diagnosed with fibromyalgia, or chronic muscular pain, as a teen. There are medications for

both these conditions, but not all are safe to take while breastfeeding. For many years, I have continued to live with the constant pain and headaches, because I prioritise breastfeeding. This isn't the right choice for everyone – and several doctors tried to convince me otherwise – but it was right for me, and I have learned to find more comfortable positions and to try to listen to what my body needs at that moment. It's also been useful for my children to recognise that my body is not their property and that sometimes I need to move or even to take a short break from feeding, even if they wish I didn't. It's helped them understand that breastfeeding is a relationship between us, not only something for them.

– B.J., England

Diverting Busy Hands

If whatever your baby is doing while nursing doesn't bother you, and you're pretty sure it won't, you don't need to do anything. If you find those curious fingers irritating, though, it's worth taking action now, before fiddling with your hair becomes something he *has* to do as he falls asleep. Here are some possible alternatives for your baby:

- Give him something else to play with: a scarf, a chunky necklace, a silky label on a piece of cloth, or a small, soft toy.
- Gently hold, stroke, kiss, or play with his hand.
- Cover a mole or skin tag with a plaster.
- Distract or soothe him with stroking, talking, or singing.
- Encourage him to explore lots of different textures when he's *not* nursing, to satisfy his need to touch.

Recognising limits during nursing is one of your baby's first lessons about respect for other people's bodies, and a first step in gentle discipline – as Allison describes:

Today we put up our Christmas tree and I was nervous that my almost walking, definitely into everything ten-month-old would pull off the ornaments or pull down the whole tree! We decided to practise touching the tree and ornaments without pulling. As soon as I said, "Gentle!" she seemed to understand and started gently touching with one finger. I realised we had been practising this, since she would try to grab at my necklace or

face or clothing while nursing and I would say, "Gentle." I had heard that nursing is a foundation for discipline, or gentle guidance, but I suddenly saw it in practice. I was so proud of how our breastfeeding journey was informing the rest of our communication and her perception of the world.
– Allison, North Carolina, United States

The key is to redirect your child's energies into behaviours that meet his needs – in this case, to play and explore – something you will be doing many more times in the years to come.

Easing Up

Your baby now can be more patient about breastfeeding. She can be distracted, and her needs can be met in other ways. She might be happy (at least for a few minutes) with a snack, a change of view, someone else to play with, or an object to investigate. If you need to be away from her, that's usually easier now.

If you've had low milk production and needed to use donor milk or formula, you may find as your baby starts eating more family foods, you can gradually reduce the milk supplements. For how to do this, see Chapter 18, Supplementing. Many parents who've had a difficult start with breastfeeding find that during these months, it gets easier – the fun part is beginning!

If nursing still feels like a struggle, or you've run into new difficulties, reach out for the support you need. La Leche League Leaders are trained to listen, and LLL groups are a safe place to talk about how you're feeling.

Zigzag Progress

If your four- to nine-month-old baby could talk, he might say,

- "I can roll over! Now I keep waking myself up by practising in bed."
- "I really want to sit up/crawl, and I can't *quite* do it – it's *so* frustrating!"
- "I love what my new teeth can do. But my gums are really sore."
- "Look at me standing up! Oops – I fell over again."
- "I can roll/crawl/shuffle/stagger/walk/run all the way over here.... Help, where are you?"

For a baby, these changes are a lot to master, a lot to savour, and a lot to think about, day and night. It's no wonder babies of this age go through patches of increased neediness. The rapid development of these months is full of minor setbacks (which seem major to him!). And nursing makes most things better. Expect your baby to check in with you often for help with frustrations, bumps, and scares. All those little here-and-there nursings keep your milk production strong, too.

Concerns You May Have Between Four and Nine Months

If your questions aren't addressed here, you may find them in Chapter 18, or on LLL websites. Or contact a La Leche League Leader for information and support, as Rieko did:

> I was worried about my third baby's weight gain. There was no group nearby, so I called a Leader to discuss the situation with her. When my baby turned six months, I really wanted to try a meeting, so I took a two-hour train ride to get to one. The meeting had a very comfortable atmosphere and I felt that it was worth going even if it was far away. I've continued to participate in the meetings every month since then, and the LLL philosophy is having a lot of positive influence in my life, not just in the area of parenting.
>
> – *Rieko, Gunma Prefecture, Japan*

How Often Can I Expect My Baby to Nurse?

It's both normal and healthy for a baby this age to nurse frequently throughout the day, and at least once at night, maybe much more often. If you're separated from your baby during the day, she might need to get most of her milk – and your company – during the night. Her body is still growing fast, and so is her brain. The frequency of feedings will vary depending on how quickly and easily your baby is able to fill her tummy, her personality, her sucking needs, and what else is going on in her life.

Some babies naturally begin to cut back the number of nursings between four and nine months, especially once they're eating a lot of other foods. Unless you're aiming to wean your baby soon, there is no need to rush it; all babies wean in their own time (see Chapter 16). Some mothers find that holding back on nursing leads to weaning before they planned (see the next section).

Is My Supply Dropping?

If your healthcare provider is concerned about your baby's slowing weight gain, make sure they're using the World Health Organization's 2006 (or later) growth charts. The WHO charts are based on a large group of healthy, breastfed babies from around the world. Many older charts were based on small groups of mostly formula-fed babies. For more about weighing and growth, see Chapter 18, Weight Gain Worries.

If your milk really has decreased, here are some possible causes:

- feeds were inefficient or limited (for whatever reason) in the early months
- starting hormonal contraception
- a new pregnancy

Of course, once your baby is eating family foods, the amount of milk you're making becomes less crucial. She can make up for any shortfall in milk by eating more of other foods, while continuing to enjoy nursing. Consider the types and amounts of food your baby is offered, as well as your milk production. For more on family foods and nutrition, see Chapter 13.

Is My Baby Weaning?

Eight or nine months is a common time to call La Leche League saying, "Help! I think he's weaning, but I want to continue nursing!" Most times, it's just that the baby is distractible. Some of the ideas in the earlier section titled The Yo-Yo Baby may help refocus him on nursing.

Sometimes the fabric of a nursing relationship has become weaker over time, and if we want to keep it strong, we need to do some repairs. If breastfeeding has become a businesslike arrangement with your baby, he might have less incentive to continue now that he has alternatives.

If it feels like your baby is losing interest in breastfeeding, could it be because nursing comes with conditions? Here's one way to think about it. Imagine that you eat at your workplace cafeteria every day. It's open only at set times, which don't always fit with when you're hungry. When you go to the counter, they quiz you about why you want to eat. You put up with it because the food is really good, plus the café is the only place you can eat. Then one day they put in a second counter. This other counter is open all the time, and when you ask for food you get it, no questions asked. Which counter will you go to?

It's similar for a baby who's always told,

- "You can't be hungry yet; it's only been an hour and a half!"
- "You're probably just tired. Let me rock you to sleep."
- "Not now. Here's a dummy."

Then one day, he gets a bottle to hold on to or a spoonful of food that he's praised for eating. He may soon prefer the bottle or family foods over the breast. Not because he doesn't love to nurse, but because the alternatives are more readily offered. Scheduled or limited nursing may also have reduced your milk supply. When milk production is low, your baby has to work harder for less reward. Eventually, he may become discouraged.

If you feel you're losing your nursing relationship and you don't want to wean yet, it's not too late. Make nursing fun and spontaneous if you can. Nurse in the bath, take naps together, offer to nurse for no reason. Make it silly: sing, play with his toes and hands. If low milk production is frustrating your baby, more frequent nursing (and maybe some expressing) might nudge your supply back into the satisfaction zone (see Chapter 18, Low Milk Supply). It can take time, but you can turn a faltering nursing relationship into something you both enjoy for months or years to come.

For how to keep nursing and your milk supply going when you're away from your baby, see Chapter 14.

Should My Baby Take Naps?

Every baby is different. Some four- to nine-month-old babies nap frequently and easily, some resist sleep but do nap at some point each day, and some barely nap during the day but wake up only once or even not at all at night. Basically, whatever your baby is doing is normal for her.

Babies who are carried for much of the day usually sleep when they need to, dozing while their parents or caregivers move about. Jen's easygoing baby fitted his naps around the rest of the family:

> My LLL Leader, Jen, used to carry her baby a lot – she was one of the first people I had ever seen who did this (we lived in a city community where

everyone used a stroller). I thought it was pretty weird at the time, but he seemed happy. She could nurse him to sleep, put him in bed upstairs, take him out of bed still asleep, put him on the back of her bike, cycle to school to collect his brother, cycle home, and put him back into bed – without waking him up. All that carrying didn't seem to stop him becoming a deep sleeper (maybe it even helped!).

– Jayne, UK

Being put down for a nap works fine for some babies and not at all for others. Many babies at this age still sleep well only when they're carried, or held, or sleeping next to an adult. The least stressful approach right now may be *sharing* that nap when you can. This stage won't last forever. Whatever you do (or don't do) about sleep now, when your daughter's a teen, you will probably have to coax her to get out of bed before noon.

During the first year, most babies "consolidate" their naps, gradually going from lots of little sleeps to fewer, longer ones. Every baby goes at his own pace, and some back-and-forth is normal. Your baby may be cranky for a few days each time he shifts his nap pattern. Some parents find if their baby naps late in the afternoon, he's not tired enough to sleep at his usual bedtime (though others find their baby sleeps *better* after a long afternoon nap). If bedtime is taking forever, you could experiment to see if napping earlier, or cutting short his nap, makes any difference. Babies in childcare will often take longer naps than at home, and that might mean, for now, bedtime is later. There are few things more frustrating than trying to wrestle to sleep a baby who's less tired than you are! For more about sleep, see Chapter 12.

Lark or Owl?

Many people have a built-in preference (known as "chronotype") for when they sleep and wake up, and when they are most alert. Some are "morning people" (larks), and others are "evening people" (owls). Some don't have a preference either way. Babies have these preferences, too, and your baby's may or may not match yours.

When Is My Baby Ready for Family Foods, and How Does Eating Affect Nursing?

Great questions! The short answer is most babies show you when they are ready for family foods and eating doesn't usually affect nursing very much, at first! We cover these topics in Chapter 13.

Does My Baby Need Water?

Exclusively breastfed babies can get all the fluid they need from your milk, whatever the weather. If your baby is having formula as well as nursing, you might offer cooled, boiled water in very hot weather (or if your baby is mostly breastfed, just nurse more often).

Once babies start eating family foods, their kidneys have to work harder, and they need plenty of fluids to keep their digestion running smoothly. Some babies will be reaching for your cup or water bottle about the time they start on family foods. Others prefer to nurse when they're thirsty. Many babies enjoy experimenting with bathwater, too! If you're worried your older baby isn't drinking enough (maybe because it's really hot, or she can't nurse as much because you're at work), juicy fruits, slushies, breastmilk ice lollies, and ice can also help her stay well hydrated.

How Long Will My Baby Be Teething?

We wish we knew! On and off, for quite a while – most toddlers get their last baby teeth at some point between two and three years old. First teeth erupt (appear through the gums) at any time from birth to over a year, though six to twelve months is the most common time. And you might notice signs of teething months before a new tooth pops through.

Your baby is born with all his baby (and adult) teeth already formed in his jaw. On his own timetable, the first teeth start to move upward through the gums. Ouch! If you remember getting wisdom teeth as a teen or adult, you probably remember how uncomfortable it can be. The urge to bite down can be overwhelming. Your baby can't tell you what's wrong, and of course he has no idea himself. He just *hurts*. Here are signs of teething you might see:

- fist chewing
- gum rubbing
- drooling
- crankiness
- more night waking

Teething really does cause a lot of misery for some babies. That's the downside. The upside is that it's such a wonderful excuse! "Well, he's teething" can last for many months and explain away many fussy times.

How can you help? Many teething babies get a lot of comfort from nursing. Older babies may like frozen breastmilk ice lollies. One thing to avoid: teething medications that contain numbing agents can also numb your baby's tongue, making it tricky for him to nurse well. The U.S. Food and Drug Administration recommends not using any topical teething medications and frozen items for babies. Try rubbing your baby's gums with your finger or giving him a hard rubber-type teether that's been in the fridge.

When some babies start actively teething, their saliva seems to increase and even become more acidic. This can cause a rash on both their faces and their bottoms as well as on your breasts. Gently wiping both breast and face a few times a day can help.

If your baby has a fever or seems ill, contact your healthcare provider.

My Baby Has Her First Tooth!

Isn't it adorable? It's quite a milestone! Teeth appearing are part of a baby preparing for family foods, but they aren't necessarily the *signal* to start eating.

The biggest change that tooth makes from the moment it appears is in what you give your baby to teethe on. A single little tooth can nip off something that the rest of the baby's mouth isn't ready to grind up, like a piece of raw carrot. Stick with a cold, wet washcloth or safe teethers from now on.

Now, let's talk about what you probably *thought* we were going to talk about....

Will He Bite Me?

Many babies never bite, some bite once or twice, a few go through a true biting phase. It was a one-off for Sara Diana:

> My first son bit me when he was about seven months old. I did not expect it, and I screamed from the shock and pain. He cried for a few minutes. I felt like the worst mother in the world, but the truth is that he never did it again.
> – Sara Diana, from Barcelona, children born in Mexico

If your baby is under about eight months old and is obviously in discomfort from teething, he's probably not trying to bite you – he would just do *anything* to relieve his sore gums. Try offering a teether or something cold and hard to bite down on before nursing.

Older babies will occasionally bite for other reasons. It could be because of an earache or a stuffy nose. One mother discovered a small piece of a paper tissue stuck to the roof of her baby's mouth. For some reason, it made him want to bite. Or a bite might just be an accident.

The interesting reaction a baby gets when he bites can encourage him to try it again. You can often tell when a baby is biting deliberately, because he looks at you with a little gleam in his eye just before he does it. We know it's *much* easier to say than to do, but try to stay calm if your baby bites while nursing. Even a telling-off can be amusing (or frightening, for sensitive babies). Biting is usually an annoying but short-lived phase. Call an LLL Leader or other breastfeeding helper if biting becomes a problem.

Discouraging Biting

If you've ever been bitten while nursing, you definitely won't want it to happen again! These tips can help discourage biting:

- Take your baby off the breast right away and set her down gently, breaking all physical contact. Then pick her up again and offer to nurse. This sends the message that the nursing has ended because of the biting; you will start a new nursing now.
- It's okay to say, "No," "Gentle," or "Don't bite!" You're the best judge of whether this will deter, scare, or encourage your baby. Or

just say nothing; show her that nothing interesting happens when she bites.
- Make sure she's positioned well for nursing, with a wide-open mouth and her head tipped back. You can show your older baby how to do a big, wide "Aaah!"
- Sometimes babies clamp down on the breast if they feel like they're falling off. Try cuddling your baby in closer, or using your body, legs, or cushions to stabilise her.
- If your baby tends to bite at the start, try a little nipple stimulation or breast compression to speed up that first milk release and start her swallowing.
- Remember that your baby can't bite if her tongue is in the way. If you feel her tongue shift, either take her off or say her name to distract her.
- If your baby tends to bite at the end of the nursing session, just stop a little sooner for a while, or switch sides. Or keep a finger positioned right by the corner of her mouth, ready to slip in between her gums.
- If your baby bites because she's bored and doesn't want to nurse (this is more likely in babies older than about eight months), let her ask to nurse when she wants to, rather than offering. Some families find it helpful to teach their older baby the word for "milk" in sign language, or make up a sign of their own.
- If your baby bites or clamps down and won't easily let go, pull her in closer, which makes it harder for her to breathe, so she'll open her mouth and let go.
- Some sippy cups have a "bite valve" to prevent spills; the cup works only if the baby bites it while drinking. Not a good idea for nursing babies! You might also want to avoid or limit bottles or dummies if they're getting chewed. Otherwise, it's hard for your baby to keep things straight: *this* sucking source can be chewed all I want; *this* sucking source can't.

What Do I Do If My Nipples Get Damaged?

This doesn't happen often, but if it does, it's important to know how to take care of it. Unlike newborns, older babies put everything in their mouths, so hygiene is extra important. Here are some ideas to try:

- Wash your nipple once a day with plain soap to reduce the risk of infection.
- Brush your baby's teeth or encourage him to drink water before nursing.
- Rinse your nipple with water or a saline solution (half a teaspoon of salt in a cup of cooled, boiled water) after nursing.

If you see any signs of infection, such as swelling, colour change, crustiness, or yellow ooze, or you feel worsening pain *between* feeds, contact your healthcare provider. You might have an infection that needs treating.

Usually, you can keep nursing while the nipple heals, but if you need to take a break from nursing on that side, express at least enough milk to keep yourself comfortable. It may hurt less to use your hands rather than a pump. Don't forget pain relief if you need it! There are lots of options that are safe while breastfeeding (see Chapter 18, Medications, or check with your healthcare provider). For more about caring for damaged nipples, see Chapter 18, Sore Nipples.

Will Night Nursing Cause Tooth Decay?

By itself, no. You'll find a fuller discussion of this question in Chapter 12, but the gist of it is that research shows human milk itself rarely contributes to tooth decay and actually has tooth-strengthening properties. For various reasons, including genetics and what happened during pregnancy, some children have weaker teeth that are more prone to decay. A good children's dentist can help you keep your baby's teeth in the best possible condition while supporting you to breastfeed.

My Baby Suddenly Stopped Nursing. Is It a Nursing Strike?

True weaning happens gradually (and very rarely before eleven or twelve months), and the child seems happily done, satisfied, and ready to move on. An abrupt, unexpected pause in nursing is probably a "nursing strike." Usually, the child seems cranky or miserable. Something has caused his favourite activity to become scary or distressing. That's not the same as wanting to give it up for good. Almost all nursing strikes end happily, but not instantly. It can help to stay in touch with a breastfeeding supporter who can suggest ideas to try. Zoe's baby went on strike after a biting incident:

> My eight-month-old had a breastfeeding strike after she bit me and I screamed! No matter what I did, she refused to latch back onto my breast. I had exclusively breastfed her, but at that point I had to pump to be able to get her to take any breastmilk. After forty-eight hours I contacted my local La Leche League and they started giving me tips and tricks. They kept me sane and comforted me during her entire feeding strike. It took five days until she finally latched back on again. I ended up breastfeeding her for another five months. I never would have been able to get through that time without the support from La Leche League.
> – Zoe, British Columbia, Canada

We have a fuller discussion of possible causes and strategies in Chapter 18, Nursing Strike.

How Do I Nurse in Public Now?

It's both easier and more challenging now that your baby is older. You've probably worked out nursing in all kinds of positions, from sitting cross-legged on the floor to nursing-on-the-move. And your baby has a bit more patience and stomach capacity than she did before. She can probably get through outings that would have required at least one nursing a few months ago. Once your baby is eating lots of family foods, you can share your own food with her when you're out and about, or add some healthy, baby-friendly snacks to your changing bag or backpack. On the other hand, your baby may be more active when nursing, lifting up your shirt or letting go to smile at you!

Audrey felt awkward at first about nursing away from home:

> I wear baggy clothes because I'm self-conscious about my body and scared to show it off. So it was hard for me to breastfeed without a cover, but I also found the cover cumbersome because she would pull it off sometimes. By my second child I was less worried about what the public had to say about my breastfeeding. I did it in corner booths and dark corners at first, but then I would just do it anywhere. I had also found the two-shirt method online, and that was a tremendous help! I had a tank top underneath, so when I pulled my T-shirt up, and the tank top down, I had zero skin exposed as he fed. I felt proud and confident. I didn't have anyone say anything to

me, but sometimes a facial expression would show how they felt. I would look down at my child and take comfort in him. He made me so proud to breastfeed.

– Audrey, Texas, United States

If you've been using a cover-up, now you may risk having your baby fling it off, so it might be time to put it away. Holding your baby's hand while he nurses can help settle him, and of course he's finished sooner these days. You're helping future parents by nursing in public, making it easier for the next person to do the same. By the time she had her third baby, Audrey had become a powerful advocate for nursing in her community:

I had to take Raizel out a lot because she was born hard of hearing so we had loads of doctor appointments. I didn't care who was in the room, I fed her. If people stared, I glared right back. If someone smiled, I smiled back. I have twice at Walmart encountered an associate while I fed my child on the floor tell me I had to go do that in the bathroom or my car, and both times I told them that by law, I was allowed to feed my child wherever I was allowed to be. And their company policy states the same thing and they are not allowed to approach me to tell me to move because it can be a terminable offence. I used each encounter as a breastfeeding teaching moment. I truly hope they learned and did look things up!

– Audrey, Texas, United States

Do You Have Any Travelling Tips?

Nursing is the ultimate in portable food. Samantha worked out early on that breastfeeding was no barrier to travelling:

I have breastfed in several countries: England, Scotland, Italy, Singapore, Malaysia, and on a number of Indonesian islands; on planes, trains, buses, boats, microlets [small vehicles], tuk tuks [three-wheeled bicycles with seats for passengers], horse-drawn carriages, and in the car; in parks, airports, cafés, restaurants, school assemblies, supermarkets, birthday parties, the circus; on mountains, beaches, rivers; in forests; and everywhere in between. Almost everyone in the world has seen my boobs (no mean feat for a shy introvert) and no one has ever, ever challenged me about breastfeeding. Luckily for them!

– Samantha, from the UK, living in Bali, Indonesia

This may be the easiest age for taking trips with your baby if he's not yet on the move. He has enough interest in his surroundings that you can distract him when he gets bored. If he's already eating family foods, you can share your own food with him. He might still get a reduced fare, or even travel for free. And he's still small enough to nurse in a limited space. Take that trip now, before he starts walking! For more travel tips, see Chapter 8.

Am I Still Protected Against Pregnancy?

If you're concerned about getting pregnant again, you can read in Chapter 8 about the lactational amenorrhea method (LAM), which gives more than 98 percent pregnancy protection for the first six months. After six months, protection remains extremely good if both of the following are true:

- Your periods haven't returned.
- You rarely go more than four hours between feeds during the day or six hours at night.

Many couples do choose to add another method of contraception at six months or before.

Occasionally, a nursing mother becomes pregnant before her first period. More commonly, when your period first returns, you'll have low levels of certain hormones, reducing the odds of conception. However, once your period returns, you should consider yourself potentially fertile. If you're using a natural family planning method, you can begin charting your temperature and other signs and see for yourself when ovulation returns. If your favourite method of birth control is hormonal, it's less likely to affect your milk supply after the first six months.

Periods During Breastfeeding

If you're exclusively breastfeeding, your period is unlikely to start before three months (though it can happen). For those nursing day and night, the average time before your period returns is thirteen to fourteen months, but there is lots of variation. The timing depends on many factors: hormone levels, how often you nurse, your diet, and more. Once it's happened for your first baby, though, it's likely to follow a fairly similar pattern for any subsequent ones.

You might get spotting on and off for a few months before your period comes back properly. Sometimes you can have spotting just once and then nothing for months. And the periods and cycles themselves may be shorter or longer than they were before you were pregnant. For more about nursing and milk production during your cycle, see Chapter 10.

My Baby Is Too (Choose One) Clingy/Irritable/Placid/Other

Most likely, whether your baby is sticking to you like glue or trying to climb the furniture, what you're seeing isn't a problem but a personality – your baby is showing you who she is. Many babies who didn't seem to enjoy being newborns are much happier by this stage, as Guajirita Alquizareña found:

> Although the first months were difficult because my son suffered from colic, after four months I felt that everything was getting better by the day. He was laughing a lot, giggling, trying to sit up, babbling. . . .
> – *Guajirita Alquizareña, from Cuba, living in the Netherlands*

Any parent of more than one child – even identical twins! – will tell you that however hard you try to treat them the same, they end up different. You may be able to help your baby adapt a bit, but it works best to accept your child for who she is, trust her to let you know what she needs, and follow your own instincts. Some babies definitely need much more support (and patience) than others. The "fit" between you and your baby may also make it harder, or easier, to meet her needs. If you have a high-need baby, look for supportive people who understand – they're probably *not* your friends who have one very placid baby! La Leche League groups can be good places to meet all kinds of babies. If you're finding it hard to understand or feel connected to your baby, reach out for help. Both you and your baby deserve it. For more about baby temperament, see Chapter 7.

How Can I Make My Baby More Independent?

Does a shy baby now mean an insecure adult if you don't start pushing him towards independence? Not at all! Independence comes from feeling secure, and your role right now is to continue to provide that secure base, just as you have been doing. Some babies simply need a secure base longer. Wise parents have often said, "Meet the need, and the need goes away. Ignore the need, and the need remains." Spoiling is still not a possibility at this age. Now's the time when you *get* to hold your baby a lot. He may not be looking to be held as often when he's older.

What Do I *Do* with My Baby?

Babies expect to *fit into* our busy days, not to be the centre of them. Most babies in human history have been born into busy households. Babies love to watch what adults and older children do – it's how they learn. Go places, meet people, do the things you need to do, and enjoy doing – and include your baby. A walk outdoors, a conversation with a neighbour, or just doing chores will teach him more than any toy – as Guajirita Alquizareña found while she was parenting alone:

> His dad went on a trip when our son was eight months old and that stage was very difficult for me. However, being alone with the baby allowed me to enjoy him more every day and learn more about the process. We played a lot, I sang to him a lot, he was doing all the housework with me, and me explaining everything to him.
>
> *– Guajirita Alquizareña, from Cuba, living in the Netherlands*

If you're longing for more excitement, or more company, maybe your baby feels just the same. We've often heard mothers say, "But my baby fusses and cries *all the time* at home!" while the baby sits happily in her mother's lap enjoying an LLL meeting. Many babies love to belong to a group.

However, some sensitive babies get overwhelmed with noise and activity. Their life works better with more quiet times at home. Teresa's daughter Lisa was like this, and for several months Teresa had to lead La Leche League meetings from a different room or in the hallway because Lisa couldn't handle being in the same room as all the parents and babies.

Finding balance can be harder if you and your baby have very different personalities. Maybe your partner, a relative, or your super sociable best friend could party with the baby while you enjoy an hour or two of peace!

My Baby Is Too (Choose One) Small/Big

Most breastfed babies slow down their growth from around four months old. If your baby is on the chubby side at this stage, don't worry. You don't need to restrict his nursing at all. When he's ready to start eating family foods, get advice from your healthcare provider or other reliable sources about healthy foods (see Chapter 13). Let him decide how much to eat and see how it goes.

If you're concerned about your baby's size or growth, check out Chapter 18, Weight Gain Worries, and talk to your healthcare provider.

How Do I Handle Criticism?

For the last two generations, in many countries, breastfeeding has been increasing. This means that many parents of today's babies were breastfed, and many of their parents were, too. In La Leche League (founded 1956), we're proud of the part we've played in this trend.

Joan shares how nurturing at the breast has been passed on to her grandchildren:

> As a former LLL Leader in Canada with three sons, all living far away, I can die happy (fingers crossed) because I have three cherished daughters-in-law who are wonderful mums to six grandchildren (in total, not each!), who have given each child the gift of a nursing relationship to start off their lives. For me, it has been a lesson in trying to be the affirming and positive person I yearned to be and to put myself in their shoes, not to linger with criticism and wondering why they don't do things exactly my way. It seems to have paid off – overcoming various nursing challenges and seeing both the mothers and the fathers grow through their parenting. I really feel that their breastfeeding journeys and the unconditional love they offer their children have given us so much to be thankful for and so much to celebrate.
>
> – Joan, Ottawa, Canada

Coming from a breastfeeding family can have its own complications, though. If you're having difficulties and thinking twice about it, you might feel pressure to keep breastfeeding. And although babies haven't changed much over the generations, in some ways the breastfeeding landscape has.

Today, very premature babies are much more likely to survive – and they can be tricky to feed. Many more mothers have had fertility treatment, or breast surgery, which can affect milk production. Much of the tech used in breastfeeding now (new kinds of pumps, supplementers, etc.) has changed beyond recognition or didn't even exist a few decades ago. Approaches to holding babies and helping them attach at the breast have changed, too – we think for the better! (see Chapter 4). If you run into difficulties, your mother-in-law's or grandmother's experiences might or might not be helpful.

Even if you were breastfed, if you're in a high-income country, chances are it was for a few weeks or months rather than the two or more years our ancestors nursed. Mary's mother did amazingly well to breastfeed her at all:

> My mum had me via C-section and at the time in the eighties had persevered with breastfeeding despite discouragement from hospital staff, who believed it was "crazy" to attempt to breastfeed after a section. One showed her the hospital "milking machine" and allowed her to overstay her allotted time with it (since it wasn't being used by anyone else). She carried on for three months until she returned to work.
> – Mary, UK

Now that your baby is older, you might already have "outgrown" your family's or community's breastfeeding norms. And maybe your family setup looks different from local norms in other ways, too. B.J. describes how it felt to be on the receiving end of questions about her family life:

> I found some of the questions and comments we were receiving challenging. There was the usual nonsense about breastfeeding in public, which I tried to ignore. Worse than that for me was the fact that some people found the idea of a two-mother family intriguing and believed they could ask anything. Some of their intrusive questions were about how we made our baby, but others were specifically about breastfeeding. They questioned me: "Doesn't your baby get confused about there being two pairs of breasts?" and "Isn't

your wife jealous that you're breastfeeding and she's not?" and "Shouldn't you give a bottle so your wife can feed the baby?" It was as if, just because we were not the average family, all our decisions and feelings were public property.

– B.J., England

Being seen as different is uncomfortable. It can feel safer to fit in, even when you know you're doing your best for your children. Seeing you do things differently can feel uncomfortable to others, too:

- Your parents might feel as if you're rejecting their ideas – or them – if you're not parenting the way they did.
- Your partner, if you have one, may feel caught between their family's norms and the way you're doing things together. They may worry that you're making things harder for yourself – and them! – by your parenting choices.

Older generations may honestly think that starting family foods after six months or nursing past a year is dangerous. Over time, those close to you will get used to how you parent, whether or not you talk about it. As your child grows and thrives, you may quietly change people's minds without saying a word.

Responding to Criticism

If you find yourself on the sharp end of other people's critical comments, what can you say? These ideas have been shared by families at LLL meetings:

- **Ask to hear their stories,** in detail. Sometimes a relative or friend will lose interest in *your* story after having a chance to tell theirs. Their criticism can be a cover for sadness. Many grandmothers weep when recalling how hard it was to hear their baby crying for "feeding time," or how painful it felt not to be supported to breastfeed when they wanted to.
- **Offer information.** Share a news article, book, or health guideline with your doubtful friend or family member. Or invite them to accompany you to a La Leche League meeting!

- A good response to the question "When are you going to wean?" is **"We're working on it."** This is true – though the process might take years!
- **Turn it around.** "Are you concerned? Why do you ask? Are you familiar with breastfed babies? Don't you think he seems happy and healthy?" (Choose one!)
- **Preempt the criticism.** "I know the way Alex and I are raising Casey is different from the way you raised Alex. It means everything to me that you're so understanding."
- **Agree to differ.** "I know this doesn't fit with your own child-raising ideas. We're doing our best, and this is what's working for us."
- **It's your call.** "My partner and I [or just I] have found that this works best for us."
- **Find some way to agree.** Focus on what you value about the relationship. Over time, early parenting differences tend to become less important than they feel right now.

Take Your Time

You don't have to respond right away if you don't want to. It can be pretty shocking and upsetting to be criticised – it's okay to take time to think about how to respond. For now, it might help to take a few deep breaths or cuddle your baby. You might want to talk to someone you trust, and maybe role-play how you could handle a similar situation in the future. LLL meetings can be a good place for this.

Any activity is easier when people around you value what you're doing. If that's not your family and friends, it can make a huge difference to get support and encouragement from somewhere else. Whether it's an LLL meeting, a playgroup, or an understanding family member, having people who can "refill your reservoirs" makes a big difference.

B.J. has the last word:

> I feel so lucky to have had this gamut of experiences; even the challenging ones have been beneficial. One of the key things that I have learned . . . is that support is vital. I could never have done all this without my amazing wife, who has always encouraged me to do what I felt was best, both for

myself and for our children. Fi ensured we got help when it was needed, she washed and set up my pump, she made me untold numbers of drinks and snacks so I was hydrated and fed while breastfeeding, she shrugged off silly comments, she kept me safe and loved, and so much more. I wish that other people had that much support and love in their lives.

– B.J., England

Want to know more?

You can find extra resources for this chapter at the "Art of Breastfeeding" tab at www.llli.org.

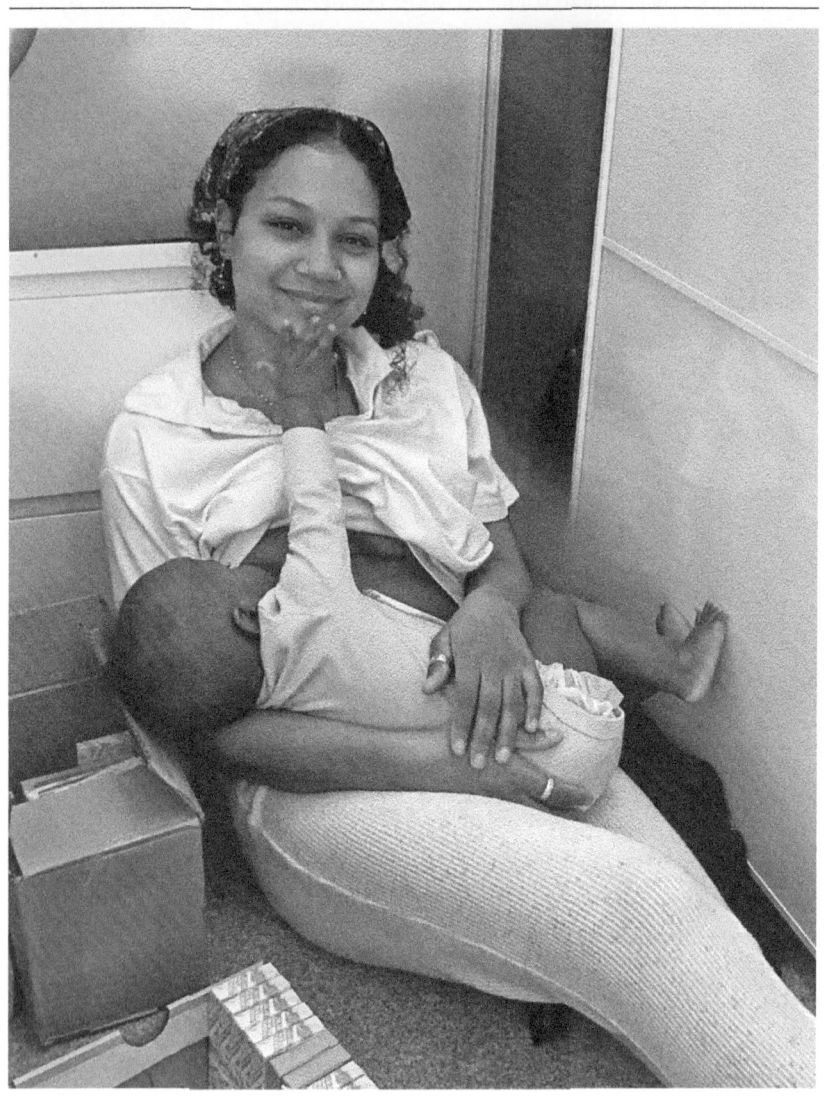

TEN

Nine to Eighteen Months: On the Move

> Although we are just nursing a couple of times a day now, it is still something we both enjoy. Before naps and bedtime we cuddle up in the rocking chair and he eagerly latches on. He has a little superhero toy in his hands at all times of the day, and while we nurse is no exception. That little toy is often being dug into my neck or scratching my tummy as he tucks it under my shirt. I love these still moments and cuddles in what is otherwise a day filled with a toddler who doesn't stop. He feels heavy to pick up now, and he's so long his legs hang off the side of the chair, but when he's nursing, he feels weightless against my body. In that moment I feel like I did when he was a tiny baby. He returns to my body that once grew him, birthed him, fed him, and continues to and will always comfort him.
> — *Olivia, Canada*

Not long ago your baby could get around only with your help. Now he can probably crawl, and by eighteen months most babies will be walking, even running. He can sit alone and play with toys. He can pick up tiny bits of food with his thumb and forefinger and pop them into his mouth. He might be saying words like *duh* or *buh* or *hah* – don't be disappointed if that first word isn't *mama*.

Guajirita Alquizareña's baby started walking and talking around the same time:

> He said his first words, started to crawl, and finally to walk just when he turned one year old. It was very, very cute.
> — *Guajirita Alquizareña, from Cuba, living in the Netherlands*

Some babies seem to prioritise one or the other, chatting in sentences before they start moving, or being too busy walking and running to work on talking! Every baby develops at her own pace. If you're concerned your baby isn't doing what you'd expect, talk to your healthcare provider.

Nursing Now: Nine to Eighteen Months

I *loved* our journey so far of the last eleven months and I'm not thinking about quitting.
— Lynn, Turnhout, Belgium

Fifteen months on and I am still breastfeeding. Each time is a wonderful moment to bond with my son: the cuddles, the laughs, passing on antibodies. It can also be a great time to sit quietly and regroup while I feed.
— Denise, UK

Your nursling has opinions on breastfeeding now, about when, where, and which side. He might announce "Side!" when he's decided it's time to switch. He may joke with you about nursing, playing peekaboo with your shirt or pretending to have his toy dinosaur nurse.

Your child's reached Olympic levels of nursing gymnastics, able to nurse in any position. Naps and bedtime still rely mostly on nursing to sleep, but you can add books, stories, prayers, and songs.

By nine months, most babies are eating some family foods. But while some are eating three meals a day, others are mostly finger painting with the foods offered. Your baby is still getting many of her essential nutrients from your milk.

During this time your milk also changes: fat and energy levels increase, and so does the concentration of some immune components, protecting your baby from the viruses and bacteria she meets in everyday life. No other food can do that. Your milk is adapting to her changing needs, ensuring that she benefits to the very last drop... whenever that comes.

Just before my son's first birthday, my husband and I were working hard to finish up the house that we were renovating. My son was staying at his grandparents' but was getting iller throughout the day.

He ended up spending his first birthday in hospital, diagnosed with the flu. Luckily, I could stay with him in hospital. I was so glad that I could help him through this horrible time, with not only cuddles but the magic of breastmilk. The first night he immediately started drinking my milk again, and by the second day he was transformed into a happy baby. We got to stay an extra day for observation, but the impact of the breastmilk was almost miraculous. Better than any medicine. I'm grateful for the medical care in the hospital but I'm convinced that breastmilk was the reason he improved so fast.

– Liesanne, Belgium

Food: Staying on Course

Part of La Leche League's philosophy from the beginning has been about eating food "as close to its natural state as possible." Now that family foods are becoming more important in your baby's diet, you might be noticing that many of the foods marketed for babies are actually ultraprocessed. And current research suggests these products can negatively affect your child's health now and in the future. Stick to real, unprocessed food as much as you can: food that doesn't contain unnecessary colours, flavourings, or preservatives, and comes in different textures, shapes, and sizes. It might take a little more time to prepare, and yes, it is more likely to "go bad" if you don't eat it in time, but food preparation for babies doesn't have to be complicated, especially if you adapt whatever you're eating so your baby can share it.

For more on ultraprocessed foods, and the shift from milk to family foods, see Chapter 13.

Beyond Water

You've probably introduced water by now, along with your baby's first foods, but what about other drinks? You might wonder whether you need to use any of the following:

- **Formula.** As long as your child is still nursing, there's no need to introduce formula now. (How much nursing is enough? Nobody knows.) Formula is heavily marketed to parents of older babies and toddlers, but these drinks are ultraprocessed and can replace more nutritious foods. The World Health Organization advises that *none* of these "follow-on" or "growing up" formulas are necessary. If babies need formula because not enough human milk is available to meet their needs, then a standard infant formula is appropriate, from birth to twelve months. After a year, formula isn't needed at all.

A mother called the other day about her breastfeeding toddler's diet. She asked, "When am I supposed to stop breastfeeding him, so he can drink normal milk?" She meant cows' milk. Then she laughed, taken aback at what she'd just said. How were we persuaded that the milk of another species is "normal" for our babies and young children, even when they're still breastfeeding?

– La Leche League Leader, UK

- **Animal milks.** It's fine to use animal milks once your baby starts family foods, as long as he can tolerate them. However, they aren't suitable as a baby's main drink until after twelve months. Is drinking cows' milk essential for toddlers and children? No. Humans in some parts of the world began taking milk from animals just a few thousand years ago. Even today, most adults lose the ability to digest milk. And nursing toddlers and children of any age don't need any other milk besides yours.
- **Plant-based drinks** (soy, almond, rice, coconut, etc.) are also often called milks. Like animal milks, these can be used in cooking, but again, nursing babies and toddlers don't need any milks to drink.
- **Fruit juice.** Whole fruits are a better choice than fruit juice because they provide more fibre and nutrients. There's a lot of sugar in juice, too. If you want to give your baby juice, wait until he's at least a year old. Older toddlers can occasionally drink juice as part of a well-balanced diet – you may want to dilute it with water.
- **Sweetened "fruit drinks"** aimed at babies and toddlers have more sugar and fewer nutrients, so are best avoided.

As babies pass the one-year mark, their rate of growth slows down. Toddlers often have small appetites, and filling them up with other milks or juice can mean they have less interest in eating more nutritious foods.

Concerns You May Have Between Nine and Eighteen Months

Here are some nine- to eighteen-month issues that often come up at LLL meetings. If your questions aren't addressed here, try Chapter 18 or LLL websites. You might also contact an LLL Leader.

Slowed Milk Release

Many of us notice our milk release gets slower as the calendar pages turn, probably because the volume has decreased. It was so ready to spill forth in the checkout line at six weeks – but now your toddler has to wait a little longer. Think of it as an early lesson in patience.

Slowed Weight Gain

Towards the end of the first year, breastfed babies begin slowing down their weight gain even more. Children who are not breastfed may continue growing faster – and are at increased risk for overweight. The World Health Organization growth charts reflect these normal changes in the growth rate of breastfed babies. If your doctor raises a red flag about weight gain, check to make sure she's using the WHO charts, or charts based on them. If your baby's growth really is concerning, you'll want to review her overall nutrition and ways to increase calories (see Chapter 18, Weight Gain Worries).

My Period Has Started Again

Fertility often returns between nine and eighteen months. Ovulation can happen before you see your first period. Your periods may be different from before: longer or shorter, or trailing into view over a day or two rather than starting in full force. Breasts and nipples may be sensitive around the time of ovulation. The length of your cycles can change, too – you might have been a regular twenty-eight days before, but now forty-five days isn't unusual.

Sometimes milk supply seems to dip for a couple of days during each cycle. Your baby may object to a change in taste or get frustrated if the milk releases more slowly. For a healthy baby who's growing well, this is a temporary nuisance rather than a problem that needs fixing. You might notice that he eats more family food on those days, or wants more water as well as nursing.

My Period Still Hasn't Come Back, but I Want to Get Pregnant

> I had thought that I wanted my children close together in age, like my sister and I had been. When my son was nine months old, I began asking the mothers at my La Leche League group when I could expect to get my period back. I said I wanted my children less than two years apart. They said, "Just let your body decide." So that's what I decided to do.
> – Cecily, Ontario, Canada

Most women who've conceived naturally before can conceive again while nursing. If you're not ovulating yet, try gradually increasing the longest gap between feeds. Once that gap is longer than about six hours, fertility often kicks back in. The gap might be overnight, or it might be during the day, if you're away from your baby. If six hours isn't enough, stretch that time some more. At some point, your period will make a welcome return. Some women have to wean completely, though.

Once you get pregnant, the balance of milk supply and demand gives way to pregnancy hormones, meaning milk production may go down or even dry up entirely at some point. If your baby is still under a year old, you might need to supplement with formula.

> My breastmilk production stopped when I was sixteen or seventeen weeks pregnant with my second child. My oldest, who wasn't yet two, was still breastfeeding, and decided that dry nursing was an acceptable alternative to not being at the breast at all. He continued to dry-nurse all the way through the rest of the pregnancy.
> – Shoko, the Netherlands

Nursing an older baby is very unlikely to pose any extra risk to a healthy singleton pregnancy. You won't have to wean your baby if you don't want to. Weaning does sometimes happen during pregnancy, either because a drop in milk production discourages your baby or because nursing becomes too uncomfortable for you. For more on nursing and pregnancy, see Chapter 16.

If you're planning fertility treatment, check with your clinic about their policy on treatment during breastfeeding. There are two possible concerns: that medications will affect your nursing child and that nursing will reduce your chances of getting pregnant. Many clinics recommend weaning in advance, as B.J. found:

> My wife and I decided to try for a second child. The fertility clinic we used was adamantly against breastfeeding through treatment, claiming the drugs weren't safe and that breastfeeding lowered our likelihood of success. They told us to return once I'd weaned our daughter. We did our own research and found that neither of those statements was true in our case (there are some drugs that are not safe when breastfeeding, but none that I was taking). We returned to the clinic a few months later, didn't mention breastfeeding, and commenced treatment. I breastfed through multiple rounds of IUIs and IVF, and my breastfeeding relationship with my daughter sustained me through the months it took to get pregnant.
> – B.J., England

For more on nursing and pregnancy, see Chapter 16.

Monique's Story: Tandem Nursing an Adopted Baby

There is more than one way to grow your family! Monique adopted a newborn when her youngest child was nine months old and nursed both babies:

My fifth child, A, was still an infant when a friend of mine told me that her teen daughter was expecting a baby. Since I had also been a teen mum, she asked me to talk to K about the options she had. I was happy to and supported her when she decided on having the baby adopted.

All the same, I was surprised when she asked if my husband, Adam, and I would adopt her baby. How could you say no to that? However, the timing was going to be a challenge.

A was nine months old when baby M was born. I had breastfed all my children, so of course I would breastfeed this one. I talked to a La

Leche League Leader about what I could do to have enough milk for both A and the newborn. I took some supplements and started to pump. I stored the milk I got, just in case the new baby needed it.

I also met with K to see how she felt about me breastfeeding the baby. She was actually quite enthusiastic about it!

I went with K when her labour was induced. Her parents were there, too – the room was full of love. Labour went slowly, and the baby wasn't born until after midnight. I stayed overnight in the hospital room with K and M, and I nursed the baby through the night. Some of the nurses made negative comments, but the hospital lactation consultant was very positive and encouraging. While K left the next morning, I stayed in the hospital with my new daughter for several days because the paperwork hadn't been completed to allow us to leave together. That extra milk I had pumped turned out to be helpful for A, not M, because A was only allowed into the hospital as a visitor.

A was a bit bewildered the first time he saw the new baby nursing – kind of "Where did she come from?" – but it didn't take long before they were happily sharing. I was quite a good milk producer, and in fact the amount of milk was pretty overwhelming for a newborn, who would normally be getting just small quantities of colostrum. I learned to nurse A first to help with that, but then M wasn't gaining weight as fast as expected, so I had to adjust again and make sure she was able to get more. We worked it out.

And I don't know if it was the nursing together or the fact that they are so close in age, but they have been best friends ever since. They even both weaned at the same time, when A was four and M was three.

– Monique, Alberta, Canada

I Feel Terrible When I Nurse!

Nursing aversion or agitation might make its first unwelcome appearance between nine and eighteen months. It can be related to menstruation or a new pregnancy, as it was for Liz:

> Then we found out we were expecting our second baby. Feeding through my milk drying up came with many challenges, including the start of aversion. I have struggled with aversion on and off since then. My heart and body want two different things.
>
> – Liz, UK

Nursing aversion happens when the act of nursing triggers strong negative feelings. You might feel an overwhelming restlessness, like your skin is crawling (this is the **agitation** part) or want to scream or walk away. The first time this happens can be very distressing. It can feel like your nursing relationship has suddenly gone terribly wrong. But it's not your fault, and you're not alone. Humans are a complicated mix of body, mind, biology, and culture. And many of us are parenting under pressure, with little support. It's not surprising that sometimes, a fuse seems to blow.

If aversion doesn't seem connected to your monthly cycle (and you're not pregnant) it may be a signal of overload. Exhaustion, old emotional wounds or trauma, trying to meet everyone else's needs while ignoring your own... all these can cause tension to build up, and something needs to change. Some mothers decide to wean, but many find a way through it. La Leche League groups are a safe space to talk about these feelings. Whatever you choose to do, we're here to help.

My Baby's Not Nursing Very Often. Is She Weaning?

By eighteen months, some nursings are probably just a few minutes long, and family foods may be greeted with enthusiasm. Breastfeeding continues to be important nutritionally and emotionally, though. The World Health Organization recommendation to nurse for at least two years is based on good evidence. Your one-year-old still doesn't have a mature digestive system, and her immune system is still incomplete. While she can manage without human milk, she isn't really ready to.

And things change. As your baby learns to crawl and walk, she might wake more at night. If your baby has busy, exciting days, she may need to fill up the tank at night.

So how can you keep breastfeeding going with one of these busy babies? Remember that "don't offer, don't refuse" is actually a way to wean. Your baby may not think to ask to nurse. If she's fussy or cranky, or you just feel she hasn't had a snuggle or a snack in a while, make the offer. You'll probably get in several more quick nursings a day this way; they're good for your relationship as well as your milk supply. Make room for a few more leisurely nursings, too. Early morning, naptime, and bedtime are often good choices.

Some older babies or toddlers stop nursing at night all by themselves. As long as your baby nurses often during the day, she'll be fine. If you're away from your baby some of the time, make the most of being together. You can pack plenty of nursing into evenings (or whenever you're off work), weekends, and holidays. Just as with a toddler's often random diet, think about averaging out your nursing over a week or a month – not just a single day!

Babies Who Really Do Wean

A small number of babies wean themselves around or just before a year. They're often exceptionally busy, active babies who've always had a businesslike approach to nursing. Sometimes there have been extra stresses on the nursing relationship, such as a lot of separation or low milk supply. But occasionally, early weaning just happens, as it did for Georgie and Trixie:

> I ended up mixed feeding with Trixie as I was still in school and also working part-time. I cherished nursing and always nursed when we were together. When Trixie was eleven months old, we travelled as a family to visit my family in California. Travel is always hard on young children, with the disruption of regular schedules and the excitement of travelling. We were staying at my parents' house and I tried to nurse but Trixie wanted nothing of it! I thought the travel had just been stressful, so I would use quiet rooms, leaving my breast out while we cuddled and encouraging her to my breast.
>
> She refused to nurse again and again. This was it. Trixie was just not going to have it and was done. I felt grief. I felt loss. I felt guilt about the bottles she had gotten as a result of my time away from her. I was worried that the relationship I wanted to have with her was not going to happen.
>
> At the same time, I respected my baby's signals. I remembered hearing about the "dance of weaning" at an LLL conference. That has stuck with me because dancing takes two partners. If one partner does not want to dance, dancing will not happen.
>
> Having a child wean at eleven months felt scary to me, but I can see now that my mothering is still infused with the principles of mothering through breastfeeding. I value touch and "people first." I am passing those values to my children.
>
> – Georgie, New Jersey, United States

A baby who seems unhappy is more likely on temporary nursing strike (see Chapter 18). A baby who is weaning himself usually seems happy about it. When a baby signals, "Thank you, Mama, but I am really done with nursing!" that is a communication to listen to. Weaning, whether or not you wanted it, can bring a strong mix of emotions. We talk about this in more detail in Chapter 16.

She's Nursing Like a Newborn!

> My daughter was exclusively breastfed until she was nine months old, because until then she didn't accept solid foods. When we started complementary feeding, she did not reduce her breastfeeding – she continued with more than seven feeds a day, and up to five feeds at night. After a year, she started with her three meals a day, but still several feedings of breastmilk. At this point she was already pronouncing many words, among them "chichi, mama," and she would try to pull my clothes so that I would give her her beloved "chichi."
>
> – Gisel, Mexico

We often hear similar stories at LLL meetings, especially with babies twelve to fourteen months old. This seems to be a common time for increased nursing. It's not surprising; getting up on two feet and learning to talk are huge changes, and nursing helps your toddler recharge. Usually, nursing will calm down again in a few days. Some extra carrying could be an alternative way to meet your toddler's need for connection. A back carrier might be more comfortable now that she's bigger, and it will keep her away from your breasts for a while!

Some toddlers seem to head for the breast at the first inkling of discomfort, hunger, or boredom and refuse any other offers. This might be partly a matter of temperament – the world can be overwhelming for more sensitive children, and nursing is their safe place.

You can gently encourage other options:

- Offer a healthy meal or snack *before* your toddler asks to nurse.
- Change up your usual activities: go out more (or less), find some different toys, books, or company.
- Find some new ways to help your toddler relax and unwind: warm water, massage, dance, playing with dough or sand, blowing bubbles, stroking animals.

Nursing will still be important to him for a good long time yet.

If you feel like you're getting into a tug-of-war with your toddler, it may be a sign that he's not quite as ready for change as you are. This is how it can go:

- Your toddler needs extra reassurance – maybe he just learned to walk or moved into a different room at nursery.
- You feel irritated by the extra nursing and cuddling. You back away a bit.
- Your toddler feels you distancing from him, feels more stressed, and steps up his demands. You are more irritated and back away more....

This little loop is no fun for either of you and it can lead to an unhappy relationship. To interrupt the pattern, try to relax into it. Recognise the real needs behind your toddler's clingy behaviour. "Fill him up" with a day or two at home, cuddling and nursing as much as he wants. Wear him in a sling, take a bath or shower together, go for a slow walk together. Satisfy the need, and it goes away. To do this, you may need to take care of unsatisfied needs of your own – your annoyance at your toddler might be a sign that you're running on empty, too. See How Can I Find Time for Myself? later in this chapter.

If your child has additional needs, listening to your instincts about what she needs may be even more important, as Laura found:

> My daughter was diagnosed with autism at seventeen months old. After receiving that knowledge, I was able to look back at our breastfeeding journey with a new perspective. I did everything in my power to hold on to that for as long as possible. I learned to not give one single thought to the opinions of others about my breastfeeding journey. To just do what feels right in my mama heart no matter what. It has been such a journey and I'm so grateful for all that I have learned and how much I have grown alongside my daughter.
>
> – Laura, United States military

My Toddler's Still Fiddling with My Nipple!

Lots of toddlers continue to want to twiddle the nipple they're not currently using, play with your hair, or pinch that loose skin on your elbow. Let your toddler know that these things are not okay and look for other options. If she likes to twist your hair, see if she'd accept a doll with long hair or a blanket with a silky binding to keep her hands busy. A small, squeezable toy in her hand might keep her from twiddling or pinching. You might have to experiment a bit! Eventually she might bring the toy over to you when she wants to nurse.

My Baby Is Scared of Strangers

Clever baby! A sense of "stranger danger" helps protect your newly mobile baby from harm. He won't toddle off with anyone he doesn't trust.

Sometimes a person your baby previously tolerated – Grandma, for example – will now be put in the "scary stranger" category. Your baby may cry and protest if she tries to pick him up. You can reassure Grandma that this is temporary! Try giving Grandma a hug, which might reassure your baby. Or let him sit safely on your lap while you talk to the "stranger," giving him time to warm up.

Your toddler may be wary of new places, too. The wise toddler knows he isn't very wise yet and errs on the side of caution. "I don't know this place. Maybe it's not safe!" You might be sitting on the floor while your baby crawls around, staying fairly close to you. Then he spots the cat leaving the room and crawls after him. Minutes later, he comes back to nurse. After just a few sucks he heads out again – to investigate the shoes in the hallway. If you leave the room without telling him while your baby is exploring, he may be really upset. It's okay for him to crawl away from you, but not at all okay for you to leave!

These "touching base" nursings are part of normal milk maintenance, and for your baby, they're part of playing it safe. Every time he touches base with you, his sense of security gets a little stronger. One day, the shy toddler who hides behind the sofa when his grandparents visit will venture not just into the next room but to a different city, or across the world.

What About Nights and Naps?

> As soon as my son turned one, people started saying things: you're not still breastfeeding him, are you? When are you going to stop? He's one now, for goodness' sake. It's no good for his teeth, you know, feeding him at night. Even the muttering of having created a "rod for my own back" – a phrase so outdated it almost feels amusing. Well, I said, there we have it. Bring on the rod, glue it to my spine. I rock this rod. I'm styling it out. Also, the World

Health Organization recommends breastfeeding up to the age of two, you ignoramuses.

Except, of course, I didn't say any of that. Instead, I wasted time worrying. I devoted whole evenings to worrying that I was failing some vital test of parenthood by continuing to nurse my one-year-old to sleep, and by making half-hearted attempts to get him to sleep in his new cot, rather than embrace bed-sharing with guilt-free gusto. No pacing the floor, no desperate beseeching him to go to sleep, or to get back to sleep when he woke up. He would just turn his head, reach for me in the bed, his mop-like mass of feathery hair tickling my nostrils, latch on, and then we'd both instantly drift off again.

Feed beyond the age of one, and your baby is more responsive, even more alert and engaged, and sometimes hilariously assertive at the breast. And, oh, I miss how easy it was to get him to nap during the day, the two of us curled together on my bed, and his jaw eventually growing slack. Peeling him off my nipple, and then reaching for my flask of tea (preparation is key!) and secret stash of biscuits, and reading for an hour or so while he snoozed alongside me. I think these feeding-to-sleep naps are what I still treasure most about breastfeeding my son between the ages of one year and eighteen months. It was as if this superpower that we'd worked so hard to acquire now really came into its own. He'd start sucking and then, soon after, ta-da: welcome to your precious naptime window, Mama! What a tool in my mothering arsenal, I now realise, what a handy mechanism breastfeeding could be. All that, on top of the constant, giddying headrush of love.

– *Kate, UK*

Your nine- to eighteen-month baby's naps may be more predictable now (unless she's one of the babies who never does a day the same way twice!). She might take two naps, one in the morning and one in the afternoon. Or maybe she takes only one nap in the afternoon. Or has catnaps throughout the day. Whatever her pattern might be, most babies (not all) do need daytime sleeps through the second year. Savour them while they last!

Does nursing to sleep create a bad habit? Not at all. It's a normal way to go to sleep when you're still small. An older baby may want nursing and a book or a song. Older still, and the book or the song is enough. Falling asleep on our own happens naturally in its proper time, no "training" needed. Many families find that their child can fall asleep for someone else without nursing if Mum is out but really needs to nurse if she's in the house. No need to rush a child out of naptime and bedtime nursings. For more about naps and nighttimes, see Chapter 12.

How Can I Find Time for Myself?

> I feel that every day I like being a mum more and more, even though sometimes I don't have the same time I had before for myself. I do see that I have learned to make better use of my time, that I am now able to enjoy much more with less, that I can do several tasks at the same time, in a more efficient way.
>
> – *Guajirita Alquizareña, from Cuba, living in the Netherlands*

Sometimes, building an entire child from your milk and a few scraps of toast just doesn't feel like enough of an achievement.

Remember those early days, when you could barely eat a snack because taking care of your baby took up all your time? Some days you might want your newborn back, but other days you'll wish he was fifteen and didn't need you constantly. (Spoiler alert: he will still need you at fifteen, but he won't be home as much.)

When he was a newborn, you often put your needs aside for the tiny person who couldn't wait. Now, the balance is shifting. Remember how on planes you're told to put on your own mask first and then help others? That applies here.

Here are some ideas, picked up from LLL meetings:

- **Prioritise one thing** a week to accomplish from your own list of goals: listening to a podcast, making a piece of art, attending a martial arts class.
- **Recognise your need for solitude.** Some mothers need a little alone time, some need a lot. One mother took a bath, alone, once a week. The rest of the week, whenever she felt under pressure, she would imagine herself in that bath!
- **Take advantage of times when your toddler is playing.** It's not about multitasking, it's about seeing what you can do (including relaxing) while she explores.
- **Plan ahead for meals.** Dinnertime can be tough – tired kids, tired parents. Try to prepare or at least start dinner in the morning. In the evening, you'll just have to reheat it or take some final steps. Or cook in bulk once or twice a week.

- **Choose your company.** Spend time with people who leave you feeling good. This could be having a regular call or coffee date with someone who's a great listener or attending a club where everyone shares your interest. La Leche League meetings can help meet this need. But maybe what you *really* crave is a couple of hours talking about football!

Do I Need to Start Setting Boundaries for My Baby?

As your child begins to grow, the simple days of needs and wants being the same thing can change. Your toddler really wants to nurse to sleep. Is that a need? Yes, nursing to sleep covers several needs: for milk, relaxation, closeness to you. Your toddler really wants to stick a screwdriver into the electric outlet. Is that a need? Of course not! But what if he really wants to play on his toy xylophone and his sister is sleeping? Substituting a safe object for an unsafe one, distraction, and removing the baby from the scene will cover most situations at first. Sometimes it's about changing the environment: older children can be encouraged to play with their toddler-unfriendly toys on a table.

If you find yourself getting angry with your baby (or can't bear to deny him anything, even if he's causing chaos), see Chapter 11.

My Baby Is a Biter. Of Other People!

Maybe it's teething, or stress, or experimentation, or just frustration. Whatever her reason, it can be upsetting to discover that your child has taken to chomping on playmates or siblings. You might even feel embarrassed – but this is a common stage many toddlers go through and doesn't mean you've done anything wrong. At this age, biting isn't prompted by meanness or bullying tendencies.

Other children may not bite but might hit, push, scratch, or kick from time to time. These behaviours, too, are totally normal for a baby who is just learning to live with others. But the others might not always appreciate this! And sadly, children are not all treated fairly. Behaviour may be judged differently, depending on cultural background or gender.

Your best strategy may be to remove your child from potentially stressful situations before the biting starts. Tiredness, hunger, or overwhelm are often triggers. You can ask other parents to help you by stopping your child and calling you over if needed. Biting or hitting really is a stage, and it really will end. For now, quick action and distraction are your best tools.

I Suddenly Have Sore Nipples!

You've been nursing your baby happily for close to a year or more, and now you have sore nipples. At this stage, there are several possible causes. Check out this list, and if nothing on it fits, talk to an LLL Leader or other breastfeeding support person:

- Maybe your toddler's been **pulling at your nipple without breaking the suction** so that it pops or smacks loudly when she releases it? Yowch! The same solutions suggested for biting in Chapter 9 may help end the game of "pop goes the nipple."
- **Thrush (yeast infection).** A yeast infection is more likely if you've had antibiotics lately or if anyone in the household has a yeast infection. The pain is usually intense, in both breasts, after and between feeds (see Chapter 18, Yeast, and LLL websites).
- Is your **period back?** Nipple tenderness is common for part of each cycle.
- **Could you be pregnant?** It's possible to conceive even if you haven't had a period yet. For more on nursing during pregnancy, see Chapter 16.
- Is a new (or chipped) **baby tooth** causing nipple pain? Babies sometimes don't quite know how to latch with a new tooth – they have to get used to it. Encourage your toddler to open her mouth wide and come to the breast chin-first, so her top teeth can't dig in. If she's teething, giving her something cold and hard to gnaw on before nursing may also help. Baby teeth chip easily, but the razor sharpness that can result can be smoothed away with a nail file. Your toddler may appreciate the result as much as you do!
- If you have any **food sensitivities,** and your toddler decides she'd like a little nursing for dessert after eating something you react to – peanut butter, citrus fruits, and dairy products are common irritants – you may end up with an uncomfortable rash. Try asking your toddler to have a drink of water before nursing, and use a damp cloth to wipe her face before nursing and your breast afterwards.
- If you have a skin condition such as **eczema,** it's probably fine to use your regular treatments on your nipples and breasts as needed.

Check with your healthcare provider if you're not sure (see Chapter 18, Medications).
- Do you have a **white or yellow spot or blister on the tip of your nipple?** It could be a bleb or milk blister. These can be extremely painful and can sometimes block milk from coming out of part of the breast, giving you mastitis (inflammation) symptoms, too (see Chapter 18, Blebs, Mastitis).

Is Anyone Else Still Nursing?

After crossing the "magical" line of twelve months of breastfeeding (after which breastfeeding is far less socially acceptable), we realised that same-aged children were already weaned and we came across the "Are you *still* breastfeeding?" question more and more often. I read all the books on long-term breastfeeding that I could find and started to visit a La Leche League breastfeeding support group.

– Christina, Germany

The hospital where my daughter was born encouraged breastfeeding. Some of my friends with parenting experience suggested that I could breastfeed her until she was one or two years old. Two of them said that their children had loved breastfeeding and said it was their best childhood memory.

– Janedy, Taiwan

There are many communities where nursing eighteen-month-olds is as normal as the sun rising every morning. In others, few babies are nursed past six months. If that's your community, you might hear: "If your baby can ask for it, he's too old to be nursing," "A baby with teeth is too old," "You're making your baby too dependent on you," "There's no value to human milk after [choose one] three months, six months, a year...." And the classic "Mothers who nurse past a year are doing it for themselves," which usually gets a hollow laugh at LLL meetings!

A simple "Thanks, but this is right for us" may be your best response. Your nursing relationship is your own and your child's, and no one else's. The world's leading health organisations are on your side. For more thoughts on handling criticism, see chapters 9 and 16.

Many find La Leche League for the first time when their babies are older than a year. As one mother put it, "I love it here, because it's the one place I feel completely normal, nursing my toddler. And I can complain about the irritating bits without anyone saying, 'Well, what do you expect, you're still breastfeeding'!"

What's Ahead?

> Now my baby girl is no longer a baby but a sixteen-month-old toddler. She is still breastfed. I do not think it will finish anytime soon, as we both enjoy it.
> – Asia, UK

> I thought, *We'll see what this new adventure will bring*.... And look at us now. She's thirteen months old and still loving her quiet time on the breast. But we wouldn't have got this far without the advice from La Leche League.
> – Sien, Belgium

By now, you might have nursed longer than many or all of your friends. Healthcare services are often geared to supporting the beginning of breastfeeding, but providers may just look confused when you ask questions about toddler nursing! It can feel like you've gone off the map. But in LLL, you're in good company. We're here to support you until the end of your breastfeeding journey, whenever that might be.

Want to know more?

You can find extra resources for this chapter at the "Art of Breastfeeding" tab at www.llli.org.

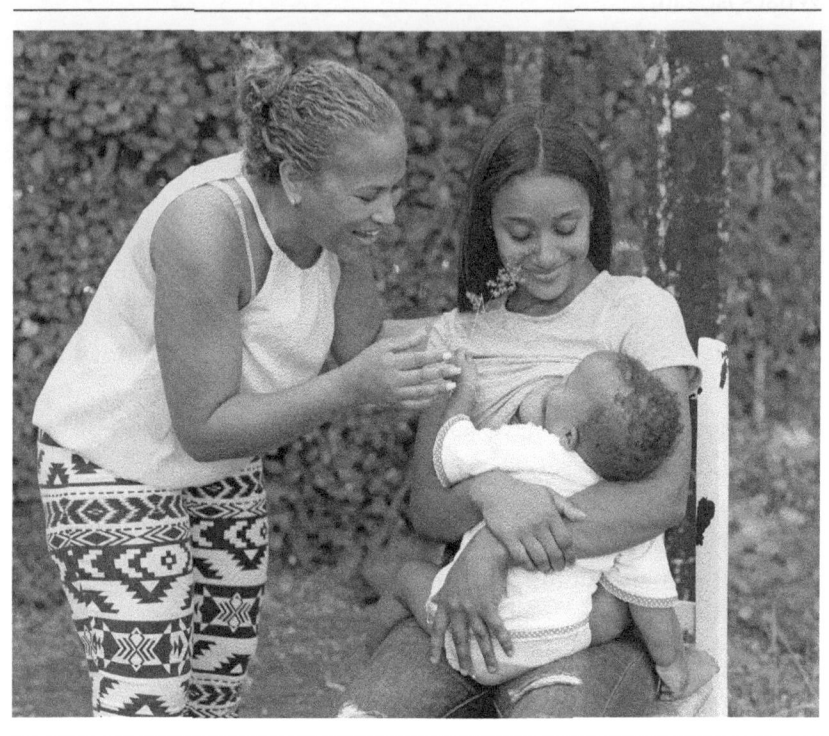

ELEVEN

Nursing Toddlers and Beyond: Moving On

> I'm not sure I ever imagined the extended breastfeeding journey, but my son and I both really enjoy it and benefit from it, so we are continuing. Through what has been a very challenging few years as we face unknown viruses, overcrowded hospitals, less accessible healthcare, and very ill children, it feels like a lifesaver. Motherhood and the breastfeeding journey have changed my life, deeper than anything. I hope that the years we have spent gazing into each other's eyes while he nurses and holding him while he falls asleep are imprinted in his emotional being, forever. To know that he is always safe, that he is always loved, that his needs matter, and that he is always enough.
> – Natalie, Ontario, Canada

Toddlerhood can be the Golden Age of nursing. Your child is eating other foods, so if your night out with friends lasts a little longer than expected, your baby's tummy and your breasts can handle it. Nursing now is not just food and drink, but communication and connection, comfort and pain relief.

Nursing came to the rescue when Lindsay's daughter broke her arm:

> I awoke to the sound of my two-year-old daughter fussing and felt her reaching out for me with her arm that wasn't in a cast. I looked at the clock – 3:00 A.M. As I lifted my shirt to let her latch, I started wondering about other mums of breastfeeding toddlers doing the same. I had night-weaned my daughter a few months earlier, but after she fell and broke her left arm, she would wake up in so much pain we decided to return to the one comfort

she had since birth, the breast. Like magic, my sweet girl could sleep again! What a gift! My daughter is all healed now, and back to only daytime breastfeeding. I look back on all the wakeful nights with such a grateful feeling; so thankful that I could always provide what she needed.

— Lindsay, Texas, United States

Maybe you never dreamed you'd find yourself nursing a child old enough to walk up and ask for it. But days turn into weeks, weeks turn into months, months turn into years. One day you realise your tiny baby has become a busy, active toddler.

Maybe you're not at this stage yet, and you're wondering what it will be like. Nursing a toddler might seem impossible to imagine. Keep an open mind. As Cecily found, it's different when it's your own child:

I had hoped to breastfeed my son until he was at least one year old. I saw a two-year-old breastfeeding at my first LLL meeting, when I was seven months pregnant. This child did look awfully big at the breast. But time went by, and now I was the one breastfeeding the two-year-old and it didn't seem strange to me at all.

— Cecily, Ontario, Canada

Is It *Normal* to Nurse Past Eighteen Months?

Absolutely! Anthropologists (scientists who study humanity, including our biology, culture, and societies) and other researchers have analysed ancient texts about weaning and the chemical composition of bones from the past. This research has shown that the normal time frame for ending breastfeeding for humans ranges from two to seven years. For more about weaning, see Chapter 16.

It's not unusual to hear stories like Laura's:

I was breastfed until three years old, so I wanted to do the same with my babies.

— Laura, Colombia

Is It *Important* to Nurse Past Eighteen Months?

Absolutely! Your child may be in no hurry to wean, and there are many good reasons to continue to nurse as long as you and your child wish:

- Continued breastfeeding promotes normal **development of the jaw and palate** – making enough space for the teeth that are still coming in.
- The **toddler brain** is going through a time of rapid growth. Human milk promotes brain growth like no other drink can, and you naturally interact, talk, and cuddle while nursing, which also helps brain development.
- Although your toddler may take less milk from you, the **immune factors in your milk** become more concentrated, giving important protection while your child is putting rocks in his mouth, kissing dogs, and picking up germs from other kids.
- **When your child is ill,** breastfeeding really comes into its own, as Kat remembers:

I breastfed my first child into her toddler years. This was an amazing blessing when she was hospitalised with double pneumonia after a mild bout of chicken pox. I was allowed to room with her. This children's unit prided themselves on Toy Therapy as a gentle distraction to treatments, but they soon learned that nursing therapy was far superior!

– Kat, United States, babies born in the UK

- Young children's digestive systems are still not fully mature. Breastfeeding provides **good nutrition** while they gradually add family foods to their diet. However picky your toddler or preschooler's eating, breastmilk is available as a backup. You can read more about family foods in Chapter 13.
- Nursing can make **bedtime** – and dealing with **night waking**! – much easier. (One toddler we know calls it her "magic sleepy milkies.")
- Nursing is a **time to reconnect** with an on-the-go child, especially helpful when you're working or separated for any reason. The connection you build through nursing long outlasts the nursing itself, as Fernanda describes:

I continued giving milk until he was two years old, and it was the best thing I've done for him. Today he has such a great affection and love for the breast that it's even funny.

– Fernanda, Brazil

The World Health Organization, based on good evidence, recommends that all children are breastfed for *at least two years*. With all these reasons to continue, "he's too old" isn't a very logical reason to stop. For more about breastfeeding through the second year and beyond, see Chapter 16.

Children should continue to be breastfed, while receiving appropriate and adequate complementary foods, for up to two years of age or beyond.
*– The Innocenti Declaration,
Alliance for Transforming the Lives of Children*

Nursing toddlers are generally pretty clear about how important breastfeeding continues to be for *them*. What about *you*? Often, as Kirsten found, it's not only the child who values it:

> At the time I am writing this, my daughter is almost two years old, and we are both still enjoying our breastfeeding experience.
> *– Kirsten, from the Netherlands, living in Austria*

Breastfeeding helps you soothe, calm, and comfort a child who's having trouble coping. B.J. explains how nursing helped her and her daughter:

> I eventually got pregnant again, only to get hyperemesis gravidarum [extreme pregnancy sickness] again. At its height, I was vomiting twenty-five times a day. Confined to bed or the sofa, I couldn't be the mother I had been before. I couldn't play or go for walks. I felt sad and guilty. But I could hold my girl, I could read to her, and I could breastfeed her. And tucked against my breast, she felt safe enough to express her fears about my illness and about what the new baby would mean for her.
> *– B.J., England*

Nursing can provide an instant emotional reboot. As one mother said, "Sometimes I feel as if a wall goes up between me and my child for some reason. When we nurse I feel the wall come down again. I know she feels it, too." Without this powerful tool, parenting may be more difficult, childhood can be more challenging. Xiang let her child lead the way:

> I know you, you are a highly sensitive child, you have shown this side of your character in many situations, and I wanted you to be the one to decide to leave the breast when you felt ready to handle all those emotions and needs that drive you to seek my contact and my breast for comfort or, as you used to say all the time, because you like Mummy's milk.
> – Xiang, from Nanjing, China, living in Padua, Italy

However long you nurse, LLL is here to support you.

Nursing Now – Eighteen Months and Older

By now, you know your child's personality. Maybe she's sociable and enjoys new people and new situations. Or maybe she's sensitive and slow to warm up to anyone new. You also know the role that breastfeeding plays in her life: food, comfort, a way to check in, a way to fall asleep.

Sara Diana's son didn't nurse often at age three, but it still mattered to him:

> When he was about three years old, people were surprised that he was still nursing. I was surprised that many thought he was breastfeeding as often as a newborn. Actually, the nursings were really rare (compared to his first month!). He would nurse before bedtime (not nursing to fall asleep, as I would nurse him, then he would let go and snuggle next to me), for naps, and when something disturbed him so much that he needed Mummy's cuddle.
> – Sara Diana, from Barcelona, babies born in Mexico

How often will *your* toddler or preschooler nurse? While separation can be a factor, your child's personality is probably even more important. And your next baby might be very different. Children with allergies, especially allergies to common foods such as dairy, may continue to breastfeed longer for nutritional reasons.

Your milk supply will dwindle depending on how often your child nurses. Yet many children continue to cherish their time at the breast, as Gisel's daughter did:

> Her feedings decreased a lot. She was already eating very well, but I didn't pressure her. As she was drinking her "delicious chichi" (that's what she calls it, with her bright eyes looking at me), I felt calm because she was still getting breastmilk.
> – Gisel, Mexico

Human milk is a wonderful and nourishing food and gives irreplaceable immune protection for as long as your child nurses. But it's the *relationship* of breastfeeding that usually matters the most to the child. Ask anyone who's nursing a toddler or preschooler about breastfeeding, and they won't list antibodies and nutrients. You'll hear about how breastfeeding connects mother and toddler.

The infrequent nurser will probably increase feeds if she is ill, as Anna found:

> One of my daughters got sick at thirteen months with stomach flu (gastroenteritis). The only fluid she tolerated was breastmilk. After two days, I noticed that my toddler's stools reverted to the yellow newborn breastmilk poos.
> – Anna, Texas, United States

Your child doesn't know it, but your milk's beneficial bacteria and immune factors help her recover faster when she's ill. By the time she's feeling better, you may have a lot more milk! Expect to be a bit uncomfortable for a day or two until your supply adjusts again.

Toddlers under stress also nurse more often. Maybe your toddler has started nursery or moved to a new nursery, or you have had another baby, or you're moving to a new house. Or maybe you're travelling, as Rosie and Megan were:

> Rosie's first flight happened early in the morning when she was two and a half. She woke up strapped in her car seat screaming in pain when the plane began to descend. I offered her snacks, and she refused them all and continued to scream. I leaned over as far as possible and offered my breast. She immediately latched and nursed and got relief from the ear pain. It worked so well I repeated nursing her on the following flight and the return flights. Breastfeeding my toddler gave me an option that saved us from a traumatic first flight.
> – Megan, New England, United States

Toddlers can be stressed by small things, too. A scary encounter with a dog, a day when you were extra busy, a bad dream, or visitors coming over might mean your toddler needs more comforting at the breast. Even mastering a new skill (like learning to walk or jump) can disrupt normal sleep patterns and make her want more nursing and cuddling. Breastfeeding is a great way to give your child the reassurance she needs.

Bottom line: don't expect toddler nursing and weaning to be a straight line. Sometimes your little one will want to nurse as much as when she was a newborn. Sometimes you wonder if she's about to wean, because she even forgets the bedtime nursing she's loved all her life. This is normal. Life at this age is as exciting and up and down as a roller coaster – it's not surprising that nursing changes fast, too.

For breastfed children, nursing becomes part of play. Your child may bring you toys to nurse. Or she may nurse her own dolls and stuffed animals, as Diane recalls:

> I had a large window van with three bench seats. As I'm driving along, I see in the rearview mirror Robin playing with her doll. Jennifer was beside her. Robin very methodically laid her doll across her lap. Then she very carefully rolled up her shirt so she can see her little nipples. Then she picks up her doll and very carefully lines up the doll's face, so it is right opposite her nipple, and proceeds to nurse her doll. Jennifer says, "What are you doing?" Robin says, "I'm breastfeeding my dolly, you know it's just not that easy." She must have been listening at all the LLL meetings she attended with me!
>
> – Diane, California, United States

Imagine how much easier breastfeeding will be for them, compared to what it was like for those who hadn't seen it before. And your children will understand how and why to help their partners. By nursing as long as you and your child both want, you're mending the breastfeeding chain that was broken in the twentieth century in many countries and communities.

The Fun (and Foibles) of Older Nurslings

It's important to feed a two-month-old when he shows feeding cues so he gets enough milk, but with a toddler, nursing can often be negotiated: "Hang on just a minute," or "Wait until we get home," or "I'm sorry we can't go to Grandpa's today – do you want to nurse while I read to you?" Negotiations and compromise can give you new flexibility. You're continuing to respond to the changing needs and maturity of your child. There is more give-and-take…but there's also more need to consider your child's feelings and personality. Mothering through breastfeeding increasingly includes understanding feelings and emotions as much as noticing signs of hunger.

From the Mouths of Babes

Nursing a toddler or preschooler gives you a new perspective on nursing: theirs.

Your milk tastes like melted ice cream. It's the best thing.
– *Teresa's daughter, Ontario, Canada*

He tells me he likes that my body is warm. He asks: "How does your body get so warm?" And then he rubs his cheeks against my skin, smelling it.
– *Uyen Tran, from Vietnam, living in the United States*

I remember with great amusement the forcefulness of their answers when someone asked them inquisitively why they were still breastfeeding: "Because I like it," said Violeta, and "I really like to eat the teat," said Ciro. With so much clarity in their arguments they always awoke smiles in the questioners.
– *Susana, Argentina*

Yeah, don't worry, one day I'm going to self-wean and I won't need "titita" anymore. Something like when I'm eleven . . .
– *Karla's son, Mexico*

When I told my five-year-old twins that it was time to stop breastfeeding, they replied to me: "Mum, we're not ready." We agreed that we would stop at the age of six, and we did.
– *Vanesa, Catalonia, Spain*

Relaxed Physical Ties

One of the joys of nursing a toddler or preschooler is that you have more say over when and how. You don't have to nurse every two hours, or spend forty minutes sitting on the sofa for each feed. You might not need to express at work. The foods you eat, the medicines you take, the way you arrange your day – all of it is much less connected to your child's needs.

Mixed Feelings

Nursing an older child isn't always a garden of delights. Sometimes you may feel pure joy at being able to relate to your child this way. Other times you may wonder if it's ever going to end. It's natural to go back and forth on how you feel about nursing your toddler. La Leche League meetings are safe places to talk about both the pleasures and the frustrations. For more about mixed feelings, see Chapter 16.

> One thing that helped me was my "blue notebook," where I would write down cute things they said so I wouldn't forget them. One day it struck me that many of them were about nursing. Reading over the pages reminded me of how special that relationship is.
>
> – *Teresa, Canada*

"I Want Boobies!"

In societies where breastfeeding beyond a year is commonplace, parents don't feel self-conscious or judged about nursing. In other places, it's harder. You and your family are the ones to decide what you're comfortable with. A tip – if you even *suspect* you might end up nursing a toddler, you might choose to use a word for breastfeeding or breasts *now* that you'll feel comfortable hearing your two-year-old yell across the room at a family reunion or in the supermarket! Popular ones are variations on *milkies, nummies,* and *nursies.*

> When her speech became very clear, I taught her to say *nummies*. Our secret word!
>
> – *Diane, California, United States*

> I loved when my kids asked for "milka," my son's word for breastfeeding/breastmilk that my daughter also adopted.
>
> – *Leah, Ontario, Canada*

Sometimes parents or children choose words that have no obvious relationship to breastfeeding, such as *tea, side, uzzerside, cuddles, eeshies,* or *yum-yum*. The toddler who used *nite nite* impressed her relatives, who thought she was asking to nap. Uyen Tran's son had a unique phrase:

> He used to call the inside of my shirt his *house*, and he used to call it *going inside my house* for nursing.
> — Uyen Tran, from Vietnam, living in the United States

Some families use signs as well as, or instead of, spoken words. Babies can often sign well before they can talk. The American Sign Language sign for milk looks like a person hand-milking a cow, and some parents teach toddlers this for nursing. Or you could make up your own sign – Teresa's grandson Xavier signaled *nurse me* by patting his own little chest.

You can also explain to your nursling where you're comfortable nursing and where you'd rather not. As your toddler grows, he'll (sometimes!) be able to wait until you arrive somewhere you're happy to nurse. See What About Nursing in Public? later in this chapter.

Tandem Nursing

Tandem nursing means continuing to nurse your older child after the birth of a younger sibling, so that you're nursing both your "older baby" and your new baby. Sarah writes:

> I haven't always enjoyed tandem feeding, but there's been times where it has truly felt like the perfect setup. And those moments I will treasure for a lifetime.
> — Sarah, UK

Many families report finding it helpful to transition the older child into the new role of big sister or brother. The older child who asks to nurse after a new baby arrives may be seeking reassurance that there is still a place for her. Breastfeeding can be a special way to provide it, as Kat remembers:

> I knew I didn't have much milk in the later stages of pregnancy, so it was probably more of a comfort thing for her, but the day after the baby was born, the toddler came in and asked to breastfeed. I let her and heard that

lovely sound again of gulping. She stopped for a moment and looked up at me, a trickle of milk dribbling out of her mouth, and said, "Mimi milky." It was probably one of the most profound memories of my whole life!

– Kat, United States, children born in the UK

Others feel that three's a crowd and encourage the toddler to wean before the new baby is born. There's no wrong approach to this. For more about tandem nursing and nursing during pregnancy, see Chapter 16.

Toddler Nursing and Working

In many ways, nursing while you're employed is much easier at this age than when your baby was younger. Your toddler isn't dependent on your milk. As Leah found, you may not need to express while you're separated:

She was fifteen months old when I went back to work full-time. I hated pumping even more by then, so I went "cold turkey" as they say. No pumping during the day and a nice long feed when I got home. My body regulated quickly to the lower demand, and we went on to breastfeed until she was almost three years old. I am so happy I didn't assume that I had to wean when I went back to work.

– Leah, Ontario, Canada

Sometimes a toddler will be happy nursing in the morning before you go to work, when you get home, and before bedtime. Others will want to nurse throughout the evening and perhaps during the night as well. Some toddlers keep their work-week routines even at the weekends; others seem determined to make up for lost time (and missed nursings!) by asking frequently when you're around.

If you work remotely from home, you might find that nursing breaks still work well, to reconnect with your child and (if needed) relieve your breasts. On the other hand, once your child is old enough to operate a door handle, you might need to review your working arrangements! Some families opt for childcare at this stage – or maybe you'd prefer to move back to your work base, if you have one, or take your laptop to a library or coffee shop while your toddler and caregiver play at home.

Questions from Eighteen Months and Older

Here are some of the topics that often come up at LLL meetings from families with children eighteen months and older. If your questions aren't answered here, see Chapter 18 or LLL websites. And always feel free to contact an LLL Leader, locally or anywhere!

What About Nursing in Public?

Many of us, when our children reach a certain age, choose to nurse at home. You might just feel more comfortable on your sofa or in bed, or you might be avoiding unwanted comments or questions:

> Around two years in, people began to ask that irritating set of questions: "Are you still feeding? Why? When will you stop?" They thought it was weird and had no compunction in telling me so.
> – B.J., England

If you want to, you can start to set limits on where you nurse, as Sara Edith did:

> We made some adjustments to avoid the comments; for example, I did not breastfeed him when we went to the grandparents' house or to some social gatherings. We resisted all that and managed to strengthen our desire to continue. Of course there were always people who supported us.
> – Sara Edith, Mexico City

Choosing where and when to breastfeed gets easier as your child becomes better able to understand and negotiate. Your child, like Diane's son, might even figure out for himself who's fine to nurse around and who's not!

> Eric would sometimes wander up to me when there were people at our house and whisper, "Mummy, are these La Lechegg people?" If I said yes, he'd climb up into my lap to nurse. If I said no, he'd nod philosophically and wander away again.
> – Diane, New York, United States

Nursing is a relationship that needs to work for you, too. Sometimes, things don't go according to plan. Maybe your toddler's having a tough day and asks to nurse more than usual, or cries when you ask her to wait till you get home. You may also need to set aside your usual limits when she's ill. You can roll with it, knowing that when she's well again, or having a better day, her needs will settle down and her patience will increase.

Some situations are especially tricky: your toddler suddenly wants to nurse in a queue at a shop, or around friends or family who really aren't comfortable with you nursing. You may need to think on your feet. Maybe you could find a fitting room for privacy or announce that your child needs a nap *right now*, then head into the bedroom (or go home). It's entirely up to you how much you choose to tell. You may decide to gently educate people, letting them know that your child is still nursing.

La Leche League meetings and playgroups with other like-minded families can be especially helpful – and fun – at this stage. As one mother said, "I look forward to those meetings as a monthly breastfeeding oasis in a mostly dry world." Some LLL groups offer special toddler meetings. Some welcome partners, who may have their own questions about nursing beyond the first year.

Is It Okay to Limit Some Nursing Behaviours?

We've already talked about setting some gentle limits about when and where you nurse. What if your toddler wants to pinch your arm, twist your hair, or twiddle the other nipple while nursing? Every relationship is different, and you know your child best.

Beth came up with a creative solution to a common nursing irritation:

> My milk supply decreased during pregnancy, much to the frustration of my twenty-two-month-old daughter. She insisted on twiddling my nipple, which was very uncomfortable for me. My last effort to change it before I felt like I would have to wean for my sanity was to ask if Dolly needed milk, too. "Tandem nursing" Dolly instantly fixed the problem.
> – Beth, United States

Playfulness and humour can often diffuse tensions before they escalate.

If you're feeling frustrated, take a deep breath... and consider what your child *really* needs. She's not deliberately trying to annoy you, that's just a side effect of whatever's going on for her right now. Maybe she's overly tired or hungry – the most common causes of toddler meltdowns. Nursing gets her back on an even keel (and down for a nap). Maybe she's frustrated because she's learning a new skill, or because you've been extra busy and she's missing your company. Maybe she's just bored and needs a distraction. Once you've worked out what the need is, you're more than halfway to figuring out what to do about it.

If you find yourself clashing with your toddler a lot, you may need to rethink the limits you've set. You wanted to wait until after you got home from nursery to breastfeed again, but she's telling you that she needs to nurse right away. Maybe she's had a bad day and craves that extra reconnection. Flexibility is important in your relationship with your child. Remember this for the future, too – it's good to be able to say to your child, "I didn't realise how strongly you felt about that, let's try it that way," or "I think I made a mistake; I apologise."

If Setting Limits Is Hard

Some of us love the newborn period, when you're the centre of your baby's universe and can meet all his needs. (Some of us find that stage much harder, and that's okay, too!) If you're a natural "newborn person," you might find it harder as your baby becomes a toddler, getting into everything. You can't just give him what he wants all the time now. He needs limits, as well as love.

Some of us have experienced "limits" to be punitive, restrictive, unfair, or even dangerous. We're determined not to inflict that on our children. But children need both love and limits. Gentle boundaries are a normal part of learning to get along with others.

Grandma Teresa was swimming with her grandkids, ages seven and five. The five-year-old kept splashing her in the face, something he found hilarious. Teresa told him that she didn't like it and asked him to stop. He did, for about two minutes, then went back to splashing. Teresa got out of the pool and started to pick up and organise the pool toys. After a few minutes, the little boy swam over, apologised for splashing her, and asked her to come back in and play. She did, and he didn't splash her anymore.

Limits don't have to be harsh or unreasonable. Good ones teach respect for people, property, and the planet. How you treat your child is equally important. Children learn by watching, so if we want them to treat people with consideration and respect, we need to model that behaviour.

What they see us do is much more important than what we *say* – or any techniques we use. Nursing toddlers, with their strong connection to you, usually have a strong desire to copy you, and to get along with you.

If these ideas about gentle, respectful parenting are new to you, LLL groups might be one place to find out more.

What If My Toddler Is High Need?

If your child was a high-need baby (as described in Chapter 7), she may still be one. She's the toddler who screams where other toddlers whine, and who is just more sensitive and intense than others. Friends and relatives may be saying that you give in too easily, that you're spoiling your child, that she needs to learn to soothe herself. But you're the one who knows her best. You can be reassured by the experience of countless parents: following our instincts rarely steers us wrong.

Nursing is a very useful parenting tool for calming and mellowing extra intense little people. And as they grow, you'll have more options for meeting their needs.

What If My Child Still Needs Extra Tending to Blossom?

Your sensitive newborn baby probably wanted to be nursed almost all day long and was only calm in your arms or sling. He got really upset about things other babies seemed to take in their stride: a bubble of gas, an unexpected noise, a new place, too much company.

That sensitivity doesn't end when your baby becomes a toddler. The world seems a scarier and more overwhelming place to him than it does to many other children his age. For now, he may prefer to sit with you on the bench at the playground, watching the others play. A sensitive toddler may want to nurse more often and longer than others, too. This doesn't mean he has a problem, it's just the way he is. Like a plant withering in the glare of the sun, if he finds the world too harsh, he may withdraw even more. If he's nurtured now, he will bloom splendidly *when he's ready*. When needs are met, even the most sensitive children can grow into independent and adventurous people – like Sarah's daughter:

> Suddenly, my three-and-a-half-year-old daughter (once a Velcro baby and cautious toddler) acquired a burning desire to explore the world

independently. I was overjoyed that we continued to breastfeed her. At this age we had already discussed (and agreed on) breastfeeding her once a day for sleep. It's the only opportunity I have today to hold her, stroke her hair, and take a good look at her perfect little face.

— *Sarah, UK*

Have we mentioned how good your instincts are?

What About My Toddler with Special Needs?

If your toddler has additional needs, nursing may present unique challenges – and provide unique support for his development. Nursing is so much more than just nutrition. It helps your child thrive physically. Melissa's son Andy had low muscle tone (floppiness), and breastfeeding helped maximise his potential:

> When we had left the hospital with Andy, we really thought, *Phew, that was a close one.* We thought his problems were all behind us. No one mentioned any problem at regular checkups, but when he was around nine months old, I began to question his development. We decided to take him to a neurologist and for the first time heard the word *hypotonia* or low tone; eventually he was diagnosed with cerebral palsy. Andy nursed for over two years. Breastfeeding was a haven of normality for us both. He wasn't able to eat solids easily for quite a while. I am convinced that extended breastfeeding and the need to use facial muscles helped his speech. He is able to speak and communicate with most people. His speech has not kept him back from performing on stage. Today, Andy is studying music at a prominent music school in Israel.
>
> — *Melissa, Tel Aviv, Israel*

Nursing helps strengthen your relationship, as Eliana describes:

> I first began attending La Leche meetings when my oldest was a nursing two-year-old. I wanted to meet other mothers and was also worried about my son's development. The Leader said, "So what if he doesn't talk – see how much love he has!" That sentence stayed with me a year later with the diagnosis of developmental delay, two years later with his diagnosis of ASD (autism), and at every milestone since. He continues to be extremely loving and lovable.
>
> — *Eliana, Israel*

Raising Children with Love and Understanding

There are hundreds of books and websites and programmes out there with advice on raising children. Discipline programmes and approaches that give you cookie-cutter techniques to deal with every situation often don't take into consideration different personalities and situations. If you respond in the same way to a sensitive, intense child as to a laid-back, go-with-the-flow toddler, you won't get the same results. You know your child better than anyone else. Knowing what your child needs and what's underneath his behaviour means you can provide loving guidance that teaches appropriate behaviour within the limits and capabilities of your unique child.

Nurturing Our Children – Nurturing Ourselves

Big toddler feelings can be contagious, and you might find yourself starting to lose it along with your child. This may happen more easily if – like many of us – you didn't get loving support with your feelings when you were small. Having your own child gives you an opportunity to learn more about yourself, and the motivation to make changes. Some of us, like Clare, find we need a little extra help:

> When my first baby became a toddler, I found myself losing my temper more than I ever had before. She was actually a pretty easy toddler – my anger was out of proportion to the behaviours that triggered it. One day, hearing myself shouting at her for some small accident I can't even remember now, I realised how frightening and out of control I must seem to her. I'd learned about gentle parenting in my La Leche League group, and I knew this wasn't the mother I wanted to be. I didn't want my child to be scared of me, like I had been scared of my mother.
>
> I found a counsellor to talk to. Over a few sessions, she helped me understand that, when things went wrong, I was hearing the critical voice of my mother in my head, and it overwhelmed my ability to cope. Those sessions were among the best investments I ever made for my family. I learned not to "beat myself up" when things weren't going perfectly. It's made a huge difference.
>
> I learned a lot of helpful things from the friends I made in my LLL group, too, especially those with older children. They gave me new models for how I wanted to parent. I'm learning to be as gentle and understanding towards

myself as I try to be with my children. Breastfeeding has led to all kinds of transformation I couldn't have imagined when I started out.
— Clare, UK

People often say that it's important to be consistent when you're raising a child. But in family life, flexibility is equally important. What works one time may not work at all the next time. Your child keeps growing and changing, and so does your family environment. Shoko saw this when she became the mother of two:

> I never shouted at my eldest when he was my only child. Now that I have a baby as well as a toddler, loving guidance has taken on a whole new meaning for me and my parenting. My eldest is nearly three, and I know that his brain is going through tons of amazing neurological development that is so often coupled with meltdowns, regardless of whether there's a baby brother in the picture or not. Although the presence of the baby brother does, I'm sure, trigger some of the behaviour that's led to me having to let go of my no-shouting record.
> — Shoko, the Netherlands

Like breastfeeding, raising children is truly an art, not a science. "I honestly don't know what to do," one mother confessed to her children during a heated sibling debate. "This one just isn't in the instruction manual."

Children are people, with feelings, capabilities, and limitations that vary from child to child, month to month, moment to moment. If we work within those changing strengths and limits and look for the need that drives the behaviour, if we show love and consistency, if we respect our children as people who are trying their best to adjust to this strange planet they find themselves on with us, *if they know they are loved*, everything will probably come out fine in the end, no matter how much we stumble along the way.

> I experienced most opposition to breastfeeding from family and friends when he was nine to eighteen months old. Their fear that breastfeeding would make him clingy and lacking in confidence to engage with the world wasn't realised, and he grew into an emotionally confident child because his needs for comfort and safety were met.

We still talk about the time he breastfed. His overall memory is of feeling comfort, love, and safety in a challenging world.
– *Helena, London, UK*

Lisa, an experienced mother of seven very different children, expressed it this way:

> I've watched neighbours who didn't really hold their children close at first, who realised, once they had preteens or teens, that things were out of control. They clutched a lot tighter then, but all it caused was more unhappiness. It was too much, too late. I've seen my job as holding my children very close at first, and gradually relaxing my hold as they mature, until when they're ready to leave home it's almost as if they've already flown from the nest. [As she spoke, Lisa formed a loose, containing circle with her hands, raising her arms as she widened the circle. She ended with her arms wide and outstretched, gently releasing what she had contained.]

My son is almost two years old and I can't believe it. Our breastfeeding relationship is still strong, and I'm so beyond grateful. I'm angry at the noise impacting breastfeeding rates and relationships. It's the most beautiful thing in the world and has absolutely changed my perspective on life.
– *Monica, United States*

Want to know more?

You can find extra resources for this chapter
at the "Art of Breastfeeding" tab at
www.llli.org.

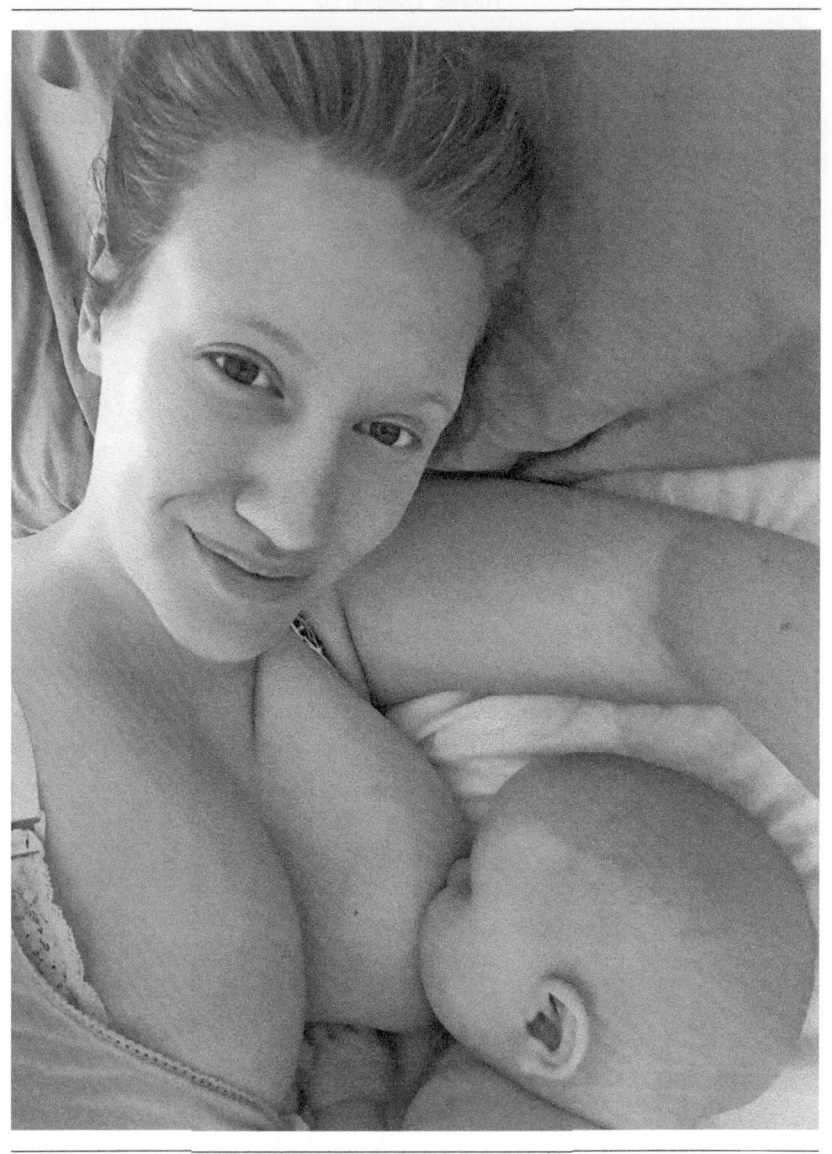

TWELVE

Sleeping Like a Baby

Co-sleeping has been such a big part of my family's life for all three of my boys. Dexter struggled with breastfeeding at first, and co-sleeping allowed me to help my wife with supplementing with donated milk. Having the baby in the bed with us just made everything easier. And there was nothing better than seeing the smile on his face when he woke up in the morning, stretched his arms, and opened his eyes to see Mummy and Daddy both there.

One time I was travelling for work, so I missed bedtime for a few days but got an early morning flight home on the Friday. I was able to sneak into bed before Dexter woke. When he opened his eyes and saw me, he kept signing "Daddy!" over and over, with a big smile.

As our sons got older, we continued to use co-sleeping as we transitioned them to their own room. Once our second child was born, I would lie with Dexter in his bed until he fell asleep, then go back to my bed. This continued with the older two, once we had our third. Having a parent in the bed lets my children feel safe as they fall asleep, and bedtime is less of a struggle. It's not always easy, but it's been the right choice for us each step of the way.

– *Dan, Ontario, Canada*

If this was the year you were hoping to maximise your rest, having a baby will probably mess up those plans. People sometimes still talk about "sleeping like a baby" as though it means a deep and peaceful slumber, but "sleeping like a baby" really means waking up frequently through the night and needing to be nursed, snuggled, walked, or rocked.

Being a parent is a twenty-four-hour-a-day job, and a lot of those hours are during the time when most of us are used to sleeping. Olivia explained:

> When the nights are hard I remind myself – he's crying for me, not at me. I am his comfort, his warmth, his safety, his home. His needs for those things don't stop when the sun goes down.
> – *Olivia, Canada*

Feeling sleep-deprived and exhausted is one of the most common complaints new parents have, no matter how they feed their babies. Unrealistic expectations about normal baby sleep make it worse. Being tired is one thing. Being tired *and worrying you're doing something wrong* is much more exhausting. Every baby is different. Ask almost any parent of more than one baby: even if they did exactly the same things, their babies just slept differently.

Communities where formula-feeding has become widespread may have little experience of normal baby sleep. Sadly, there is lots of money to be made from convincing families that their babies have a sleep problem that needs fixing. Thousands of books, programmes, websites, social media feeds, and practitioners offer strategies to get your baby to go to sleep alone, sleep longer, and put herself back to sleep when she wakes up. And formula advertising plays into parents' concerns, suggesting that fussiness and night waking are symptoms cured by formula.

> Many people would call her a "bad sleeper," but I think she sleeps exactly how she needs to. No one would call me bad if I had to wake up every couple of hours or needed my partner in bed with me to sleep well. She may not sleep in a way that is convenient for my sleep, but I didn't become a parent for the convenience of it! I cherish our 12:00 A.M./3:00 A.M./5:30 A.M./7:30 A.M. snuggles, and know I will miss them when they are gone.
> – *Allison, North Carolina, United States*

The reality: your healthy baby doesn't *have* a sleep problem. She's not suffering from insomnia or sleep disorders. She's just behaving the way babies around the world have behaved since time began. It's not normal, or safe, for young babies to sleep very deeply, or for long stretches at night. Just as babies sit, walk, and talk when they're ready, they reach "sleep maturity" in their own good time. Trying to force a sleep pattern your baby isn't ready for is a recipe for stress. That's not to suggest that there's nothing you can do to help your baby sleep, or to get the rest you need – you can find plenty of ideas in this chapter. But understanding what babies really need for sleep, and finding ways to adapt to the baby you actually have, results in happier parents and babies, and smoother breastfeeding.

What's Normal for Babies When It Comes to Sleep?

There's a huge range of normal sleep, especially in the first few months of your baby's life. Books and websites list expected hours of sleep for babies of different ages – but these might not fit *your* baby. Just the fact that a study shows, for example, the average baby sleeps for fourteen hours out of twenty-four doesn't mean that sleeping fourteen hours is *better* than sleeping eleven hours (or twenty hours, for that matter). It's just maths – not a target to aim for. Recommendations on how long babies "should" sleep are often very different from research findings on how babies *really* sleep.

Some babies are very regular in their sleep patterns. By the time they're six or eight weeks old, you can predict when they will be tired and ready to doze off. They might have long(ish) daytime naps or short catnaps, but they are consistent. Others are not. They might fall asleep for a nap at 9:30 today, 10:45 tomorrow, and 8:55 the next day. They might sleep so long one afternoon that you start to worry, and then wake up, ready to play, after half an hour the next day. They are just irregular by nature. Some adults are also like this! If you and your baby are very different – you love schedules and your baby never does the same thing two days running, or the other way around – it can be a challenge. But just understanding your differences can be very helpful. For more about baby "temperament" (inborn nature, or personality), see chapters 7 and 9.

Where Should Babies Sleep?

Our ideas about sleep are formed by where and when we live. Separate bedrooms, cribs, and even beds have only been around for a relatively short time in human history!

Babies can sleep in a safe crib in a separate room. But during the first six months, sleeping in a separate room increases the risk of sudden infant death syndrome (SIDS) and makes breastfeeding harder.

Babies can sleep in a crib, or a sidecar-type bed, which is attached to or set up next to your bed. These setups are called room sharing, or co-sleeping.

Babies can sleep in bed (a raised bed or a floor bed) with one or both parents. This is bed-sharing (also sometimes called co-sleeping). Nursing parents get the most sleep when bed-sharing, and when the Safe Sleep Seven guidelines are followed, this is also a safe arrangement. Check the following illustration for information on how to sleep safely with your baby.

It is not safe for a baby to sleep with an adult on a sofa, armchair, or recliner.

Setting the Scene for Sleep

What helps your baby fall asleep and stay asleep, or get back to sleep quickly and easily once he wakes up? Being close to you. He feels secure and relaxed, with milk close by in case he wakes up hungry or thirsty.

> Before I had my baby I was determined to never, never allow myself to fall asleep with her in my bed. I took the warnings to heart and I was afraid of what might happen. Then I had my baby and I learned in my bones that we are mammals and we are supposed to lay down with our babies.
>
> *– Tina, United States*

Your baby relies on you (or his caregiver) to keep him stable and feeling secure, day and night. When he's alone, his heart rate, breathing, and temperature are less stable. He's more likely to go into a deep sleep in a way that's not normal or healthy. His stress level increases. At night, babies expect to stay close to you, waking as needed to nurse or reconnect. Keeping your baby close at night and letting him nurse to sleep meets his physical and emotional needs.

Having a reliable way – breastfeeding – to encourage a tired baby towards sleep is also an incredibly helpful parenting tool. Hannah,

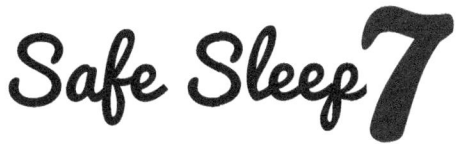

Safe Sleep 7 — SMART STEPS TO SAFER BED-SHARING

IF YOU ARE BREASTFEEDING, MEET ALL SEVEN FOR SAFER BED-SHARING.

 **1 NO SMOKING**
In the home or outside

 **2 SOBER ADULTS**
No alcohol
No drowsy meds

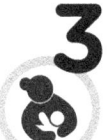 **3 BREASTFEEDING**
Day and night

 **4 HEALTHY BABY**
Full term

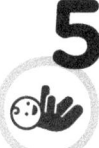 **5 BABY ON BACK**
Face up

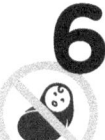 **6 NO SWEAT**
Light clothing
No swaddling

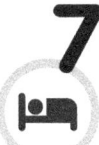 **7 SAFE SURFACE**
No soft mattress, no extra pillows, no toys, no tight or heavy covers. Clear of strings and cords. Gaps firmly filled: use rolled towels or baby blankets.

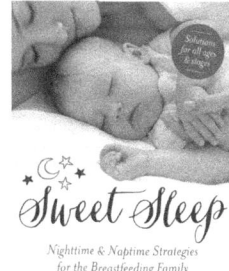

Sweet Sleep
Nighttime & Naptime Strategies for the Breastfeeding Family

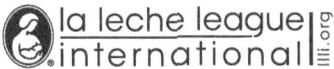

who has severe hearing loss, found that keeping her babies close at night meant she was alerted when they needed her:

> I have four children, whom I have breastfed into toddlerhood. The first two (now teenagers) I breastfed without a disability. The younger two I have breastfed with a severe hearing loss. I am lucky that I found La Leche League with my two older children, and so keeping my babies close was already something I was used to. With the younger two, keeping my babies close

> became a necessity to ensure their safety. One silver lining of hearing loss is taking my hearing aids out at night and not being able to hear anything. Not so good with a small baby, though, as I also cannot hear if they need me. It was important to be able to sleep with a hand on my baby's body so that I could sense the rise and fall of breathing, and the vibrations of crying.
> – Hannah, UK

Since about 1900, however, parents in some cultures have been advised to make their babies sleep separately and not wake during the night, starting as young as possible. Why? Here are some reasons for this:

- Medicine began to understand the role of bacteria and viruses in causing illness: doctors worried that parents would pass germs on to their babies by sleeping close to them. Of course, they were not aware that breastmilk provides antibodies and important protection for babies.
- Behavioural psychologists were suspicious of physical contact between parents and children. They thought that cuddling children leads to an unhealthy dependency. This belief led to some very unhappy babies (and parents). We now know that loving interaction with caregivers is vital for healthy development. True independence happens when a baby's needs are fully met, on a timetable that varies from baby to baby.
- Some parents worry that having a baby in bed with them will interfere with their sexual relationship. This doesn't need to be the case! For more ideas about keeping intimacy going, see Is This the End of Sex? later in this chapter.

This focus on making babies sleep alone, against biology, has made breastfeeding difficult and caused many parents considerable stress. Our aim in this chapter is to give you information about normal, safe sleep for babies, so you can figure out what works for you in your specific situation. If we ask ten families at an LLL meeting what their sleeping arrangements were last night, we're not surprised when we get ten different answers! Many of us take a while to find a way of sleeping that works for our family – as Allison did:

> I was exhausted from labour/recovery but could *not* fall asleep. After a few nights of suffering through what I thought was the "right" way for us to sleep,

I was so sleep deprived that I had to do something. So I put our queen-size mattress on the floor, kicked my partner (who was totally happy to play musical beds as long as it got us sleep!) out of the bed, and snuggled up with my baby. It wasn't perfect – the learning curve was steep, and my little one needs to reconnect every two hours – but it got me the sleep I needed to survive.

– Allison, North Carolina, United States

The Sleep-Breastfeeding Connection

It turns out that breastfeeding and sleep are connected in more ways than we knew:

- **Your milk varies in composition through the day and night.** Nighttime milk has more of the "sleepy hormone" melatonin (which isn't in formula). This, and other subtle changes in milk, help the baby's internal clock to develop. This is another reason why expressed milk is not *quite* the same thing as milk directly from the source.
- **If you sleep with your baby, you're more likely to breastfeed for longer.** Could this just be because communities where it's normal to breastfeed for longer also tend to practise bed-sharing? Or maybe, if you're already committed to "longer" breastfeeding, you're more likely to join breastfeeding support groups and learn about bed-sharing? Maybe. Research also suggests that bed-sharing (or not) can affect how feeding ends up going, right from the start. One study found that babies randomly assigned to sleep in cribs separated from their mothers in the first few days post-birth were about half as likely to still be breastfeeding at four months as those who slept in the bed with their mothers. Babies who slept in sidecars attached to the mothers' beds were somewhere in the middle. Why the difference? Frequent nursing in those first few days helps milk production. Babies sleeping separately from their mothers tend to nurse less often – not helpful for getting breastfeeding off to a good start.
- Many assume formula-fed babies sleep "better" (with less waking up), but **if you bed-share with your baby, you may actually get more total sleep than if you sleep separately,** despite spending more time nursing. Researchers can now measure (via a device like a wristwatch) how much parents *really* slept. A study that used this method showed exclusively breastfeeding mothers got

more nighttime sleep than those who were using formula. But wait – if bed-sharing babies feed more at night, how come their mothers get more sleep? Babies in their own beds have to wake and fuss to get your attention. They take longer to settle once fed. You have to wake up, too – you have to hoist the baby out of the crib, feed her, then put her back. It takes both of you more time to settle back to sleep. So you lose out on breastfeeding time but don't get any extra rest.

To Track, or Not to Track?

Staying with the topic of measuring sleep: how much sleep you *feel* you get can affect your mood. You might find you feel better if you turn the clock to the wall, turn off your phone, and stop counting or timing wake-ups. And think twice about whether sleep tracker apps are doing you any favours. Many are designed to make money rather than support your family's well-being. Again: being tired is one thing. Being tired *and worried about it* can make life a whole lot harder. Asia makes an important link between sleep and mental health:

> I believe breastfeeding can be easier than bottle-feeding. Since we started co-sleeping, I never had to get up to pick up a baby. Anytime she would wake up, she would quickly fall asleep while feeding. And sleep is important for one's mental health, which can in turn affect the whole family – positively or negatively.
>
> – Asia, UK

As Teresa found, being woken at night doesn't necessarily *have* to be a big deal:

> We travelled to my in-laws' house for baby Matthew's first Christmas. My sister-in-law was also there with her new baby, James. I had Matt sleeping in the bed with me and my husband, and my sister-in-law had brought a port-a-crib for James, who was bottle-fed. A couple hours after we all went to bed, James woke up crying. I could hear his mum get up, pick him up, and carry him, still crying, down to the kitchen to warm up a bottle for him. She fed him, then came back up to the bedroom and put him in the crib again. He started to cry again. They let him cry for a while, but eventually picked him up and he stopped. Back in the crib. This time he only cried for a short time before falling asleep. Whew.

Not long after, I felt Matthew stirring in the bed next to me. I snuggled him in close to my breast, he latched on, and we went back to sleep. In the morning my sister-in-law asked me: "Is Matthew sleeping through the night already? I didn't hear him at all last night." She was surprised to hear that he had nursed several times during the night. But nobody knew except me and Matthew.

– *Teresa, Ontario, Canada*

If you're struggling with the amount of sleep you're getting, see But I'm *Really* Exhausted! later in this chapter.

Is Using a Co-Sleeper Crib Beside the Bed the Same as Bed-Sharing?

Yes and no. A sidecar right next to your bed makes for easier nursing than having your baby sleep farther away. Your baby can hear you moving and breathing, which is important. Babies under about six months of age who are near enough to hear their caregivers breathing and moving have less risk of sudden infant death syndrome (SIDS). This is why experts recommend that babies sleep in the same room as you for at least the first six months.

Room-sharing without bed-sharing is a bit different for your baby – and for you. A very young baby only really knows you're there if he can *feel* you, if he's snuggled against the curve of your body, feels the weight of your reassuring hand, or senses your heartbeat. And as we've already mentioned, nursing is a bit more complicated if you have to move the baby in and out of bed (or get up to sit in a chair) each time. Bed-sharing is the simplest way of meeting a baby's nighttime needs. However, it isn't safe for every baby, and it doesn't suit every family. There are options for all situations. Stay tuned!

Sleep and Milk Supply

My supply remained strong from all the little sips and drips throughout the night.

– *Christine, Utah, United States*

Christine puts it beautifully! For some of us, night feeds are especially important for overall milk supply. We all have different "storage capacities" in our breasts; while most can make enough milk for our babies, the amount we can *store* (and therefore give to our babies in a single feed) varies a lot. That means some need to feed more often than others – and skipping a feed or two during the night might mean the baby won't be able to get enough milk overall. Stopping night feeds too soon can jeopardise milk production and your nursing relationship. It can also trigger your period to come back earlier, especially once the longest gap between feedings gets to about six hours.

You may have been told that your baby wakes at night because you aren't producing enough milk or that your milk isn't good enough quality. But unless a baby is showing other signs (such as low weight gain), night waking is not going to be caused by lack of milk. Babies have many reasons to wake besides hunger. If your baby is not gaining well, talk to your healthcare provider and see Chapter 18, Weight Gain Worries.

So Where Should My Baby Sleep?

> I was amazed at how attuned my baby and I were to each other. But that quickly turned to dismay as three . . . then four . . . then five nights passed with very little sleep for me and my husband. The YouTube videos and Instagram accounts said that laying my baby down in a bassinet was normal, and so that's what I did. But my baby just seemed to want to be with me. And by "with me," I mean *on* me, and nursing frequently. I'd heard about La Leche League from my mum and older sisters, so I read *Sweet Sleep*. I wept when I learned about sharing sleep with a baby being one of the great unsung pleasures of the flesh, and immediately brought my baby into our bed. We were safe and cozy.
>
> – Christine, Utah, United States

Christine, like many of us, found herself torn between her baby and her instincts and the expectations of her culture. In many parts of the world, this isn't even a question – babies sleep next to their mothers, as they have through most of history. Cribs and cots were invented in Western countries in the 1600s, and they became almost universal in these countries a few decades ago, when breastfeeding rates were very low. As nursing began to increase in popularity again, so did the idea of the "family bed." No surprise; having your baby close to you at night makes breastfeeding easier.

As Glenys found:

Breastfeeding is tiring; we began co-sleeping out of sleep desperation and never went back.
— *Glenys, United States*

That doesn't mean your baby has to be *in* your bed to breastfeed. But keeping your baby close to you – in a crib in the same room, in a cradle or crib beside your bed, in a "sidecar" attachment to your bed, or actually in your bed – will make it far easier to respond to your baby quickly, with as little disruption as possible to your own sleep.

Room-Sharing with Your Baby

He had slept in our bed since birth, and night nursing was where we all got the most sleep. When he was four months old our doctor suggested I move him to a crib. For one week I went to his room in the middle of the night to feed him. I was completely exhausted. I said to my husband, "I can't do this. I am more tired now than I was when he was a newborn." We brought him back into the family bed and went back to getting all the sleep we needed.
— *Cecily, Ontario, Canada*

Cecily's doctor's well-meaning suggestion not only robbed her of sleep but (we now know) also increased risk to her baby. The safe sleep recommendation says your under-six-month baby needs to sleep in the room where you are. This applies to naps as well. It might mean moving the crib into your daytime living space or having a second baby bed set up there. Many parents find it's easiest to have their babies nap in a sling, pram, or pushchair during the day, giving them the freedom to move around while keeping the babies close.

When your baby is in your bed, you nurse, she falls asleep, and you can just close your eyes and go to sleep yourself. If she wakes a little, she'll be comforted by your breathing (the breathing she listened to for so many months in your womb) and your smell. She can touch you if she needs extra reassurance, wriggling a little closer if she feels she's too far away.

If you want your baby on a separate sleep surface, try nursing her on a small towel, pad, or receiving blanket. Once she's asleep, pick her up, pad and all, and transfer both. The warm surface goes right along with her – no cold bedding and strange smell when you lay her down elsewhere.

But Is Bed-Sharing Safe?

> We muddled through the haze of newbornness with my son sleeping in our room but in his own bassinet, since everyone told us bed-sharing is dangerous. Sleep deprivation was getting extreme.
> – Monica, United States

Like Monica, you might have heard warnings against having your baby in your bed. That's scary. The thought that you might be a danger to your baby can make many new parents outright terrified. Let's look at the concerns more closely:

- You might be surprised to know that **how safe your baby is in your bed depends in part on how you're feeding her.** Babies who are formula-fed are twice as likely to die of SIDS than those who are breastfed. Yet, as Lara found, parents are often advised:

> "Your baby will sleep better if you give them formula before bed." Not true.
> – Lara, London, England

- Researchers observe that a formula-feeding mother who sleeps with her baby tends to keep the baby up near her face, or even on the pillows (which puts the baby at risk of suffocation) and will often sleep with her back to the baby. **A breastfeeding mother usually sleeps with her baby near the breast.** Many spend most of the night facing their babies. Some move up one leg and create a protective "fort" for their babies with their arm above the baby's head. (The La Leche League sleep book, *Sweet Sleep*, calls this position "the cuddle curl.")
- Researchers tickled both breastfed and formula-fed babies with air jets under their noses while they slept (something you'd think few sleep-deprived parents would volunteer for!). The **formula-**

fed babies were much less likely to wake up in response. The researchers speculate that this might be one reason formula-fed babies are at a higher risk of dying of sudden infant death syndrome (SIDS): they just don't wake up as easily when something goes wrong.

Breastfeeding reduces the risk of sleep-related infant deaths, and while any human milk feeding is more protective than none, two months of at least partial human milk feeding has been demonstrated to significantly lower the risk of sleep-related deaths.
— *American Academy of Pediatrics*

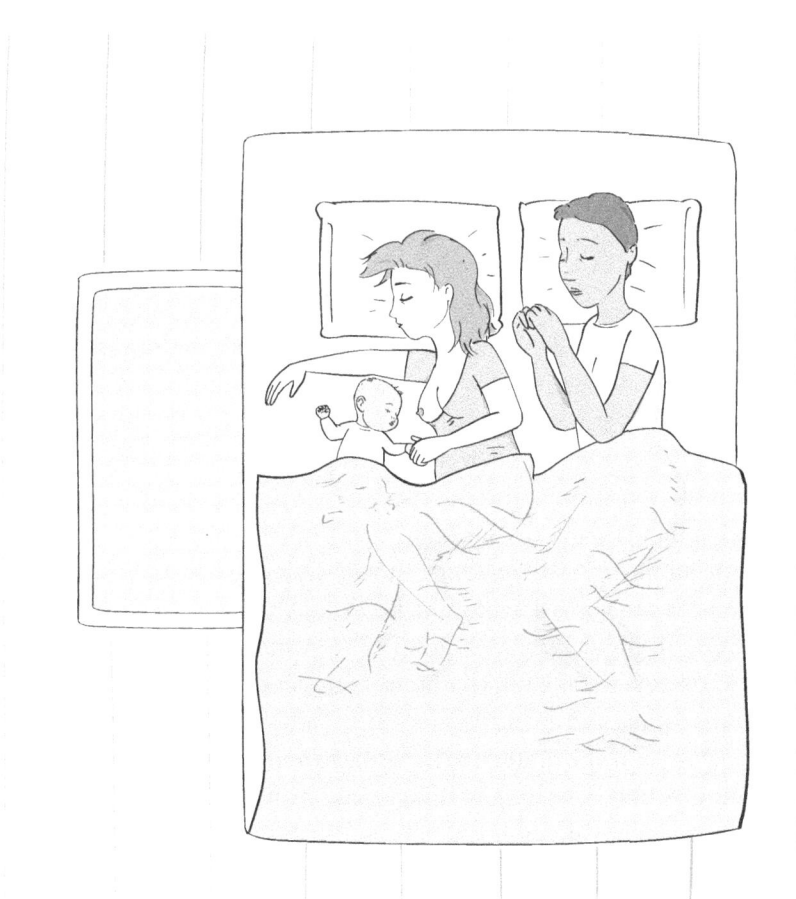

Your "cuddle curl" protects your baby

How About Communities Where Bed-Sharing Is Normal?

If bed-sharing itself is dangerous, you'd expect there to be more baby deaths in cultures where bed-sharing is common. This is not the case. Other factors, such as high levels of smoking or alcohol consumption in some communities, also play a role in baby deaths. Some experts thought that differences in death reporting might make data unreliable. In 2012, one researcher compared families that immigrated from South Asian countries to those born in the UK and living in the same city. Immigrant families were much more likely to bed-share, to breastfeed, to be non-smokers, and to avoid alcohol. The rate of SIDS in that group was significantly lower than that in the families born in the UK. Same community, same death reporting process.

Recognising the importance of breastfeeding, many national health authorities are revising their advice on bed-sharing. Instead of the single message "don't bed-share!" they're providing information on how families can keep risks to a minimum.

The authors of La Leche League's book *Sweet Sleep* created **the Safe Sleep Seven** – an easy way to remember the factors that make it safer to bed-share with your baby.

The first three factors relate to the parent:

1. **Breastfeeding.** As mentioned, formula-feeding increases the risk of SIDS and affects how you position yourself and interact with your baby. What if your baby is only partially breastfed? Or if you're expressing for a baby who can't nurse? We don't know. Nobody has studied these situations yet. But if your baby tends to naturally position himself at the breast when sleeping next to you, and you curl around your baby, that probably works.
2. **Non-smoking.** We've long known that exposure to cigarette smoke is a major risk factor for SIDS, and being close to a smoking parent all night increases that risk – even if you never smoke in bed, or never smoke in the house. Smoke clings to your hair and your clothes and is in the air you breathe out. So bed-sharing is much safer if the adults in the bed are non-smokers.
3. **Being sober.** Anything that can make you less aware of the baby in your bed – alcohol, recreational drugs, or some prescription medications – will increase the risk.

The next three factors relate to the baby:

4. **Healthy and full-term.** Premature and low birth weight babies are at higher risk of SIDS no matter where they sleep. A baby who is ill may be too weak to cry for help or to move himself when needed (a minor cold or illness is not a concern in a baby who is basically healthy). When is it safe to start treating a premature baby the same way as a full-term one? Again, we simply don't know. It's going to depend on the individual baby: one who was born very early and still needs extra oxygen at home is more vulnerable than a baby who was born at thirty-six and a half weeks and is robustly healthy. This is a conversation to have with your healthcare provider.
5. **On his back.** Of course, when your baby is actively breastfeeding, he'll usually be lying on his side, but once he falls asleep, it's helpful to gently move him onto his back. (Once he's able to roll from front to back and vice versa, sleep position is no longer an issue.)
6. **Lightly dressed and not swaddled.** Overheating has been found to increase the risk of SIDS, and a baby sleeping next to you will be warmed by your body heat. So dress the baby in light clothing. Swaddling not only makes the baby warmer but restricts his movements, so it's not recommended for babies who are bed-sharing. There's more on swaddling later in this chapter.

The final factor relates to the bed you're sleeping on:

7. **A safe surface.** This is important even if you don't plan to bed-share, because most breastfeeding families end up with the baby sleeping in the adult bed at some point, even if they never intended to.

Breastfeeding is relaxing for both you and your baby; if you bring her into bed to nurse, the odds are high that you will both fall asleep. Trying *not* to fall asleep while breastfeeding is fighting against biology. Soothing babies (and mothers) off to sleep is one of the many functions of nursing. It can also feel... *right,* as Monica describes:

> I ordered the LLL sleep book at 3:00 A.M. from my nursing chair as I sprayed myself with water to stay awake as my son slept latched on me. It arrived

within a day, and right away we made our bed safe and our son began sleeping with us. We felt rebellious, as if we gave up, according to the sleep training culture. But in fact, it was the absolute best decision we ever made. We were all safe and loved.

– Monica, United States

A study in England found that more than one in five babies slept in an adult bed on any given night. An Australian study found that nearly half of babies slept with a parent – and more than half of bed-sharing was unplanned. It's *much* safer if you plan and prepare for bed-sharing, as Tina did after discovering it by accident:

I had a very hard birth, and then my family had several emergencies in quick succession and my body and emotions were hammered. I really wanted to breastfeed so I pumped and I fed and I cried around the clock. Between the physical recovery, the stress, the never-ending lack of sleep, and the postnatal depression I was out of my mind. I don't even remember doing it, but I woke up with my baby next to me in a cuddle curl. I don't know how long we had been asleep like that, but after that little bit of rest I felt like I could see in colour again! I moved her to her baby bed, and we resumed our untenable routine.

The second time I did it on purpose. I was fearful and guilty and ashamed but also desperate. I fell asleep with my baby on my breast in bed and it was so easy and right. The more I gave in and took her in my bed at night, the more my baby and I got in sync with each other. My body was able to rest and start to recover. My milk gradually caught up to her needs. We both got real restful sleep. I was able to tune in to her gentle sounds and she didn't have to cry to get my attention. It was like bed-sharing was some kind of cheat code for being a new mum. Then I found *Sweet Sleep*. I was already pretty much doing the Safe Sleep Seven instinctively, but hearing some rules and some supportive data was amazing. Maybe it was just the hormones, but I cried reading this book.

– Tina, United States

Making Your Bed Safe for Your Baby: A Recipe for Safe Bed-Sharing

If you've taken the Safe Sleep Seven into account and decide to have your baby sleep in your bed, here's what you'll need to set it up safely:

- a bed with a firm mattress (no waterbeds or thick pillow tops)
- minimal pillows
- no heavy duvets or comforters
- no gaps between the mattress and bedframe, or bed and wall, where the baby could be trapped

You could use several light layers of bedding, which can be adjusted according to the room temperature. If it's cold where you are, you might want to wear an extra layer or two of clothing so you can keep the bedding farther down the bed without getting chilly. See the following section for more tips.

Different Sleep Arrangements

Different things work for different families at different times, as J.D. describes:

> As a light sleeper I found co-sleeping with a noisy, snuffly newborn very difficult, combined with general sleep deprivation at the time! With my eldest baby, my husband slept with the baby in a next-to-me crib and called me (from the spare room) for night feeds – this was the only way I'd get any decent sleep. I always did the night feeds in the rocking chair in the baby's bedroom, and moved her into her own room around five or six months. With my youngest, I managed with the next-to-me crib and fed him lying down in our bed. He also moved into his own room at a similar age, but we continued a morning wake-up feed lying down in our bed until he self-weaned at three years and three months!
> – J.D., UK

Maybe you have one or more of the risk factors that make a family bed less safe: you have a preemie, you or your partner smoke, or you have a waterbed, for example. If you can't or don't want to nurse lying in bed, it's still important to think about safety. Exhausted parents sometimes fall asleep in places more dangerous than a properly prepared bed. *It is never safe to sleep on a sofa, couch, armchair, or recliner with a baby,* because he can become trapped between the seat and the back cushion. Falling asleep on a chair is also hazardous; you might slump over the baby, or he could roll off your lap onto the floor. One mother we know was so exhausted that she fell asleep at the wheel of her car.

Fortunately she and her two young children were fine — but being dangerously tired is a warning sign that something needs to change.

If you move your older baby to another room, consider using two baby monitors or phones — one with the speaker in your room so that you can hear the baby, and one with the speaker in the baby's room so that he's stimulated and reassured by your sounds. Some families put a bed (or mattress on the floor) in the baby's room, so the baby can be nursed lying down, with the option to return him to his crib.

Is It Safer for My Baby to Go to Sleep with a Dummy?

Research suggests that babies who go to sleep regularly with a dummy may have some protection against sudden infant death syndrome (SIDS) compared to when these babies are put to bed without a dummy. Why? It's normal for babies to *nurse* to sleep — to go to sleep sucking. Nursing to sleep probably has the same protective effect; and it doesn't come with any downsides, such as ear infections or misaligned teeth. If you can't or don't want to nurse to sleep, then a dummy might be an alternative to consider.

Nursing Your Baby to Sleep

You may hear that letting your baby fall asleep at the breast creates a "bad habit." That's just not true. Even if you nurse every night and nap, your baby will eventually outgrow the need, as Allison found:

> I have nursed my baby to sleep for every nap/bedtime/night waking since day one, and I know it was the right choice. She falls asleep for my partner and my mother, who do not nurse her, and now that her birthday is this week, she has started pulling off the breast to drift off all on her own.
> – *Allison, North Carolina, United States*

Soothing babies to sleep is one of the many useful functions of nursing. Babies tend to fall asleep when they have a full tummy, feel warm and secure, and are tired; you don't teach them this. Breastfeeding provides the full tummy, warmth, and security, and boosts the baby's sleep-inducing hormones. Falling asleep at the breast is what most baby mammals do.

Some suggest that the baby should be taken off the breast while still awake but drowsy, and put down by herself. This might work for some babies, but for many it makes feeds stressful. You'll need to watch your baby closely, to make sure she doesn't fall asleep. If her eyes start to close, you have to break the suction and remove her, and she might cry and protest. Some babies will anticipate this after a few times and clamp down or bite.

When you leave a baby alone in a room, she's not capable of thinking, "Hey, no worries, the grown-ups are just down the hall watching TV." She knows she's helpless to go and find you if she needs food, comfort, or a fresh nappy. For all she knows, you've been eaten by a sabre-toothed tiger. Being left alone can be very scary, and the only thing your baby can do is cry for you.

As children get older, they understand that when you're out of the room you still exist. She can call you, and when you answer, "It's okay, I'm just in the kitchen," she is reassured by your voice and explanation. A still-older child won't even need to call you because she'll know you're there.

Nursing to sleep won't last forever. At first, your baby will probably fall asleep at the breast most if not all the time. But as she gets older, you'll find she begins to fall asleep in other ways as well. If you want to encourage the process, you can deliberately begin to add other things that help her doze off, like singing a lullaby or reading a story as you nurse her to sleep. Then you can sing her that same lullaby sometimes without nursing, as you rock her in your arms or pat her back. If you have a partner or supporter, they might come alongside and share the singing or reading. It can be a gradual process.

But a baby? She's growing faster than she ever will again, and sleep helps with growth. Falling asleep after her meal is natural and healthy. All it really causes is ... a nap.

Nap Nursing

When your newborn baby naps, you might be tempted to set him down immediately so you can finish the dishes, but chances are he'll wake up again as soon as you do. Young babies who have just fallen asleep at the breast are usually in a lighter phase of sleep and are easily woken. If you can hold your baby in your arms for a few more minutes, you'll see him relax into a deeper sleep. At that point, being moved to another location is less likely to wake him up. Another strategy: nurse in a sling. Then once your baby is asleep, you can adjust your clothes and do whatever you need to do. Your movements as you move around the house will help keep him asleep. You won't have to rush to get things finished before he wakes up.

Your older baby is less likely to fall asleep at every nursing. Sometimes he nurses, lets go on his own, and is ready to interact or play. If you think he's sleepy, you could try nursing him lying down on a blanket or pad on the floor. Many of us have discovered the "oozing away method" (also known as the "ninja move"). You nurse until your child is asleep and lie there another few minutes. Then, toe by toe, bone by bone, you slink away, holding your breath and trying not to disturb the molecules in the air. Or you could just enjoy the nap with your child. Sleep if you want, listen to a podcast, read a book.

Some toddlers can enjoy a quiet time alone, falling asleep if and when they get sleepy, but many still want to nurse to sleep. Naptime and bedtime nursings are often the last ones a child gives up. It makes sense: nursing is such a simple way to convert the daytime's buzz into quiet and calm. Why not use it while you have it?

If you're going to be away from your child, for work or study, you don't need to stop nursing him to sleep in advance. Even young babies understand that different adults care for them in different ways – they won't expect to nurse to sleep when you're not there. For more on work and other separations, see Chapter 14.

To Swaddle, or Not to Swaddle?

It's natural for babies to move during sleep, as Pomme describes:

When my son was born, we practised bed-sharing, for the closeness that it brought us and because it enabled me to rest, despite the night feeds. Between one and two months, I discovered a skill in my son that I did not suspect: he could move towards me to come and nurse. What a distance he travelled every night! I discovered that babies can actively breastfeed, but they must be allowed the necessary proximity. When he was napping, belly-to-belly, on my bare chest, suddenly he'd raise his head, eyes closed, peck a few times on my chest until he got it right, and start to suck . . . while sleeping.

– Pomme, Ardèche, France

Swaddling is intended to fool a baby into thinking she's being held. In bed with you, she doesn't need it. But swaddling means she can't easily move – no poking you if you get too close or rolling into a more comfortable position. What babies want isn't tight wrapping, it's you nearby. Swaddling with legs straight can also cause issues with hip development.

Swaddling may help some babies who, for whatever reason, can't sleep close to a parent. For more on swaddling, see Chapter 5.

Burping the Baby at Night

Many parents of nursing babies just don't. Babies tend to gulp in less air while nursing compared with bottle-feeding. However, some breastfed babies do need to burp after nursing. Try draping your baby over your hip while you're still lying on your side, or sitting him upright and rubbing or patting his back. *You* don't have to sit up. Once he burps, you can nurse him back to sleep on the breast you just used.

Too Much Milk?

If you have a lot of milk and rapid flow, you might find nursing your baby to sleep is more challenging. Just as she seems to be falling asleep at the breast, you have another milk release. Your dozing baby gets a mouthful of milk. She might cry and let go, wide awake again. You might be able to solve this by following some of the tips on slowing down milk production (see Chapter 18, Oversupply) or by switching her back to the less full breast. Some babies who have to deal with firehose-style milk ejections may come to prefer falling asleep in a sling, or by being rocked or patted.

Night Nursing and Tooth Decay

Your toddler has tooth decay and the dentist recommends night weaning. Is it really necessary? There is no evidence that nighttime nursing *by itself* causes cavities. Other mammals with teeth nurse day and night, and they don't get cavities. Nursing is not equivalent to drinking formula from a bottle – though some dentists may assume it is. For example, milk doesn't pool around the teeth while nursing. Cavities are prevented by some of the components in human milk. Human milk also strengthens teeth by depositing calcium and phosphorus on them.

The best way to prevent toddler cavities is to wipe or brush your child's teeth thoroughly at least twice a day. Encourage him to swish with (or at least sip) water after eating family foods. Avoid sugary foods or carbohydrates after the bedtime teeth cleaning. But there's generally no need to keep your child from nursing at night.

Nursing children do sometimes get cavities, even if they have their teeth brushed often and well and haven't eaten after brushing. Why? Some evidence suggests the mother's health, her diet during pregnancy, antibiotics used during pregnancy, and genetics may play a role. Our modern diet also has many more cavity-inducing foods. Human milk is no match for cookies, dried fruits, fruit juices, or even crackers, and those cute little O-shaped cereals that turn into sugars. It's often impossible to get all those sugars off a squirmy child's teeth. Certain bacteria can cause cavities, and babies can pick them up from adult carriers who share food, utensils, or mouth kisses with them. With all these factors, night weaning is unlikely to solve the problem.

If your child has cavities, work with a dentist to help you come up with a plan that protects both their teeth and nursing. Remind your dentist that breastfeeding affects the development of the face and jaw. Children who aren't breastfed are more likely to need braces to correct misaligned teeth.

Dressing *for* Bed . . . and Dressing *the* Bed

Your bed-sharing baby needs no more than a nappy and a light shirt. You could wear a T-shirt, maybe cut short to keep your shoulders warm and breasts accessible. Pyjamas or a nightie with a front opening work well. If it's cool in your room, and you need to keep the bedding away from your baby, you might want a cardigan as well. If you've got larger breasts, a loose sleep bra can provide support without constriction.

A stack of **nappies,** some wipes, a bin, maybe breast pads (or a cloth nappy) to catch drips, and a change of clothes for both you and the baby near your bed will save time. Depending on your baby's skin sensitivity, you may be able to skip midnight nappy changes after the first few weeks, but keep the nappies handy.

Some nursing mothers' breasts don't leak milk at night; others produce lakes. If **leaking** is a problem for you, waterproof mattress protectors, incontinence pads, or similar items can protect your mattress. Or make a pile of bath towels so you can put down a dry one as needed and drop the damp one onto the floor until morning. Leaking is more likely to be a problem in the first few weeks; you may also leak again for a while if your baby starts sleeping for a longer stretch at night. Leaking usually stops being an issue eventually, although the timing varies.

A **nightlight** can give you enough light to nurse or change a pooey nappy by, yet be dim enough to sleep with. Avoid the blue light emitted by most phones and screens – it interferes with the brain's sleep rhythms. **Phones** can steal sleep, but they are also a great way to connect with support people when you're awake in the small hours!

Musical Beds

Many bed-sharing families, like Annalee's, go through a whole series of sleeping arrangements:

> We used a bassinet for our first baby from Day One, as that's what everyone around me did. At six months we went to move her to her own room in a crib, and I realised this was *not practical* at all! From this day on, she jumped into bed with us and stayed there until I was halfway through my pregnancy with our second, when she switched to a mattress on the floor in our room. Our second baby lay next to me in bed from Day One, and we will never go back! We all get sleep and there are hardly any tears at night from anyone (including us!).
>
> – Annalee, Canada

Here are some ideas that work for other parents:

- If your partner has an earlier wake-up time, it may work best for them to sleep separately at first. Or they may start the night with you and the baby, then move elsewhere later in the night. Or vice versa.
- You could have the baby sleep separately in the same room, then bring him into bed for a leisurely early morning cuddle and nursing.
- An older child may start out in his own bed and trot down the hall to his parents when and if he wakes. Or he may crawl in with his older brother across the room.
- Some families have a daybed or twin mattress on the floor next to the parents' bed for nighttime visitors.

These musical bed arrangements, which may change many times over the years, have one main goal – to give the most people the most sleep... *tonight.*

In an **emergency situation,** you might need to get really creative, like Cecily did when she found herself in hospital overnight with two children:

> When our son was three years old and our first daughter was three months old, I took the children to visit friends in our former town, about one and a half hours away. My son was recovering from a minor cold and was getting better, so I was surprised to hear his raspy breathing that night. I decided to take him to the hospital. That meant taking my little baby to the hospital, too.
>
> The doctors suggested that we stay the night. The room contained a single adult hospital bed and one children's hospital crib with tall, barred sides. At home we all slept in one king bed on the floor, with me in between my two children and my husband on the other side of my son.
>
> I realised the single adult bed would have to do. I put my son with his head at the top of the bed and raised the rail to protect him from falling, and put my daughter at the foot of the bed. I lay down beside her with my head at the foot of the bed, my arm around her. The nurses checked in on us, but they left me to care for my children in my own way. When my son woke up, I got up, nursed him, and then returned to my place beside my little girl. I went back and forth as needed all night long. It wasn't the best sleep of my life, but the children were perfectly content. When morning came, my son was much better and we went home.
>
> – *Cecily, Ontario, Canada*

A simple arrangement (one many families adopt when their babies get mobile) is to take your own bed off its frame and set the mattress on the floor. Falling out of bed is no longer an issue, and all the cracks and crevices are gone. You can also add a twin mattress to create a wall-to-wall bed if you want.

Is This the End of Sex?

Never underestimate the creativity of people who want to have sex – many children who bed-shared have younger siblings! You can move the baby temporarily to another sleeping surface – a crib or cradle or crib if you have one near the bed, or a blanket on the floor. Or just leave the baby in the bed, asleep. *The baby doesn't care* what you're doing, so long as *he* feels safe and comfortable. Expect to be interrupted sometimes, though.

With an older baby or toddler who can safely be left alone in your bed, you can just go to another room for some intimate time together. One father who slept in a separate bedroom while his partner was bed-sharing with their baby renamed his room the Boudoir of Seduction, and that became their special place for intimacy. Every home is full of horizontal (and vertical) surfaces. Get as creative as you need to. Some parents arrange for a friend or relative to take the baby for a walk for an hour in the evening (or morning!). If parents choose to sleep separately when their children are very young, it's only for a while. Rested parents get along better (and probably have more sex).

But I'm *Really* Exhausted!

We hear you. Looking after babies and young children, especially if you don't have a strong network of support, is the most tiring thing most of us ever do. What can you do when you're exhausted and your baby keeps on waking up? Here are some ideas that have worked for other families:

- If you haven't already, **try bringing your baby into your bed.** (Assuming you can do so safely – see the Safe Sleep Seven earlier in this chapter.) Breastfeeding puts you in a hormonal state that facilitates sleep. You can relax, knowing your baby is safe. Your sleep states sync with your baby's, meaning you often wake just before or as the baby does – you're not dragged out of deep sleep. You don't have to wake fully to meet your baby's needs. Teresa remembers her husband asking if the baby nursed during the night. Teresa felt her softened breasts and answered, "Apparently." The reality is that new parenthood usually involves a sleep deficit for a while, regardless of how a baby is fed or where she sleeps. But keeping your baby close can make nighttimes easier. If you aren't sure how to nurse lying down, practise in the daytime first, when you're alert and can see what you're doing.
- As much as possible, **sleep when the baby sleeps.** Turn off the phone and get into bed, even if it's 11:00 A.M. or 7:30 P.M. If you're

feeling pressure to get things done while the baby sleeps, try adding "Sleep" to the top of your to-do list. You don't have to do the same every day – every bit of snatched sleep helps.
- **Nurse lying down** as much as possible. Even if you don't sleep, being horizontal helps enormously to give you rest.
- **Pay attention to your nutrition.** Often when we're tired, we resort to caffeine and sugary foods to keep up our energy. These may work in the short term, but they end up making us even more drained. A reasonably healthy diet will maximise your energy and ability to cope with interrupted sleep.
- **Get all the help you can.** Help with the baby, help doing household tasks, help with older children – any of these will let you get more rest or sleep. If help just isn't available, you may need to let some things go until you're less tired.
- **Limit visitors** (other than the ones who are helping with laundry, groceries, house cleaning, cooking, etc.!). If people do come over, stay in your pyjamas or nightie so they get the message that you aren't really ready for visitors; plus, already being in pyjamas may encourage you to go back to bed as soon as they've left.
- **Go to an LLL meeting and complain!** It's a safe place where people *won't* respond with "Well, what do you expect if you're breastfeeding/expressing/bringing your baby into bed?" You'll almost always get useful ideas. You'll *absolutely* get solidarity, and reassurance that this stage is temporary.
- **Get outside** for at least an hour every day; this really seems to make a difference in how well babies (and older children) sleep at night. The fresh air, change of scenery, and gentle exercise are good for you, too.
- Most newborns seem to have their days and nights mixed up at first – they sleep well during the day, then are wide awake at night. Some persist in this unfortunate preference for months. You can encourage change by **offering to nurse more during the day** (babies will often latch even if they're half-asleep) and keeping them in the main living areas of your home so they'll be stimulated by noise and activity. Keep lights low and avoid blue light at night.
- Or **keep that reassuring noise and activity going at night,** in the form of "white noise" – a fan or air conditioner, say, or a radio set to a quiet station or to very soft static. Babies in the womb are surrounded by noise all the time. If you're using a white noise

app, make sure it's not too loud or too close to your baby, and don't run it all day long.
- **Take turns** with your partner or another support person in getting extra sleep while the other person tends to the baby – like Audrey and her partner did:

> At home, the nights are for me and the mornings for Dad, and that's fine. I enjoy my two hours of sleep in the morning when Dad takes over; it's my time, their time. We have found a balance.
> – *Audrey, France*

Maybe you could get up with the baby on Saturday, leaving your partner to sleep late, but on Sunday you could sleep in while your partner tucks the baby in a sling, makes breakfast for you, brings the baby in to nurse, and then goes out for a walk with the baby while you keep sleeping. If you don't have a partner to help, consider collaborating with another mother – one of you looks after both babies while the other takes a nap.
- **Have a sleep angel.** This is a doula or supporter whom you pay to stay near your room at night *and who expects to be wakened to help you with nursing* or anything else. They might take your awake-but-fed baby for a while, bringing him back to nurse. Knowing that your sleep angel is just a room away, ready to come and help in any way you need at any time you need, can help you relax and get to sleep. Sometimes just a night or two with a sleep angel can give you enough sleep to change your outlook. If you're really lucky, someone who loves you might do this for free.
- Ask your partner or see a massage therapist to help **relax your tired muscles** by giving you a back rub or a foot massage. Some of your tiredness may be related to aching muscles from carrying your baby and sitting in less than comfortable positions.
- **Eight straight hours of sleep isn't based in either biology or history.** Our no-electricity ancestors had *much* longer nights than we have today. They often had a period of sleep, a rather lengthy middle-of-the-night period of wakefulness, and another period of sleep. Lengthen your "night" by going to bed early and staying in bed in the morning. You're sharing your wee-hours wakefulness with not only your ancestors but with other families around the world.

- **Remember, this is temporary.** On about day four, you may feel that life as you know it has sunk into a fog of sleepless chaos. But this is absolutely temporary, and it's absolutely survivable. Get help where you need it, knowing that ending breastfeeding won't help. This is just normal life with a new baby.
- If you find that you can't sleep (even when your baby does), and are getting increasingly anxious or depressed, **talk to your healthcare provider.** Not being able to sleep when you're really tired can be a red flag for low mood or anxiety. Lots of us have been there; you're not alone, and you can get better. For more about postnatal mood disorders, see Chapter 18.

Do I Need to Train My Baby to Sleep?

You don't have to train your baby to sleep – just as you don't need to teach her to walk by holding her upright. She'll get there in her own time. A lot of sleep training is based on the hope of a magic fix for tired parents. And often, there's money to be made by promoting it.

Most sleep training involves responding less to your baby at night. But it's not normal or safe for young babies to manage alone at night. Shared sleep is the norm for babies: sudden infant death syndrome (SIDS) risk is increased for a baby who sleeps separately before six months, and milk production can suffer, too. Most sleep experts (and experts on infant mental health) warn against using these approaches at least in the first half-year.

But how about older babies and nursing toddlers? The risk of SIDS is much lower after six months, and milk production is usually settled and robust. So is your baby ready to sleep longer and go back to sleep without nursing or cuddles from you?

Maybe. As time goes by, many babies nurse less and call for their parents less often through the night. If you've got one of those easy babies... enjoy the sleep! And try not to judge those of us who don't. A sizeable proportion of children continue to need help at night, though, and sometimes well beyond the first year. This isn't because their parents are doing anything wrong – they're just different babies. (Lots of us have had both kinds.)

Sleep training can work in the sense that babies may, at least temporarily, ask for you less at night. Research finds that babies who are sleep-trained still *wake* about the same amount at night, but have given up calling out to their parents for comfort and reassurance. This "self-soothing" comes at a cost to the babies: their stress levels may still be high, even though they don't cry. Is it worth it? In the context of a warm, secure relationship with you, sleep training may be tolerable for some babies, especially when balanced against other needs within the family – for example, the exhaustion of a parent who is back at work, depressed, or ill.

Many parents report that sleep training doesn't make any difference. If it does, it may need to be repeated several times. Parents often find it really upsetting, feeling that the baby's trust in them has been damaged. And the effect doesn't last – no long-term gains have been found in how children sleep. In other words, children who were sleep-trained end up sleeping just as well (or badly!) as children who weren't.

Fortunately, classic sleep training, such as cry-it-out or controlled crying/comforting, is not the only approach. Recent research on the biology of sleep has led to some great resources on how to work with, rather than against, the grain of your baby's development. You're the best judge of whether your baby can cope with some gentle nudges towards more independence at night. And even if you do nothing at all, a healthy child *will* eventually manage without you all night long. One day, you'll be lying awake on your own in bed, wondering where she is and what she's up to.

Would Solid Food Help?

Parents are sometimes tempted to give the baby solid food such as cereal before bedtime to encourage him to sleep longer. Research has found adding solid foods doesn't help babies sleep more – in fact, for some it caused more night waking because of digestive problems or allergies. Starting family foods early increases the likelihood of overweight. Many babies do start to sleep longer around the usual time for starting solids, probably just because they're getting older.

I Don't Want Her in Our Bed Forever!

Tina loves her sleeping arrangement:

> My baby is now six months old and we all sleep eight hours a night. She loves going to bed snuggled with me, and I love waking up snuggled with

her. There is no stress around sleep – we just enjoy it. If things need to change later on we will do something differently, but for now and the foreseeable future, my baby and I stay together and it has made all the difference for our little family.
– Tina, United States

Some parents worry (or are told) that if they bed-share now they'll *never* get the baby out of their bed. We promise: your sixteen-year-old isn't going to be sleeping in your bed. But the process to independent sleep is often two steps forward, one step back, and it's different for every baby. One day your baby *will* sleep four or five hours straight. You might be surprised, as Allison was:

Now that my little one is a year old, she sleeps for two four-hour stretches, and we have found a new normal.
– Allison, North Carolina, United States

A week later she might wake up miserable from teething. Then the four hours will stretch to six or seven hours without waking, then a short nursing and another two or three hours of sleep. In time, her nighttime hours of unbroken sleep will increase, and so will yours. (And when your baby is a teenager, she'll sleep like a log and you'll find you can't drag her out of bed in the morning....)

If you move your baby or toddler from your room before she asks for her own room, do it gradually and with love. You could try a crib, or floor mattress, or bed in the new room as a site for naps first. Try a white noise source, or relaxing music, in your room before the move and then take the noise source to the new room. Or get a baby monitor and use it backward, piping your nighttime noises into the other room to provide comfort. If possible, move the toddler in with an older sibling. Some parents find a separate room cuts into their sleep at first; calls for nighttime company increase temporarily while the little one adjusts. (If you find that nightmares, night terrors, or head-banging begin, you may want to return to co-sleeping for a while longer.)

You can experiment. Try bringing your child into bed with you at the first waking, or start with her in your bed, then move her to the new room after the first nursing. Maybe have your partner do the back-to-sleep soothing. Let your little one sleep with your partner but without you and see how that works. If your child is unhappy, go back to what was working before and try moving towards separate sleep again a few weeks or months later. If your child is ready, the next step is often easy, as Cecily found:

> When I asked him to stop nursing during the night at age two years and three months, it went very smoothly. I said, "Mokies are sleeping. You can have it when the sun comes up." He was sad and cried and complained for five minutes and then drifted back to sleep beside me. That was it. With night nursing over, I was happy to carry on nursing during the day.
> – Cecily, Ontario, Canada

The age of readiness for separate sleep varies hugely. One mother *finally* convinced her high-need five-year-old son to try sleeping in his own room. As soon as his two-year-old sister saw the new arrangement, she wanted her own room, too!

Many parents, like Lindsay, find they miss having their children in their bed:

> I look back on all the wakeful nights with such a grateful feeling, so thankful that I could always provide what she needed.
> – Lindsay, Texas, United States

Important conversations with our teens and even with adult children still take place with a child lying on our bed: "Mummy, guess what Ayesha said today!" or "Mum and Dad, what do you think I should do about football?" or "I've met this boy . . ." Family beds can be flexible. They can last a lifetime, changing form over and over to meet your family's ever-changing dynamics. Nighttime nurturing and family closeness might become, as they did for Anna, some of your child's happiest memories:

> Visits from relatives were such happy events, especially when our grandmother Birdie visited. Birdie was a ruthless game player who would not let you win at Sorry, Dominoes, cards, or any other game. She was also a great storyteller and reader. My sister and I would squabble to get to sleep with Grandma Birdie. She would lull the lucky child to sleep with reading stories, then telling stories in the dark. They were mostly folktales, Bible stories, an occasional poem, knock-knock jokes. Scary stories were no

scarier than "It floats... it floats... it floats..." "What floats, Grandma?" "Ivory Soap floats!" What timeless, wonderful memories all these years later, when I myself tell my grandsons stories in the dark.
– Anna, Texas, United States

Want to know more?

You can find extra resources for this chapter at the "Art of Breastfeeding" tab at www.llli.org.

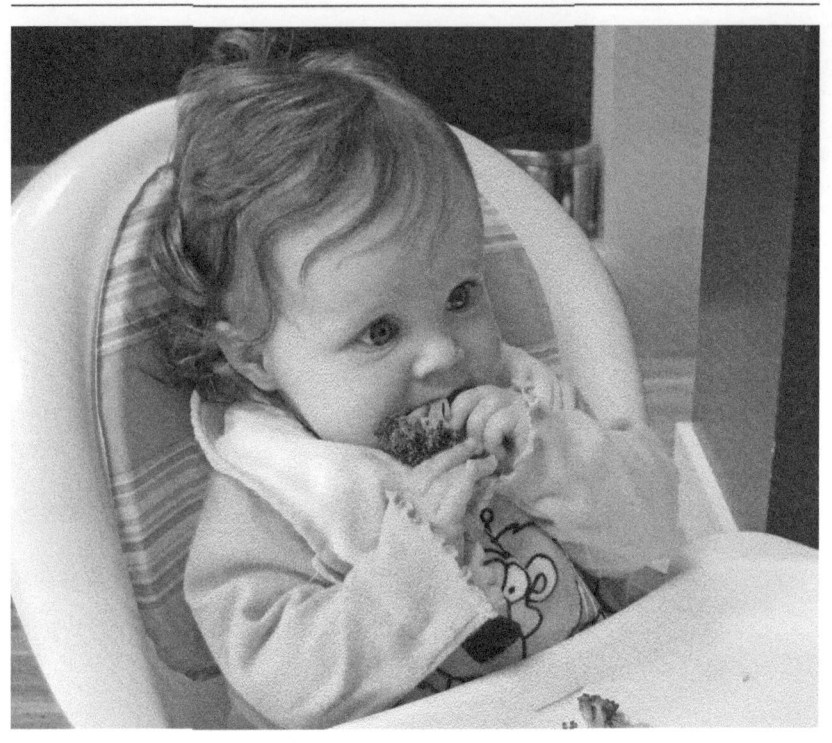

THIRTEEN

Beginning Family Foods

> Because I strongly believe my milk is the best thing he can get, I was a little skeptical about introducing solid foods. Or should I say I was a little jealous? We are now in the experimenting phase, and I must say it's not as bad as I thought. It is funny to see how he learns to eat.
> – *Luisa, Switzerland*

It can feel like just when you've got breastfeeding working, people start asking when you're going to start family foods (often called solids or complementary feeding). You may be looking forward to this next milestone – or dreading it! Either way, there's no rush, and you can let your baby lead the way.

Long ago, before there were baby food manufacturers or even spoons, nursing babies ate what their parents ate. Not whole nuts and tough meats, of course, but whatever family foods they could handle. Most likely no one had the time or interest to feed a baby who wasn't already reaching for someone else's food, typically around the middle of the first year.

In the first half of the twentieth century, there was a dramatic shift away from breastfeeding in some parts of the world. Parents were given recipes for making "formula" for their babies, but they were crude, and babies sometimes showed signs of malnutrition after just a few weeks. Doctors sought solutions to this man-made problem. For example, three Canadian physicians developed Pablum, a processed cereal intended to be a nutritious, easy-to-prepare food for small babies. It added some nutritional elements missing from the homemade formulas, and soon many parents were told to start using it within the first six weeks. Early introduction of solids became common in many places.

Solid Changes

That remained the situation as late as the 1980s, even though newer commercial formulas were less nutritionally deficient. Then researchers began to identify links between the early introduction of solids and a range of health problems, and the recommendations changed.

Multiple public and government health organisations now follow the 1991 World Health Organization recommendation on infant feeding.

Infants should be exclusively breastfed for the first six months of life to achieve optimal growth, development and health. Thereafter, to meet their evolving nutritional requirements, infants should receive nutritionally adequate and safe complementary foods while breastfeeding continues for up to two years of age or beyond.
—*World Health Organization*

Of course, grandparents and others might not be aware of these newer recommendations. You might have relatives who really think your baby will starve if solids aren't part of his diet early on.

People look to solid foods for other reasons, too. Maybe you're wondering whether other foods would help your baby sleep through the night. Not according to the research. In fact, your baby might sleep *less* well because of the indigestion that too-early solids can cause. Babies sleep for longer stretches when they're ready – which sometimes does happen around six months, but not because of solids. For more on sleep, see Chapter 12.

So What Makes a Baby Ready for Family Foods?

It's a matter of development. Normally, the baby's *insides* are ready once her *outside* has developed enough to eat them on her own. If she can't pick up food, get it in her mouth, and swallow it without gagging, she's probably not ready for solids, and her tummy probably isn't, either.

Sure, you can get food in her mouth sooner. But she may just push it back out with her tongue – a reflex young babies have to protect against choking. What if you put the food farther back? Now you've bypassed her defences – something she wouldn't do herself – and while she's more likely to swallow, she's also more likely to choke. And you're putting foods into a digestive tract that probably isn't ready for them.

Babies are also protected by being unable to pick up small items until around eight or nine months, when they develop a "pincer grip" using thumb and forefinger. Until then, your baby is not likely to get anything tiny (like a raisin or pea that might cause choking) into her mouth.

If your baby was born prematurely or has a developmental delay, your time frame may be different. Work with your healthcare provider to figure out your baby's individual timetable.

Signs That *Don't* Mean Your Baby Is Ready

Normal developmental changes might leave you – or other people! – wondering if your baby's ready for solids. But do they really mean that? Not usually. Here are some examples:

Frequency Days (Growth Spurts)

Does your baby suddenly want to nurse a lot more than usual? What you may be seeing is a "frequency day," sometimes called a growth spurt. These intense phases tend to last a couple of days – sometimes leaving you with full breasts that take another few days to settle down. Is it because your baby needs solid food? If there aren't any other signs of readiness (see the following sections), probably not. Frequency days are common throughout the early months. Getting your baby weighed will usually confirm she's doing fine. If you're worried your milk supply might be faltering, see Chapter 18, Weight Gain Worries and Low Milk Supply.

Distractibility

Around four months, babies start noticing the big, bright world, and it can be hard to get them to focus on nursing. This doesn't mean they're outgrowing it – they just haven't developed the skills to plug in to both their surroundings and the breast at the same time. Until his multitasking improves, your baby may nurse more often at night, when life is less exciting. For more about distracted babies, see Chapter 9.

Night Waking

Many babies wake more around four or five months, but not because they're hungry. Their wakefulness is more likely related to what's going on in their brains than in their stomachs. Your baby may be too busy to nurse much in the day and may get disturbed by practising new skills (like rolling) in his sleep. Sore gums may also bother him. For more on sleep, see Chapter 12.

Fascination with Eating

Around five months, many babies become fascinated by *your* eating. Your baby's eyes may follow your every mouthful. She may make a grab for your utensils, or your food. Does this mean she's ready to eat? Not by itself, no. At this age, she's fascinated by *everything* you do – it's how she learns. She's probably curious when you drive the car, too, but if you hand her the car keys, you know they're just to play with! Try giving your baby safe versions of your eating utensils; they might be all she wants, for now. Many babies practise with the tools for a few weeks before they're ready to eat family foods for real.

Starting Out

Your baby can join the mealtime fun even if he's not quite ready to eat yet. Beginning whenever he can sit on his own, he can sit in his own chair next to you, or on your lap. Give him a spoon, maybe some water in a sippy cup, and let him play Dinnertime.

Is your baby reaching for the food on your plate? Put some baby-suitable food in front of him and see what he does. Babies who aren't ready for solids may play with food, even taste it, but they won't get serious about eating it.

The day will arrive when the food makes it into his mouth and down the hatch. You don't have to control the amount. Your baby will take care of that, just as he does when he nurses.

Different Babies, Different Stories

Just as babies crawl and walk at different ages, they're not all ready to start eating on the dot of six months. Every baby has their own timetable, and style, as Anna describes:

I went by the book with our first child. We started him on commercial baby foods at six months. I noticed that he gagged on finger foods and small cereal pieces. I found La Leche League with our second child, and learned about family foods as socialisation and fun, not a firm and fast requirement. We tried bananas at five or six months, which she promptly rejected. However, she was happy to help herself to broccoli a short time later. Our third child grabbed my garlic bread at lunch one day, around five or six months, and gobbled it down.

– Anna, Texas, United States

What if you're having porridge, or soup? Is spoon-feeding ever okay? Sure! Liquid or semi-liquid foods are much easier to offer with a spoon. The key is to make sure you're paying attention to your baby's signals. With thick semi-liquid foods, you might be able to give him the spoon to hold with some food already on it. Some parents find that, with more liquid foods, putting the spoon right at the tip of the baby's mouth will encourage him to lap up what's being offered. Another strategy: offering the side of the spoon rather than the tip. The goal of spoon-fed foods is to introduce new tastes and textures in a fun and relaxed way that keeps your baby in control.

What Should My Baby Eat?

Although advertisements suggest otherwise, babies don't need "baby food." If you've waited until your baby is ready to start eating, she won't need to eat mush (purée) – she can enjoy a range of textures from the start. If your family eats a reasonably healthy diet, all you need to do is adapt your usual meals a bit so your baby can safely join in. Find information on safe eating, allergies, and foods to avoid later in this chapter. You may have been told to avoid fruit because it "will give your baby a sweet tooth." Don't worry; *nothing* tastes sweeter than your milk!

The sour face? That's common with any new food. It isn't necessarily that your baby doesn't like it; she's just never tasted it so strongly before. But she *has* tasted it! Although formula always tastes the same, your milk has traces of whatever you eat, so these first tastes of family foods will probably seem familiar to your baby. In fact, research shows that formula-fed babies don't accept new tastes as readily as breastfed babies.

Your baby will signal that her meal is over when she starts finger painting with her food (or throws it on the floor).

Some Simple Starter Foods

Your family or community may have traditional first foods. In your locality, other foods may be more appropriate. La Leche League groups can be good places to talk about healthy local foods for babies and children. If you have no idea what foods to start with, here are a few possibilities:

Meats – cooked, shredded, or slivered (chicken can be served on the drumstick, with any skin, cartilage, and small bones removed)

Fish – small pieces of cooked, flaky fish; feel for and remove any bones

Fruit – ripe to the point of being slightly mushy, cut in baby-fist-size chunks
  Banana
  Mango
  Melon
  Avocado
  Apple or pear – no chunks – peeled and grated, or lightly cooked
  Peach

Vegetables – cooked and limp, or cooked and mashed
  Beans – very soft or mashed with a fork
  Hummus – offer on your finger! Or spread on a cooked carrot slice or rice cake, or in a small bowl so your baby can scoop it out with his hands
  String beans – cooked and mashed
  Sweet or white potato – big chunks or mashed with water or your milk

Grains
> Whole grain breads (very dry or toasted)
> Whole wheat breadsticks
> Rice cakes
> Sticky rice
> Cooked barley, millet, etc.

Some proteins and fats for the vegetarian or vegan baby
> Seed butters (such as tahini) as dips or spreads
> Nut butters
> Well-cooked beans, lentils
> Seitan cut up into small pieces

If you're raising your baby vegan, don't forget his need for supplementary vitamin B12 once solid foods become a bigger part of his diet. Your baby's healthcare provider can advise.

For more about drinks for babies, including formula, water, and juice, see Chapter 10.

A Breastfeeding Approach to Starting Family Foods

One of the things people sometimes see as a disadvantage of breastfeeding is that they can't tell how much milk the baby has taken, or how much milk is still left in the breast. It turns out that this is an important *benefit*.

Researchers compared breastfed babies with those who'd been fed formula or expressed milk by bottle. When they became toddlers, those fed by bottle tended to drink everything in their cup and eat all the food on their plate. Those fed at the breast ate and drank only what they wanted – no "Clean Plate Club" for them!

If the baby drinks, for example, 90 or 120 ml (3 or 4 ounces) from a 180-ml (6-ounce) bottle, many parents and caregivers will jiggle the nipple in the baby's mouth, encouraging him to take "just a bit more." It's understandable: expressed milk is precious, and formula is expensive. But maybe he's had enough. Do we really want to encourage him to take more than he needs?

Responsive feeding means trusting your baby to know his own appetite. When nursing is going well, the strategy is simple: you offer the breast, and the baby takes as much or as little as he wants. That same strategy creates a healthy eater as your baby starts eating solids. Your job is to offer nutritious food, prepared so the baby can safely eat it; it's his job to decide how much to eat. For more tips on how to avoid overfeeding, see Chapter 18, Weight Gain Worries.

Some babies have medical or other issues (Type 1 diabetes, for example) that mean you need to manage how much they eat. Work with your healthcare provider if this is the case for your baby. An LLL Leader may be able to connect you with other families whose children have similar issues.

Safe Eating

Babies and young children should never be left alone when they're eating. It's much friendlier to eat in company – and someone needs to be on hand in case of choking. True choking is rare, but can be very dangerous, and it's important to know what to do if it happens. Some parents take a first aid course so they're well prepared. If your child is in nursery, or being looked after by someone else, check their first aid knowledge, too. For more on choosing alternative caregivers, see Chapter 14.

Choking – or Just Gagging?

There's a big difference between choking and gagging. Here's how to tell one from the other:

- When a child **gags** on food (or her own saliva), she coughs and splutters. The food gets worked to the front of the mouth and spat out, and the baby is okay. *Gagging is noisy.* It might be stressful to listen to – but the noise means the baby is coping with the food. You can safely watch and wait to see what happens.
- **Choking** is when food gets lodged in the windpipe (trachea). With food stuck in the way, a baby can't get air into her lungs. *Choking is silent* – the baby can't make a noise, because her airway is blocked. This is why you need to be with your baby, and paying attention – you can't hear choking when your back is turned, you're distracted by your phone, or you're in the next room.

Choking Hazards for Babies and Toddlers

Whole nuts

Raw carrots, apples, and similar hard foods that can break off in chunks

Grapes (unless cut up into small, elongated pieces) and blueberries (okay if cut up small)

Popcorn

Hot dogs, unless cut up into *very* small pieces

Soft breads and rolls

Balancing Family Foods and Breastfeeding

You can relax about the balance between family foods and breastfeeding if you let your baby lead the way. Family foods don't usually have much impact on nursing at first, because most babies start by eating very little. Servings may be tiny – one or two bites each. As he becomes more skilled, your baby will be able to get more food into his mouth. Eventually, maybe well after a year, he'll be getting more of his calories from other foods than from your milk. Each child goes at his own pace.

It generally helps at first to nurse your baby before you both sit down to eat (if you get a chance). It doesn't need to be right before – that's not very practical if you're the one preparing the meal! – but a ravenous baby is probably in no mood for dinner, as Shoko found:

> My eldest was happy to be fed solids and showed interest in a variety of foods from around six months on, but he always wanted breastmilk first at mealtimes. It seemed like he needed to know that his familiar "comfort food" that had (almost) been his sole food for months wasn't going to be taken away, and only when he had had his fill of breastmilk would he be calm enough to try what was on the table.
>
> *– Shoko, the Netherlands*

When you've both finished eating, you can offer to nurse again. Your baby may fall asleep at your breast and take a nap, or he may not; that's fine. As he gets older, you can do what feels right – feed him before, after, either, or neither. Some meals will eventually replace nursings, and some feedings will happen instead of meals. No calculator needed!

If you've needed to use supplements of expressed milk or formula, it may be possible to reduce and even stop these during the next few months. Family foods can gradually take up the slack and provide the extra calories (see Chapter 18, Supplementing).

She Wants to Eat off *My* Plate!

Smart baby! She knows not to trust her own judgement yet. Maybe babies are programmed, for their own safety, to want only what they see the grown-ups eating. You could try putting her food on your plate first.

What About Salts and Spices?

Many of us are accustomed to more salt than we need. Leave the salt off when you fix your baby's food. Salt is hard for little kidneys to deal with. Babies can enjoy surprisingly spicy and flavorful foods, but it is better to start out without them. As your baby gets used to eating, you can experiment to see how much spice he enjoys – you might be surprised!

Our Family Eats a Lot of Ultraprocessed Foods

UPFs are convenient, often cheaper, and children (and adults!) tend to love them. They're also heavily marketed, including to young children. The same product from the same brand looks, feels, and tastes identical, no matter where you get it. This predictability appeals to many people, including toddlers, and children with sensory processing issues (if you want to read more about sensory processing disorders, see Chapter 7, Why Is My Baby Nursing Much *Less* Than My Friend's?). Some brands make health claims for their products, persuading even very well-informed parents that ultraprocessed food is a good alternative to (or even better than) real food. The rapid spread of UPFs has been the biggest revolution in eating for thousands of years. In some places, it's hard to get anything else.

What Are Ultraprocessed Foods?

Not all "convenience foods" are ultraprocessed. The key is to look at the list of ingredients. If a food contains ingredients you've never heard of, or wouldn't find in a home kitchen, you can assume it's ultraprocessed.

The problem is that ultraprocessed foods are not a healthy way for a baby or young child (or anyone else, for that matter) to eat. They are made by industrial processes new to human eating. They often contain large amounts of salt and sugar to make them palatable and fats that don't occur in nature. Where ultraprocessed foods have become widespread, so has obesity. Evidence is mounting that links them to all kinds of health problems (see Chapter 10, Food: Staying on Course and Chapter 18, Weight Gain Worries).

Our bodies do best with real food – food your ancestors would recognise. This includes fresh food that has been frozen or tinned. Food frozen soon after harvesting, preserving its nutritional value, may even be healthier than "fresh" food that's sat around for a good while. When you choose foods closer to their natural state, you and your baby will get necessary nutrients in their natural proportions.

If you'd like to make changes to how your family eats, here are some ideas. If you're eating a lot of convenience foods (many of them probably UPFs), the thought of doing more food preparation might feel overwhelming. Where you live, real food might be harder to get and more expensive. Maybe you're not used to cooking from basic ingredients, or don't have the equipment or time to do it. Other family members, including older children, might resist change.

You're unlikely to transform how your family eats overnight. But small changes towards healthier eating can add up to a big difference, continuing the good start you've given your baby by breastfeeding.

Ideas for Healthy Food on a Budget

- **Shop at the end of the day** when shops are selling off older food for less. Some places also sell off perfectly good but "wonky-looking" fruit or vegetables.
- If you (or someone willing to share) have freezer space, or room for tinned goods, **buy or pick surplus produce in season and store it.** This can be a good project for a team of family or friends. Get seasonal recipes and storage tips online or from gardeners.
- If you've got storage space, see if you can **find a whole food co-op** in your community. In a co-op, households join together to buy tinned and dried foods in bulk from a whole food provider – items like beans, nuts, or flour – for less than buying on your own.
- Find out about places in your neighbourhood where you **can pick vegetables or fruit.** Gardeners might be happy to share surplus produce.
- Look into safely **foraging** – harvesting food that grows wild.
- If you have any outside space, a windowsill, or even room for a tray of wet paper, **you can grow food.** If they grow it, children may be more likely to eat it. Even a few leaves of fresh herbs can help nourish taste buds and cultivate an interest in where food comes from. Some cities have community gardens or allotments families can join. Experienced gardeners are often generous with knowledge and plant cuttings.
- If it's **hard for you to access any healthy food,** your healthcare provider, local government organisations, food banks, or charities may be able to help. Many communities are coming up with creative ways to avoid food waste – like making leftover, still-in-date food from big stores available through co-ops.

Hacks for Taking the Stress out of Food Prep

- Find **instruction videos online** for making any food you might think of, from cooking an egg to preparing a wedding banquet!
- **Experienced cooks are often delighted to share recipes and tips.** Grandparents and older community members might be honoured to pass down favourite recipes for your children. Or try **skill-sharing** with friends: they teach you how to cook their favourite recipe; you or your partner mend their bike or update their website!

- **Start making dinner at breakfast time.** Evenings can be the worst time to cook if you've got a frazzled baby, and maybe a tired toddler. Start chopping the first ingredient in the morning and do bits here and there throughout the day. By the time everyone's hungry, you'll nearly have something ready to eat. Or use a slow cooker – you can set up dinner while your baby takes a morning nap, or maybe even before work.
- If you're careful, you can **cook while carrying a baby or toddler in a sling.** Try carrying your baby on your back as soon as she's old enough.
- **Get children involved in food preparation.** With supervision, even a toddler can cut up a mushroom or banana with a blunt knife or put dry pasta in a pan (if you don't mind some mess!).
- Save time by **batch-cooking** and freezing extra meals. Cooking several in one go cuts energy bills, too.
- If you're in a rush in the morning, **set the table the night before.** Check online for healthy no-cook breakfast recipes (like soaked grains with fruit) that you can put together in a couple of minutes and leave overnight.

How to Encourage Cautious Eaters

- **Eat together.** When you're throwing food in the microwave, it's easy for everyone to eat what they want, when they want. When you're cooking a meal, you want people there to eat it, and everyone to eat the same thing (maybe with a little adaptation). Children learn by watching. If they see others enjoying a food, they may be more likely to try it. If work or school schedules make it tricky, try having dinner together at weekends. Or eat breakfast together before work.
- Some parents join together with one or more families, or people living alone, to **share a regular meal and take turns cooking.** If other children in the group are more adventurous eaters than yours, that might be a bonus!
- **Give dishes names that make sense and sound simple,** focusing on the ingredients your wary child is already familiar with. "Yellow Chicken" sounds fun and reassuring; you don't need to list the spices. You could name dishes for people ("Auntie's Rice") or stories ("Magic Porridge Pot Porridge"). One creative parent of a hesitant eater came up with "Tractor Chicken" –

complete with a toy tractor on top, plowing the mashed potato "field"!
- **Cultivate a culture of "give it a try."** Unless you really love being a short-order cook, don't give free choice of alternative options (especially if you've got more than one child). Have an alternative meal for your little selective eater that takes minimal prep. If you keep offering a range of foods, expecting them to be tried – but not making a fuss if they're rejected – over time you'll probably build a confident eater. If your child is so selective that you're concerned about her health, and it's not improving with time, talk to your healthcare provider.
- If necessary, **start with just one meal or day a week** when you make food from scratch. Maybe breakfast, if you eat lunch at work. Starting is the hardest bit. Every small change helps.

Is There a Window of Opportunity for Introducing Family Foods?

Babies don't come with an instruction book, so it's unlikely a child will fail starting solids because his parents missed that page. It *is* true that some children have difficulty with chewing and swallowing and need a specialist's help. Maybe the notion of "a window of opportunity" first came from children who didn't start solids "on time" and who went on to have difficulties, but these children may have been late starting because they *couldn't* start earlier. If your baby is running on his own timetable – because he was born prematurely, say, or has developmental delays – work with your healthcare provider to figure out the best timing for him. And let your healthcare provider know if he seems to struggle with the mechanics of eating (gagging or choking a lot) or gets upset about food.

Are There Specific Times to Introduce Specific Foods?

Recommendations on when and how to introduce specific foods change as research develops – check with your healthcare provider for up-to-date guidelines.

You might have heard about delaying introduction of **gluten** (a protein found in wheat, rye, and barley) to prevent **coeliac disease,** a digestive and immune disorder that damages the small intestine. It can be triggered by eating gluten-containing foods. Gluten-free diets have become popular in some places – but only 1 to 3 percent of the world's population has true coeliac disease. (Some countries and regions have higher rates than others.) Unless your child has been diagnosed with coeliac disease, there's usually no need to avoid these foods or wait to introduce them. Consult with your healthcare provider if you have any concerns.

It is important to delay introducing honey until your baby is at least twelve months old, because it may contain botulism spores, which can cause serious illness in babies.

What About Allergies?

For many years doctors in some countries recommended babies avoid some of the more allergenic foods – such as peanuts, shellfish, eggs, and wheat – until they were twelve months old. The hope was not only to avoid having to deal with an allergic reaction in an infant but to prevent the development of allergies. But then experts noticed that in countries with these guidelines, *more* children developed allergies. Studies comparing early and late introduction of allergenic foods suggest that it is actually helpful to introduce these foods at the start rather than delaying them.

Where children have a family history of allergies, parents may now be advised to offer these foods from six months, or even as early as four months (and then to keep on including them as part of the baby's diet). This can be a concern for parents whose babies are just not interested in or ready for solids that early. If your baby is in this category, work with your healthcare provider.

Unless your family has a history of allergies, you don't have to make a big deal about waiting a few days between each new food. Odds are, your baby isn't going to have a problem. If she does show signs of a reaction (rashes on her face or bottom, for instance), she may have a sensitivity to a particular food. If she's eaten several foods at once, you may need to offer one kind of food every few days to find the culprit.

As Noémie found, having an allergic child can be very challenging and requires plenty of support:

> By sharing my story with a close friend, Allergies Quebec, La Leche League, and a support group for breastfeeding mothers with babies with intolerances/allergies, I realised that I was not alone in feeling helpless in the face of what my baby was experiencing. Over time, I was able to be accompanied by a nutritionist specialising in breastfeeding mothers and

people with allergies, and to remove the problematic foods from my diet. I did slip up more than once along the way; it was not easy at times. The improvement in my baby's general condition with the removal of each problematic food confirmed that my decision was the right one.
— Noémie, Québec, Canada

Occasionally, an allergic *mother* gets a rash from her baby's saliva after the baby has started eating family foods. If this happens to you, try wiping your breast and nipple with a damp cloth after nursing.

Check out LLL websites for more on food sensitivities (allergies and intolerances) and breastfeeding, or contact an LLL Leader.

Signs of Food Allergy

An allergic reaction to a food usually happens within a few minutes of eating it. Reactions can include the following:

- sneezing
- runny or blocked nose
- red, itchy, watery eyes
- wheezing and coughing
- a red, itchy rash
- asthma or eczema

Most allergic reactions are mild. But if your baby has an allergic reaction the first time he eats a food, he could have a more severe reaction the next time.

A severe reaction known as **anaphylaxis** or **anaphylactic shock** is a medical emergency. These are some of the signs of anaphylaxis:

- itchy skin or a raised, red rash
- swollen eyes, lips, hands, and feet
- swelling of the mouth, throat, or tongue, which can cause breathing and swallowing difficulties
- wheezing
- abdominal pain, nausea, and vomiting
- collapse and unconsciousness

— *Adapted from NHS (National Health Service), UK*

Such severe reactions to food are rare. If your child is at risk of anaphylaxis, you can carry emergency treatment (an auto-injector of epinephrine) with you. It's important to make sure the medication is up to date and always with your child (including when your child is not with you).

She Feeds Herself and It's *Messy!*

Babies don't know messes are work to clean up – they just know they're fun!

> The food introduction stage was a lot of fun. He would get all messy. I did not want him to make a mess and now I laugh a lot thinking about it; all babies make a mess!
> – Guajirita Alquizareña, from Cuba, living in the Netherlands

Here are some ways to keep the mess down and the enjoyment up:

- In warm weather, **outdoor meals** are ideal. You can just hose down the highchair afterwards. Or put the baby on the floor and have a picnic.
- Use a **plastic tablecloth or washable shower curtain** under your baby's place at the table as well as on the table so you won't have to look at the carpet years later and say, "Yep, that's where Sophia sat."
- **Keep her cup at your own place.** If your baby's cup is some distance from her, she'll learn to reach for it when she wants a drink, and there'll be less spillage. But do offer water. Many babies are slower to get interested in water than in food. You can encourage your baby by offering sips from your own cup. If you use a no spill cup, consider removing the valve. There may be more spills, but without the valve the cup will be easier for your baby to manage, and better for learning how liquids work, which means less spilling in the future. For more about drinks for babies, see Chapter 10.
- **Keep a flannel handy** to mop up spills, hands, and face at the end of the meal. But don't be too zealous. Imagine having your dinner interrupted six times by a cold, wet cloth across your mouth!

- If you don't use a dining table, **your baby can sit with you** on the sofa or floor and cruise the furniture during dinnertime once she's older. Later, you might find yourself using a table after all because it creates a space where everyone is facing each other and the family is literally together.

The Power of Family Meals

Busy schedules and electronic devices mean fewer families share a regular meal. It's worth taking the time to eat together if you can. Research suggests regular family meals are linked to better grades, reduced risk of obesity and eating disorders, and even reduced risk of substance abuse in the years ahead. That's a lot of benefit for a few minutes sitting around a table!

- More than one of us has **put a child in the (dry) bath or on the floor of the shower** to eat something especially messy. If you strip off most of your baby's clothes before she eats, you can save on laundry and wash the mess right off afterwards.
- Dogs can be excellent floor cleaners when there are children at the table.

A Healthy Eater

Will letting your baby feed himself lead to a healthier attitude towards food? Maybe. Individual differences may also be important, but there are numerous reports of children whose parents controlled their meals who rebelled in the only way they could – by refusing food, sometimes to the point of ill health. Directed feeding – whether it's "Clean your plate!" or "That's enough!" – and preventing exploration and self-feeding may not be in a child's long-term best interests.

You've given your baby an excellent start towards a healthy diet by following his appetite cues during breastfeeding. A little mess as he learns the textures, tastes, and delights of family foods is just another part of that healthy start.

What If I'm Working?

You may want to wait until you're with your baby to offer family food for the first time, so you can enjoy the experience and make sure she's truly ready. At first, offering solids only when you're both home will be enough. When your baby is ready to eat regularly, talk to your caregivers about what to offer, and how much. Let them know your preferences about allowing your baby to feed herself. If you have any choices for caregivers (see Chapter 14), look for one who's supportive of responsive feeding. The caregiver provides the "what, when, and where," and your little one decides "how much and whether" to eat. Instead of buying baby foods, it can be cheaper and healthier to provide leftover finger foods from your own dinner when you pack her lunch.

What If He's Not Interested at First?

It's not a big deal. Your milk can keep him going for quite a while longer, providing a nice, wide comfort zone. It's a complete blend of nutrition, vitamins, minerals, electrolytes, and fluids, not to mention anti-infective, anti-inflammatory, and immune system–boosting factors. Your "late starter" or "long-term dabbler" isn't missing any developmental milestones. He may still need to develop his chew-and-swallow skills. He just needs a few more days, weeks, or months. And if there's a *particular* food he doesn't like? Keep offering it, and he'll probably be happy to try it again later.

There are some caveats here. Term babies, if their umbilical cords are cut after they stop pulsating (see Chapter 3) are normally born with a good amount of iron. That stored iron can begin to run low around six months, and babies need iron from other sources, too. Human milk doesn't have a lot of iron (though that iron is in the best form to be absorbed by the baby). Make sure you offer some iron-rich foods as part of your baby's diet (for example, red meat, cooked lentils, chickpeas, black beans, dark green leafy vegetables, and egg yolks). Pairing plant-based sources with foods high in vitamin C can help your baby absorb the iron.

Iron can become more of a problem if the baby is also getting cow's milk to drink. Cow's milk can cause tiny amounts of bleeding in the baby's intestines, meaning that he is regularly losing iron. If the baby is not eating much by way of solids, there is a risk he could become anaemic, which can lead to health and developmental issues. Check with your baby's healthcare provider if you're concerned. If necessary, your baby's iron levels can be tested, and he can be given iron supplements.

She Eats Anything I Give Her. Is She Going to Wean?

Some babies think solids are the greatest thing since, well, sliced bread. Even babies can have surprisingly sophisticated tastes, as Teresa describes:

> When my son Jeremy was about eleven months old, we were attending a party – one of those relaxed get-togethers with food set out on every horizontal surface. Jeremy toddled over to a coffee table with a platter of devilled oysters (*not* on my list of toddler foods). He picked one up, took one bite, and happily ate it, then went back for more. The adults were laughing at his delight in this new flavour. To this day, he's a very adventurous eater!
>
> – *Teresa, Ontario, Canada*

Make sure you give plenty of opportunities to nurse for comfort as well as for food, and your baby probably won't ignore you in favour of cooked carrots (or devilled oysters). If she's self-feeding nutritious foods, you don't need to limit her family foods, but watch the sweets and ultraprocessed foods. Your Eager Eater won't know they exist (for a while) if they're not on the menu.

Is It a Good Idea to Restrict Certain Kinds of Food?

Maybe not, according to research, because of the lure of forbidden fruit. In other words, if you ban or ration particular foods, your child is more likely to crave them. This makes sense. As children get older, you have less control over what they eat; you want them to develop self-control, and they get this by practising.

You can probably keep your one- or two-year-old away from cake or ice cream if you're determined. By the time she's three, though, she might eat it at other people's homes. It may be better if she knows from experience how much to eat.

It's probably wise to be cautious about ultraprocessed foods. Because they're not normal foods our bodies are adapted to cope with, they don't give us the usual signals that we're full. (Some experts describe them as addictive.) If young children don't eat them often, they may be more likely to grow healthy bodies that know when to stop eating. On the other hand, some research suggests that babies encouraged to feed themselves choose to eat fewer of these foods. Talk to your child about different kinds of foods and how they affect us. You're preparing her – in a world flooded with unhealthy food – to decide for herself what to eat.

My Toddler Hardly Eats a Thing!

Many toddlers go through phases when they seem to live on air. That's completely normal. Your toddler can get plenty of fuel from your milk for months to come. If babies kept gaining at the typical infant rate (remember, most babies *triple* their weight in the first year!), even the most petite baby would become gigantic in no time. Toddlers often grow very slowly for a while, and slow growth in a small body means not very much food required.

It is possible, though, for some toddlers to get stuck in a loop, where they ask to nurse the moment they feel any discomfort, including hunger. They sometimes need encouragement to think beyond nursing. This may be more likely when children have additional needs, like autism. If you have concerns about your baby's transition to family foods, consult with your healthcare provider.

Family Foods: The Big Picture

Feeling a bit overwhelmed by the whole topic of food? Just like with breastfeeding, it can help to zoom out your focus on family foods and look at the big picture. Feeding your child isn't just about grams or ounces of this or that, or this or that vitamin or mineral. It's not about formulating a perfectly balanced diet – if there even is such a thing – and ensuring your child eats it (if you figure out how to do *that*, please let us know!). Like breastfeeding, eating family food is about bodily satisfaction, pleasure, and relationships. It's about exploring what our amazing planet and biology can provide. We know healthier eating can be far from easy – many of us live in places where the food culture is very messed up. But if you're feeling lost, it can help enormously to know where you'd *like* to go.

Having a baby gives many of us the motivation to reassess what food means to us and the relationship we'd like to have with it. Maybe you want to eat a little (or a lot) more healthily, or want to pay closer attention to appetite. Perhaps you want to develop skills and enjoy the processes of preparing food – maybe growing it, too. Or maybe you want to waste less and help make nutritious food cheaper and easier to find in our communities. Perhaps you want to push back against an industrial food system that values profit over health. Almost all of us want to relish the pleasures of sharing food with people we love.

Want to know more?

You can find extra resources for this chapter
at the "Art of Breastfeeding" tab at
www.llli.org.

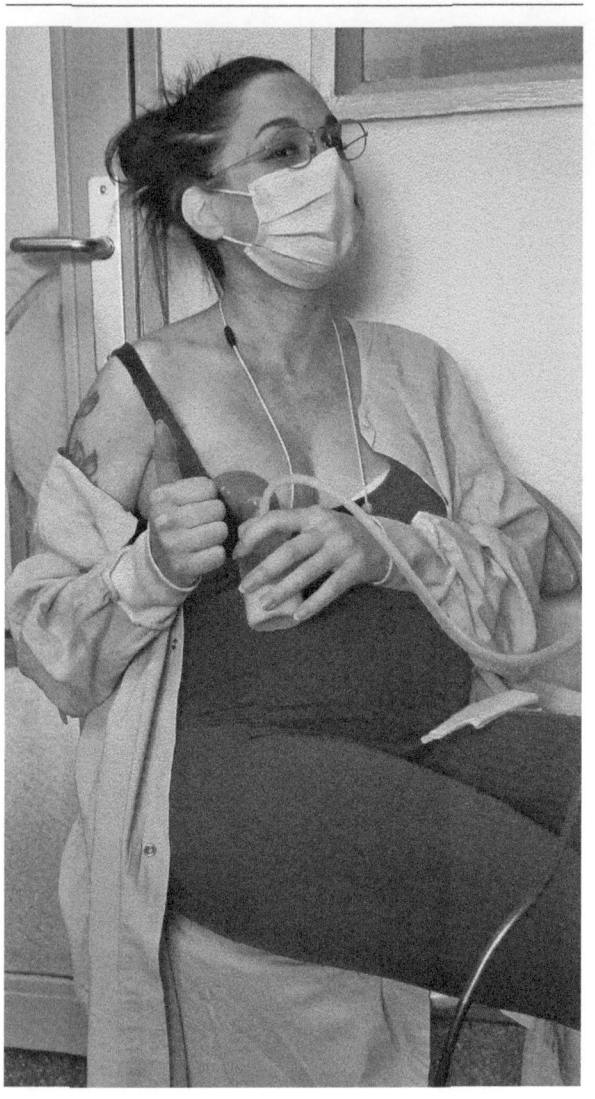

FOURTEEN

When You're Away from Your Baby

A week before my baby turned two months old, I returned to work, and my baby stayed with my mother. I had to adapt to the role of a working mother, and to a series of changes in my job, while organising myself to pump twice during my eight-hour day. In the afternoon I would come home and my little one and I were together again, carrying (in a sling) and feeding on demand.

At nine months, it was time to go to nursery; despite having been bottle-fed my milk for so long, he started firmly rejecting the bottle! The girls at the nursery insisted they would offer him formula, but I gave them a resounding "No!" My son didn't need it, because before I went to work, I would feed him, and as soon as we got home, he would be eager for Mum's taste and warmth. After a year, I only pumped once at work, and after a short time I stopped expressing altogether.

What was the secret? To inform myself, trust myself, and surround myself with a community that understood and gave me the support I needed. Breastfeeding and working is possible!

– Haydee, Coahuila, Mexico

Babies normally nurse frequently, day and night. Their brains and bodies are growing rapidly, and nursing provides comfort and protection against illness. That's our basic biology.

But many of us, from necessity or choice, are separated from our babies – an hour here and there, many hours a day, and sometimes even for several days. Can breastfeeding continue? Almost always – but it may take some extra effort and planning. Biology is bendable, but only so far, which is what this chapter is about: Bending biology where it can bend, and bending to it where it can't.

Returning to Work or Study

Is it worth continuing to breastfeed? Yes! All the reasons to do it are still important, and some are even more important now. For example, babies in childcare are exposed to many germs and tend to get ill more often than babies at home. Your milk helps your baby fight those germs and recover quickly if he gets ill.

What you might find matters even more is the continued connection that breastfeeding gives you and your baby. Knowing your baby is drinking your milk helps you take care of him even when you're apart.

Are you looking ahead, like Rosie, wondering how on earth your baby will manage without you?

> For some foolish reason I thought it would be a good idea to apply for a full-time master's [programme] while I was pregnant. Nine days after my daughter was born, I received my acceptance letter and thought, "How's this going to work?!" I couldn't see through the newborn haze how it would ever be possible for me to leave my baby with anyone for more than five minutes so that I could study. She ate constantly! She needed me!
>
> – Rosie, England

Work comes up often at LLL meetings. When asked what they'd tell someone who's worrying about it, experienced mothers say, "It works out, somehow. I wish I hadn't spent my maternity leave worrying!"

This was Rosie's experience:

> Autumn came around and she was seven months old and refusing a bottle. I tried pumping and giving her milk in a cup but in the end found that it was more trouble than it was worth. When I wasn't around she was quite happy to go without milk for a few hours and then have a feed during my lunch break. Studying while taking care of a baby is a huge challenge, but the feeding side of it was far more straightforward than I could have imagined.
>
> – Rosie, England

La Leche League has decades of experience supporting families to breastfeed through every kind of separation. We can support you, too.

Planning Your Maternity Leave

The longer you can be with your baby, the easier it is to get breastfeeding established and keep it going when you're apart. Maternity leave varies hugely from country to country.

The International Labor Organization, an agency of the United Nations, recommends at least fourteen weeks (preferably eighteen weeks), paid at two-thirds of previous earnings (preferably 100 percent).

There's also a global trend towards parental leave available to either parent or reserved for the parent who didn't give birth. Depending on where you live and work, a solid maternity/parental leave might be your reality or only a dream.

Going back to work is harder when maternity leave is shorter. But whether your leave is measured in days, weeks, or months, continuing to breastfeed is still doable.

Another question is when to *start* your leave. Research shows that having a longer leave *after* birth enables longer breastfeeding. But research also shows that those who start their leave a few weeks *before* birth are less likely to have a caesarean birth or a premature or low-birth-weight baby.

Even if the law or your employer doesn't provide for more than a few weeks of leave, it's sometimes possible to get an extension. This may be unpaid, or paid at a lower rate, but planning ahead may make it possible to stretch out your leave.

Planning Your Baby's Care

The most important preparation for a return to work is choosing the best possible caregivers for your baby. You'll need to think about these things:

- what's available in your area
- your budget
- your work schedule

- the kind of setting (childcare type) that you think will work best for your baby

Some couples work different shifts, or from home, to minimise the time their baby spends in childcare. Some are lucky enough to have family members or friends who can help out. The dynamics of sharing a child's care can sometimes be challenging for the adults, but this kind of care has real benefits for babies.

What Does Research Say About Different Types of Childcare?
Research from many countries shows the same thing: babies and young toddlers (under two years or so, and definitely under a year) thrive best in a home setting, cared for by people who love them. Unless circumstances at home are unsafe or extremely difficult, babies do best with their parents, and next best with a relative or someone close to the family.

Grandparents – A Special Bond

All over the world, grandparents help care for babies and young children.

I need to make money, and now Isha is five months old. I'm going to look for a job. My mother can help. I can still nurse and give Isha bottles.
– *Fatmata, Freetown, Sierra Leone*

I have doting grandparents who could not wait to spend time with my baby. My father's retirement coincided with my return to work, and he was in his element at the thought of being a hands-on granddad. He told me that the love you have for your children is wonderful, but the love you have for your grandchildren is second to none.
– *Ausilia, UK*

In some communities, it's traditional for grandmothers to nurse their grandchildren while caring for them, as Nicole learned from Rebecca:

As most mothers who have breastfed know, the easiest way to calm a baby is to put the baby to the breast. When trying to calm her grandson,

Rebecca instinctively offered him the breast. Within a few days she noticed that her breasts were producing milk! This was the beginning of many months of breastfeeding him while her daughter was at work. I was so amazed at this special bond between this grandmother and her grandchildren that I hope to be there one day when my own daughters need a backup.

– *Nicole, South Africa*

For more about babies being breastfed by more than one person, see Chapter 18, Milk Sharing.

When relatives are not available, any home-based care may meet babies' needs better than a larger group setting with a professional caregiver.

This makes sense. The more adult attention to go around, and the closer the relationship, the better. Even the most amazing caregiver has only one pair of arms! By the age of two or three, though, many children start to enjoy the company of other children, so group care may work for them.

Research also shows that not all settings of the same type are equal. Some nurseries are much better than others. Another important factor is the amount of time spent at nursery. The outcomes for babies who spend a few hours in nursery a couple of days a week are more positive than for those who are there full-time.

Long, regular separations can be hard for both of you. Research shows that a baby in nursery all day has raised levels of the stress hormone **cortisol**. Cortisol levels are usually higher in the morning, falling through the day. Cortisol levels of children in nurseries stay high through the afternoon. (On weekends, when they're home, cortisol goes down.) It isn't always easy to tell how children are doing at nursery; a child who seems calm may have higher stress levels than one who cries and protests.

Some effects of long hours in group childcare seem to last. Higher levels of behaviour problems are seen into adulthood. Long-term studies show increased risk of overweight in children who were in group childcare in their early years.

Our intention is *not* to make life even tougher for families who already have difficult choices to make. But knowing this information can help as you assess your options, even if they're limited. Liz chose different care for her second child with more knowledge (and a very different baby):

> I wish I'd been able to stay home for longer, but it just wasn't possible. If I'd had more information about the impact of different types of childcare, I would have made different choices. I was so focused on how very hard being apart was going to be, and the logistics of continuing to breastfeed, I think I assumed it wouldn't matter to my baby where they were. We didn't have any family or friends to help, and our workdays weren't flexible, so that made things harder. My eldest child settled well at nursery — he was always with his key worker, and they were happy to cuddle him to sleep and hold him as much as he needed. But my second child was utterly miserable until we could move them both to a childminder. Now I realise nursery was just too busy for him; he was sad to be separated from his brother and he didn't have one consistent caregiver. Both children thrived much better in a home environment. Knowing more about what babies need helped me choose what was right for my children.
> – Liz, UK

The economic priority is to get women back to work – as if mothers with their babies are doing nothing. Research on the first thousand days of life has clearly shown the importance of good early care for children's well-being. Yet the value of spending time with (and breastfeeding) your own young children is not even considered by most economists.

> **Breastfeeding is work. It takes time, effort and skill, and it has immense economic value. Yet breastfeeding women aren't being recognised as contributing to the economy, whereas formula is.**
> – Dr. Phillip Baker, a health and nutrition policy expert in Australia

---

In many countries, good-quality childcare is expensive. We're too often forced to choose between our own needs and our babies'. This isn't okay for anyone. Whatever you have to do, the LLL community is here to support you.

I returned to work after all my babies. For me personally, I feel it made me a better and more well-rounded mother. I sometimes feel guilty that I didn't want to be with my small person 24/7 but remind myself that nuclear families aren't how we are designed to live. That said, I still wanted to meet my baby's needs as well as my own, so we purposely chose a childminder and nanny over a nursery.
– Rae, UK

It was time for me to return to work. I loved breastfeeding, and so did my son. I was so mad that it was so hard to continue with the structure of our society – I would have been away from him for nearly ten hours a day, five days a week. With virtually no childcare options (nannies costing over half my salary, nursery wait lists, etc.), I quit my job to stay with my son, and I am overwhelmed with gratitude that we were in the position to be able to make that decision.
– Monica, United States

Choosing Caregivers
Here are some things to think about when you're choosing caregivers:

- Good caregivers know that **babies need to know and trust them.** They offer settling-in time, their staff turnover is low, and they have enough adult attention to go around. Caregivers are warm and reliable, and they quickly figure out each child's unique personality. They respect parents as the experts on their own children. (You are!)
- **You know your baby best.** Temperament plays a big part in how children cope with separation. A sensitive, slow-to-warm-up baby may be overwhelmed by group childcare, even if his placid big sister seemed fine. Children who have already experienced big separations – like being placed for adoption or having a parent move out – might especially benefit from consistent care from someone they trust.
- If you don't have a family member to help, or a nursery option at work, **consider finding a nursery closer to work than to home.** This means less time away from your baby. (When you're bursting with milk, that half-hour commute seems very long!)

Some Questions You Might Ask

I'LL BE LEAVING MY MILK FOR MY BABY. HOW WILL YOU STORE AND HANDLE IT?

Experienced caregivers may already have a procedure for storing and handling mothers' milk. If not, they should be willing to follow the steps you give them. You can find guidelines on LLL websites and from national health authorities.

WHEN WILL MY BABY BE FED?

Breastfeeding works best when babies are fed responsively (see Chapter 7). Most childcare providers have a schedule, but some are more rigid than others. You can ask for a more flexible approach. It's not helpful if your baby's fed right before you arrive to pick him up. It's frustrating to have full breasts out of sync with a full baby!

CAN YOU SHOW ME HOW YOU WOULD BOTTLE-FEED MY BABY?

There are ways to feed from a bottle (or cup) that help support breastfeeding and reduce the risk of overfeeding and ear infections (see Chapter 18, Supplementing, Weight Gain Worries). Good care providers make eye contact with the baby and pay attention, checking to see if they're going at a comfortable pace. They pause when she needs a break, and don't encourage her to take more than she wants. Feeding comes with cuddles and conversation; it's not just a task to rush through.

WHERE CAN I NURSE MY BABY WHEN I COME TO PICK HER UP?

Nursing when you pick up your baby can be a great way to reconnect after time apart, as well as to relieve full breasts. It also gives you a chance to pick up some of the germs in the setting so you can produce antibodies for your baby. It helps if her schedule's arranged so she's ready to nurse when you arrive. (Of course, you'll call if you're running late!)

WHAT DO YOU DO TO HELP A CRYING BABY?

The answer tells you about the caregiver's philosophy; you want it to match yours. If you carry your baby and respond quickly to crying, you'll want someone who will do the same. Childcare providers can seem intimidating. But you're paying for a service, and you have a right to request whatever your baby needs. If you don't have confidence in a caregiver, maybe your baby won't, either. Visit the settings you're considering. Watch the children, chat with other parents. Ask questions and follow your instincts. Local LLL meetings and online groups can be good places to find out about childcare.

Planning Your Milk Supply

Older Babies

If your baby will be older than about eight or nine months when you go back to work, you can probably skip this section. The older babies get, the more flexible breastfeeding becomes.

Babies who already enjoy family foods often manage without milk while you're at work.

Leah's and Louise's babies were both twelve months old when they returned to work:

> I always hated pumping, and never really had much success with it, so my goal was to pump as little as possible just for comfort, to make it through the workday. For the first week back at work, I pumped twice each day. When I picked up my son from nursery and we got home, he would have a nice long breastfeed. We still breastfed to sleep and during the night. For the second week I pumped only once a day. By the third week I didn't need to pump at all. We went on to breastfeed for another two years!
> – Leah, Ontario, Canada

> With eleven hours apart, I anticipated needing to pump to keep my breasts comfortable but was pleasantly surprised I never needed to. Despite being a frequent breastfeeder, he managed fine when we were apart, requiring no expressed milk, or any other milk.
> – Louise, UK

On the other hand, Rosie continued expressing through her baby's second year:

> Some people don't express at all at work, particularly after twelve months. Others do! I still express five ounces at lunchtime, at twenty months. It's okay to do whatever is best for you!
> – Rosie, UK

Babies who've started family foods but aren't eating much yet may eat more when you're away. You might want to leave some milk for peace of mind, but (unless you already know your older baby likes expressed milk) there's no need to spend much time and energy expressing in advance.

If you've got unused milk, see Chapter 18, Milk Sharing. Some milk banks accept donations up to a year after the milk was expressed.

Younger Babies

If your baby is still fed entirely or mostly on your milk, expressing ahead of time can ease the transition back to work. It builds up your milk supply, too – an insurance policy in case of difficulties. The easiest way to do this is to express once or twice a day, beginning a few weeks before you start work, or (if you're going back to work soon after birth) once nursing is running smoothly. Even if you express just once, first thing in the morning, when the flow is often fastest, you'll soon build up a freezer stockpile. You could express before, during, or after nursing – experiment to see what works best. You don't need to fill your entire freezer, or even a drawer. You just want enough for a bit of a cushion against emergencies. Most of the time, you'll give your caregiver milk you expressed the day before.

When Ausilia lost her milk stash, it wasn't a disaster:

> I used to waste hours trying to pump to build a freezer "stash" and lost it all when our secondhand freezer broke down. I was quite pragmatic about it and decided that I would just pump at work each day for the following day.
> – *Ausilia, UK*

You'll be adding plenty of breastmilk as you go – and fresh milk is better than frozen. Expressing and storing milk are covered in Chapter 15.

Starting to Express

Don't worry if you don't get much milk when you first begin expressing. You're just telling your body to make extra in *addition* to nursing. You should start to see the results in a couple of days. When you're expressing *instead* of nursing, you'll get much more!

How Much Milk?

Between one and six months old, breastfed babies normally take about 60 to 120 ml (2 to 4 ounces) of milk at a feeding. If you'll be away for nine hours, your baby will probably need about six 60-ml (2-ounce) containers. You might want to send more milk at first, so the caregiver has plenty on hand. Over time you can adjust up or down. Use small containers until you have a feel for how much your baby needs; that way your caregiver won't waste precious milk.

If you don't express enough on a particular day, or your baby routinely drinks a bit more than you pump at work, pumping on the weekend puts you ahead again.

If you run into nursing challenges during your maternity leave, get help quickly, while you're still at home. This is the time to line up your support (see Chapter 2). Employed members of LLL communities are generous with ideas and encouragement.

Do I Need to Drop Feeds in Advance of Going Back to Work?

If your baby can eat solids while you're away, you might wonder about reducing feedings in advance, so you're no longer nursing during what will be work hours. This isn't usually necessary, as long as you can express for comfort at work.

Some people prefer to get their baby, and breasts, used to nursing just in the morning, evening, and overnight, so they don't have to deal with uncomfortable or leaking breasts at work. If this is your goal, reduce feeds gradually, allowing your breasts to be a little full (which slows down milk production) but not too uncomfortable. You can reduce your milk supply in the same way if your caregiver will be feeding your baby formula. Part-time nursing is very doable, especially after the early months.

On the other hand, as one mother put it, "I wouldn't cuddle my children less just because I'm going back to work. I cuddle them more while I can! Why would I breastfeed less?" You could nurse as normal right up to the day you go back to work, making the most of your leave. This is what Hannah did:

> To start with I needed to express a little for comfort, but it soon became apparent that he didn't want to take expressed milk at nursery, and we quickly settled to a pattern where we'd feed as normal when we were together, and the days I was working he would have water and cow's milk. I was glad not to need to express at work because alongside the pressures of returning from maternity leave and needing to leave on time ("early"!) to do nursery pickup, it felt like another obstacle.
>
> – *Hannah, UK*

Do you and your baby have to adapt to some kind of "breastfeeding routine"?

No. Babies and breasts don't have to do the same every day. You can nurse as much as you like on evenings, weekends, days off, and holidays, and less on workdays. It makes more sense to your baby that she can't nurse because you're not there than for you to mysteriously refuse to nurse her when you are! Plenty of nursing when you're together keeps your milk production strong.

Andrea's baby was more adaptable than she expected:

When I had to go back to work, my baby drank milk either from the breast or from the bottle as if it was the only thing he had ever drunk.
– Andrea, Mexico

Do I Need to Stop Nursing My Baby to Sleep Before I Go Back to Work?

If your baby usually nurses to sleep – as most love to do – you might worry that he'll be upset when you're not there.

Don't panic! Babies find other ways to go to sleep when they're with other people. You can make it clear to your caregiver that you don't want your baby to be left to cry.

Creative caregivers have lots of ways to help babies fall asleep: rocking, patting, singing, wheeling a pram or stroller, using a sling....

Audrey says:

[My partner] developed his own codes, his own tricks, with a baby who usually suckled every hour at night in my presence. He sang, rocked, played, and rocked again. In the end, he spent the most cumulative time alone with Liam.
– Audrey, France

Baby Laveen had two mothers caring for him, so he could still nurse while Kendra, his birth mum, was at work:

I am so grateful I was able to nurse Laveen, and that Kendra gave me this opportunity. It also made the transition for Kendra going back to work significantly easier.
– Cyndel, Ontario, Canada

As long as your baby's safe and happy, it doesn't really matter how he and his caregiver get through the day (or night). Their way may look very different from what you usually do! Enjoy nursing your baby to sleep as much as you like – you can trust him and his caregiver to find their own way. For more about sleep, see Chapter 12.

Planning Your Expression Schedule

When to express at home. When you start expressing, it can feel like you're stealing milk from your baby. Just remember, she *will* get the milk, just not right away!

As your first workday approaches, you might want to build your freezer stash faster. One way is to put the pump near where you often nurse and do a few minutes of pumping after several nursings each day. Another approach is to put the pump somewhere you pass often and do just a few minutes' pumping whenever you go by. For guidelines for storing milk, see Chapter 15.

When to express at work. During a nine-hour separation from a young baby, plan to pump three times to start with, and then experiment. How often you'll need to express depends on how much milk you're making and your breasts' milk storage capacity. Express often enough to keep your breasts comfortable or to meet your day's expression target.

This is real life, of course, so your pumping schedule won't be set in stone. Neither will how much you get when you pump. As one experienced mother said, "Put in your pumping time, and don't fret about the amount you got. It's going to vary. If you see a change over time, that's when to take action. But not after one bad session. Bad sessions happen."

Here are some possibilities for ensuring a steady supply of milk while you're working:

- Nurse first thing in the morning and again right before leaving home, or when you arrive at your baby's nursery.
- If you have a hands-free pump, you might be able to pump while commuting.
- If you have time, express for a few minutes as soon as you get to work.
- The next chance to express might be mid-morning, then lunch, then mid-afternoon.

- If possible, find out whether your child is likely to be awake when you arrive to pick him up. If so, you may want to nurse him before you head home.
- If your child's asleep, express before you leave work or while you're on the way to pick him up if you can't wait until you arrive at nursery or get home.
- Nurse whenever your child likes in the evening and before bedtime.

Nurse at least once during the night, too, if your baby wakes up for it. Extra waking is common at first. Night nursing can help keep milk production strong, and it gives you extra time with your baby. Louise recalls:

> For a few months after I returned to work, he wanted to feed more at night, which was a strain, but it soon settled back to our old normal. Sometimes, though, those added night feeds weren't about milk at all. He would wake and want me, and whilst I always offered the breast, all he wanted was to sit there in the semi-darkness, looking me intently in the eyes. We drank each other in at those times, making up for lost time.
>
> – Louise, UK

Emergency Milk Kit for Work

You might not need any of these items to help you express at work, but it's good to be prepared!

- **Photos or videos** of your baby nursing or looking especially cute, or **a piece of her unwashed clothing** to sniff to help your milk release while expressing. (Or it might work better to think about something else.)
- **Breast pads** – even if you haven't needed them in a while.
- **Spare bra and top,** in case of milk leaks.
- **Silicone breast pads,** to prevent leaks if you have an important meeting or class where leaking would be a disaster. It's probably best to use these sparingly, though, allowing the breast its natural "overflow." Try pressing the heels of your hands firmly against your breasts if you feel a leak starting (this can be done discreetly at a

desk – it's harder if you're standing up!). If you leak a lot, it may be a sign that you need to express more often.
- **A sweater, jacket, or scarf** to temporarily cover any damp patches.
- **Nonsteroidal anti-inflammatory medication** (one you would normally use) in case your breasts get very full and expressing doesn't quickly sort them out. See Chapter 18, Engorgement, Mastitis.
- **A couple of clean flannels** for cold or warm compresses to ease discomfort or help milk flow while expressing.
- The **phone number of an LLL Leader or breastfeeding helpline** in your contacts!

Making the Most of Time Together

It can be tempting to ask someone else to give your baby another bottle after work while you make dinner or help older children with homework. As much as possible, though, when you're at home, aim to nurse. Frequent "conversational" nursings keep a milk supply – and a nursing relationship – in good shape. Babies who associate the breast with comfort and pleasure as well as food will usually keep right on nursing, however much you're separated.

Customising Work and School Arrangements

> I was a midwife working in a clinic. I gave birth to all three of my children at the clinic where I worked and was already back at work from the second week after giving birth. Before my babies could lift their heads up, I would assist the birth of other mothers' babies while my children slept in the labour room. Later, I used the onbuhimo (back-carrying sling), which made it possible to work whilst carrying the baby. Breastfeeding between deliveries, breastfeeding together with a new mother whilst explaining to her how to breastfeed her baby, breastfeeding in front of pregnant women at an outpatient appointment! Everyone was always surprised, saying, "Oh, wow, babies want to breastfeed so often!" I learned that it is possible for breastfeeding to become a natural aspect of daily life, with the support of one's employer and the system.
> – Akiko, Japan

Throughout history, women have been creative about combining motherhood with other commitments. You might be short on options, but one or more of these might work for you:

- **Take your baby with you,** like Akiko in her midwifery clinic. Maybe we can stretch our ideas of what is possible!

My boss told me even before my son was born that I could bring him to work. He gave me the choice to have a fenced-in play area or to have him in my office. We removed a table to accommodate a bouncing chair. I was able to nurse, take care of, and enjoy him while I worked.

– Sara Diana, from Barcelona, children born in Mexico

- **Reduce your hours, or job-share.** Sometimes, once childcare costs are factored in, shorter hours actually mean better income.
- If you're studying, **take courses part-time or online.**

I was apprehensive when I found out that I was pregnant while at university. I had my baby girl in July and decided I would take an interruption year so I could fully focus on her. Now she's older I find I have longer periods of time that I am able to get things done, including some studying. When I go back to university, I plan to see if I can do some study from home so I am still available to her, although the days I do need to be in I plan to enroll her in the nursery on campus so I am close by and can be available to her in my breaks.

– Kia, Manchester, England

- **Work the same number of hours but on a more flexible schedule.** Maybe you could do your work in four longer days rather than five, so you'd have less total time away from your baby. Taking the middle day off (for example, Wednesday if you work Monday to Friday) means you're only away two days in a row.
- **Do some or all of your work remotely.** A caregiver in your home could help as needed, while you are still able to be available to your baby.

Working from Home

What mothers say about working from home:

No one admits it, but it is totally normal and common to work from home with a sleeping, feeding baby or toddler on your lap!
– *Rosie, UK*

I could go for a walk with my baby whilst being on a work call and, for online meetings (with the camera on), I would usually either be carrying my baby on my front or on my back with him asleep, or I would be breastfeeding him. I never asked for anyone's permission to breastfeed my baby on camera, and I never received any comments (apart from positive ones whenever I showed my baby on camera, usually near the end of the meetings).
– *Shoko, the Netherlands*

She fed until twenty-two months and mostly through every Zoom meeting I had once she got tall enough to reach the door handles!
– *Ausilia, UK*

If you can't change your work or school schedule, maybe you can customise your breastfeeding arrangements:

- **Return to work on a Thursday or Friday** to minimise the initial separation. It will be like a trial run with a two-day holiday before Monday rolls around. If you can, take the next two Wednesdays off. You'll work no more than two days in a row for a full two and a half weeks, allowing you and your baby a gentler transition.
- **Go to your baby at lunchtime** or have him brought to you. Half a day is easier to manage from your breasts' point of view! Childcare near your workplace helps make this possible. Some babies find it harder to cope with two separations a day, though.

> When I went back to work, my husband took a six-month parental leave, with my encouragement. I would rush home to nurse her at lunchtime.
> – Janedy, Taiwan

- **Use formula when you're at work and breastfeed at home.** If you're feeling overwhelmed by the thought of pumping, using formula while you're at work and breastfeeding when you're at home may be an option. Any amount of breastmilk your baby gets is beneficial. Nursing as much as possible when you're together helps make combining formula-feeding and breastfeeding work.

> I went back to grad school while Fred was a baby and ended up doing a mix of formula and nursing because I couldn't pump enough. I did bring him to class when he was small enough to not disturb my classmates, but as he got older and more mobile, he had to stay home.
> – Georgie, New Jersey, United States

Talking to Your Employer About Expressing Milk at Work

You might feel a bit uncomfortable thinking about expressing at work, especially if your country doesn't give you a legal right to breastfeeding or expression breaks. But it doesn't have to be a major conversation. You just need to clear the use of a clean and private place.

If you have a desk job, maybe you could pump while you work (for more on hands-free pumping, see Chapter 15). Otherwise, you'll need to take a couple of twenty-minute breaks each day – about the same amount of time most smokers take – in addition to your lunch break (which could be another opportunity to express). If taking the breaks is an issue, you could offer to work a bit later to make up the time.

> I went back to work (part time) when she was three months old and pumped at work. Eventually I got wearable pumps, as I work in theatre and cannot always be gone for thirty minutes at a time during shows/rehearsals. The freedom they give me is amazing! I don't like

pumping and always prefer nursing, but wearable pumps have been a game changer.

– *Allison, North Carolina, United States*

It's to your employer's advantage to help you continue breastfeeding. You're likely to need fewer days off work to care for a sick child. Your own health risks are minimised, too. Studies have shown that nursing parents – and other employees – feel more positive about companies that support them in continuing to breastfeed. So you're not asking for favours – it's in the interest of the organisation!

You might worry about bringing all this up before the baby's born. But that's easier than having to figure it out when you come back to work. It's often helpful to talk to colleagues who've done it – they'll have been-there-done-that tips and can help you in getting what you need. Your human resources department may also be able to help.

If there just aren't any private spaces where you work, perhaps you could borrow someone else's office or an empty meeting room. More than one employee has turned her back to the door or rigged a curtain across a cubicle opening. Not ideal, but these are all approaches that have worked for others. A "Baby's Lunch in Progress" sign can let colleagues know they shouldn't barge in. Some last-ditch options include your car or the bathroom (which might need an extension cord if there's no outlet, and which isn't a legal option in all countries). Ausilia ran into some challenges but was able to make it work:

> I had to arrange for my work to put aside a clean room I could use at the same time each day. It doubled as the prayer room and an office. Trying to explain that I'd need the window blocked out was painful, so I resorted to doing it myself. And let's not talk about the time I spilled my milk or forgot my cool bag (hurrah for a supportive team!). Sorting a room on the odd occasion I worked from a different office was strangely easier, with one receptionist insisting on standing outside my door as I pumped to ensure I wasn't disturbed!
>
> – *Ausilia, UK*

If it's hard to talk to your employer about breastfeeding arrangements in person, an email might be easier. When writing, you can take your time, point out why breastfeeding is important, and run your words past a few friends. Explain why you'll be doing it and what you'll need rather than asking permission. You're well within your legal rights almost everywhere in the world, as Audrey discovered:

> I work in retail, and I worked overnight as a stocker from 10:00 P.M. to 7:00 A.M. At our workplace, we would have two fifteen-minute breaks and one one-hour lunch. When I said I would like to express milk while at work, they told me I had to do it within my allotted break times. It takes five minutes to set up, five minutes to dismantle, which meant, by their terms, I only had five minutes to pump. They would not budge on this. So I would use my whole hour lunch to pump everything I possibly could. Several weeks of this and my body decided that the baby must not be needing the milk, so it diminished. Crying and dejected, I finally gave up. It hurt my heart a great deal to make the decision, but I was too tired to fight anymore.
>
> It wasn't until a year and a half later I found out the company policies and laws that my workplace broke. I was so angry. [With] my second child I came back with the policy and Texas laws printed, and highlighted the areas that stated how they have to provide a place and how it is an offence to make me express milk in the car or bathroom. They couldn't argue anymore. When I came back from my leave, they had altered a fitting room with an electrical outlet that could be mine to use.
>
> During my [next] pregnancy, our store was going through a remodel. They added a mothers' room! The one thing I would tell first-time mothers is about the laws: keep printed copies of the laws and their workplace policies with them, so they don't spend their time arguing.
> – Audrey, Texas, United States

Health and safety laws may help you if your country has no legal protection for breastfeeding or expressing. You can point out that not being able to express at work could lead to mastitis.

Storing Milk Expressed at Work

A fridge or insulated cooler with ice packs will keep your milk cold at work. If you work a standard work-week, when you pick up your baby you can give your caregiver the milk you expressed today to be used tomorrow. Milk pumped on Friday can be stored in the fridge until Monday. For more on milk storage, see Chapter 15.

Variable Schedules

Whatever your schedule, there's almost always a way to combine breastfeeding with your job. Breastfeeding is more of a challenge if you do shift work, but it can be done:

> When Amalya was six months old and Indi two and a bit, I went back to work part-time as a nurse. I was out of the house for fourteen hours at a time, and my husband and our mums were taking it in turns to care for the girls. Amalya wasn't the slightest bit interested in the milk I pumped for her, preferring ham sandwiches, Granny's cake, and an abundance of fruit!
>
> – Samantha, from the UK, living in Bali, Indonesia

> I went back to work when my baby was eleven months old. My job is almost entirely twelve-hour shifts, including night shifts, and it was a forty-five-minute drive away. My biggest worry was how my baby would cope at night without me. My husband felt we should night-wean to prepare, which we did. I have colleagues who didn't, and I'm not sure it was necessary. For the first few months I had to pump at work at least twice [a day] for comfort – it was too painful to put my seatbelt on otherwise! My baby didn't take a bottle, so I wasn't pumping for the milk – in fact, I donated it to my local milk bank. After a while I was able to just pump once a shift and then not at all. When I was home my baby would still feed what felt like a hundred times a day, and continued until three years old, so it certainly didn't shorten our breastfeeding relationship!
>
> – Ilana, UK

Military Mothers

> I was able to breastfeed as an Active Guard & Reserve soldier in the Mississippi Army National Guard. Doubt began to rear its ugly head when I was offered a promotion to sergeant first class in a city that was three hours from my home. If I refused the promotion offer, I would lose my full-time job and be removed from the AGR programme. I left not only my son, who was sixteen months at the time, but the only unit that I had known for the last twenty years of my military career. I had a stash of milk and was reassured by my husband, Rahshaad, that everything would be

okay. I was pregnant, driving back and forth for doctor appointments, without a fridge at my unit, making at least two trips to the store for ice, driving a round-trip of two hours between the unit and Camp McCain so that I could sleep at a safe place, having to deal with a male-dominated unit, and all while being in one of the most racist areas in Mississippi. This unit was the total opposite of my previous unit, and they were not too accommodating when it came to my having to pump and store my milk.

I would be gone for almost two weeks on at least two separate occasions, and it was not looking good for my milk supply. I remember thinking that the military had destroyed my breastfeeding journey and ruined my relationship with my son. I now fully understood the feelings that military mums have about leaving their little ones at such impressionable ages. I became a lactation education counsellor and later a military lactation counsellor in hopes to continue to educate civilians and the military in Mississippi on the importance of breastfeeding education. I want to give everyone the tools and the will to fight for their right to breastfeed.

– *Montoya, Mississippi, United States*

Being both a mother and a member of the military can be one of the most challenging work situations, especially if you're on active service. Maternity leave, sometimes called convalescent leave, is often short, and schedules and pumping don't always mix, plus sending milk home for your baby may not be possible. Temporary or partial weaning is sometimes necessary, though some manage to maintain their supply by pumping, even when they can't get their milk to their baby. Some military policies require that mothers be given a space to pump, although that may mean sitting on the edge of your cot in a tent or converted supply closet.

Though it may be stressful, preparing for the first postnatal weigh-in and fitness test probably won't affect your milk – breastfeeding may even help you lose weight (see Chapter 18, Diet and Weight).

Deployment deferment after birth varies widely by country and branch of the military. Despite the obstacles, many mothers have found ways to make breastfeeding work while they're on active service. But if it's all just too much, services may allow for separation due to parental hardship both during the pregnancy and after birth.

Introducing Bottles (Or Not)

If you return to work when your baby is older, family foods and water may be all he needs to keep him fed and hydrated while you're away. Health professionals recommend that all babies, including those who have always been bottle-fed, stop using bottles by eighteen months (some advise twelve months) because of their effects on teeth, weight, and iron levels. If your older baby is already drinking from a cup, these are good reasons not to introduce a bottle at all.

But if you're going to be separated from a young baby regularly, you'll probably be using bottles. They're the most common, convenient, and usually easiest way to feed a small baby away from the breast, and they're what most caregivers expect.

There's no magic window of opportunity for starting bottle-feeding. If you can, wait until nursing is going smoothly. There's no need to introduce bottles long in advance; enjoy nursing while you and your baby are together. Some parents have their caregiver introduce bottles, with no practice beforehand. Others start offering bottles at home a couple of weeks before returning to work.

Don't be surprised if, like Ausilia's baby, yours won't take a bottle from you!

> As the time got closer for me to return to work, I kept being asked whether I'd started pumping for my baby, and what if she doesn't take a bottle, and it wasn't a good idea to keep breastfeeding because how would anyone else settle her. I'd try her occasionally whilst I was still on maternity leave, and she'd never take it . . . but why would she, when the boob was in eyeshot!
> – Ausilia, UK

You could try going out for an hour or so and having someone else make an attempt. If that doesn't help, see If Your Baby Won't Take a Bottle later in this chapter. We know it might be hard to believe right now, but your baby won't starve – even if, like Lynn's baby, she doesn't eat much while you're away:

> My daughter could drink from the bottle, but preferred the breast a lot. She would drink some at the nursery but kept this to a minimum to get through the day.
> – Lynn, Turnhout, Belgium

Allison and her partner found a novel solution when their baby started refusing bottles:

> My little one had a bottle strike for a month (around four to five months old) and would not drink any milk while I was gone. I kept pumping at work to keep my supply up, and my partner kept offering my breastmilk; then we nursed on demand at home as well. Eventually we introduced a straw cup. Not sure if it was some negativity to the bottle specifically, or what, but she is now great at drinking breastmilk, and water, from her straw cup.
> – Allison, North Carolina, United States

If necessary, your baby can get those daytime feedings in during the evening and nighttime instead, in a pattern called "reverse cycling." At one LLL meeting, mothers described their babies sometimes sleeping eight or nine hours at night. Other mothers were concerned that their babies might not be eating often enough while they were at work. Hey, if a baby can go that long at night, she can go that long during the day. But she really can't do *both*! Night nursings are a big help to your milk supply if you're away during the day, as Sorrel and Ausilia discovered:

> Co-sleeping and breastfeeding through the night enabled me to feel connected to my son when I returned to work. My hours were long and I was exhausted, but we all got more sleep, plus he got my milk without my needing to pump during the day.
> – Sorrel, London, UK

> My pumping yield was low, and I found that my baby wouldn't drink it, so I gave up, as my baby was hitting all her growth milestones. And she was okay. There was some reverse cycling, but I didn't notice it too much, as we also bed-shared, so the bar was on tap throughout the night anyway.
> – Ausilia, London, UK

For more about easier nights, see Chapter 12.

If Your Baby Won't Take a Bottle

Be patient and creative if your baby refuses a bottle. Something almost always works! Here are some ideas you can try:

- **Have someone else offer.** If someone else is used to giving bottles, the baby may pick up on their confidence.
- Offer the bottle as just one more interesting thing when the baby **isn't hungry.** Let him explore it and find out for himself that there's – cool! – something he recognises in the bottle. Squeezing a drop onto the tip for him to taste may help.
- **Dance and sing** while you offer the bottle – make it part of a dinner show.
- Offer the bottle **when your baby's sleepy,** either just waking up or drifting off, when he's running more on instinct than on intellect.
- Try **different types of bottle teats** to see if there's one he'll accept.
- Offer **a plain cup or a sippy cup.** Older babies might think it's exciting to drink from a cup like their big brother's, or yours. Nobody said milk has to come from a bottle!
- **Warm the milk** (but not in a microwave, which can create hot spots).
- **Hold the baby close,** mimicking a nursing position, to make bottle-feeding feel more like nursing.
- Use **lots of cuddling** and cooing.
- **Wrap the bottle in something of yours.** One father wore his partner's robe when he offered their baby the bottle. It worked! (This is just to get things started; your nursery provider won't have to borrow your clothes.)
- See if yours is a baby who'll **learn bottle-feeding better from you** than from someone else.
- Offer the bottle **tucked underneath an adult arm** so the baby feeds from it in a breastfeeding position, with the bottle nipple close to where your nipple would be.
- Bottles can be given in **skin-to-skin contact.** Some babies will accept a bait and switch with a little milk from the breast beforehand to take the edge off their appetite. Again, this is just to get your baby started. Your caregiver won't have to take off their clothes – though dads and co-parents might enjoy snuggling their baby skin-to-skin!

If those don't work, see if you can make bottle-feeding different from nursing:

- Hold the baby in a **totally different position,** facing away from you, or in an infant seat.

- Offer the bottle in a **new setting,** in your sitter's home or riding in a sling.
- **Distract your baby,** and offer the bottle when he is watching people walk past a window or children playing in a park.
- **Chill the bottle and milk;** teething babies may especially appreciate this.
- If your baby is older, **make taking the bottle a game.** Have fun in a shared bath with a water-filled bottle. Sprinkle the water over each other, laugh, suck on the bottle, be goofy with it.
- Offer a **"milk slushy,"** partly frozen milk from a spoon. Nobody said milk had to be liquid!

Help! My Caregiver (Not Necessarily the Baby) Wants More Milk!

Here are some things to investigate before you put your pumping into overdrive.

Could It Be the Setting?

Your baby might be drinking more than she needs at nursery. **Babies don't need more and more milk over time** – their peak milk intake is usually reached around one month after birth. Some babies do take more milk per feed as they grow, but this is balanced out by taking fewer feeds – they don't need more milk overall.

- **Watch the baby, not the bottle,** to know when the feed is over. Your caregiver can always put more milk in the bottle if your baby needs it, but encourage them not to start with too much. You could send in mostly 60- or 90 ml (2- or 3-ounce) portions, with a few 30 ml (1-ounce) portions for top-ups.
- **Offer a dummy** if your baby's well fed but still needing to suck.
- **Offer attention and holding** as well as food. Your smart baby might have learned that she gets held when she's fed. Some caregivers may be willing to use a sling or soft carrier to give your baby the body contact that means as much to her as food.
- If your baby's already eating family foods, **replace some milk feeds** with meals, snacks, and water.

For more on how to avoid overfeeding, see Chapter 18, Weight Gain Worries.

Could It Be a Frequency Day (Growth Spurt)?
Maybe your baby really does need more milk for a while. Mothers who are with their babies full-time have days when the baby wants to nurse more. At work, try to pump an extra time or two during the day while this phase lasts. Or add an extra expressing session at home, maybe during the night, knowing that it's temporary. You could also dip in to your freezer stash and rebuild as you go.

None of the Above Seems to Be Enough?
Here are some things that can also be playing a role:

- **How's your pump working?** Parts wear out and need replacing. See Chapter 15 for troubleshooting tips for breast pumps.
- **Has your period recently come back?**
- Could you be **pregnant?** A gap of six hours or more without nursing or expressing may trigger the return of fertility.
- Are you taking any new medications – maybe **contraceptives or decongestants** – that can sometimes reduce milk production? For more about hormonal contraception, see Chapter 9 and Chapter 18, Medications.

If you're not sure, a breastfeeding supporter can help you figure out what's going on.

Missing Your Baby, Your Baby Missing You

> When my then-fourteen-month-old began attending nursery, she carried little bags of breastmilk down the hall with her, and I pumped in my office at work, missing her at every moment.
> – B.J., England

> So, the day comes for my office return, and I have to say I skipped into work. I was in my element, and I needed to be back. I know it's not for everyone, but it was the right decision for me.
> – Ausilia, London, UK

Going back to work can be stressful, especially if you live where maternity leaves are measured in weeks. No matter how well you have all your resources lined up, no matter how much you've missed your job, or the income, or your colleagues, separating from your baby might be one of the hardest things you've ever done. Even thinking about leaving your baby can feel overwhelming.

You might also feel relief. In some communities, life at home with a baby is a lonely experience. You might have so many strong, contradictory feelings that you wonder how your heart can take it! While some want to return to work fairly early, and certainly have the right to, many would love to wait longer. So what can you do, if you can't stay with your baby as long as you (and your baby) prefer?

Helping Your Baby Manage Separations

Here are some ideas other families have used to help their babies through the working day:

- **Take time to help your baby get to know your caregiver** in advance. If you'll be taking your baby to nursery or someone else's home, try to spend some time there – maybe an hour or two a day over a week or more – with your baby before you start work. That way it'll be a familiar place when he's first left without you.
- Leave with your baby some items that have **your comforting scent** on them – a T-shirt you've slept in, maybe.
- **Try to arrive early enough that you don't have to rush off.** Maybe you can nurse your baby one more time before leaving. Or hold him while the caregiver talks to him or plays peekaboo. It's hard on all of you when you dash in and drop off a crying, protesting baby.
- **Don't rush in and scoop up your baby** at the end of the day. Sit beside him, or near him, until he's ready to come to you. Babies sometimes protest being picked up as much as they do being dropped off. Take time to help your baby through this transition.
- **Ask your caregiver for a daily update.** This will help you understand your baby's needs – if you know he didn't nap well that day, or ate more than usual, you can adjust your evening plans.
- When you get home, try to **clear some time to focus on your baby** before starting on chores. Older children may need to wait a little longer for your attention.
- Be prepared for some **marathon nursings during the night** – on- and-off nursings that last for several hours. They're a way of reconnecting, building up your milk, and giving both nutrition and immunities to your baby.

- **Consider using a sling** or soft carrier when you and your baby are together. It allows you to get other things done while meeting your baby's need for contact.

In the future, if you have the time, money, and energy, do what you can to advocate for legislation that supports mothers and children, so that our children, when they become parents, aren't faced with these dilemmas. For now, you're working enormously hard to meet both your child's needs and the requirements of the workplace. Continuing to breastfeed will help buffer both you and your child against life's stresses. The support of others who have been there can help you get through this intense stage of life, too. You aren't alone.

Changing Your Mind

Many of us find that there's a gap between pre-baby plans and the reality of life with our babies. Priorities change in ways we couldn't have imagined. We're not quite the same people we were before. It's okay to change your mind, and your plans – and to change them again. A lot of parenthood in the years ahead is going to be about adapting to your changing world, and your family's changing needs, like Guajirita did:

> In my family, it was always emphasised that everyone should try to achieve economic independence, especially if you are a woman. The society in which we live is more unfair to women, so a woman must always be, or try to be, independent of her husband, if she has one, and fight for her professional goals at all costs. These mixed feelings, this contradiction, dominated my breastfeeding.
>
> My constant frustrations about work made me reject or want to stop breastfeeding. My conscience, my reading, the breastfeeding groups, the information I was looking for, made me continue. It was very difficult.
>
> I tried to do everything well, and I could not. I felt that I was not taking good care of the baby, even though all day long I was with him. I also felt that I was not doing well with my thesis because I was only taking care of my son.
>
> I could not take it anymore. I decided to stop breastfeeding. It was abrupt, it was not respectful at all. Then the baby got sick, and we spent a week in the hospital. I felt guilty for everything, absolutely everything. I

decided, when the semester in Cuba was over, to come with my son to where his father is and start another life in the Netherlands, look for a job, learn the language, but above all give lots of love to my son and free myself from so many pressures that made me not enjoy this process to the fullest, as I would have liked.

– *Guajirita Alquizareña, from Cuba, living in the Netherlands*

Making the Most of the Time You Have

You and your baby need time together in the early weeks. You're recovering from birth, discovering each other, and beginning one of the deepest and most meaningful relationships you'll ever have. Many communities recognise the first month or so after birth as protected time, enabling the new mother to rest and focus on her baby.

Some of us can only dream about this kind of support. We're expected to provide service as usual almost immediately after birth and, in some countries, to leave our babies a few weeks later. If you're feeling caught between competing demands, it's not because you're in any way inadequate. We're bending biology a long way.

Some of us, consciously or not, harden ourselves to the reality of an early return to work and try not to "melt into our babies" during maternity leave. While it's understandable to try to protect your heart, most of us are happier in the long run if we give our hearts freely to our children – even though doing so seems to make the transition back to work tough at the start. And our babies need us to.

If you're finding it difficult to feel a connection with your baby, there's no shame in reaching out for help. It can be harder to connect with your baby if you never had the experience of a mother who enjoyed spending time with you. Many of us have had to learn about mothering and nurturing for the first time while doing it ourselves. For more about unmothered mothers and unnurtured parents, see Chapter 7.

A baby who feels well loved at home knows how to relate to other caregivers when she needs to. You'll both find ways to manage separation at whatever stage it happens. Nursing – though the logistics might seem complicated right now – can help you stay connected even when apart, as well as protecting you and your child from stress and illness. A strong relationship with your child outlasts any job you'll ever have.

Other Separations

Work isn't the only reason you might need to be away from your baby, of course. Maybe you're wondering how to manage a social event or just go for a run. We have plenty of experience of managing these times away and more.

Microbreaks: Exercise, or a Few Minutes Alone

If you've recently given birth, exercise may be the last thing on your mind! Or maybe you're keen to get your walking or running shoes back on, or return to your gym, pool, or exercise class. Perhaps you're just longing for a few minutes of solitude. Here are some tips for taking a microbreak:

- If you have a choice about when to go on a microbreak, know that **mornings can be the easiest.** Many young babies are most relaxed and sleepy in the morning and most unsettled in the evening.
- **Nurse right before you leave,** to "tank up" your baby and get your breasts comfortable. Your baby might even choose to nap the whole time until you get back.
- **Slings or baby carriers** are a great way for caregivers to keep babies happy without milk. You could leave some expressed milk just in case (but try to make sure your baby's not fed just before you walk in the door!).
- Another option might be for **your caregiver to come with you** and stay nearby so you can easily get together if your baby needs you or if your breasts need relief.

Here are some exercise ideas:

- A **home workout** with a video or app can be great if you can't or don't want to leave the house. Your baby might enjoy watching!
- Some communities have **postnatal exercise classes** designed for both you and your baby.
- **Running pushchairs** enable energetic parents to take their babies along for the ride.
- **Outdoor walking** is excellent exercise, and most babies love to be

walked. You can find "buggy-fit classes" in many cities if you'd like a trainer and some company. Younger babies will usually sleep in a sling or pushchair on the move. Walking can be an ideal opportunity for some uninterrupted thinking time, favourite podcasts, or conversation.

Minibreaks: Weddings, Hen Parties, Holidays, and More

Occasions that used to be a lot of fun can suddenly seem complicated when you've got a baby to consider. With a little planning, though, you can still have a great time. Young babies are very portable (many of us realise this only when it's a bit too late!).

You might have more options than you think:

- Sometimes, you might decide that, on balance, while your baby is very young, **it would be less stressful simply not to go.** Evening events or overnight stays can be especially tricky. There will be other opportunities, when your baby is older and can manage more easily without you.

> I decided to take part in a dance competition in another city. I brought my baby and my mother with me, to get her to bed while I was supposed to be dancing. I only left her for four hours, between 8:00 P.M. and midnight, but they were the hardest four hours of my life. I was on the phone texting my mother most of the time. I didn't dance well, and my baby got tired and cried. When I got back, I took her in my arms, and she started breastfeeding. She soon seemed happy again. I still think about it and wonder what I could have done differently so that she would have had a better experience.
>
> – Aphrodite, Athens, Greece

- Could you **take your baby along?** A young baby in a sling is rarely any trouble and (if awake) may be a star turn.
- If your baby can't stay with you, maybe **someone could look after him nearby.**
- If you need to be away for a longer period, you can find lots of information on **expressing milk** in Chapter 15. Remember that not only will your baby need milk, you'll need to express often enough to keep your breasts comfortable.

- **What you wear** affects how easily you can nurse or express. Glamorous nursing clothes are available for every budget – or wear separates for easy access.
- You can find information on **breastfeeding and drinking alcohol** on LLL websites.

> I took my eleven-month-old to a wedding on what turned out to be the hottest day of the year. It seemed like a good idea at the time to wear a dress that zipped up the back. Even though she often went several hours without nursing, that day she was really thirsty. We spent a lot of time in the bathroom with the dress unzipped!
>
> – Clare, UK

If it's **your own party or wedding,** you have more flexibility with the arrangements. You'll probably want a helper to look after your baby at key moments. Plan for nursing breaks to keep both of you relaxed and your breasts comfortable. When you're choosing your outfit, factor in your changing shape and size. If your baby is young and fully or mostly breastfed, shapewear with underwires can put pressure on full breasts, causing discomfort and swelling. You might want to plan a final fitting shortly before the big day, leaving enough time for adjustments. Remember to allow enough room for your breasts at their fullest!

Hospitalisations

Hospitals used to keep parents away, until they saw how badly that separation worked out for their little patients. Now they usually welcome parents, which makes continued nursing much easier. Some hospitals also enable you to keep your baby with you if you're the patient – perhaps with another adult to help take care of the baby.

The biggest challenges can be figuring out nursing before and after surgery, or keeping up your milk production if either you or your baby is too ill to nurse. A hospital stay can also be challenging if you've got more than one nursing child, or the child you need to be with in hospital is not the one who is nursing.

For more information, see Chapter 18, Hospitalisation and

Medications, and LLL websites. Your local LLL group may have useful info about hospital policy, helpful staff, availability of pumps, and layout.

Coming Back to Your Baby

All close relationships are dances of rupture and repair. You move along smoothly together until a misstep interrupts your flow. Then you find your way back together, until you're in sync again.

Relationships with our children are full of subtle back-and-forth moves, too. For example, your baby is tired of peekaboo and turns away. You wait for him to turn back to you before engaging with him again. He protests when you leave the room. Returning, you take a moment to reassure him.

Longer separations need more substantial repair. As Olivia realised, it's worth taking the time to do this well:

> When I would get home from work he would nurse as soon as possible. Even though it wasn't ideal, since I needed to get dinner going and I felt there were tons of things to do, I would sit and nurse him. We connected and I slowed down after a busy day. During times of change and transition, nursing was our constant.
>
> – Olivia, Canada

When you come back, your baby might sometimes turn away and refuse to nurse. He might cling to his caregiver. The hours apart have felt very long to him. He didn't know where you'd gone or when you'd come back, and he's letting you know he's not happy about it. Let him come to you when he's ready. If he still refuses to nurse, you can find information on nursing strikes in Chapter 18 or talk to a breastfeeding supporter.

With every repair, your relationship gets a little stronger. Finding ways to fix the little glitches now builds the skills you'll need to sort out bigger ones as your child grows. Continuing to nurse, or provide your milk for your baby, helps keep your unique relationship strong, as Louise describes:

> I remember fondly the anticipatory "breast tingles" when reaching the road his nursery was on. The mutual contentment of the first feed together

after a long day was almost worth going to work just to experience.
– Louise, UK

Want to know more?

You can find extra resources for this chapter at the "Art of Breastfeeding" tab at www.llli.org.

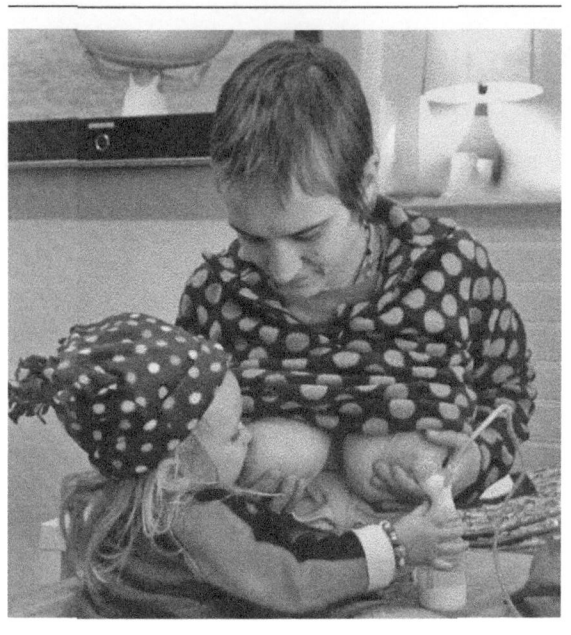

FIFTEEN

Milk to Go

Sebastian was born eight weeks early, and they whisked him off after only a couple of minutes. My doula helped me hand express, reminding me that if Sebastian had been full-term, I would have put him to the breast right away. I didn't get a lot of milk, but it was reassuring to see that I had something to give him. I kept on hand expressing for the next few days, and when my milk came in, I switched to using the hospital's electric pump. I pumped every three hours around the clock until he had grown enough to breastfeed. During his whole hospital stay, he never had anything except my milk.

– *Esmaralda, Ontario, Canada*

- Kristina collected colostrum during pregnancy, knowing her daughter would be born with Down syndrome.
- Brie's twins were born at twenty-nine weeks.
- Fauzia's baby didn't latch for two months.
- Denise returned to work when her baby was nine months old.
- Hannah was admitted to the hospital without her baby.

What do these mothers have in common? They all needed to express milk.

There are as many feelings about expressing as reasons for doing it. A few people decide from the outset to pump rather than nurse directly – a huge labour of love. For more about exclusive pumping, see Chapter 17. For most, expressing is a necessity rather than a choice, and may be connected to a difficult time: your baby is too small or weak or sick to nurse, or you're ill yourself.

Olivia found purpose in expressing when her baby was in the NICU:

> It was just me and my pump in the quiet, empty [hospital] nursery. It would have been so easy to choose to sleep on those first few nights. Nevertheless, I pumped every couple of hours until he was home in my arms. I couldn't soothe him during his night wakes, but I could fill his belly with liquid love when we were apart.
>
> – Olivia, Canada

If you're expressing at work, your feelings might be mixed. Expressing takes time out of your busy day, and you might miss your baby – but feel proud she can still have your milk though you're apart. Whatever your reasons for expressing, we can support you.

It's probably going to be a three-part process:

- **milk out** (of your breasts)
- **milk stored** (until your baby receives it)
- **milk in** (to your baby)

Part One: Milk Out

When your baby can't nurse, or isn't with you, expressing not only keeps him fed, it keeps milk production going. Some expectant mothers buy a breast pump in advance, or get one as a baby gift. Depending on where you live, there may be a bewildering variety of pumps to choose from. How do you know which pump to get? Do you need one at all...?

Hand Expression

Before pumps were invented, if you couldn't nurse, you expressed milk by hand. In many places, this method is still common. It's how Hedi turned things around for her sleepy newborn (for why he was yellow, see Chapter 18, Jaundice).

> My son was born in 1980. The next day he was yellow and sleepy, and I was told he needed two ounces of formula every two hours. I had the [LLL] Leader's number and I wanted to check out this plan. This sweet Leader told me, "Well, I can't tell you not to do that, but let me teach you hand

expression!" Remember, this was forty-two years ago! No FaceTime or Zoom. She described how to get the milk out and cup-feed.
– *Hedi, California, United States*

Hand expression is free and needs no equipment (except maybe something to catch milk in). In the first few days after birth, it's usually the best approach. Amounts are small initially, and colostrum is *sticky*. It likes to cling to the pump, making it easy to lose most of what you've pumped.

On the other hand (pun intended), hand expression takes practice, and it can feel awkward at first. Once you get the hang of it, though, it can be quick and simple. One mother could hold a coffee cup under each breast with her fingers, express with her thumbs, and be done in five minutes!

Why Learn to Hand Express?

- If for any reason your baby can't nurse right away, you'll be able to **get your milk moving.**
- If your breasts feel full and **engorged,** you can express a bit to soften them, making it easier for your baby to latch (see Chapter 18, Engorgement).
- There may be times when **your baby sleeps extra long,** leaving you uncomfortably full.
- Even if you depend on expressing (for work, or a baby who can't nurse), a **pump failure or power cut** isn't a disaster with hand expressing as your backup (see Chapter 18, Feeding in Emergencies).

You can learn to hand express before your baby arrives or afterwards. Collecting colostrum before birth (see Chapter 1) may be especially helpful if you have diabetes or are likely to be separated from your baby.

How to Hand Express Before Birth

When you hand express during pregnancy, amounts are usually tiny: from nothing at all to a few drops. A few people get more. How much you get now *doesn't* predict how much you'll make later!

- The most practical way to store colostrum (your first, rich milk) is usually in a tiny (1 ml) oral syringe. Your healthcare provider might supply them, or they can be bought online or in a pharmacy.
- You can either syringe the drops directly off your nipple (you might need a helper for this!) or express into a teaspoon and use the syringe to suck up the drops.
- Put the syringes in the freezer, in a bag or box labelled with your name. If you're having your baby in a hospital, take the bag of syringes with you, or have it brought to you – ideally in an insulated cooler with ice packs.

How to Hand Express After Birth

What equipment do you need to hand express? To practise, you may want a big bowl on your lap and a towel. That way, you don't need to aim carefully and can mop up any drips. Or just express in the bath or shower and don't bother about collecting the milk yet. Once you get the hang of it, you can express into any clean container. In the first couple of days, when amounts are small, a teaspoon can work well. As amounts increase, you could try a jug or a flexible bowl that lets you form the edge into a spout. You could use a pump flange or regular funnel attached to a bottle or bag. Or, like the coffee cup mother, you can learn to aim carefully!

What about hygiene? You don't need to sterilise your equipment – just wash it thoroughly. Unlike formula, which is a highly processed product, your milk is a living fluid, packed with immune cells that attack germs. The most important hygiene precaution (if you're planning to use the milk, not just practise) is to wash your hands first.

What else do you need to do before you start? You might want to lock the door, put your phone on silent, or find another way to say "Do not disturb." Now you're ready to go!

STEP 1: WAKE YOUR BREAST
Even though there's no baby there, touch tells your breast to get ready. Try the following:

- Gently massage your breast.
- Knead, shake, or tap your breast.
- Gently tug or roll your nipple.

You might feel tingling, or even get drops of milk.

STEP 2: COMPRESS YOUR BREAST

Here's how:

- Hold your breast with your fingers and thumb cupped around it in a C shape, an inch or so (2 to 3 cm) back from your nipple.
- **Compress** the breast by moving your fingers and thumb towards each other. *Don't* drag your fingers or thumb across the skin of your breast – the friction can make you sore.
- **Release** the pressure.
- **Repeat,** in a regular rhythm.

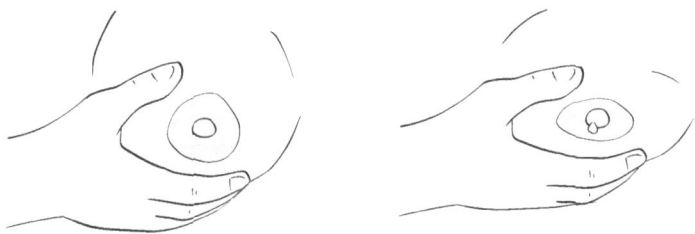

Hand expressing (compress/release)

Move your hand to a different place around the breast after every few compressions or whenever milk flow stops. Then switch to the other breast.

You won't usually get milk right away, but neither does an expertly nursing baby. That's a good thing – this "milk delay" keeps you from spurting milk every time someone brushes against you!

Hand Expressing: Optional Extras

- **Warm your breast and/or hands.** You could use a warm cloth or warm water.
- **Adjust your hand position.** A fraction nearer to or farther from the nipple makes a big difference. Find your personal "sweet spot."
- **Find your rhythm.** Babies usually start with short, shallow sucks, moving into slower, deeper sucks once the milk releases.
- **Push your hand back towards your ribs** just before you compress your breast.

- **Use your other hand as well.** Even touching the breast with one extra finger can encourage faster flow.

Every breast is different – there's no single technique that works for everyone. The key is to experiment and practise. See also Tips for Pumping later in this chapter.

Breast Pumps

Once you've got more milk, pumps have some advantages over hand expression. They're easy to learn, they move the milk directly into a container, and you may be able to multitask while pumping. If you need to express a lot of milk (say, for a baby who's not nursing at all or to increase low milk production), a pump is usually the most practical option.

The kind of pump you need depends on some variables:

- **how often** you expect to pump (occasionally, once or twice a day, or full-time)
- **how long** you expect to be pumping (days, weeks, or months)
- **where** you'll be pumping (if your pump needs to be portable and if there is an electrical socket)
- **what you can afford** (consider if the cost will be covered by insurance, and remember to factor in pumping accessories, which are later in this chapter)

Comparing Pumps

Type	Cost	Effectiveness and Durability	Adjustable?	Notes
Hospital-grade (also called rental-grade)	Most expensive, usually rented out. You'll need to buy the milk collection kits.	Very effective, designed for years of use.	Can usually adjust speed, intensity of suck, pattern of suction.	May have a programme of fast, short sucks at the beginning to stimulate milk release. Most can be used on both breasts at the same time. Are "closed system," so milk can't get into the motor, reducing risk of infection.
Single-user electric pump	Medium price, though a wide range of brands and types. In some countries may be covered by medical insurance.	Generally less durable, but can be expected to last a year of part-time pumping (less if you're doing a lot of pumping).	Most can be adjusted to some degree.	Some can pump both breasts at the same time. Some have batteries so you don't need an electrical socket. Most are "open-system."
Wearable (hands-free) pump	Prices vary, can be expensive.	Quality is improving as they become more popular.	Varies.	You can move around while you pump. Probably not the best option if you need to express a lot of milk, unless used in addition to a larger pump.
Manual pump	Low price.	Less durable, may be better for occasional, short-term use.	You are doing the pumping, so can adjust as you choose.	Very portable. Can be tiring if used frequently.

Squeezy silicone "milk collector"	Low price.	Not a pump in the conventional sense, though can apply gentle suction if squeezed.	Collects milk passively (with no suction or suction is controlled by squeezing).	Very portable. Can be useful for collecting milk on one side while you nurse on the other, or if you just want a small amount of milk. If overused, might encourage oversupply.

What About *Used* Pumps?

Virtual (and some face-to-face) communities are full of ads for secondhand pumps (which may be third- or fourth-hand). Or friends may offer to pass on theirs. The trouble is, **single-user electric pumps aren't built to last** much more than a year, the average length of time you might pump for one baby. When pumps start to wear out, they may not suddenly stop working. The suction and cycling mechanisms can slowly break down until you eventually realise you aren't pumping as much milk.

Most single-user electric pumps aren't "closed systems" like hospital-grade pumps. This means that milk or moisture can enter the mechanical parts, where it can grow bacteria, mould, or viruses. Is this a genuine risk? The companies all say so, of course, but there just isn't good research either way. Our best suggestion is to consider the source, use your best judgement, and at least buy a new pump kit.

Pumping Accessories

Pumps often have parts that can be purchased separately. It's worth taking time to choose well: if pumping is more comfortable, you'll get more milk, too.

Choosing Breast Flanges/Shields
What if pumping is uncomfortable even though the pump is good quality? The most likely problem is a poor fit between your breasts and

the pump **flanges** (or shields), the funnel-shaped pieces. Too small, and they can rub. Too large, and too much breast tissue is pulled in – either way, a mismatch can result in pain and swelling. The standard size that comes with your pump may not fit – or may fit one breast but not the other. Here are a few things to consider:

- Some pump manufacturers have a **range of flange sizes** in their kits – many make them available as accessories.
- There are now many **parts-only manufacturers,** making flanges that can be used with many common pump models. Check to make sure the parts you choose will fit your pump.
- You can also get **inserts to fit inside the flanges,** giving more options for finding a combination that fits well.

To know if you're using the right size flange for your nipples, you can measure their diameter – depending on the brand, the size may be indicated on the packaging. It's even more helpful to look at what happens *when you pump*. You should see the nipple moving easily in the tunnel, pulling your areola *slightly* with it. Look at your nipple immediately after you pump. It will almost certainly be bigger but shouldn't be swollen, and it should be completely comfortable during and after pumping. Let comfort and milk flow be your guides.

You might have to try a few flanges to get the best size. You may even find that eventually you go back to a size you tried earlier and rejected, since breasts and nipples can change over time. Any leftover flanges can be recycled as kitchen funnels or water toys.

Hands-Free Pumping Bras

These allow you to do other things while pumping. They work better for some people than for others. You could buy one – or make your own:

- One option is to get an inexpensive sports bra that zips up the front and fits snugly over your nursing bra. Put it on with your inner nursing flaps down, adjust your breasts normally, and using small scissors,

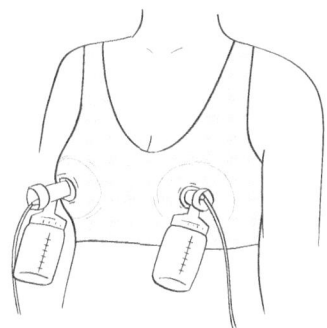

Homemade hands-free pumping bra

cut increasingly large holes at your nipples in the sports bra until the holes are big enough for you to work the flanges through but small enough to hold the flanges firmly and evenly against your breasts. Voilà!
- Another option is to skip the nursing bra and just use any sports bra. Cut holes out of the fabric at your nipples for the flanges.

You can find more hands-free pumping hacks online.

Extra Kit(s)?

If you need to pump several times a day, you'll want to wash or at least rinse the flanges and collection cups and let them air-dry in between uses. If you can afford it, consider getting extra kits so you don't have to wash the parts every time.

Tips for Pumping

For either pumping or hand expressing, these tips will make things easier:

- **Set up an expression station** at home or work with everything you need (water, TV remote, books and toys for older children, phone, laptop, headset...).
- **Open your clothing.** A cardigan or shawl can keep you warm.
- **Find a comfortable position.** Being relaxed helps milk to flow.
- **Wake up your breasts** by massaging, shaking, lifting, stroking, or tapping. Tug or roll your nipples.
- **Look at or think about your baby.** One dad made his partner a video of their baby nursing and looking especially cute, to watch while expressing.
- **Or distract yourself,** as Sara Diana did at work:

> One day my boss came into my office and asked to discuss some results. I asked him if he had a problem with me pumping while we reviewed the data. He said, "Of course not." I activated the pump discreetly. Within five minutes I started to notice leaking. I asked my boss for a second, stopped the pump, peeked through the collar of my blouse, and saw that in those five minutes of total distraction I had managed to fill a cup. I had never been so fast before!
>
> ~ *Sara Diana, from Barcelona, children born in Mexico*

There are a number of other distractions that might work for you:

- Watch or listen to something that makes you **laugh** – great for milk release!
- **Visualisation.** Maybe think of a fountain, waterfall, or geyser!
- **Touch.** Ask your partner or supporter for a shoulder or foot rub; or wrap a shawl or scarf around your shoulders, like a hug.
- **Smell.** Sniff your baby's head. Or smell a piece of your baby's clothing; the scent may help your milk to flow.
- **Sound.** There are guided relaxation tracks designed for expressing. Or experiment to see what kind of music works best for you.

An ICU nurse at my hospital struggled with her milk production because it's a difficult job to leave and go pump. One time she was pumping while soothing music was playing on my computer. She looked down at how much she had pumped and was amazed. She had pumped twice as much as usual!

– *Anna, Texas, United States*

Here are some ideas for pumping:

- **Warm the flanges** with a little warm water, if available.
- **Centre the flanges on your nipples,** top to bottom and side to side (the angle may be different on each breast).
- **Cover the collection bottle** so you can't see what's happening. A sock does the job nicely.
- **Make yourself comfortable.** The flanges don't need to be pressed hard and you don't have to lean forward. Use pillows, a footstool … whatever you need.
- Begin on the **starter setting,** which may be faster and gentler than your "keep it flowing" setting. If your pump is controlled manually, start fast and light, settling into a slower, deeper rhythm when the milk releases.
- As you pump, try **breast compressions** (see Chapter 6) or **gently press the flanges towards you,** hold for two or three seconds, release the pressure, and repeat.
- Take a break midway to **massage your breasts.**
- **Single pumping** (first one side and then the other) makes it easier to massage while you pump, but it takes longer than **double**

pumping and may not yield as much milk. Experiment to see which works better for you.
- **Pump one side while your baby nurses on the other,** to take advantage of the milk releases triggered by your baby.
- If you're working to boost milk production, after pumping, tip the flange down and **spend a minute or two hand expressing** a bit more into it. This helps "strip out" milk the pump couldn't get.
- When you've finished, unless you're pumping for a premature or sick baby, **just rinse the flanges and set them aside for the next pumping, washing them every six to eight hours.** Washing in hot, soapy water is fine for healthy, full-term babies; you don't need to sterilise every time, or maybe at all (for more information, see Pump Hygiene later in this chapter). If your baby is in hospital, follow the hospital's guidelines.

With practice, you may be able to get your double-pumping routine down to a total of ten minutes, including setup and rinsing. Don't worry if it takes much longer than this at first.

How Often?

If your baby is newborn and you're expressing instead of nursing, to bring in a full supply you'll need to express at least eight to twelve times in twenty-four hours without any long gaps (more than five or six hours) in between. Expressing is a big investment of time and effort for a big payoff – plenty of milk – in the months to come.

For more details on how to increase milk production, see Chapter 18, Low Milk Supply.

How Long?

To replace a whole nursing, expect to spend fifteen to twenty minutes expressing both sides at once or ten to fifteen minutes per breast if you're single pumping. Sometimes it's worth expressing a bit longer to see if you can get more milk. Or take breaks in between, doing several stop-start sessions instead of one longer one (usually the best approach if you're trying to increase milk production).

Intensive Expressing to Increase Milk Production

Here are some tips from pumping pros:

- Aim for ten, work for eight, and never go under six.
- Don't think "every three hours" or you won't get eight sessions in. Three hours will stretch to three and a half, and by the end of the day you'll have done only five, with no way to catch up. Instead, think – and *do* – eight.
- Put eight to twelve treats in a dish or on a shelf, and eat one each time you express. By the end of the day, they should all be gone.
- Don't worry about spacing out your sessions evenly – babies don't! Just do them whenever you can. It's fine to take a few hours off to go out, or sleep – you can make up for it by expressing more the rest of the day.
- Instead of setting an alarm to pump at night, try drinking a tall glass of water before bed – your full bladder will wake you up!
- Find podcasts, videos, or TV series that you enjoy and treat yourself to episodes while you express.
- Your pump may track pumping sessions for you, or you can get an app to remind you if needed.
- Use an app or spreadsheet to calculate your daily total, or just write down the number of sessions and add them up. If you've got a competitive streak, each day aim to beat your personal best!
- Don't worry that you'll be doing this forever – you won't! Think of it as an experiment, and set short-term goals, like three days at a time. Review how it's going and decide what to do next.
- If one day doesn't go well, learn from it and move on.

Milk Maintenance

Once your milk supply has settled down (usually by four to six weeks), how often you need to express depends on how much milk you need and your breasts' storage capacity. Remember: you make milk fastest when your breasts are emptiest – the pressure of milk in the breast slows production. So, breasts with larger storage capacity (and no, that can't be judged by looking at them!) can go longer between expressions. Breasts with less storage space need to have milk removed more often.

Experiment to find out the minimum number of times you can express while still getting the volume you need. If you start getting less total milk, increase the number of sessions until you're getting as much as you need.

When to Express (If You're Also Nursing)

- **Expressing after nursing.** Removing some of the milk your baby leaves after nursing helps drain your breasts thoroughly and keep up your supply if your baby is not nursing efficiently. If your baby is nursing well, you may not get much milk by expressing afterwards, but that's okay – you're telling your breasts to make more. If your supply is low, your baby may be too unsettled after nursing for you to express. Try offering him the rest of his meal by supplementing – followed by a little "dessert" at the breast if he'd like – and then express.
- **Expressing between nursing sessions.** If you're trying to increase milk production, expressing between nursing sessions (maybe while your baby naps) is also helpful because it gives your breasts more reminders to make milk.
- **Expressing before nursing.** If your baby wants to nurse soon after you've expressed, there may be less milk available in your breasts, but it will be high in fat – like an extra dessert. If you feel like you're "stealing" milk from your baby, remember he'll be getting it all in the end – and the extra expression boosts your overall supply.
- **Do you need to express at night?** It depends on your situation. Is your baby nursing well? You might just want to nurse at night and fit any pumping you need to do into daytime hours. If you're on an intensive milk-increasing plan, you'll probably need to express at least once at night to fit enough in.

Bottom line: you don't need to get too hung up on exactly *when* you express – during, after, or between nursings, day or night. The key thing is the *number of times* – you can flex expressing sessions around other things you need to do.

For expressing while away from your baby, see Chapter 14.

Keep Going

How much you sleep (or eat) won't affect your milk production, but it might have a huge impact on how you're feeling. Intensive expressing is hard work, and you need to look after yourself while you're doing it.

Better still, be looked after by other people. This is not a one-person-size job! Ideally, family or friends will keep you well fed and hydrated, and help take care of everything else. La Leche League groups are always happy to be your cheerleaders.

Troubleshooting Expressing Problems

Problem: Getting Less Milk over Time

COULD IT BE YOUR PUMP?

- Are all the parts **properly connected?**
- **Are any parts frayed, worn, clogged, or soggy?** Discs and membranes can tear, tubing can get pinched and broken, dried milk can prevent valves from sealing, membranes can get wet. Starting at the flange end, carefully check every part, all the way back to the motor.
- Even if your pump is working fine, it might no longer be working well for *you*. It can sometimes be helpful to **change to a different kind of pump** – maybe a larger one – or add a wearable pump for extra on-the-go pumping.

COULD IT BE HOW YOU'RE EXPRESSING?

- Have you been expressing **as often or for as long** as you used to? If you express fewer times than your personal minimum (see How Often? earlier in this chapter), your milk production may gradually go down. You'll need to express more often again while you catch up. If you're just too busy, could you multitask while expressing? If a wearable pump isn't within your budget, maybe a hands-free pumping bra is. But if you really can't express any more than you're doing now, know that any amount of expressing is valuable.
- Have you stopped doing **the "extras" you used to do to encourage milk release?** It may help to try some of the pumping tips in Intensive Expressing to Increase Milk Production earlier in this chapter.

COULD IT HAVE NOTHING TO DO WITH PUMPING?

- Are you **expressing less milk because your baby is older?** If your baby is eating family foods now and nursing less overall,

your milk supply will naturally be lower. Nothing to worry about.
- Have you taken **medication that can reduce milk production?** Hormonal contraception (see Chapter 9) or over-the-counter decongestant medication (see Chapter 18, Medications) can affect your milk production while you're taking them. Talk to your healthcare provider about your concerns.
- **Has your period come back, or is there any chance you could be pregnant?** Many of us notice a brief supply dip for a couple of days during each cycle. If milk supply reduces because of pregnancy, it may be irreversible – though you can keep on breastfeeding if you and your baby want (see Chapter 16).

Problem: Pumping Hurts
We've already covered finding flanges that fit well in Choosing Breast Flanges/Shields earlier in this chapter. Here are some extra ideas for possible solutions:

- **Start with rapid, light suction.** This mimics what babies usually do. If you can, programme the suction on your pump to ease your nipples into the process.
- **Use lower suction overall.** A pump provides the most milk when set at the upper end of fully comfortable. Find your ideal suction level by turning it up until it's a *tiny* bit uncomfortable, then turning it down a fraction.
- **Add lubrication.** Coating the flange or your breast with a bit of olive or vegetable (not corn or nut) oil may provide just enough lubrication to make pumping comfortable. But if pumping is painful, you'll need to do more than this. See Choosing Breast Flanges/Shields earlier in this chapter.
- **Adjust the sucking speed.** Nipples need intermittent breaks in suction – exactly as a baby does while nursing.
- **Make sure the pump is set up correctly** for the way you're using it. For instance, using the double-pumping setting while single-pumping can cause soreness.
- **Check for infection.** Yeast and bacterial infections can make pumping painful. You might notice swelling, colour changes, and pain when you're not pumping. Your healthcare provider and breastfeeding supporter can help.
- **Check for allergic reactions.** Occasionally, sensitive skin reacts

to the material used to make the flange (or to something else the breast is in contact with).
- **Change to a different pump** if possible.

If none of these ideas helps, contact a breastfeeding supporter, a friend who's a pumping pro, the place where you bought the pump, or the pump company's customer service.

Part Two: Milk Stored

Your fresh milk is very different from formula. Even after being frozen, it offers anti-infective qualities no formula has. So it's worth storing your expressed milk in a way that maximises its immunity-boosting power.

What to Store Milk In

Milk for healthy full-term babies can be expressed into any clean container. For convenience, many people opt for bottles or bags (single-use plastic or reusable silicone) designed for human milk storage. But these aren't essential. To reduce plastic usage and keep costs low, you could repurpose any food-grade container with a tight-fitting lid: preserving jars, ice cube trays, food storage boxes. For safe storage, consider these points:

- To avoid possible toxins, **use bisphenol-A (BPA)-free containers.** In some countries it's identified with a 3 or 7 recycling symbol.
- A safer alternative is **polypropylene,** which is soft and semi-cloudy and in some countries has the 5 recycling symbol and/or PP.
- **Glass** is a good option. It's easy to clean and may be better at preserving active components in the milk.
- **Silicone** has some advantages over plastic. Silicone is BPA-free, more durable, and preserves breastmilk nutrients better than plastic.

How much? If you're not sure how much milk your baby is likely to need, try storing 60 ml portions, to start with. These labelling tips can help you:

- Put **the date you expressed the milk** on the container so you can use the oldest milk first.
- If your baby is in hospital or goes to nursery, **add her name** to the container label.
- A tip learned the hard way: if you use bags, it's much easier to write the date on an *empty* bag, not a full one. And use waterproof ink!

How to Store Your Milk

Once your milk is in your chosen containers, you'll be doing one of three things:

- giving it straight to your baby
- putting it in the fridge
- freezing it

The fresher the milk, the more nutritious and disease-fighting ingredients it has. Just-expressed milk (at body or room temperature) has the most. Refrigerated milk has more of those ingredients than frozen milk. And milk frozen for two weeks has more than milk frozen for two months. It's best to refrigerate or chill your milk straight after expressing if it can't be given to your baby in the next few hours. But even long-term frozen milk is far superior to formula. (For context: vulnerable babies in the NICU are fed on donated milk that's been frozen *twice* – once in the donor's home and again after heat treatment in the hospital!)

Pump Hygiene

It's vital to wash and sterilise all equipment used to prepare and feed formula – bacteria love to grow in it. But you can be much more relaxed about handling your own milk. Fresh human milk is full of live cells that kill almost all bacteria, viruses, and fungi it encounters, so it's not necessary to sterilise pump and bottle parts when you're pumping for your own full-term, healthy baby. Just wash thoroughly with hot, soapy water (or in a dishwasher).

Some people choose to sterilise occasionally (maybe once a day, or once a week) for peace of mind. If you plan to do this, check which parts can be sterilised.

To dry the tubes quickly, stand well away from people, pets, and furniture and shake them in circles. Centrifugal force will push the water out of the ends. If a small amount of moisture remains, you can dry it by connecting the tube to the pump and turning it on.

Milk Straight to Your Baby

Your milk will stay fresh for four hours at room temperature (approximately 77° F/22° C), or up to six to eight hours at lower temperatures. The hotter the day, the shorter the time; but for a healthy full-term baby, there's no need to rush to put the milk in the fridge. If you're planning to use it at the next feed, you can just leave it out – sealed tightly in case it gets knocked over. (Whoever said, "Don't cry over spilled milk" had clearly never expressed!)

Milk from your before-work pumping can be given to your caregiver to use in the next few hours. If you have a commute of more than half an hour, it may be a good idea to put your milk in an insulated cooler with ice packs. Not because it won't last that long, but just in case there are any travel issues, such as the trip taking longer or the milk being exposed to a higher temperature.

Milk to the Fridge

You can combine the milk from several expressing sessions in one container. Chill the newly expressed milk separately first, so you're adding cold to cold. Your milk is good for four days in the fridge. Put it in the back, not in the door, where the temperature tends to vary most. Any unused milk can be frozen after four days.

HOW TO WARM REFRIGERATED MILK

- Hold the container under warm running water for several minutes, or stand it in a pan or jug of hot water.
- *Don't* heat the milk directly on a stove – you may overheat it, damaging some of the active components.
- *Don't* use a microwave – it can cause hot spots in the milk, which could burn your baby badly.
- If you're out and about, you could take a flask of hot water to warm your milk. If you're in a café or on a plane they'll probably be happy to provide hot water.
- Bottle warmers, designed to heat formula, can also be used to

warm your own milk – although because it's so quick and easy to warm milk using hot water, there's probably no point getting one just for this purpose. Follow the manufacturer's instructions, and heat the milk only as much as your baby needs.
- Heat your milk to a comfortable feeding temperature, which is usually what feels warm, but not hot, on your wrist.
- Some babies are happy to drink milk at room temperature, or even chilled. (If your baby is teething, she might also appreciate a chilled bottle teat.)

WHAT'S MILK MEANT TO LOOK LIKE?

Don't worry if your milk is separated into two layers. All freshly expressed milk separates, including fresh cow's milk. (Most milk in stores is homogenised to prevent separation. The fat globules are broken up under pressure so they disperse evenly through the milk.) The top layer is the cream, which just means it has more fat. Swirl your milk gently, and don't worry if it doesn't look totally mixed.

Don't worry about the colour of your milk. Milk can look different depending on when and how it was expressed, and what you've been eating. Just remind yourself, *If my baby got this milk directly at the breast, I'd have no idea what colour it was!* If the milk looks red or pink, search "blood in milk" on LLL websites or contact a breastfeeding helper.

Storage of Fresh Human Milk for Healthy Full-Term Babies					
Milk Storage/ Handling	Room Temperature (50–81°F/ 10–27°C)	Insulated cooler bag (5–39°F/ –15–4°C)	Fridge (39°F/4°C)	Freezer compartment of fridge with separate doors (0°F/–18°C)	Deep freezer (–4°F/ –20°C)
Fresh	Up to 4 hrs. (optimal); 6 to 8 hrs. if at the lowest temperatures.	Up to 24 hrs.	Up to 4 days (optimal); 5 to 8 days if very clean conditions.	Up to 3 months (optimal); up to 6 months (okay).	Up to 6 months (optimal); up to 12 months (okay).
Frozen, thawed	Up to 4 hrs.	Up to 24 hrs.	Up to 24 hrs.	Do not refreeze.	Do not refreeze.

| Fed (the container of milk has already been offered to the baby) | Do not maintain at room temperature. | Up to 1 or 2 hrs. | Up to 1 or 2 hrs. | Do not refreeze. | Do not refreeze. |

Adapted from *Breastfeeding Answers: A Guide for Helping Families* (Nancy Mohrbacher, 2020) and *Core Curriculum for Interdisciplinary Lactation Care* (2019).

Milk to the Freezer

- Milk expands as it freezes, so leave some space at the top of the container.
- You can add refrigerated milk to frozen milk; think, *Add cold to cold*.
- Store milk in the middle of the freezer – temperatures fluctuate more at the sides.
- Double-bagging reduces the likelihood of leaks. The outer bag needn't be designed to hold human milk. Keeping frozen milk inside a second bag or container can also reduce long-term "freezer taste."
- Lay bags flat to freeze them. Once they're solid, you can stand them in rows or stack in piles (alternating the direction keeps your pile even).
- Make a "filing system" so you can use older milk first. One way is to put new milk at the back.

See the previous table for maximum recommended freezing times.

Power Cut!

If you're reliant on frozen milk, a power cut could be your worst nightmare. But you may be able to save all or most of your milk in some situations:

- Your milk is probably okay for up to two days if the freezer is full (one day if it's half-full). If your freezer is a compartment inside a fridge, it may defrost faster.

- Packing foods close together helps them stay frozen longer.
- Adding any available ice to the freezer will help the milk stay frozen longer.
- If it's below freezing outside, you can store your milk in snow or deep shade – but don't leave it exposed to the sun.
- As long as it still has a frozen core, it's okay to refreeze partially defrosted milk.

THAWING FROZEN MILK

It's safest to thaw milk in the fridge overnight or hold it under cool running water, gradually increasing the water temperature. Heat thawed milk as described earlier in How to Warm Refrigerated Milk. But maybe you don't need to heat your milk at all – just like big kids, some older babies are happy to drink cold milk.

Strange Smell?

Does your expressed milk smell or taste soapy or fishy after thawing or standing for a while? This odour is caused by the breakdown of milk fats. It's often said that this breakdown in expressed milk is the result of higher levels of lipase enzymes (normal substances that help the baby digest fats). Research *hasn't* shown higher lipase levels in milk that smells soapy – but milk does seem to behave differently in storage depending on who's expressed it and how.

Strange-tasting milk is completely safe, and most babies will still drink it. Milk banks will usually accept milk that tastes unusual, which tells you a lot about how safe it is! The breakdown of fats helps protect the milk against microbes. But if your baby turns her nose up at it, all is not lost:

- **Keep storage times as short as possible.** Fat in milk breaks down over time.
- **Double-check your storage procedures.** It might help to switch to a different kind of container, freeze the bottle or bag in an extra container, store the milk in a colder part of the fridge or freezer, or turn down the temperature.
- **Try turning down the speed and suction on your pump.** Some experts think adjustments while pumping can help preserve milk better.

- Some parents find that their babies will accept the "soapy" milk if it's mixed with fresh milk. Experiment to find a ratio your baby will drink.
- If nothing else works, you can try to stop the fat breaking down by "deactivating" the lipase. Heat freshly expressed milk to scalding (bubbling around the edges, but not boiling), then quickly cool and freeze it.

STORING THAWED MILK

Thawed milk can be kept in the fridge for up to twenty-four hours and at room temperature for up to four hours. Don't refreeze completely thawed milk. See Power Cut! earlier in this chapter for how to deal with partially defrosted milk.

Real-World Milk Handling

There's very little research on the day-to-day problems of milk handling, so guidelines tend to err on the side of caution. Here are some answers based on common sense and on the fact that your breastfed baby has, essentially, your immune system:

- In general, what works for **handling and storage of your own food** works for breastmilk for your baby. Don't forget to wash your hands!
- It's okay to **reheat leftover milk** refrigerated after a previous feeding as long as it's then used within one to two hours.
- You can pump and **put the whole pumping kit (flanges attached to containers) in the fridge,** in a lidded container or bag, until the next pumping session. The cold flanges might also feel pretty good on your breasts when you go to pump the next time! (If you prefer warm flanges, run hot water over them before pumping.) Clean the whole setup after six to eight hours.
- There are many little ways to push the envelope, but **don't combine too many of them.** If milk stood at room temperature for six hours, was partially consumed, then refrigerated for a day, then frozen, then went through a freezer failure and was refrozen, um, *we'd* throw it out.

What About Travelling?

If you're expressing all or most of your baby's milk, planning ahead makes travel doable. Here are some things to keep in mind:

- As long as you express enough times in twenty-four hours, it doesn't matter exactly when you do it. You can **shift your sessions around** to fit your travel plans.
- Milk is okay at room temperature for up to six to eight hours (see the previous table) or twenty-four hours in an **insulated cooler** with ice packs, enough time to get most places.
- If you're making a long journey, **pack enough collection bottles and bottle teats.** Plan for possible delays.
- If you're flying, **check your airline's rules** about carrying milk on board. Some require frozen milk to be carried in hold baggage. Don't be surprised if you're asked to drink a bit of your milk to prove it isn't poison. It also may be necessary to prove that your pump isn't a detonation device; bringing the instruction book should help.
- **Travelling without your baby?** In some countries, milk can be shipped home if it's packed in dry ice. Wrap the frozen containers in newspaper, pack them close together, scatter chipped dry ice around them, and seal the package tightly. The milk should last this way for several days. Or carry frozen milk home in your luggage. If you're travelling away from your baby and you can neither save nor ship your milk, you'll have to discard it, knowing it isn't going to waste because every bit you express makes it possible for your baby to have that same amount when you're back together.
- If you need to **pump on the move,** you'll need a manual pump, a battery-powered or wireless pump, or a car adapter. Some pumps may feel underpowered on battery power compared with being plugged in.
- It's possible to **express hands-free while driving.** Make sure everything is in place before you start, and drive safely, with your seatbelt positioned correctly. It's much easier if you're a passenger! A car sunshade can be attached to the inside of your window for privacy.
- Be sure your pump is compatible with the **power supply** at your destination – take an adapter if necessary.
- If you're going to be away for a while, consider taking **spare pump**

parts – or a spare manual or smaller electric pump. La Leche League Leaders around the world get frantic calls from mothers who have suffered a pump malfunction far from home. Hand expressing works anywhere.
- Pack **hand sanitiser or wipes** if you won't easily be able to wash your hands.

So, you've expressed it and you've stored it. Now for the last step: offering the milk to your baby.

Part Three: Milk In

This part of the process is covered in detail in Chapter 18, Supplementing. The method you use will depend on your baby's age, the reason for supplementing, and the amount of supplement needed. A breastfeeding supporter can help you find feeding tools that work well for you and your baby.

Putting the Parts Together

Whether you chose to express or needed to do it because of separations or feeding challenges, it's a gift to your baby, giving him his normal food when direct breastfeeding isn't possible. The availability of new types of pumps makes provision of expressed milk a realistic option for many more families. Whatever your mix of nursing and expressing, expressed milk or formula, we're here to help.

Want to know more?

You can find extra resources for this chapter at the "Art of Breastfeeding" tab at www.llli.org.

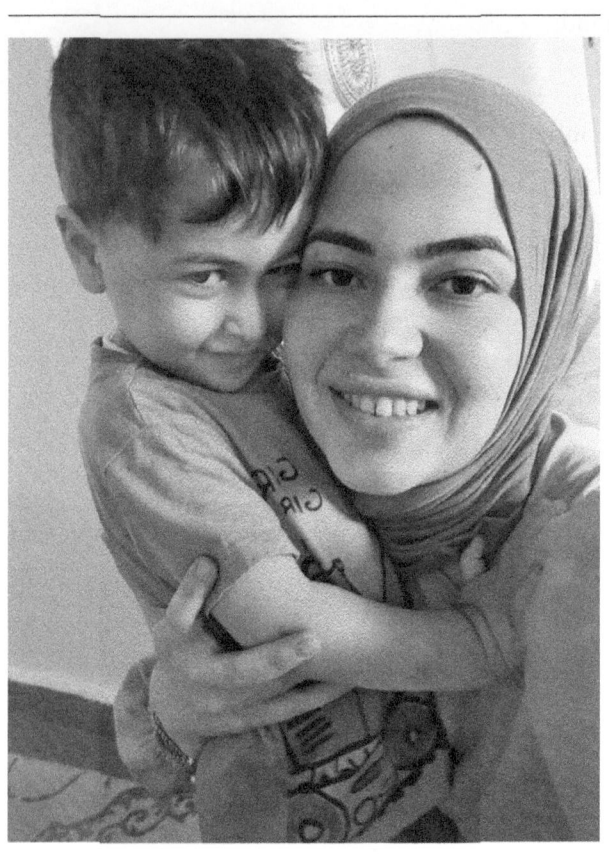

SIXTEEN

Everybody Weans

When I was pregnant the first time, I made up my mind to breastfeed for six months. But by the time Matthew was six months old, everything was going so smoothly that it seemed a pity to quit – and I didn't want to have to go out and buy formula. Maybe I'd keep going for another three months. At nine months, he was enthusiastically eating solids, but still nursing quite often, and again weaning seemed like more trouble than it was worth.

When I found out that I was pregnant again, I thought, *Well, I'll have to wean now*. My doctor reassured me that it wasn't necessary, and I was so tired during early pregnancy that continuing to breastfeed just seemed easier. After the new baby was born, I was too busy to contemplate weaning, and I was glad I still had this easy way to soothe and comfort Matt.

But when he was about two and a half, he began to lose interest. His favourite nursing had always been first thing in the morning. One warm summer day he woke up and started to nurse, then let go and asked (pointing to my breast), "Can you make juice?" "No," I said. Clearly disappointed, he climbed down from the bed and led me downstairs to pour him a cold cup of juice. That was the beginning of the end of our nursing relationship.

– *Teresa, Ontario, Canada*

The word *weaning* can mean different things. Some say the first swallow of anything other than human milk is weaning, so using formula or starting family foods is weaning. Some use *weaning* to mean ending breastfeeding completely. We think weaning involves both. From the first time your baby eats or drinks something other than your milk, weaning has begun. It ends the last time your child nurses or drinks your milk. And that means weaning can take days, weeks, months, or years.

If you're loving breastfeeding, you may hate to see it end, and if you're not having such a great time, you might be looking forward to it ending. One thing's for sure: Breastfeeding *does* end eventually. For *everyone*.

Who Leads Weaning?

Many people think of weaning as something the parent does to the child. But this isn't the only way. You could also allow your child to lead the way and continue breastfeeding until she outgrows the need. Often it's a combination – both of you working your way towards weaning, sometimes one leading, sometimes the other.

If I Leave It Up to My Baby, When Will Weaning Happen?

As in so many things, every child is different. What we *can* tell you, based on research and experience, is that if your baby could choose, he'd probably want to nurse for at least a couple of years. The most common weaning age, worldwide and throughout history, is somewhere between two and a half and four years. The span of possible weaning ages is wide, though – anything from a few months to seven or eight years.

> Before 1500, we nursed until the children stopped asking, sometime between three and seven years of age.
> – Stephanie, Six Nations of the Grand River, Ontario, Canada

---

Beyond a certain age (which varies from family to family), nursing often disappears from public view. You probably know more nursing toddlers and children than you think!

Some societies, including much of North America and Europe, expect babies to wean around a year, or earlier. But this belief isn't in step with our biology and isn't what most humans do. As Gisel puts it, the expectations are a *rush* to wean:

> Overall, breastfeeding has been such an enriching experience, so unique, so wonderful as well as exhausting. She is the only daughter we planned to have, so there is no rush for weaning.
> – Gisel, Mexico

There are plenty of reasons why parents feel rushed – life is often so fast-paced we can barely catch our breath. And we may not have the family and community support parents have always relied on. But if you can, it's worth slowing down a bit where weaning is concerned.

When babies learn to walk, we match our pace to theirs so we can walk together. Rushing with a toddler in tow can be miserable for all concerned (you see it in supermarkets every day!). When you go at your toddler's pace, you don't get there as fast, but there's time for conversation, new perspectives, and getting to know each other better. When we slow down *weaning* to our child's pace – just like a toddler-speed walk in our local area – there are benefits we'd have missed if we kept rushing.

What Do Health Organisations Say?

Breastfeeding continues to support children's nutrition, immunity, and development throughout their early years. There's so much research showing this that leading health organisations including the World Health Organization, UNICEF, national health bodies, and paediatric societies recommend breastfeeding for *at least* two years.

A common concern is that breastfeeding for two years or longer could make a child more clingy or dependent. But personality differences aside, research indicates that children who are weaned early tend to be somewhat *less* secure and independent.

For children with additional needs or health challenges, like Alma's, nursing may have extra significance:

> All three always found the comfort they needed, and they remember it as something very nice, it calmed them so much. I still think that if it had not been for extended breastfeeding, they would have accumulated a lot of stress in their life situations as autistic children.
> – Alma, Mexico City

Emily, who has an autistic child and is herself autistic, found the same:

Breastfeeding my autistic child was one of the most intense experiences of my life, but it included so many positives. Aurora started stimming [repetitive movements or noise] whenever her emotions were heightened, meaning if she was excited, happy, frustrated, or sad she would stim seemingly uncontrollably. Breastfeeding helped, as she would relax her entire body, letting her snuggle up and rest.

Aurora's behaviour became very challenging, too. She would try to run away and get very upset in busy or enclosed spaces. Breastfeeding became an excellent coping strategy. Aurora would sit in her sling and latch on, keeping one eye open calmly watching what was going on outside of her very safe and enclosed sling space.

Another common issue is food. A child with sensory-based eating (and sometimes drinking) issues may struggle to eat, with children often ending up being fed by a nasogastric tube. The magic of breastfeeding means a breastfed child can continue to sustain themselves, and breastfeeding has prevented hospital admissions for my child and many others. Of course, a child over six months needs complementary foods, but breastfeeding can provide a lifeline during extraordinary times.

I never imagined when I was pregnant with my first child that I would have breastfed for over six and a half years, but I'm so glad we did as it became my best parenting tool for my special needs child.

– Emily, Norfolk, England

What's the Advantage to *Me* of Continued Nursing?

More than you might think! Nursing is work, of course, but so is every aspect of caring for a toddler or preschooler. Nursing can make life easier:

- **Nursing is an instant peacemaker.** Toddlers typically have big energy, and even bigger feelings. Unless you have a lot more patience than we do, there will be moments when you'd give almost anything for a few minutes' peace. But tears and tantrums often melt away with the offer to nurse. And a nursing "reboot" can often reset an overwhelmed toddler, averting a meltdown.
- **The hormones released by nursing help soothe a child into sleep.** As one tired mother put it, "Nursing is the nearest thing my toddler has to an off switch!"

- **Nursing might be the only time you get to sit or lie down** while your busy toddler is awake. As Christina puts it,

  Breastfeeding means little islands of calm.
  – *Christina, Germany*

- **Nursing calms us,** too. Clare reports,

  I was a nicer, mellower person when I was still breastfeeding. At least, that's what the rest of my family said, after our youngest weaned!
  – *Clare, UK*

  You can find more in the "Refilling Your Tank" section.
- **Illnesses tend to be milder** and easier to manage. You have on tap an effective pain reliever for your child with no negative side effects. Nursing provides comfort, and your milk may be all she can keep down. No manufactured electrolyte replacement fluid also has nutrition *and* anti-infective agents *and* growth hormones that help children get better faster.
- **Travelling is more convenient** if you don't need to worry about formula. When your child's main attachment is to you (and your breasts), you don't need to panic if her favourite toy or blanket gets left behind. Your child feels instantly secure wherever she is, because her "home base" is still there.

Nursing is an all-purpose tool that makes a whole lot of parenting – from tantrums to flu – a whole lot easier. And the health impacts of breastfeeding continue as long as nursing (or expressing) does.

Human infants (aged up to 12 months) and young children (aged 12–36 months) are most likely to survive, grow, and develop to their full potential when fed human milk from their mothers through breastfeeding, due to the dynamic and interactional nature of breastfeeding and the unique living properties of breastmilk. Breastfeeding promotes healthy brain development and is essential for preventing the triple burden of malnutrition, infectious diseases, and mortality, while also reducing the risk of obesity and chronic

diseases in later life in low-income and high-income countries alike.
– The Lancet *(one of the world's leading medical journals)*,
Breastfeeding Series

The impact of breastfeeding on children's health is well known, but what about on our health? It turns out that nursing longer isn't good just for toddlers. Breastfeeding helps protect us against chronic diseases, too, including some of the most common risks to women's health: cardiovascular disease, breast and ovarian cancers, and type 2 diabetes. It helps space pregnancies, maintain a healthy weight (see Chapter 18, Diet and Weight), and manage stress.

Does nursing a toddler still seem strange? Many who end up doing it never started out planning to nurse a child who could talk. We just found it worked. And once you spend time around nursing toddlers and preschoolers, it no longer seems weird. It's just... normal, as Christina recounts:

We grew into long-term and tandem breastfeeding; we never planned to do so in the beginning. Before I became a mother, I was one of those women who found breastfeeding toddlers strange.
– *Christina, Germany*

If your baby is young, there's no need to worry about weaning now. Just know that there's no reason to stop before you're both ready, and the longer you breastfeed, the better it is for both of you.

The Normal Pace of Weaning

A child's pace of weaning is typically a two steps forward, one step back process. It's often so gradual that you may not even know the last time you nursed.

Telling your child, "Just a minute while I finish the dishes," is part of weaning. We respond quickly to a newborn; we're slower and more likely to negotiate with an older child, all part of gradually putting on the brakes. Impatience may creep in: "It's irritating when she fiddles with my other nipple even though I thought it was cute when the baby did it." Gradual spacing of nursings and a decrease in nursing time are all part of the normal process.

Your child might go through phases when he's not concerned about nursing at all – and phases when he's so passionate you're convinced he'll still be doing it at fifteen!

Eventually, though, your nursing relationship winds down to one or two short nursings a day (plus nursing to ease the pain of skinned knees and bruised feelings). It may taper off from there, or your little one may announce calmly that, thanks, but he'd rather have fruit. Children naturally have a tremendous desire to move on to the next stage of development: once they can walk, they stop crawling. As the wider world opens up to them, they gradually close the door on babyhood. So even if you never lift a finger, even if you never even ask him to wait, *your child will wean*. Just as surely as his teeth will come in.

What If I Want to Wean Now?

It's normal to find nursing irritating at times. Mothers are occasionally told they're nursing "for selfish reasons." This usually gets a hollow laugh when reported at LLL meetings! Yes, there are many lovely things about nursing beyond babyhood, but like any relationship, it has highs and lows. Like most toddlers, those highs and lows can be intense. If you're feeling you'd rather move to the Arctic right now than go through another day (or night) of nursing, we'd encourage you to explore the situation a bit. Maybe weaning really would make life easier. In communities where most babies are weaned before a year, it's often assumed it would. In reality, though, weaning is often more mixed. Nursing has its irritations – and its uses. It's worth counting the cost before giving it up.

I Want My Body Back!

It's not unusual to feel like your nursing toddler has taken over your breasts. If most people around you wean their child at the one-year mark, you might be feeling that normal sense of "nursing impatience" early. Early weaning does give you your breasts back, but life may not be quite as easy as you hoped. Your baby will still want to be held and carried and cuddled – maybe even more. Tantrums and illness may increase for a while, and bedtimes might be tricky. Weaning doesn't make your child need you less; it just gives you one fewer tool to meet her needs.

Partial weaning might be worth considering. Nursing becomes very flexible as children get older: it doesn't stop you from working, going away on a trip, taking up a new sport, getting a makeover... or doing pretty much anything else you might want to do. We know a mother who pumped on her bike during an Iron Man endurance race. Nursing doesn't have to hold you back. And your sex drive usually returns eventually, whether or not you've weaned.

If you want to wean, of course you can – we're happy to support you as you do it. It might be worth thinking about whether that's the *whole* story of what you need.

Wouldn't Life Be Easier Without Nursing Anymore?

Maybe. But your baby will still need to be fed and nurtured. If he's under twelve months, you (or someone else) will have to mix, heat, feed, and clean several bottles of formula a day. When you go out, you'll need to pack enough bottles and formula, and carry the used bottles around until you get home.

Ginny weaned her adopted daughter Carly during a family emergency. She doubts whether weaning made life easier:

> I'm not quite sure what happened at the end. David [my husband] was ill with the flu, and I was looking after both the children and him, running up and down the stairs. I suppose I was overwhelmed. Carly ended up weaning – easily and comfortably – by a year. I'm sorry we didn't carry on for longer, as it had been going so well. It's much harder work looking after a toddler when you're not nursing them!
>
> – Ginny, UK

And then there's how it *feels*. You might have been told that you need to wean for your own good. That's a calculation only you can make. Laura's reckoning was different:

> I suffered severe postnatal depression and anxiety. I kept hearing things like "It's okay to wean early to protect your mental health," but for me, nursing was not contributing to that at all. It was actually the opposite. Breastfeeding was one of the few things I had control over in our birth

experience. I did everything in my power to hold on to that for as long as possible.

– *Laura, United States military*

Laura's instincts are backed up by research. Nursing, when it's going well, protects mood and reduces anxiety. Weaning can cause, or worsen, low mood (keep reading for more on mood and weaning). If you're told you need to wean because of one of these conditions, or to take medication for them, it's worth getting a second opinion (see Chapter 18, Medications and Postnatal Mood Disorders).

If you want to shake off your nursling like a cat shakes off her kittens, those feelings are real. They don't necessarily mean you have to wean completely. As the saying goes, it might not be a good idea to make a big decision on a bad day. But your needs are important, and that urge to escape is a red flag for overwhelm. Are you "running on empty"? With some extra resources for yourself, your toddler might seem less demanding.

Refilling Your Tank

- Prioritise doing something for yourself every day, even if it's just listening to a podcast while your child nurses or naps. Or nap with your child!
- Mornings are often easier times to find solitude – babies and toddlers usually need their main person most intensely at bedtime.
- Find ways to get moving, get outdoors, or get creative.
- Connect with others who know what you're going through. Solidarity doesn't make your day easier, but it can change your perspective. Go to a playgroup, meet a friend, attend an LLL meeting. If you're back at work or school, some groups offer evening, weekend, or virtual meetups. And we have online communities all over the world.

If you're low for days at a time, are struggling with anxiety, or just not yourself, reach out for help. Skilled listening can make a big difference. Treatments are available for the mood disorders that are common after birth, and most mood medications are safe to take during breastfeeding (see Chapter 18, Postnatal Mood Disorders). You're not alone.

It's Just Not Working Out

Has breastfeeding been a nightmare for you? Milk supply problems, pain, an unhappy baby? Exclusive pumping? It's so, so tough when what should be enjoyable generates more stress than pleasure.

Maybe things can still get better. Chapter 18 has information on many breastfeeding problems, and you can find plenty more in books and online. Have you had much one-to-one support? There may still be people out there who can help you, even if you think you've already tried everything. Breastfeeding helpers vary. Some are more up to date than others, have better problem-solving skills, or are just a better fit.

La Leche League Leaders are available by phone, messenger app, video call, and more. Many provide help at monthly meetings. Some may even come to your home. There is never a fee. If the problem is beyond their expertise, they may be able to refer you to an International Board Certified Lactation Consultant (IBCLC) or other specialist.

If you've reached the end of your tether and decided you just can't do it anymore, *you know what's right for you*. That's how good parenting works. As Linett writes, sometimes you just reach the end of your resources:

> After so much struggle, so much fighting, and so much trying to breastfeed, I decided to give up. I understood that it was not my fault. Because I tried everything.
>
> – Linett, Mexico

Give yourself a truly warm hug for your efforts – and here's a big one from us, too. You'll find information about how to wean later in this chapter, and LLL Leaders can support you. Know that any amount of milk or nursing you provided is a lifetime gift to both of you.

Just because this breastfeeding experience was tough doesn't mean future ones will be. If you had milk supply issues, you might have more milk next time, because pregnancy and nursing both help with future supply. If your baby had difficulties, your next baby probably won't have those same issues. If your birth or hospital experience didn't go well, you've learned more for next time. In fact, your next breastfeeding experience might help heal some of the emotional pain from this one. La Leche League will be there for you, whenever you want us. There are some excellent books on breastfeeding grief – check out the extra resources that go with this chapter (at www.llli.org, "Art of Breastfeeding"). Our Leaders are always willing to listen after nursing has ended.

I'm Pregnant

Pregnancy rarely *requires* that you wean, though it's often *assumed* you need to, as Heather found:

> When I had my second daughter, Delaney, I was still nursing my first. I can remember being out with people and Presley asking to nurse. They would look at my pregnant belly and say, "I didn't know you could do that when you're pregnant."
> – Heather, Texas, United States

But there do seem to be some weaning incentives built in, for both you and your child:

- About three-quarters of nursing mothers have some **nipple tenderness or pain** in early pregnancy.

> I nursed my first until age four. I weaned while pregnant with their sister because my breasts got very sensitive and I felt touched out. My second nursed until about sixteen months, when I was pregnant with her brother and again had breast sensitivity. Fred nursed until about sixteen months, when the same things happened while pregnant with my final child.
> – Georgie, New Jersey, United States

- More than half of nursing women begin to feel **fidgety and impatient** when they nurse during pregnancy.
- Most find that their **milk supply drops significantly** when pregnant.

> When my firstborn was around fifteen months old, I got pregnant again. Everything was perfect until around eighteen to nineteen weeks. Suddenly my little girl was screaming through the night – and it took me quite some time to figure out why – turned out that my milk supply was gone due to my

pregnancy. She stopped night feedings shortly before she turned two and became a big sister.
— Sonja, Austria

This seems to be biology's way of putting the new baby's needs first. Some mothers opt to work through fidgetiness or nipple soreness, others choose to wean. Some children, like Sonja's daughter, wean but resume later:

When her brother was two weeks old, she asked if she could taste my milk — so I let her — and even though she hadn't breastfed for four-plus months, she latched like a pro at her first try. And obviously she liked what she tasted — as from that point on I was tandem-feeding both kids.
— Sonja, Austria

Samantha had expected her daughter to start nursing again, but Amalya chose not to:

I very much by surprise became pregnant again. Hyperemesis and migraines kicked in, and I had to rapidly wean Amalya, as even being touched made me vomit violently. I hadn't planned on stopping breastfeeding and it was such an emotionally hard thing to do. I always told her that when the new baby came, there would be milk and that she could breastfeed again. While I was pregnant she readily agreed, but then, when Ruhi was born and I offered Amalya milk, she laughed and said that the baby could have the milk.
— Samantha, from the UK, living in Bali, Indonesia

Feelings and responses are all over the map. You can follow your instinct and your judgement about what might work best for you and your child.

Breastfeeding and Miscarriage

Occasionally it is necessary to wean to maintain a pregnancy, but this is rare. The concern is that oxytocin released with nursing will stimulate uterine contractions and start labour prematurely. If you've got a history of premature labour, or there are signs that labour might be trying to start early, you might be advised to avoid sex, orgasm, and nursing. Research has found that nursing through pregnancy (except perhaps when pregnancies are very closely spaced, conceived during the first six months while exclusively breastfeeding) doesn't increase the risk of miscarriage.

If you are having a miscarriage, you can nurse through it, if you want to. Some mothers describe nursing as comforting after pregnancy loss. If your pregnancy lasted more than about sixteen weeks, your milk will increase afterwards (see Chapter 17, Lactation After Loss). We're here to help, whatever you decide to do.

Nursing Beyond Pregnancy: Tandem Nursing

Tandem nursing is when you nurse your older child along with your new baby. It's not very common in any known culture, but many families do it, and we have plenty of experience of it in LLL, as Jessalyn discovered:

> I am currently pregnant with my second baby. It's been so special being able to nurse my toddler while her new little sibling is cuddled in my womb close by. Today she said, "Rosie share Babas with baby!" (*Babas* is what she calls nursing.) It was very sweet to hear that she would share with her little sibling! Before going to LLL meetings, I hadn't heard much about what it was like to be pregnant while also still nursing an older sibling. I fully expect we will be tandem nursing once the baby is born.
> – Jessalyn, North Carolina, United States

Mothers who tandem nurse often report feeling that it helps with the transition, like Cyndel and her partner, Kendra:

> When Sloane was born, tandem feeding became a thing not only for myself but as Kendra was still nursing Laveen she now had the ability to nurse our youngest also. The way we chose to do things definitely helped ease a new baby into our family and strengthen sibling bonds.
> – Cyndel, Ontario, Canada

It's not always sweetness and light, of course – as Kat remembers!

> The gentle way the newborn and toddler would nurse together and caress each other's faces and hair was so adorable, and still today, at the ages of twenty-two and twenty, they are very, very close. As an aside, when number 2 tandem-fed with number 3, he would be poked by the baby and she'd pull at his mouth, so they didn't nurse together very long, and number

3 still today, at seventeen years old, is quite a bolshy [argumentative] so-and-so!

– *Kat, United States, children born in the UK*

Chetana, who adopted her second daughter, describes how putting limits on the older child's nursing can help keep tandem nursing manageable:

We tandem-nursed for almost two years as Disha was not ready to wean yet and Tamia was already with us. It was mostly manageable, as Disha's needs were not as demanding as time passed by. The boundaries I set for Disha helped me not feel overwhelmed and meet both my children's needs.

– *Chetana, Bangalore, India*

For more about tandem nursing, see Chapter 11.

I Want to *Get* Pregnant, but I Think Breastfeeding Is Preventing It

This can be a tough one. Frequent nursing is a powerful fertility suppressor, as part of a well-designed system: nursing less often signals that your baby is finally able to share his mother with a younger sibling. Throughout most of history, this coincided roughly with the mother's own recovery from the birth. The World Health Organization's review of the research finds that it takes a good two years for a woman's body to recover fully from pregnancy and childbirth, and for mother and baby *both* to be ready for a new pregnancy; survival rates for both are greater with more than two years between children. The high-need or sensitive child who nurses more frequently than average might keep his mother infertile a bit longer, to make sure his own needs are fully met.

In countries where formula-feeding became common, though, so did much shorter birth intervals. And many of us have the added pressure that we're giving birth at older ages than our mothers and grandmothers, so we need to squeeze our pregnancies into a shorter span of years. If you're feeling pressure to conceive as soon as possible, what can you do?

If your periods haven't returned and you want to get pregnant soon, you could consider night weaning, not pumping during the day, or just generally cutting back to see if that starts your periods up. Often a regular break of six hours over a few days (or nights) is enough to kick-start fertility.

Charting your cycles can tell you when you ovulate and the length of your "luteal phase" – the time from the day after ovulation until your period starts. Short luteal phases relate to high prolactin levels, which can be caused by several things, including breastfeeding.

A minority of us are unable to conceive again until we've completely weaned. If gradually increasing the longest gap between feeds isn't doing the trick, you may need to calculate the benefits of nursing against those of conceiving again. This can be a heartbreaking decision, especially as there's no guarantee of a new pregnancy. Some of us have been there. We're always willing to listen.

If you're planning **fertility treatment** and wondering if you'll need to wean ahead of time, you can find more information in Chapter 10.

I'm Going Back to Work or Study

Does it seem like nursing will be too difficult when you go back to study or work? Are there no opportunities to express? Is it an unsupportive workplace or learning environment?

Fortunately, nursing is flexible, especially with an older baby or toddler. You don't have to do the same thing every day. If you can't express during your working hours, you can still nurse when you're with your child. Any amount of your milk helps protect your baby against the germs she'll pick up if she's in group childcare. It's in your employer's best interest to support you to continue nursing if you want to. For more about how to manage work or study while you're nursing, see Chapter 14.

I Need to Wean for Medical Reasons

It's rare for a medical procedure or surgery to require even temporary weaning. Adri was told she had to wean in order to take medication:

> I had started weaning but I wanted to do it little by little. When I got sick with Covid-19, and then my baby (very sad), it broke my heart to see how she was asking me for milk, but because of the medicines I had to take for my treatment, I had to deny it to her. I even asked the doctor what he thought about giving her the milk back, to comfort her, but he forbade it. It

was very painful emotionally.

— *Adri, Querétaro, Mexico*

If you're told to wean, it can be well worth getting more information before taking a step that can have far-reaching effects (see Chapter 18, Medications).

As Hannah's story shows, many obstacles can be overcome with determination and support:

> When my second child was seven months old and her brother was four, I was diagnosed with bowel cancer. The hospital allowed me to bring my breastfed baby to the hospital while I had surgery. My husband also came and cared for her while I was recovering. It was a hard recovery, but I breastfed her straight out of surgery as soon as I was awake. I spent most of the four nights in hospital co-sleeping and breastfeeding her. Then ten days after surgery I was rushed back to hospital without my baby. Baby would visit me once a day to nurse, but since I was nil by mouth [not able to eat or drink] and had no food at all, my supply basically shut down to a trickle. Eventually I was able to eat again, and my supply started to increase as I was well enough to pump. As soon as I got home I tandem-fed my two children, and by the end of that week my supply was back to full power. I was lucky enough not to need chemo so I was able to keep breastfeeding my children.
>
> — *Hannah, Sheffield, UK*

Sometimes, weaning is not negotiable. We've supported many families to wean for medical reasons, like starting chemotherapy. If you find yourself in this situation, we're here to help (see Emergency Weaning later in this chapter).

Over time, the bitterness of a weaning you wouldn't have chosen can be sweetened by memories of the nursing relationship that came before:

> I continued to feed my toddler but it was too upsetting to not be able to feed my daughter [who had a serious kidney condition] when she could smell the milk and was still only a baby. So I stopped breastfeeding him. I don't know if I'll ever stop feeling guilty, but I look fondly on the times we did feed.
>
> — *Emma, London, UK*

I Just Can't Take the Criticism!

As Helena found, other people may become less comfortable with breastfeeding as your child grows:

> Whilst opposition may have stopped with family and friends, opposition still continued from people we didn't know well who were appalled at witnessing a three-/four-year-old child still breastfeeding. Of course, by then my son was able to speak directly to those questioning his need to breastfeed. I remember one memorable conversation where he was asked directly by a visitor to my mother's home – "How long are you going to breastfeed for?" He replied, "Until I get married – no, until my mum dies." Of course, he stopped well before these two events!
> – Helena, London, England

Maybe the critics have never been around an older nursling. Maybe they're blaming normal toddler or preschooler behaviour on breastfeeding. But this is *your* baby, *your* breastfeeding relationship. Weaning will change your life and your child's, not theirs. This is your decision.

Laura was discouraged from continuing breastfeeding by her healthcare providers:

> When she was a year old I got pregnant with my second child and I was told to start the weaning process, because I was a working mum and the paediatrician said he didn't know of any successful tandem breastfeeding in those circumstances. I found support in some family members, but most of them didn't really think it was necessary or important. Several health professionals suggested that I had to stop breastfeeding, because it was not beneficial.
> – Laura, Colombia

Telling critics that you truly appreciate their concern and that you know they're saying this because they care tends to defuse the tension. People like to think you see them positively. Humour can disarm them, too, and of course you can gently tell them that you've studied the issues and made an informed decision. B.J. was able to point to clear evidence that a health professional's concerns were unfounded:

> When a health visitor told me that I needed to wean my then-one-year-old, or else "she'd never learn to speak," I shook my head, corrected her, and

pointed out that my daughter was in fact already speaking!
— B.J., England

If none of these suggestions appease them, you may just have to agree to disagree. Groups like LLL can be havens. You need a safe space where you can feel...normal. And vent – including about the irritating aspects of nursing! Knowing you're not alone will help you feel stronger in the face of any further criticism.

If you're looking ahead and worrying that you might face criticism as your child grows, one possibility is to become more private about nursing. While it's appropriate to nurse a baby promptly, many two-year-olds and older children can wait until you get somewhere where you feel comfortable. Cecily's experience is typical:

> After the age of about two and a half or three I almost never fed him in public. He was willing to wait until we got home.
> — Cecily, Ontario, Canada

Janedy and her daughter were creative about finding privacy:

> After she turned two, we would always be looking for a nursing room when we went out, sometimes even breastfeeding while walking, with her hiding herself completely under my clothes to enjoy her nursing time.
> — Janedy, Taiwan

Continuing to nurse outside your home, though, if you feel confident, helps normalise nursing in your community. Clare found her neighbourhood more accepting than she had expected:

> I attended an event at my daughters' school, and took my youngest, then not quite two, with me. She was getting restless, so I thought about nursing her, but hesitated, as I wasn't sure whether this would be approved of. I needn't have worried; as I tried to calm my squirming child, I realised the mother in front of me was nursing her three-year-old!
> — Clare, UK

It's especially hard to continue nursing if you're not supported by those closest to you. Alexis's daughter was tube-fed at first and couldn't nurse until she was nine months old:

It has taken me two and a half years to achieve the goal of breastfeeding my daughter without a pump, nipple shields, or nursing supplementer. I am finally achieving this goal I never thought possible. People around me want to know when I am going to stop breastfeeding and why I have continued as long as I have. I lost my husband's support around eighteen months. For the last year this has been a silent journey that only my daughter and I know all the details of.

– Alexis, Maryland, United States

Breastfeeding and Child Visitation

Nursing sometimes becomes an area of conflict between separated parents. The non-nursing parent might suggest that the child needs to wean so they can have longer contact visits, like overnights, or weekends. If you're in this situation, this information might be useful to share with your child's other parent and your legal representative, if you have one:

- **Children can spend longer periods away from their main caregiver without weaning.** Many nursing toddlers and preschoolers spend whole days in childcare, or whole weekends with grandparents, and they easily pick up nursing again once they get home. It's the same with contact visits. The nursing mother just needs to keep her breasts comfortable and, if necessary, express to keep up her milk production.
- **Children understand that different adults care for them in different ways.** Just as children know which parent they play a particular game with, they don't expect anyone but their usual nursing parent to nurse them. This doesn't take anything away from their unique relationship with the other parent. The non-nursing parent needs to figure out their own ways to comfort the child and help him fall asleep – whether or not the child continues to nurse.
- **Weaning (or providing expressed milk) won't make separation easier.** If the child is upset about being separated from his mother, it's not just nursing or milk he's missing. His main caregiver is his main source of comfort and security.
- **Days and nights aren't equal.** Nighttime can be scary for small people, and bedtime is a big transition. Most babies and young

children find nighttime separations harder than daytime ones. Going at the child's developmental speed reduces stress for everyone.
- In addition to all the health impacts of nursing, it **helps provide emotional security** for children during unsettling transitions, like a parent moving out. Weaning before the child is ready just gives him an extra loss to deal with and takes away a valuable source of reassurance.

Depending on the legal system and nursing norms where you live, breastfeeding beyond babyhood might be well accepted... or seen as strange, even unhealthy. If early weaning is common in your community, it's probably more constructive to focus on the universal needs of young children. *Whether or not they're breastfed,* babies, all toddlers, and preschoolers need a secure home base. Frequent contact is the key to maintaining relationships with other important people. Visits can gradually get longer as the child becomes better able to cope with separation. The timetable is different for every child.

I Don't Want to Wean but My *Baby* Does

Some of us find, to our surprise and perhaps disappointment, that our children are ready to wean before we are.

One possibility is that nursing has had a lot of competition. If you need to use bottles because your baby needs supplements or is in childcare, these ideas may help:

- If your milk supply is low and your baby is supplemented at home routinely, make the bottle-feedings strictly business and nursings a time for cuddles and conversation.
- Try offering the bottle before breastfeeding, so the baby associates the breast – not the bottle – with the satisfaction of a full tummy. Or use an at-breast supplementer (see Chapter 18, Supplementing).
- Avoid or minimise dummies and encourage soothing at the breast. If you want a dummy for quieting a baby in the car, consider keeping it in the car.

Nursing is at least as much about communication as it is about food – feel free to use it for every reason under the sun! All those little "just because" nursings help keep your relationship strong.

What if your baby is weaning without bottles or dummies in the mix? It's worth looking at how things are going overall. See if any of these ideas might work for you:

- Take time to relax together – in the bath, at naptime, in other settings where nursing can happen with no time pressure.
- Let nursing be a source of snuggles, giggles, and silliness as well as food.
- Look for times to "use" breastfeeding – to reconnect after time apart, to calm her when a dog scares her, to keep her occupied while your partner is on a video call.
- Go to an LLL meeting and watch other mothers. Ask them when and why they are nursing. Being part of a group can answer questions you didn't know you had. And seeing other children nursing may encourage yours to ask!

Occasionally, even after the happiest, easiest nursing relationship, a child just has a different plan – like Audrey's one-year-old:

> Malachi self-weaned at eighteen months to my great sadness, because I wanted to get us to the age of four, with how easy he was. It took four children for it to not be difficult, so I had such high hopes. And I guess that's why it was the greatest heartache that he refused the breast. Because there was no medical excuse, no work excuse that led to any milk depletion.
> – Audrey, Texas, United States

It's okay to be sad when nursing ends before you expected. People around you might not understand, especially if you've already nursed beyond the typical length of time for your community. But we know that it can be a real loss of something you were enjoying, and the way you thought things would go. We're here to listen. For more on emotions about weaning, see How Weaning Feels later in this chapter.

My Baby Is Suddenly Refusing My Breast

If your older baby (most often around eight to ten months) has *suddenly* stopped nursing, it could be a "nursing strike." This *doesn't* mean he wants to wean. Something has made him not want to breastfeed right now, and it can usually be worked through, with time and patience. Common causes include earaches and stuffy noses, or a scare. A baby on a nursing strike, unlike a baby who's simply weaning, is usually miserable – you can see something's not right. For tips on how to get through this, see Chapter 18, Nursing Strike, and reach out to a breastfeeding supporter.

My Baby Has *Never* Nursed Well

There are many reasons why a baby simply doesn't nurse well. A breastfeeding helper can often make a difference... but not always. Yet even a difficult nursing journey can be a source of satisfaction and pride, as Montserrat discovered:

> Thanks to these nipple shields I was able to breastfeed my daughter. The funny thing was that she only used one breast; she did not want the other. I don't know why, but she did not want the left breast, and I only breastfed her with the right. It was very, very painful. I could only do it until she was a year old because I couldn't stand it anymore. But without a doubt it was a great experience, despite the pain. I had a very nice connection with her, she looked at me with eyes of love, she caressed my breast every time she took her milk. I was happy to be able to do it, because with my two older children I did not do it, and with her I did. Without a doubt it was something wonderful.
>
> – *Montserrat, Querétaro, Mexico*

Weaning from the breast doesn't necessarily mean your baby has to lose the protection of your milk. Audrey chose to express for a year after Malachi's unexpected weaning:

> I would pump when he wouldn't feed, until my body stopped producing in quantities worth pumping. He still got breastmilk until he was two and a half, but just not direct. So I made my peace with that.
>
> – *Audrey, Texas, United States*

If this is an option you'd like to explore, see Chapter 17, Exclusive Pumping.

Weaning from the Pump

If you've been expressing all the way through, instead of (or as well as) nursing, at some point you'll wind down and stop. If you can, do it gradually, giving your breasts time to adjust. You can do this by

- increasing the time between pumping sessions
- removing less milk when you express
- ... or a bit of both

If your breasts get too uncomfortable, you can go back a step or two and try again – perhaps more slowly – when everything has settled down. If you've been prone to mastitis, you might need to be especially cautious during the wind-down phase.

Nicola exclusively expressed for Thomas, who has cerebral palsy:

> We were racing towards Thomas's second birthday, and I began to think about what would happen then. Some days I felt like I would go on forever, others I hated it so much it was all I could do to pick up my pump. We celebrated his second birthday and I hung up my breast pump. I worked out that I had expressed somewhere in the region of 355 litres of breastmilk in those first two years. I had hated and resented having to do it for most of the time but was always so grateful to be able to on the multiple occasions that he was ill and in hospital. It gave me hope to know that breastmilk was packed full of antibodies and stem cells, good for brain and eye development. He'd had a very difficult start to life, but I had given the best possible nutritional support.
>
> – Nicola, Berkshire, UK

For more about exclusive pumping, see Chapter 17. It's the most enormous labour of love, giving immeasurable benefit to the most vulnerable children. We're here for you every step of the way.

What If "Child-Led Weaning" Won't Work for *Us*?

Breastfeeding is "dose-dependent," meaning that every bit of milk and every day cuddled at your breast increases the impact. Breastfeeding your baby for even a day is the best baby gift you could give her. A single spoonful of your own milk contains millions of live cells and other components no formula can provide. Breastmilk is potent medicine for a premature or sick baby.

If you end up nursing, or providing milk, for a shorter time than you'd hoped for (or other people thought you should), you might wonder if it was worth it. *Only you* know how much it cost you – no one else gets to judge. We've talked with mothers who never planned to nurse at all but expressed for their premature or sick baby after they learned how important it was. They're some of our heroes. The value of nursing or expressing is not measured by length of time.

We believe that every drop of human milk and every nursing deserves celebration – especially when it's been tough. Below you can see just a few things you might have achieved, from among many health impacts. And we also know that the value of nursing or expressing can't be measured just by health impact.

Breastmilk is the ideal food for infants. It is safe, clean, and contains antibodies which help protect against many common childhood illnesses.

Over 820,000 children's lives could be saved every year among children under 5 years, if all children 0–23 months were optimally breastfed.
— *World Health Organization*

As Alejandra writes, the memories last, too:

Between harvesting raspberries, bathing in the river, planting and watering the orchard, we watched the stars, picked the fruit, and learned about insects; our breastfeeding story with Leon continued for a whole year, a precious experience. It was difficult at the beginning, even painful, but then it turned into a generous and enjoyable commitment. I am happy and excited to have been able to experience this bond with my eldest son; it remains a warm memory.
— *Alejandra, Santiago, Chile*

If Your Child Weans When He Is Ready . . .

If your child self-weans, you can feel confident that you've met his physical and emotional needs in a healthy way. The World Health Organization, UNICEF, the American Academy of Pediatrics, and many more organisations strongly encourage breastfeeding through the second year and beyond. Your child's biology seems geared to weaning in the third year or later.

Scientists and researchers have added a lot to our knowledge

If you breastfeed or express milk for...

	The first few days:	• Concentrated antibodies in the colostrum protect against illness • Your baby's blood sugars will be stabilized • Your baby's gut is prepared with enzymes and healthy microbes • Your hormones help you tune in to your baby
	Four to six weeks:	• Protects your baby against diarrhoea or constipation • Protects your baby against chest infections • Helps your baby's immune system develop • Your baby is much less likely to die of SIDS
	Three to four months:	• Protects your baby against developing asthma • Protects your baby against later food allergies • Helps you lose postpartum weight • Helps to prevent postpartum depression in you
	Six months:	• Protects your baby against ear, nose, throat, and sinus infections • Protects your baby against childhood leukaemia • Helps your baby's brain develop • Protects you against type 2 diabetes
	Nine months:	• Comforts your baby when teething or getting medical care • Increased antibodies help prevent infections in your active baby • Provides nutrition as your baby starts on family foods
	One year:	• Reduces your baby's risk of becoming overweight in childhood • Protects your baby against later high blood pressure and heart disease • Your baby will have better jaw development and straighter teeth • Reduces your risk of breast cancer
	Eighteen months:	• Protects your baby from illness in childcare • Helps your baby recover quickly if they are ill • Your baby develops words for nursing such as *num-nums* • Your baby can wait to nurse sometimes
	As long as your baby wants:	• Antibodies continue to protect your baby from illness • Your baby will have experienced years of closeness and comfort • Your baby's cognitive development will be optimal • Slow weaning will help reduce your risk of mastitis

about the health impacts of human milk since the last edition of this book. But it's still not the whole story. Ask a nursing mother (or child) what they value, and they often don't even mention milk. Nursing can help shape your whole relationship, as Liz found:

> I set an ambitious goal. I knew almost nothing about breastfeeding but I was going to breastfeed for two years. This is the length of time I was breastfed for, and man, am I glad I set that goal. Because without breastfeeding I'm

almost sure I wouldn't be the mother that I am and we wouldn't have the bond we have today; because to us, it's become so much more than "just milk."

– Liz, UK

Ivannia felt her breastfeeding shaped her children's interaction with their wider world, too:

I have my medals in my heart; every time the teachers congratulated us because the child behaved with empathy and enthusiasm in the classroom, I knew that the merit was due to the skin-to-skin contact I always had with my children. That wonderful contact remains forever.

– Ivannia, Costa Rica

The end of breastfeeding is a big step for both of you. Whenever it ends, if possible, do it gradually, and with love.

Speeding Up Weaning

Whatever the situation, it's almost always possible to find ways to make weaning gentler.

Sudden, "cold turkey" weaning is sometimes recommended (and may be appealing at 3:00 A.M. when you're nursing for the umpteenth time!). However, gradual weaning is safer and kinder on both your baby and your breasts.

If you have to wean immediately, see Emergency Weaning later in this chapter. Here are some things to make this type of weaning easier:

- **Make time for plenty of attention and cuddling.** A nursing child gets these as part of the package. After weaning, you might need to be more intentional.
- **Babywearing (or carrying an older child in a sling or carrier) can be an excellent substitute for nursing.** Maybe someone else could do some of the carrying. If you're doing it yourself, back-carrying can work well: it's better for your back and keeps your breasts out of reach!
- **If you can, be flexible.** There might be days that only nursing will comfort her. That's okay. She might be teething or coming

down with a cold, or just need the reassurance that she's still your baby. You can cut back again when she seems ready.

The way you go about weaning will depend largely on your child's age. Here are some age-specific weaning strategies.

Weaning Under Six Months Old

Unless you have access to donor milk, weaning your child who's younger than six months will mean transitioning to formula. Talk to your healthcare provider about what's appropriate. The change may take some trial and error:

- If your baby hasn't had formula before, you might consider **expressing for any dropped feeds** during the first week or so, while you make sure your baby can tolerate the formula. More than one family has discovered that continuing to breastfeed is easier than the eczema, irritability, or digestive problems that may suddenly crop up. Your child may tolerate formula better if it's tried again a few weeks later. In the meantime, keeping your supply up lets you swing right back into nursing, if need be.
- Some families start by offering **just one bottle a day** for the first two or three days. If your breasts feel uncomfortable from this missed feeding (and you aren't pumping as insurance while you try formula), express just enough milk to feel comfortable but not enough to drain your breasts. You're signalling them to slow down milk production. Then add another bottle for a day or two, gradually increasing the number of bottle-feedings and decreasing the number of nursings. The last to go are often first thing in the morning, naptime, and bedtime. As your supply keeps dropping, at some point your baby will probably indicate she wants a bottle instead of your breast, even at the favourite feeds.

The whole process could take two or three weeks or more. Since breastfeeding means more than just food, your baby may not bottle-feed as often as she nursed. You can make up for the comfort feeds by giving more cuddles and attention.

Once you're down to her favourite times, you might even decide you don't have to do anything more. A couple of nursings a day may be manageable for you. They take no more time than you'd be giving to the baby anyway, they give her your milk for a bit longer, and your supply will probably be low enough that your breasts are never uncomfortable.

Weaning a Baby Six Months to One Year Old

In the past, most health authorities advised giving formula to babies between six and twelve months, if they were not breastfeeding. However, these guidelines are changing in some places, so talk to your healthcare provider about your situation.

Weaning a Baby Twelve Months or Older

It's very different weaning a child who's old enough to understand, as Leah describes:

> When my son was approaching his third birthday, I knew I was done breastfeeding. I felt "touched-out" and wanted my body back. By this time we were only breastfeeding at bedtime and during the night sometimes. I told my son that he had drunk all the "milka" and that it was all gone. He still asked for "milka" every few days for a while, but I would offer cuddles and a drink of water instead and that really seemed to help the transition. My supply was so low by that time that my body quickly adjusted.
> – Leah, Ontario, Canada

On the other hand, like Janedy's daughter, your nursling might have very clear views of his own!

> When she was two years old, I started to talk to her about weaning, but she loved breastfeeding and didn't want to give it up. She was not willing to wean until she was four years old!
> – Janedy, Taiwan

Here are more ideas about weaning older children:

- Beyond twelve months, **formula is no longer necessary** – your child's nutritional bases can be covered by a varied diet. For more about family foods, see Chapter 13. For more about animal milks, alternatives to milk, and other drinks, see Chapter 10.

- A time-honoured way to encourage weaning is **"don't offer, don't refuse."** You stop offering the breast voluntarily, but you don't refuse if he asks. It helps to avoid the places you usually nurse. As one mother put it, "If you're keen to wean, you don't get to sit down a lot!"
- **Distraction** often works, too. When your child asks for a quick nursing, offer him a drink, or a healthy snack; or find some new toys, go out more often, or invite people over to play. The idea is to offer substitutes that compete favourably with nursing.
- **Naps and bedtime** may be harder. Some mothers taper away bedtime nursings by saying they will nurse only as long as the length of a song. Or you could count to a certain number (the count can go as fast or slow as you need). Tamara knew she was pushing too hard when her toddler pleaded, "Don't count!" Try replacing the nap and bedtime feeds with other rituals that cue your child to feel sleepy. Cuddles, rocking, back rubs, lullabies, and favourite poems and stories are very soothing. You can make this a snuggly time by holding your child close, maybe letting him lean his cheek on your breast. Introduce these strategies along with nursing at first. For example, sing a lullaby while you nurse. A few days later, just sing for a while and finish with nursing. After a few more nights, the lullaby alone may work to put him to sleep. If you have a partner or supporter, it can be helpful for them to get more involved in your child's bedtime. If taking over bedtime feels like too big a step, you can ease into it by including them alongside whatever you're doing, so your child gets used to them being there.
- **Talk about what's going on** and why you need him to wean. Even a one-year-old may understand more than you expect. This was all Liz needed to do:

Earlier this week, I told Alannah we will have special cuddles instead from now on. We are both ready. She hasn't even asked for milk since.
– Liz, UK

- **It's okay for your child to be sad.** Being able to express all kinds of feelings is healthy and teaches children to manage their own feelings:

As he approached his fifth birthday, I decided it was time for him to stop nursing. I told him that Mokies would be all done on his birthday. He was sad, but I didn't notice any concerning change in his behaviour. The night before his birthday, he nursed for the last time. I was ready and I think he was, too.

– Cecily, Ontario, Canada

We've included some children's books about weaning in the extra resources that accompany this chapter (at www.llli.org, "Art of Breastfeeding").

Marking the Moment

Weaning is a major milestone in a child's life, and many families, like B.J.'s, find a way to mark it:

> My older daughter weaned when she was over six years old. This was emotional for us both, and we both celebrated and reminisced by making a breastfeeding photo album, and getting jewellery for us both made of breastmilk.
>
> – B.J., England

We've heard of parents taking a photo or video of the last feed or expressing session, receiving a piece of jewellery or other gift from their partner or loved one, writing a poem, creating a piece of art, or even getting a weaning tattoo. Some plan a "weaning party" with their child, letting her take the lead on guest list, foods, and activities, and maybe letting her choose a toy she can have once she's weaned.

Consider *not* using a birthday as Weaning Day so the excitement doesn't spiral too high. And be prepared for your child to say, at bedtime, "I changed my mind." Don't feel you have to follow through if that's how your child feels; another day can be weaning day. Parenting is full of false steps, half steps, advances, and retreats.

Emergency Weaning

For information about dealing with your milk after the loss of a pregnancy, baby, or child, see Chapter 17, Lactation after Loss.

Sometimes weaning has to be abrupt:

- When your breasts feel uncomfortably full, remove only enough milk to feel comfortable again. This will help you avoid mastitis while signalling your breasts to slow down production.

- Depending on how much milk you're making and how much your breasts can hold, you might need to express every few hours, once a day, or even less. Over time, you'll need to express less often, until you can stop altogether.
- If you've started medication that's not compatible with breastfeeding, you may need to discard your expressed milk; otherwise, it can be fed to your baby.

Will continuing to express some milk keep your milk production going? Yes, a bit – but it's safer to slow down gradually, using your body's natural "brake" (fullness of the breast) than to stop suddenly – unless you're given medication to shut down your milk production quickly.

Milk Suppression

It used to be quite common to give powerful drugs to stop milk production. These days this is rarely done because some of the older drugs had dangerous side effects. But medication is still an option, for example, if you need breast surgery quickly. It completely stops milk production within one to two days. Your healthcare provider can advise you on safe options.

To speed the process of milk reduction without those drugs, others choose to use herbs or over-the-counter medication. Talk to your healthcare provider or a breastfeeding specialist for more information. Breast binding does not speed up the process and may cause inflammation, so it is no longer recommended. However, you may find a supportive bra helps with comfort. For more on managing breast engorgement (fullness and tenderness) and mastitis (inflammation), see Chapter 18.

Provide plenty of snuggles during this sad and confusing time. An older baby may understand that your breasts are "broken" (you could even put plasters on them), but he may do better if you wear a dress or tucked-in shirt that can't be opened or lifted by searching hands. A younger baby may need a lot of walking and singing, a still younger one may adjust quickly to a bottle but will be grateful for your warmth and bare skin during his meal, and perhaps your finger to suck on afterwards.

If you're a co-sleeping family, it might help to have your partner or another close person sleep alone with the baby while a new pattern is established.

Whatever his age, your baby is losing something important, just as you are, and you both have a right to mourn. If possible, change as little else right now as possible. While leaving your baby for a weekend in order to wean may feel less stressful to you, not having the centre of his universe around for such a big change will probably make it extra hard on him.

La Leche League Leaders are always willing to listen after breastfeeding has ended.

Night Weaning

What if you just don't want to nurse at night anymore? Maybe you're hoping for uninterrupted sleep but want to keep nursing during the day. If you've been told to wean at night to **prevent cavities** in your child's teeth, you can find more information in Chapter 12.

Be aware that stopping night feeds before your baby and breasts are ready can cause problems for your milk production. If you have a younger baby, or a smaller milk storage capacity, you might need to express at least once at night to keep your supply strong and your breasts comfortable – which partly defeats the purpose of night weaning.

Keep in mind that babies wake at night for different reasons:

- Young babies rely on calories taken throughout the day and night.
- If you and your child are separated during the day, she might get most of her milk at night.
- Nursing at night is a way of reconnecting after time apart, as well as providing antibodies against germs children pick up in childcare. It's also comfort after a bad dream or challenging day.
- Night waking can also be increased by teething, illness, or allergies, or just the developmental stage your child is in.

If you think your older baby or toddler might be ready to manage with less nursing at night, give it a go. She might surprise you by being readier than you expect! She'll still wake at night – we all do – but she may quickly learn to go back to sleep with little or no help.

Replacing nursing with cuddles and lullabies as described in the section on weaning toddlers might help, though this just substitutes one way of helping your child get back to sleep with another. This may work fine if your reason for night weaning is to increase your chances of getting pregnant, for example, or if you want someone else to settle your child while you sleep. Some night-weaned babies and toddlers quickly manage without adult help at night, and some don't. If yours is one who still wakes a lot and needs help to get back to sleep, you might decide it's easier, for now, just to roll over and nurse. Only you can decide whether the energy involved in making a change is worth it, or whether you'd get more sleep if you waited a little longer.

It's always possible to make a change, if you need to, and there are many gentle strategies that can help (see Chapter 12, But I'm *Really* Exhausted!).

Eventually, almost all children manage by themselves until morning, though needing reassurance at night is still common through the preschool years. In the meantime, keep in mind these tips:

- Make sure your child **eats and drinks enough during the day and gets plenty of exercise** – this may help him sleep as much as he is physically and developmentally ready for.
- If your child is old enough to understand basic concepts, you might be able to **explain that you aren't going to be nursing at night anymore** because the [insert your own term for breasts here!] have to sleep, too.
- You could **practise shortening nursings during the day,** using counting, singing, and so on. If your child accepts this easily, you may be able to do the same at night. Once nursing is down to a few seconds, it might just fade out.
- Some families tell their children to **wait for the sun to come up** or use a clock that lights up at a time of their choosing. It may be easier to start night weaning in summer, when nights are shorter (and your child is less likely to be ill).

With any of these nudges, you'll know soon enough whether the time is right. Many a mother who was met with hysterics when she first tried night weaning tried again a few weeks later and found her child fussed a little for a night or two, then slept soundly. Or your night-weaned child might need to nurse at night again for a while when she's ill or teething. Like many aspects of parenting, weaning is often a dance of forward and backward steps.

Every child is different. If yours needs to nurse at night longer than her siblings or peers, it's no reflection on her, or on you. La Leche League groups can be good places to air frustrations. If you're responsive to her changing needs, you can encourage longer night stretches without pushing your child past her developmental limit.

How Weaning Feels

It's hard to know how you might feel about the end of breastfeeding until it happens. Nursing might have become so much part of what you do and who you are that it's difficult to see beyond it, as Vanessa found:

> I've been breastfeeding for over ten years. This is my last baby and he is now almost two. I see my journey coming to an end in the next year or so. I'm excited to get my body back, but anxious for the unknown.
> – Vanessa, Florida, United States

Mothers whose children wean after several years of nursing often feel a mix of nostalgia, wistfulness, and relief, but the emotions tend to be muted because the process is slow, and the weaned child is ready for more mature interaction. The mild looking-back pangs Natalie describes have been felt by mothers for ages before us:

> I am finding this ending bittersweet. I am no longer able to pull out my breast to make anything better. On the other hand, it is so nice to be able to buy a regular bra and not have leaky breasts leaving wet spots on the sheets or my clothes; these are the things that I am happy to move past. Sometimes, I long for the days of pulling out my breast. Other days, I am amazed by the wisdom of my growing children. I know that while my breastfeeding years have come to an end, they made me the parent that I am now and will help my family face challenges together as we grow.
> – Natalie, Ontario, Canada

The exact moment when nursing ended might stay in your memory forever... or, like Sonja, you might not even know when it was:

> I felt a bit sad that we didn't have one last, special nursing session – but it's perfectly okay now.
> – Sonja, Austria

The strength of your feelings might surprise you. Sadness is more likely if you weaned in the first couple of years, but it can happen at any time – even if, like Samantha, you wanted to wean:

> My ten-year breastfeeding journey came to an unexpected end when my then-four-and-a-half-year-old got tonsillitis and suddenly wasn't able to breastfeed because of the pain. She tried again a week later and said, patting my breasts, "There's no milky in them boobies, Mama." She had another few tries over the following days, but then quite happily stopped. I had been feeling pretty ready to finish breastfeeding, but this unexpected ending brought up so much grief.
> – Samantha, from the UK, living in Bali, Indonesia

You may revel in your non-nursing status, but also feel weepy or sensitive for a time. You might feel a sense of rejection if your child stopped too easily or weaned sooner than you wanted. It's common to experience a period of low mood or increased anxiety after weaning. It's thought this may be at least partly related to shifts going on behind the scenes, as hormones settle back to pre-pregnancy levels. These feelings may be more likely if you've experienced depression or anxiety before. Be gentle with yourself as you find your new normal, and don't be afraid to ask for help if you need it.

There Is Life After Breastfeeding

If you can barely remember life before nursing (or pumping), it might be hard to imagine it ending. It surely will – but what you learned during this time remains, as Cecily writes:

> In the end, I breastfed every day for thirteen and a half years. Then, it was done. Even after all those years, it was very emotional for me to wean my last child. As they had grown, I had grown as a woman and a mother.
> – Cecily, Ontario, Canada

Breastfeeding is not just about better health – it may feel like one of the most rewarding things you ever do for your child:

> My son is about to turn nine years old. I breastfed him for a third of his life and I can assure you that one of the things that I will treasure most about my motherhood, and one that I will miss the most, will be precisely this stage of breastfeeding; because beyond carrying life in my womb, I was able to nurture my son physically and emotionally and the looks he gave me were my best reward.
> – Haydee, Coahuila, Mexico

Weaning is an important transition – the end of a process that began at conception, and the end of a unique intimacy. But the close relationships that began with breastfeeding continue long after weaning, as Shanna describes:

> My children have reaped the benefits of our nursing relationship far beyond their nursing years.
>
> – *Shanna, Ithaca, New York, United States*

Want to know more?

You can find extra resources for this chapter at the "Art of Breastfeeding" tab at www.llli.org.

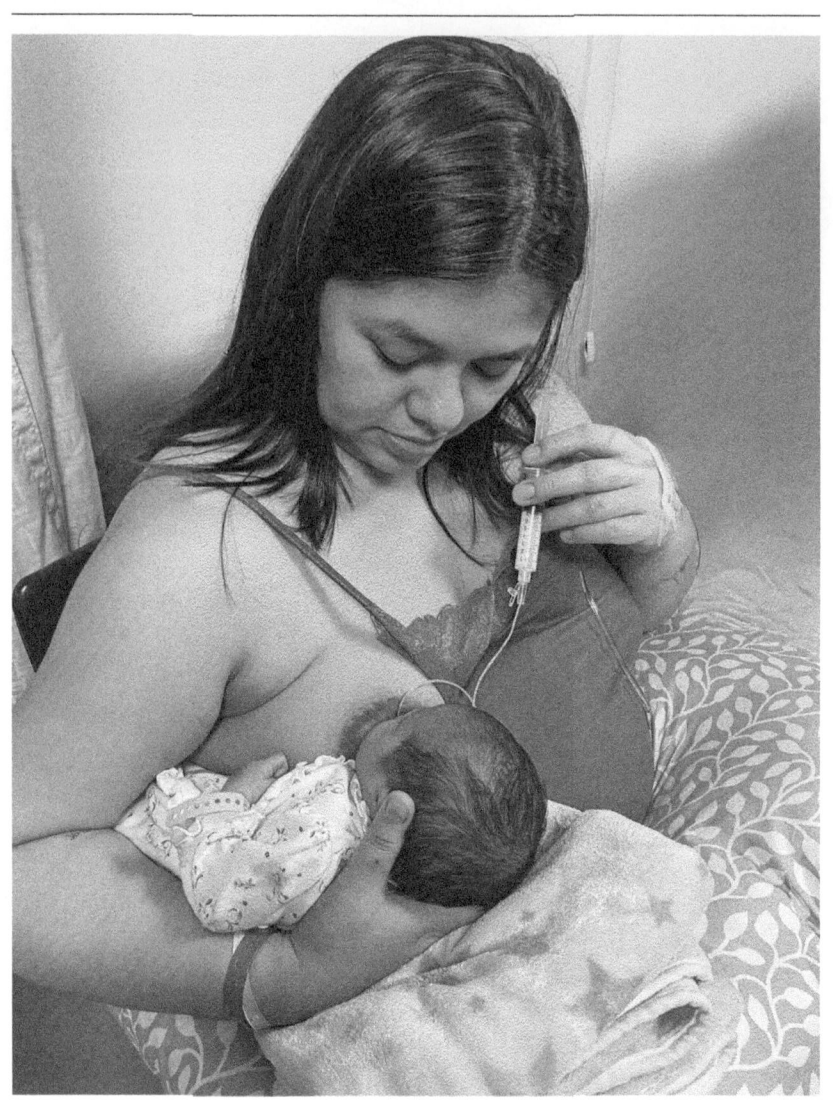

SEVENTEEN

Alternate Routes

Calvin was born eight weeks premature; he weighed just over three pounds. I was given a hospital breast pump. I couldn't hold Calvin, I couldn't even see him yet, but I could ensure that he had the nutrition he needed! What kept me sane through all of this was my ability to pump. Calvin astounded the neonatologists and the nurses with how well he tolerated his feeds. I'll never forget when he was up to two-ounce feedings, I tentatively asked when I could breastfeed. The nurse just looked at me and said, "Now." I cried; I was so happy! The nurse started walking away to find a nipple shield when suddenly Calvin popped himself on perfectly and started nursing away, no problem. Breastfeeding was a gift that not only nourished him back to health but allowed me to regain the bond with my baby.

– Faith, United States

Breastfeeding is often straightforward – common issues can be solved early on. But some of us have more complicated stories like these:

- Kristina's baby has Down syndrome. She fought hard to continue breastfeeding, with extra milk given through a nose tube, while waiting for her baby's heart surgery.
- Sandra discovered that the reason she'd had to supplement with formula while breastfeeding was that she had "hypoplasia" (see Chapter 18, Breast Tissue Insufficiency).

- Trevor, a trans man who'd had chest masculinization surgery, nursed his baby with the help of an at-breast supplementer device and donor milk.
- Willow suffered brain injury at birth and couldn't nurse. Her mother, Fee, and a group of friends expressed milk for her.

Every situation is unique, and each family has their own priorities. Yours might be nursing at the breast or giving as much human milk as possible. Or a bit of both or something else entirely.

You might have challenges that last just a short while, like Allison:

> My little one had a three-day NICU stay and a bit of a bumpy start learning how to latch. We did some pumping and bottle-feeding, as well as a small amount of formula, to get us through the first week.
> – Allison, North Carolina, United States

Or your challenges might last for the whole of your breastfeeding time. Whatever your situation, if nursing or human milk play any part in your story, we're here to help.

Exclusive Pumping

"EPing," exclusive pumping, means expressing milk *instead* of nursing directly. It's become more common as pumps have improved and the importance of human milk has come to be better understood. Most often, exclusive pumping is not the family's first choice; it's a labour of love for a baby who can't nurse – like Melissa's son:

> I just assumed that you went into the hospital and came back home with a healthy baby. I never thought of something going wrong during labour. Without getting into all the details, Andy was born not breathing. He was rushed out before I had a chance to see him. Many hours later I was finally able to visit him in the ICU. Andy was in hospital for two weeks. The hospital's lactation consultant helped me get through the first days of painful engorgement and into regular pumping. I luckily had enough milk to feed at least two more babies. It was my way to take care of him and provide for him.
> – Melissa, Tel Aviv, Israel

Is Exclusive Pumping the Same as Breastfeeding?

Yes and no. Yes, because babies are fed human milk and get immune protection formula can't provide. It's a unique connection with your baby. There are differences, too:

- Unlike the "exclusive" in "exclusive breastfeeding" (where the baby gets only human milk), in exclusive pumping the baby may get formula (or solids), too. The "exclusive" part means **all the human milk the baby gets is expressed – he's not nursing directly.**
- **Nursing is about more than just milk.** Breastfeeding is a whole-body experience for your baby. It calms, comforts, and warms him, relieves pain, and builds connection, all in a single package.
- **The "mechanics" of feeding are different.** The palate, jaw, teeth, face, and airway are shaped by nursing.
- During nursing, **immune system "messages" pass between baby and breast.** If the baby has been in contact with a virus or other bug, his saliva passes the memo along to the milk factory – which responds with custom-made antibodies in the milk a few hours later. This doesn't work quite the same way if a pump is in the picture.
- **Nursing is child-driven,** and it varies according to the baby's needs. Expressing is more likely to happen on a regular schedule.

Exclusive pumping is a huge commitment. Whether you provide any, some, or all of your baby's milk, every drop is valuable, and we're here to help.

How Often Do You Need to Express for a Baby Who Isn't Nursing?

There isn't a set number of times below which a supply will dry up. Most of us will keep making some milk, even just expressing once a day. To bring in a *full* supply, though, you'll need to express around eight to twelve times in twenty-four hours. These tips might help:

- **Think targets rather than schedules.** *How often* you express is more important than exactly *when*. You can work in expressing around other things you need to do.

- **For more milk, express more times.** Even five minutes here or there helps!
- Aim for **500 ml (17 ounces) per day by one week after birth, and 750 to 1,000 ml (25 to 34 ounces) per day by two to three weeks.** If you can get to this level, you've got a good chance of making all the milk your baby (or babies) will ever need. A premature baby may take much longer to be ready for these amounts, but if your goal is to provide all the milk he'll need, aim for these volumes early.

For more on milk production, see Chapter 6 and Chapter 18, Low Milk Supply. For more on expressing, including how to choose a pump, see Chapter 15.

Keeping Up Your Supply

When you're reliant on a pump, sustaining milk production over time is a common challenge.

- Sometimes the issue is that the baby is getting **too much milk by bottle.** For tips on avoiding overfeeding, see Chapter 18, Supplementing, Weight Gain Worries.
- **Check your pump.** For troubleshooting tips, see Chapter 15.
- **Extra stress** can make expressing harder. If you get less milk during a crisis or busy period, a few days of frequent expressing can get you back on track. You might want a temporary upgrade to a larger, faster pump, too. For more ideas, see Chapter 15 and chapter 18, Low Milk Supply.

How Often Does Your Baby Need Feeding?

Human milk is digested more easily (and therefore faster) than formula, so an expressed-milk-fed baby is likely to need to be fed more frequently than a formula-fed baby. Healthy, full-term babies are good at figuring out their own feeding pattern. If you see any of these signs – sucking on her hand, smacking her lips, turning her head towards you – it's a good moment to offer.

If your baby is premature, or has health issues, for now you might need to take more control of her eating. Aim to feed her at least eight to twelve times in twenty-four hours, and work with your healthcare provider to monitor her growth.

Babywearing – using a sling or soft carrier – is a great way to meet your baby's need for closeness between feeds.

Staying "Pumped"

It can be hard to keep going with exclusive pumping, especially if you wanted to nurse directly. It helps to find a place to belong, and friends to cheer you on. La Leche League Leaders can support you whether or not you want to connect with a group. Our groups welcome anyone who's providing human milk for their baby, whether nursing or expressing. There are also online EP communities with unmatched expertise in expressing.

Babies Who Need NICU Care

When you have a premature or sick baby, your milk is even more important. Your baby may be moved to a neonatal intensive care unit (NICU), the part of the hospital that specialises in caring for very premature or sick babies. The NICU can seem overwhelming at first. With all the tubes and monitors attached, it's easy to feel that your baby belongs to the hospital, not to you. Machines beep and alarms go off. The staff bustle about, adjusting this dial and changing that setting. You have no idea what any of it means and might feel like a spare part, even an intruder.

Even if you're familiar with hospitals, having a baby in NICU can still be difficult, as Marisela found:

> I am a licensed nurse and intensive care nurse. The hardest thing for me was to deal with my feelings of sadness and uselessness after having prepared myself so much, and on top of that being a health professional.
> – Marisela, Mexico

But even if you're feeling unsure, out of place, or underskilled, you're *hugely* important to your baby. The best NICUs recognise this by welcoming parents as partners in their babies' care.

Day by day, the NICU will seem less strange. You'll get to know the staff, the machines, and the routine. Watch closely, and don't be afraid to ask questions. It's the staff's job to help you become confident to care for your baby. You can learn a lot from parents who've been there longer, too.

Though the NICU is your baby's place of residence for now, he recognises your body as his *real* home. Research has shown again and again that babies are warmer, calmer, and more stable in skin-to-skin contact with their parents than in an incubator.

Kangaroo Care

Kangaroo Care means caring for babies skin-to-skin, on their mothers, or another close person. The baby is usually naked except for a nappy. Kangaroo Care was first developed in low-resource countries, to care for very premature babies. The evidence that babies do best in Kangaroo Care is so compelling that it's now routine in many countries. Mariana describes her experience:

> María Victoria was a tiny one-kilo premature baby. With her I learned kangaroo mother care and nursed her exclusively from my breast. She doubled her birth weight within forty days. In the beginning she nursed very weakly, but within days she gained strength.
> – Mariana, Guatemala

When you hold your baby skin-to-skin, she receives many benefits:

- Her oxygen levels and breathing rates are more regular and stable.
- Her heart rate is slightly higher.
- You automatically adjust your own body temperature to raise or lower hers.
- Her immune system is boosted; she is less vulnerable to allergies and infections in her first year.
- She's likely to breastfeed more easily, and your milk production increases.
- You feel closer to your baby – a help in healing the trauma of premature birth and separation.

Hospital policies on skin-to-skin contact vary, and your baby's age and condition will need to be factored in. Transitions between your body and the incubator can be stressful for preemies – it's easier on your baby if your sessions are at least a couple of hours long. Hospital practices can present barriers, as Marina experienced:

> The next time I saw [Noel] was eight hours later, when I could go to the NICU in a wheelchair. I could start breastfeeding him around eighteen hours after labour. I could only see him and nurse him every three hours. In addition, only one parent could come in at a time, so for days Noel's dad couldn't see him, as I was the one to go in and nurse him.
> – Marina, Madrid, Spain

Even when hospitals promote skin-to-skin, busyness can get in the way. And staff might not all be equally helpful, as Brie discovered with her premature twins:

> The nurses said skin-to-skin was important but acted like it was a hassle and would give excuses as to why we shouldn't do it. I had a nurse tell me I couldn't take my baby out to hold her because she hadn't pooed yet, but then the doctor came by and said that I absolutely could and that it would help her bowels. It was confusing receiving mixed messages, and when I asked to do skin-to-skin with the twins together, the nurses were very annoyed and made a big deal about how much work it was for them. If we didn't arrive at the right time, we weren't allowed to hold them until their next care cycle started, hours later. [We] dedicated ourselves to doing skin-to-skin as much as we could, but even then each twin was only being held once or twice a day.
> – Brie, Florida, United States

Even if you're usually good at standing up for what you need, it can feel *much* harder in the NICU. Some hospitals have patient advocates and social workers. There might also be outside NICU support organisations. A knowledgeable friend or relative can also speak up for you. At some level, most of us believe that NICU staff have magical powers to make things go well (or not) for our babies. But they don't. Staff are professionals, doing the best they can, often in difficult circumstances. The real magic is in the skin-to-skin contact between you and your baby – and in the unique protection of your milk.

Milk as Medicine

Your milk is the most powerful medicine for your premature or sick baby.

> Our teachings say that Our Milk is Medicine. Western Science has proven some of our teachings to be correct: breast crawl, skin-to-skin benefits, human milk as medicine, keeping baby close. It's funny to us that Western Medicine is catching up to us, when they said our teachings were primitive.
> – Stephanie, Six Nations of the Grand River, Ontario, Canada

If your baby is born early, your milk will be different from milk produced for full-term babies and will contain more of the nutrients your premature baby needs. Formula, even special premature formula, increases the risk of damage to your baby's immature digestive system and makes it more likely that he'll get infections and illnesses, including *necrotizing enterocolitis* (NEC), a very serious disease that damages the gut.

In some hospitals, very premature babies may have cow's-milk-based fortifiers added to their expressed milk. These fortifiers are given to increase the levels of protein, minerals, and other nutrients to help the baby develop and grow at about the same rate as they would if they were still in the womb. Human-milk-based fortifiers are now also available in some NICUs. Research continues on the best way to support preemies' growth and development.

Building Your Milk Supply

To get your milk production off to the best possible start, express early and often. For more on exclusive pumping, see earlier in this chapter and Chapter 18, Low Milk Supply.

Seeing all the milk you're pumping that your baby can't begin to use yet may make you think it isn't important to pump so much. But your little baby, who looks so tiny now, is going to grow fast, doubling his size in a few weeks or months, and before you know it, he'll need every drop of a full milk supply. It's better to overproduce in the beginning so you'll have enough later.

It's common to get temporary dips in your milk production when you've got a premature baby. Being the parent of a preemie is a stressful experience. Maybe you got some bad news about how your baby is doing, or, like Brie, you're juggling other responsibilities with being with your baby in hospital:

> My older daughter needed me at home, so I spent every day with the twins and every night with my four-year-old. Thankfully my husband and sister were caring for her and she was getting a lot of love and attention from them, but she still had a hard time not having enough time with her mama. It was so painful having to be separated from them [the twins], but I was comforted knowing they were having my milk.
> — Brie, Florida, United States

In countries without maternity leave, parents may have to return to work shortly after giving birth to save time off for when the baby comes home from the NICU.

If you're consistently having trouble making as much milk as your baby needs, even though you're pumping eight to twelve times in twenty-four hours, some herbs or medications (*galactagogues*) may help. Check your planned approach with a breastfeeding-knowledgeable healthcare provider. For more about milk production problems, see Chapter 18, Low Milk Supply.

Breast or Bottle First?

At first your baby may be fed by a tube going from her nose down to her stomach (a nasogastric tube) or a tube going from her mouth down to her stomach (an orogastric tube). After the tube is removed (or if it isn't used at all), some hospitals have policies that the babies need to be bottle-fed before they can try breastfeeding, or that they must take bottles before being discharged. The research doesn't support this approach. Breastfeeding is *less* stressful for a preemie than bottle-feeding. If your baby doesn't seem to be ready to handle the flow of milk from the breast, she can practise by nursing on your breast just after you've pumped.

If you're doing Kangaroo Care, at some point your baby may start moving down your body, heading for your breast. She may even latch on without much help from you. This is an excellent sign that she's ready to start nursing!

Nipple shields (thin pieces of shaped silicone that sit on your nipple while your baby nurses) may make it easier for a premature baby to latch on, stay on, and nurse effectively. It's certainly worth trying to nurse without a shield first, but keep shields in mind if your baby needs some extra help. If you can, work with someone who's used to using shields (see Chapter 18, Nipple Shields).

Premature babies in hospitals are often fed every three or even four hours. Preemies do need to sleep a lot. Often, though, that schedule is partly due to staffing constraints. Your baby in skin-to-skin contact may very well have the energy and interest to nurse more often. If you don't feel up to debating this with the hospital staff, you may decide to go along with their instructions. As long as you keep your milk production going, you've got lots of time to sort out nursing. As Brie's story shows, it's a long game:

> The next step was transitioning from my milk through the NG tube to only breastfeeding because I didn't want to introduce bottles before we established nursing. I asked the occupational therapist, and she told me they had never seen it done before!
>
> I suggested weighing before and after feeding to the doctor. I quickly found that the babies were getting much more than we thought, and we started reducing their tube feed by how much they got each time they nursed, just like how hospital staff normally do it with bottle-feeding. They started waking up more often and I was able to nurse them more and more.
>
> It was so exciting and rewarding seeing them get rounder and healthier from breastfeeding. It was still super challenging and stressful, but my heart would fill up with love for my babies every time they nursed. Within a week of doing weighted feeds for each session, we graduated from the NICU and began the next part of our breastfeeding journey at home. I became the first mum to leave this particular NICU exclusively breastfeeding twins.
>
> It was far from easy after we came home, yet we continued breastfeeding and established a wonderful bond through it. They met all their milestones, stayed on track for their weight gain, and now they are two-year-old toddler nurslings who aren't slowing down yet!
>
> – Brie, Florida, United States

When Your Preemie Nurses

It's normal to feel nervous the first time your preemie baby nurses. He probably still seems impossibly tiny! You might like to try a laid-back nursing position first (see Chapter 4). If you've been doing Kangaroo Care, you've likely been in this position many times: get comfortable semi-reclining, and relax with your baby tummy-down on your chest. He may move over to the breast all on his own, or with a little help from you.

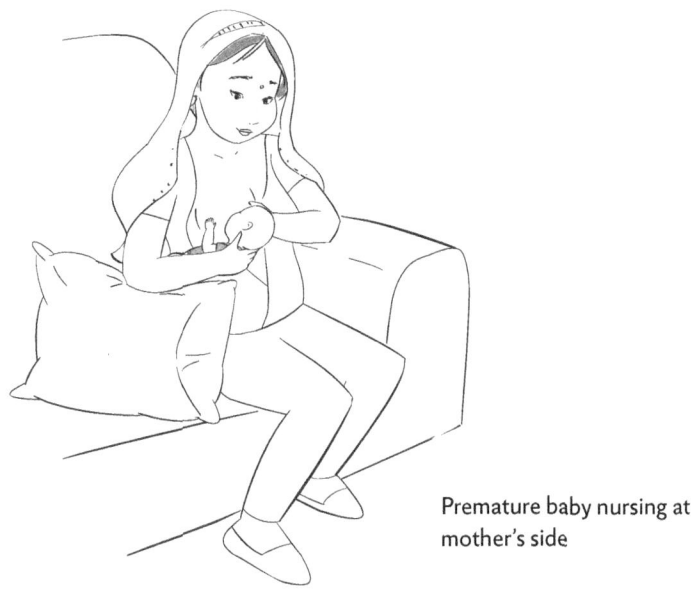

Premature baby nursing at mother's side

Good help can make a great difference, as Dawn found:

A lovely NICU lactation consultant was able to help me advocate for feeding my baby directly from the breast. She was able to be present for my first latch and also showed me how to use a nursing supplementer.
– *Dawn, British Columbia, Canada*

To start with, your baby may latch, take a couple of sucks, then promptly fall asleep. No worries. You can try again when he wakes up. Continue expressing to keep your supply strong. It's probably going to take quite a while before your preemie can do much of the work of feeding. He will get there. Time and patience are key:

The first time I nursed them I was so excited and felt like they would pick it up quickly and we'd be out of there in no time. I was very wrong. They would quickly get stressed or tired and only nursed every so often and I was devastated over and over. I learned to be patient even though it was constantly disappointing and frustrating. Weeks went by while I continued to pump, do skin-to-skin, and try to breastfeed.
– *Brie, Florida, United States*

From Hospital to Home

> Most parents who have spent any time in ICU will probably say that it's not an easy transition. Coming home is what we wait for, but being home without the schedule and the support of the staff can be quite difficult.
> – *Melissa, Tel Aviv, Israel*

You aren't the first person who has wondered if you can cope. Remember: your medical team is confident that your baby and you are ready for this.

Take your time. You may need to remind your baby to nurse for a while yet, until she's got more energy. When she nurses, she will probably have more pauses and shorter sucking bursts than a full-term baby. She's likely to tire out before she's had enough milk. Most premature babies need at least until their due date to nurse well. If your baby's been having supplements of expressed milk or formula, you'll need to reduce the supplements gradually (see Chapter 18, Supplementing). It's *so* tempting to rush it – but experience tells us that the transition from NICU to relaxed, go-with-the-flow nursing can't be hurried. Your baby's healthcare provider should monitor her weight gain closely.

Keep her close. Carrying your baby in a wrap designed for Kangaroo Care or in a sling helps her grow faster, saving energy by keeping her calm in her natural habitat. Check with someone knowledgeable about carriers and premature babies to make sure you're doing it safely.

Build your network. Having a baby in hospital can be incredibly lonely. Back home, you can draw on the support of family and friends. Most of them won't fully understand what you've been through, though, or the challenges of bringing a NICU baby home. You might want to connect with people who do. Support from her lactation consultant transformed Melissa's experience:

> I told her that it wasn't working out and that I didn't think I'd be able to breastfeed. I had given up, I was tired. Soon after, she had arrived at our home, and with her support Andy was breastfeeding! We were on our way.
> – *Melissa, Tel Aviv, Israel*

Some hospitals have NICU parent support groups, and you can

find virtual ones, too. Any LLL group will include families who've been through the NICU experience. La Leche League Leaders are here to help, before and after you bring your baby home.

Late-Premature and Early-Term Babies

> **Late premature** means born between thirty-four and thirty-seven weeks.
> **Early term** means born between thirty-seven and thirty-nine weeks.

Just-a-bit-early babies often *look* like term babies, especially if they're large for their gestational age (LGA). They usually don't need NICU care. Health professionals may treat them like term babies, assuming they can nurse easily from the start. But they often *act* like earlier premature babies and need extra help with feeding at first, as Glenda's baby did:

> He was born at thirty-six weeks, at a reasonable weight of 2,250 grams. The baby cried a lot – my mum just told me to put him to the breast and asked me if I felt him sucking. And I answered no. Once in a while he managed to suck, but the next day my baby was taken to the neonatal ward for jaundice that lasted eleven days. I survived thanks to the La Leche League Mexico group.
>
> – Glenda, Cuba

Knowing what to expect when your baby is born a bit early makes you less likely to be taken by surprise – especially if you take action to head off problems before they start.

Late-Premature and Early-Term Babies: Common Challenges

What?	Why?	What You Can Do	More Info
Gets too **cold**	Less body fat. Not as good as a term baby at managing her own temperature.	Hold your dried baby skin-to-skin in a warm room, with a towel or blanket over both of you.	Chapter 18, Hypothermia

Low blood sugar	Not as much energy stored in his body as a full-term baby, especially if small for gestational age (SGA). Blood sugar more likely to drop if mother is diabetic.	Skin-to-skin contact keeps your baby warm and calm, saving energy. Express colostrum before birth in case your baby needs extra milk. If your baby needs more energy fast, ask about dextrose gel or donor milk.	Chapter 18, Hypoglycaemia Chapter 1, Chapter 15 (expressing colostrum before your baby is born) Chapter 18, Milk Sharing
More likely to get jaundiced (turn yellow, due to buildup of the waste product bilirubin in the blood)	Liver is less mature so slower to break down extra red blood cells.	Nurse, or offer expressed milk, early and often, to flush out the bilirubin. If your baby starts to look jaundiced, contact your healthcare provider. If your baby needs more milk fast, ask about donor milk.	Chapter 18, Jaundice Chapter 18, Milk Sharing
May take more time to feed well	Gets tired faster and needs to sleep more. Can't coordinate sucking, swallowing, and breathing as well as a term baby. Might have a weaker suck. Might be smaller in relation to the breast, making latching more challenging.	Offer the breast often, at least 8–12 times in 24 hours. Keep your baby skin-to-skin to encourage interest in nursing (and so you can spot early signs of interest). Keep the room calm and quiet so she can concentrate. Express milk often, to bring in a plentiful supply. Offer your expressed milk to your baby; more energy means better feeding. If your baby needs more milk than you can express, ask about donor milk.	Chapter 15, Part 1: Milk Out Chapter 18, Milk Sharing Chapter 18, Supplementing

Helping your late-premature or early-term baby nurse:

- **Handle him gently** – his nerves are more raw than if he'd been born later. He may startle and get overwhelmed easily.
- Try **laid-back positions** to give him a nice stable base for nursing and encourage his feeding instincts (see Chapter 4).
- Or try **holding your baby to your side** (see clutch or football position in Chapter 4).

- Use **your hand cupped under your baby's chin** while nursing, to support his chin and cheeks.
- Use **breast compression and massage** during feeding to help bring milk down for him (watch carefully, and stop if the milk comes too fast!).
- **Count poos and wees.** For how many to expect at each stage, see chapters 5, 6, and 7. If you're not seeing as many as expected, let your healthcare provider know and start expressing your milk (or express more often).
- **Monitor your baby's weight.** Plan regular weight checks until your baby has a track record of gaining well (see Chapter 18, Weight Gain Worries).
- **Act quickly** if there are any signs that your baby isn't getting enough milk or your milk production is low. Talk to your healthcare provider, and find breastfeeding help (see Chapter 18, Low Milk Supply).
- **Get the support you need.** Nursing early babies can be *very* different from nursing full-term ones. The usual advice – "Nurse when your baby wants to nurse, for as long as they want to nurse" – often just doesn't work yet. Connect with people who know about the special challenges of nursing babies born a little early. La Leche League Leaders are here to help.

Multiples

The most common worries about **breastfeeding twins, triplets, or more** are having enough arms and having enough milk. We hope you'll have some help to give you a few extra arms to hold the babies, but you're the babies' best source for milk. The milk part might not be as difficult as you think. With enough breast stimulation from straight after birth, most of us can probably make enough milk for more than one baby. The biggest challenge many families face with multiples is that so many of them are born prematurely (see the previous section on premature babies).

Once your babies are home, you'll need to pay close attention to their nappy outputs and weights to make sure they're getting enough milk. Sometimes it's hard to keep the numbers straight for each baby, so it might help to have a separate colour-coded clipboard or app for each of them. Don't be surprised if one nurses better than the other(s) at first. Just like all babies, some multiples catch on faster, and some need more time. Sometimes one baby will be significantly bigger than his sibling(s). However, one of the smaller babies may be the more vigorous nurser! Alternate the breast each baby gets to keep your milk supply evenly stimulated. The tips in the previous section on nursing early-term babies may be helpful as your babies transition to nursing.

Should You Nurse Two at the Same Time?

It saves time, of course, and the babies stimulate milk ejections for each other. There's a learning curve in figuring out how to manage it, though. This can feel overwhelming at first. When you feel ready, you can try adding in a second baby after the first has latched. Pillows may be helpful – some companies make nursing pillows just for nursing multiples. But don't feel like nursing your babies together is something you *have* to do right away – or even at all if you don't want to.

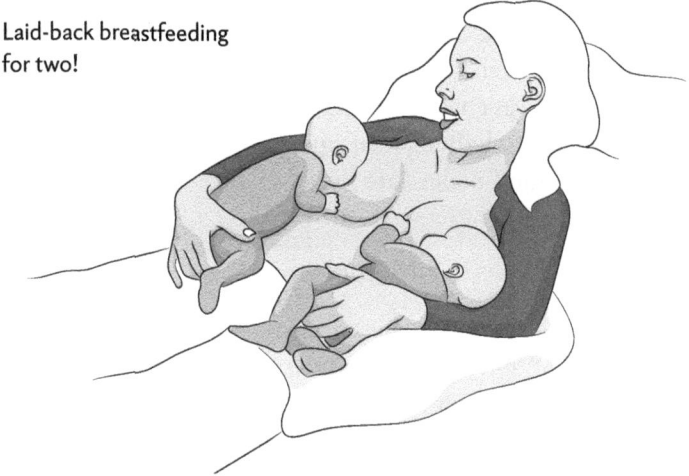

Laid-back breastfeeding for two!

As Nikki found, each baby has their own timetable:

> Did you know two babies born a mere ten minutes apart from each other can be *very different*? The older one took to nursing like a champion. She would latch perfectly, snuggle into me, eat until she was full, never spit up, and immediately fall fast asleep for several hours afterwards. The younger twin was a much different story. I became a hybrid breastfeeder – nursing the older twin while pumping for the younger and bottle-feeding her. I was able to finally nurse both of my children as they neared six months old.
>
> – *Nikki, United States military*

Positioning Options for Nursing Two Babies at Once

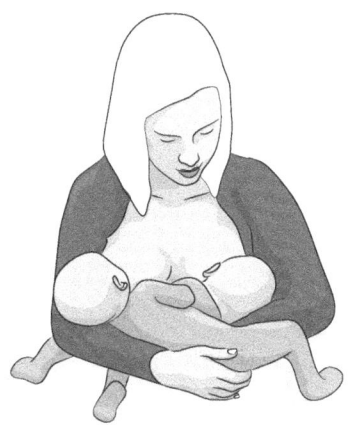

One laid across the other

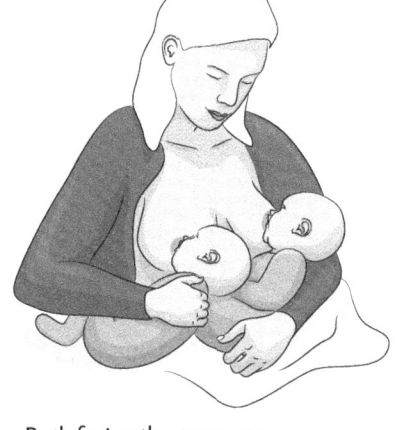

Both facing the same way

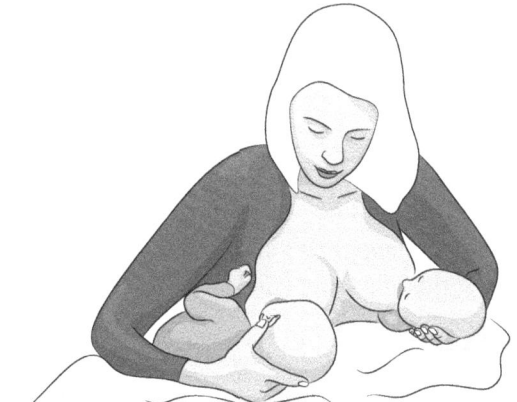

Both in the clutch position

You may feel you're glued to your sofa when you're nursing twins or more. An enlightening moment for one mother of multiples came when she met a mother of grown twins who told her, "Oh, I still remember fixing and feeding and washing all those bottles!" Feeding twins or more is a demanding undertaking, however you do it. But nursing becomes easier and more efficient over time (and usually more fun). Washing bottles doesn't.

One of the most important factors in taking care of multiples is taking care of *you:* this is a time when the support of family, friends, and community is not just helpful but essential. For ideas on building your support network, see Chapter 2.

Relactation

Relactation is the process of restarting milk production after it's been stopped for a while. There are several possible situations:

- You might have thought you didn't want to or couldn't breastfeed, then changed your mind.
- Maybe your baby really needs your milk because he's having problems with formula.
- You might be relactating to feed a child you didn't give birth to, e.g., because you're adopting.

Whatever your reason, bringing back your milk supply can be well worth the work. It's helpful to have a realistic idea of what's involved before you set out.

How Tough Will It Be?

The stronger your track record of making milk up to now, and the more recent it was, the easier relactation is likely to be. If you never had a full milk supply, or if it's been several months or more since you weaned, regaining *full* production may not happen. It's almost always possible to get *some* milk production back, though! Only you can calculate the costs and benefits.

Laura relactated for her toddler a few weeks after stopping breastfeeding:

> I let comments from friends and family members pressure me to wean before I was ready. Weaning never felt right because she loved nursing, and it seemed her sleep and behaviour got worse after weaning. When my daughter got her autism diagnosis one and a half months after weaning, I researched relactating and put her on my breast, and she took right to it like time had never passed.
>
> – Laura, United States military

Restarting Milk Production

Is your baby willing to nurse fairly well, even though there's no milk yet? If so, this alone can bring your milk back, although your baby will need to be supplemented during the process.

Keeping Your Baby Well Fed

As you work to bring back your supply, make sure your baby gets as much milk as usual. It will take your breasts time to get the message that more milk is needed. Offer your usual amount of donor milk or formula to start with. A nursing supplementer – a gadget that enables the baby to drink donor milk or formula via a thin tube as she nurses – can be an excellent tool for relactation. (You can see a photo of a supplementer in action at the beginning of this chapter, and find more information in Chapter 18, Supplementing.) If your baby can nurse efficiently with a supplementer, you might not need to express, and your baby can do all her feeding at the breast or chest.

Once you start to notice signs of milk production (see the next section), you can gradually offer less supplement. It's important to keep an eye on your baby's weight during this time.

Pumping Up the Volume

If your baby is reluctant to nurse, or won't nurse for very long, you can get things going by **using a breast pump.** Because you need the best stimulation possible, it's usually most effective to use a combination of hand expression and a double electric pump (hospital-grade if possible).

Most newborn babies need to nurse at least eight to twelve times in twenty-four hours to bring in a full milk supply. For maximum milk production, you might want to aim for this number of expressions – but any amount of expressing is worth it. For more about expressing, see Chapter 15.

The first sign that milk production is starting up again is usually tender breasts, then drops forming on your nipple when you express. These may be clear at first but soon may change colour to yellowish white, cream, or bluish white. Gradually, the volume will increase. You'll probably begin to see good results in two to six weeks.

I followed simple steps – increased breast stimulation – nursing Tamia after supplementing her, breast massage, skin-to-skin, and using the homemade lactation aid. I also consumed galactagogues to aid my efforts to relactate. We did a lot of skin-to-skin, which helped us bond and helped Tamia get more breastmilk. Although I had a double electric pump with me and I did try pumping many times, I could not keep at it in a sustained manner. Over time, I reduced the amount of formula she was getting through the lactation aid and was able to wean her off formula at about ten months.

– Chetana, Bangalore, India

For more about increasing your milk, including about galactagogues (medications, foods, and herbs that may help increase milk production), see Chapter 18, Low Milk Supply.

Enticing Your Baby (Back) to the Breast

This section may be useful if you're doing any of these:

- transitioning a preemie to the breast
- encouraging an older baby to nurse after a period of exclusive pumping
- nursing a baby you didn't give birth to

Take it gently, and get as much help and support as you need. **The younger your baby is, the more likely she is to nurse.** Newborns are strongly hardwired to breastfeed. The older the baby, the more likely he is to continue doing whatever he's used to doing. But many, many babies have started nursing after the early months.

Chetana wondered whether her adopted daughter's brief early experience of breastfeeding helped her breastfeed easily later:

We adopted Tamia when she was almost five months old. She was wet-nursed by mothers in the hospital when the nurses could take her to the maternity ward. At the children's home where she stayed most of the first few months, she was given diluted cow's milk and sometimes formula. With the lowest of expectations, but a flame of hope and a fluttering stomach, I used a nipple shield and dropped formula from a bottle into it. She latched

on and suckled for almost fifteen minutes! What may have helped is the memory of being wet-nursed. Tamia was breastfeeding like a pro.
– Chetana, Bangalore, India

After many early difficulties, it took more than six months before Marina's baby nursed well:

At five and a half months old, one day, I realised Noel's suction was stronger and it continued to get stronger and stronger after that. Around this time, Noel started breastfeeding at all times of day, awake, playing, and happy, which was incredible for me. He wasn't rejecting my breast anymore. At six months, I stopped pumping. When we went to Canada on vacation something clicked. I jumped on the plane and thought I would breastfeed Noel. To my surprise, he loved it during the eight-hour flight. We got to Canada and we went to visit Niagara Falls. I thought I would try to nurse him there, in such an inspiring place. Noel accepted and even smiled at me as he was eating. I couldn't be happier. Noel was seven months old. After that, I started nursing Noel whenever and wherever, and he would enjoy it more and more. Things just got better and better.
– Marina, Madrid, Spain

Counting the Cost

How about if your baby *never* nurses directly from the breast? The more milk there is, the stronger the incentive. But there are never any guarantees that a baby will go back to the breast (or start nursing, if she's never done it before). Even a small amount of milk gives your baby immune protection no formula can provide. But this needs to be balanced against the work involved in expressing. You might ask yourself this question at the outset: *If my baby never does go back to the breast, is this effort worth it?* Only you can answer that. We're here to support you, whatever you decide to do.

The most important thing as you go along is to be gentle and patient. You're *enticing* your baby to nurse – not *making* her do it. Chetana is an adoptive mother and LLL Leader who supports other adoptive parents to breastfeed by increasing their supply, relactating, or inducing lactation (see below). Chetana recalls her experience:

Most babies and toddlers can be coaxed to accept the breast. Depending on the baby's temperament and personality — some take to breastfeeding faster than others.

— Chetana, Bangalore, India

Bringing In a Milk Supply – What Do the Words Mean?

Relactation means bringing back your milk supply after a break. **Induced lactation** means bringing in a milk supply from a "standing start," when you haven't recently been pregnant (or may never have been pregnant). Keep reading for more on this!

Here are some ideas to try:

- **Hold your baby skin-to-skin.** Take baths together, lounge around in bed together. Some babies may prefer to be lightly dressed rather than skin-to-skin.
- **Laid-back nursing positions** (see Chapter 4) set the scene for your baby to explore the breast in her own time. If she doesn't nurse, it's still a comfortable way to spend time together.
- **Take a nap or sleep together** in a safely prepared bed (see Chapter 12). Some babies will latch when they're falling asleep, waking up, or in light sleep.

My lactation consultant encouraged me to start nursing him during the day, in the afternoons, after his long nap. I did. Later, we did the same in the mornings. She kept encouraging me.

— Marina, Madrid, Spain

- **Babywear.** Most babies love being carried in a sling or soft carrier on your front, and this is a great way to help your baby feel comfortable near the breast.
- **Encourage your baby to associate the breast with eating, and satisfaction.** If you're using bottles or cups, try feeding your baby with her cheek against the breast. She can drift off to sleep, with the breast as her pillow, when she's full and content. She might

progress to nursing as she falls asleep. Keep her away from the breast any time she's frustrated.
- **Rub milk over your nipple and areola.** The smell of your milk helps your baby find the breast and gives her an incentive to explore it.
- **Try drip-drop feeding.** Have your helper use a spoon or eye dropper to drip milk down your breast towards your nipple. If your baby has a go at attaching, keep up the flow of dripped milk to encourage her.
- Try an **at-breast supplementer** to deliver expressed milk or formula via a tube while your baby nurses (see the photo at the beginning of this chapter). This encourages the baby who's keen to nurse but discouraged by the slow flow of milk (see Chapter 18, Supplementing).

I made a lactation aid at home by watching YouTube videos. All it took was two tries for both of us to get comfortable. It is not very expensive if made at home. An infant feeding tube, a feeding bottle, and sharp scissors are all that is needed. Supplementing at the breast means that the baby gets the pumped breastmilk or formula while latched on and suckling. This helps stimulate the breast to increase the milk supply. A lactation aid helps to eliminate artificial nipples, and baby learns to breastfeed while getting adequate nourishment.
– Chetana, Bangalore, India

- Try a **nipple shield,** which fits over your own nipple but feels more like a bottle teat. You could pre-fill it with expressed milk or formula, to give your baby an instant reward as soon as she sucks (see Chapter 18, Nipple Shields).

If you want to try these feeding tools, work with a breastfeeding supporter who's used to using them, if you can.

If your baby gets upset when you offer the breast, or is older than about three months and has never nursed, you may need to be especially patient and creative. For more suggestions for older babies, see Chapter 18, Nursing Strike. An LLL Leader, an International Board Certified Lactation Consultant (IBCLC), or another breastfeeding helper may have other ideas in their bag of tricks.

Celebrate the baby steps. This doesn't have to be an all-or-nothing process; it can be a gradual shift in the direction of the breast. Maybe your baby used to cry when she even saw the breast, but now she'll tolerate having a bottle in skin-to-skin contact. Wonderful! Maybe she'll nurse with a nipple shield or a supplementer. It's a nuisance to have to deal with the equipment for sure, but she's *nursing*! Notice how far you've come, not just how far you'd still like to go.

Induced Lactation

Bringing in a milk supply without having been pregnant is becoming more common as more families realise it's possible. Chetana, an adoptive mother and LLL Leader, puts it like this:

> The anatomy of the female human is designed in such a wondrous way. The mammary glands can start breastmilk production from adequate and continued stimulation. While pregnancy and childbirth prepare the body for breastfeeding, there are induced lactation and relactation protocols available to help mothers breastfeed without giving birth. These are especially helpful for mothers who are interested in adoptive breastfeeding. Be it a newborn or a two-year-old toddler, mothers have been able to successfully breastfeed and produce milk.
>
> – Chetana, Bangalore, India

For many parents who bring in a milk supply without pregnancy, the goal is less about the milk and more about connecting deeply to their new babies. But with new advances in the science of lactation, the chances of getting a good milk supply, or even a full one, are better than in years past (see Chapter 18, Low Milk Supply).

Nursing Without a Milk Supply

If you're starting with a newborn, or an older baby who's willing to take the breast, you can begin nursing right away with an at-breast supplementer filled with donor milk or formula (see Chapter 18, Supplementing). Depending on your baby's willingness, you may also be able to entice him to nurse for comfort in between feeds without the supplementer.

Ginny, who adopted her daughter Carly, started using an at-breast supplementer right away, even though she had no milk of her own yet:

We travelled up to the foster family's home and met Carly, who was ten weeks old. We brought her home that evening. I put her to my breast while we were still there, and a couple of times on the way home. I had no milk at that stage – I'd only had a week or two to prepare, I'd taken no drugs, not done any expressing, nothing – except chat to an LLL Leader who knew from experience about adoptive breastfeeding, and read about it in LLL material.

We were still giving Carly her usual formula in bottles that first day, of course. Carly took the breast easily and got milk from the Lact-Aid [supplementer]. I fed her that way virtually all the time, knowing that frequent nursing was the best way to bring in a milk supply. I never made a full milk supply – she always needed formula as well – but we carried on like that for months. It was amazing for me to have a baby in my arms and at the breast again, and it really helped me feel that I was her mother.

– Ginny, UK

How to Induce a Milk Supply

The best approach for your situation depends on whether your baby has already been born, how old she is, and what you feel comfortable doing. You have lots of options. Ideally, you'll work with a breastfeeding supporter who's experienced in induced lactation and (if you use any medications) with your healthcare provider. You can find online communities that specialise in this area.

Stimulating the Breasts

The key to getting a milk supply started is to stimulate your breasts in a way that tells them to make milk: by frequent nursing, hand expression, or pumping. The more stimulation, the better; newborns usually nurse at least eight to twelve times in twenty-four hours, so if you're aiming to make as much milk as you can, this is a reasonable target. Starting each session with some breast massage often helps. For more tips on expressing, see Chapter 15.

You probably won't see milk for a few days or weeks. That's okay. If you've lactated before, it's likely to be quicker than if you never have.

If you're nursing with an at-breast supplementer, your breasts will eventually start making milk that your baby will get along with the milk from the tube. As your milk increases, it can be hard to know how much is coming from you and how much from the tube. One way to get an idea is to weigh both baby and supplementer on a sensitive scale before and after the feeding. Any increase in weight came straight from you – an amazing achievement! Trevor, a trans man who had chest masculinization surgery and gave birth to his baby, describes how it felt for him:

> After he was done, [the midwife] weighed him again. Looking at the level on the bottle, Ian [my husband] thought he'd had about 30 ml. The midwife did the second weigh and said, "Well, Trevor, he took in 40 ml just now. That means you made 10 ml." I jumped up and hugged her, I was so incredibly happy to hear that I had made a quarter of what Jacob just ate. This was considerably more than the nothing I had felt like I was providing.
> – *Trevor, Manitoba, Canada*

Weighing your baby every week or so can give you an idea of how much your milk supply is increasing. You can also track how much supplement your baby is taking – you'll see if the amount is going down over time. Ginny noticed some more subtle signs of increased milk production, too:

> Within a week or two, I could see that her poos were changing, to more like breastfed baby poo. I was extremely thirsty whenever I put her to the breast almost from the start, and had to have a glass of water! I also noticed that her skin was looking different – I'm not quite sure what it is, but there is something different about the skin of a breastfed baby.
> – *Ginny, UK*

If you're already nursing with an at-breast supplementer, you can pump the other side at the same time for even better stimulation. If you don't have the baby yet, hand expression or pumping while you wait for them to arrive will begin stimulating your milk production. For expressing tips, see Chapter 15.

There's no need to be so scientific unless you want to be. Nursing is a relationship. It isn't measured in units any more than love is.

Simulating Pregnancy Hormones

Some parents who have induced milk supplies find that they can build a bigger supply faster by using hormones and galactagogues. These stimulate the process that would usually build the "lactation infrastructure" during pregnancy. The general idea is to simulate the hormones of pregnancy, and then those of birth and lactation. The results depend on many factors, including how long you have to prepare before the baby comes to you. Even if you need to get ready quickly, you may still make more milk than you would by just expressing or nursing alone.

As the infrastructure develops, your nipples and breasts or chest will begin feeling tender, just as in an actual pregnancy. Hormonal treatments to build your "milk factory" suppress lactation at first, so are generally not appropriate if you're already nursing another baby.

It's important to partner with a healthcare provider if you want to use hormonal therapies to lactate. These therapies are not safe for everyone, and each situation is unique. La Leche League Leaders can support you throughout.

Reducing Supplements

Your baby is nursing now. You're noticing signs of increased milk production; she's also swallowing more often, and nursing for longer. She's growing well. How far and how fast can you safely reduce her supplements? See Chapter 18, Supplementing, and work with your healthcare provider and a breastfeeding supporter to come up with a safe plan.

Relactation can be a two steps forward, one step back process. Be prepared to take things more slowly if your baby becomes fussy or seems hungry, and reach out for support if you need it. During the transition from supplements, it's important to weigh your baby regularly on a reliable scale to make sure she's getting enough. If she isn't, you can give her more of your own expressed milk, donor milk, or formula – but don't cut down on the nursing or expressing.

Your own needs are important, too (and not just because you make milk!). If you get run down, you might not be able to hang in there for the payoff. Don't try to do everything yourself. This is a time to reach out to all your supportive friends, family, and online buddies. Line up help with household chores and older children. Gather a cheerleading team to celebrate your successes and console you on days when you're discouraged. Any LLL group would be delighted to be part of it.

The Special Importance of Colostrum

Colostrum is the milk made during the last few months of pregnancy and the first few days after birth. It gives a powerful boost to the newborn's immune system when he's meeting the world of microbes for the first time. Colostrum is sometimes known as liquid gold, for both its colour and its importance to the baby's health.

Milk produced by inducing lactation or relactation doesn't include a colostral phase – you go straight to mature milk. This milk will be appropriate for feeding your baby; any safe human milk is much more suitable for a baby of any age than formula milk. However, the *ideal* first food for your baby is colostrum from their mother, which is custom-made for the baby. No other milk can match its unique value.

For this reason, some new parents make an agreement with the birth mother or surrogate to express milk for the baby for a defined period. She may be pleased to be able to give this gift. Expressing milk has some benefits for her, too, including helping her uterus return to its pre-pregnancy size and reducing her breast cancer risk (see Chapter 1).

If you're going to be co-nursing a baby birthed by your partner (see Chapter 2), it makes sense for your baby to be fed mainly or entirely by his birthing parent for the first few days at least, to get as much colostrum as possible.

Time Period	Milk Produced
From about 16 weeks of pregnancy to 2–5 days after birth	Colostrum
From day 2–5 to day 10–14	Transitional milk (still contains some colostrum)
After day 10–14	Mature milk

Physical Challenges

If you have a disability or chronic illness, are blind or visually impaired, or are recovering from illness or injury, people might assume that nursing your baby is "just too difficult." But babies have to be fed somehow, and you're the person your baby expects to do it. Whether or not you breastfeed (or express) is your call to make. Nursing may be the most practical option, as Betsy describes:

> Another advantage of breastfeeding for a blind/visually impaired mother is that you do not have to worry about pouring formula into bottles, and the mess that would make. This is so much easier than trying to hold the baby

with one hand with a bottle in the other and trying to find the baby's mouth with a bottle in your hand.

– Betsy, Georgia, United States

When you rely on care from other people, nursing is the one thing you can do that makes it absolutely clear whose baby this is. Emotionally, breastfeeding can do wonders for your self-esteem, confidence, and connection with your baby, as Ecobavila describes:

A mother can be whatever she wants, she can be a worker, she can be a housewife, or as in my case, even without wanting it, she can be an epileptic. A neurologist told me that it was harmful to my baby, because my epilepsy treatment passes through the milk and could affect the formation of his brain . . . but this time, mum was informed, learned, and fought. The medication I have to take can be consumed without affecting breastfeeding. Mum continues her treatment and my four-month-old baby wears ten-month-old clothes thanks to breastfeeding.

– Ecobavila, Spain

These nursing tips have been shared by mothers with disabilities and chronic health conditions:

- If you're told that a **medication** you need isn't compatible with breastfeeding, it's worth double-checking (see Chapter 18, Medications).
- There's lots of **specialist equipment** that can help: pillows and wedges, devices that enable you to pick up the baby without using hands, visual or auditory sensors to alert you to your baby's movements if you can't hear or see them, and more.
- An **occupational therapist** or similar health professional might not have expertise in breastfeeding, but they may be able to help figure out adaptations for you and your breastfeeding supporter to work with.
- **There are ways of working around spinal cord injuries or other nerve damage that affects milk release.** Visualisation and/or oxytocin nasal spray can be used to trigger the milk ejection reflex if nerve pathways are blocked.
- **Baby slings and carriers** come in many types, to fit all bodies. Chosen and used well, they can be helpful for nursing and moving your baby around. You might want to add a babywearing

consultant or an experienced babywearing parent to your support team.

I have been offered various paging systems to alert me to my baby crying (a pacifier/dummy symbol lights up) because I have a severe hearing loss. I was never happy with the level of crying that would be required to trigger them. This was hard to explain to the social workers. Keeping the baby in the sling was by far a better option for me.
– Hannah, UK

- **Be clear about exactly what assistance you want from other people.** It might be bringing the baby to you, helping position her at the breast, switching sides, burping, changing their nappy, soothing. Or you might prefer to use a breast pump and share some or all of the feeding with others from your support team. Part-time nursing is very doable, especially after the early weeks.
- **Connect with relevant advocacy groups and peer support.** If you are differently abled, or whatever your health challenges, there are probably people out there who understand and can help. Support organisations can provide you with resources and tools for adaptive parenting. Your LLL Leader may know of local organisations and be able to connect you with others who've nursed with similar challenges.

Illnesses

If you're living with a chronic illness, others may assume that breastfeeding isn't an option for you. The barriers may not be as high as you think:

- The hormonal and metabolic shifts of pregnancy and lactation can **reduce the symptoms of some chronic illnesses.** These include rheumatoid arthritis, multiple sclerosis, lupus, gastrointestinal conditions, and diabetes. You might even go into temporary remission during pregnancy.
- **Many of the medications and treatments used for chronic conditions** – including ADHD, diabetes, sickle-cell disease, and thalassaemia; and autoimmune disorders such as rheumatoid

arthritis, multiple sclerosis, and lupus – are compatible with breastfeeding.
- **For some medications, additional strategies may be needed,** especially if the baby is premature or unwell (see Chapter 18, Medications).

You can find more information at www.llli.org about specific conditions, including diabetes, HIV, and cancer. We wish we had room to cover all these conditions, plus many more, in more detail! Within the worldwide LLL community, families have expertise on feeding their babies with pretty much every health challenge you could imagine. We're here to help.

Previous Breast, Chest, and Nipple Surgeries

All previous surgeries in your chest area – including cancer surgeries, reductions, augmentations (implants to make breasts larger), chest masculinisation (top) surgery, nipple piercings, and nipple inversion release surgeries – can affect future milk production if nerves and ducts are damaged or if a lot of breast tissue has been removed.

We know this might be hard to read, especially if you were assured at the time that surgery wouldn't affect breastfeeding. Or maybe babies and milk just weren't on your mind then, as they often aren't before people arrive at this stage of life.

Trevor reflects on his chest masculinisation surgery and whether he might have done things any differently:

> The most painful part of it all was to think that this is of my own doing. Just a few years ago, I had breasts that could have nourished him perfectly and I chose to get rid of them. I remember reading before my procedure that anyone who goes through such a surgery must grieve for what they leave behind. At the time, the surgery was imperative – I needed it in order to be mentally healthy. I did not experience any sense of loss whatsoever. Now my whole body ached to feed my baby and I can only describe what I felt about my failure to do so as a deep mourning. . . .
>
> Ian [my partner] later told me that at the time of my surgery, he'd wondered if we might have kids someday, and if I'd want to feed them from my body. He knew there was no way for him to suggest this to me at that time. He could see how desperately I wanted to have a body I was comfortable with. . . . I don't think I'd make a different choice even if I could

do it all again. I can't be Jacob's mother. I gave birth to him, but I am his breastfeeding dad.

— *Trevor, Manitoba, Canada*

How much will earlier surgery affect milk production and nursing? It depends on lots of factors:

- **How much tissue** is damaged or removed.
- **Where incisions are located.** Incisions around the lower, outer part of the areola are most likely to damage the nerves that affect milk release.
- **Where and why any implants are put in.** Implants below the muscle are less likely to reduce milk production than implants above the muscle. Were implants done because your breasts were different sizes? Very uneven breasts, or no breast growth, may affect milk production. See Chapter 18, Breast Tissue Insufficiency.
- **How the surgery healed.** Scar tissue may block milk from moving freely through the ducts or coming out of the nipple. Reduced sensation may affect milk release.
- **How long it's been since the surgery.** Some of the nerves and ducts can knit back together. The more time that's passed since the surgery, the more healing may have occurred. So even if you have low milk production with your first baby, you might have an easier time if you have a second (or third...) child.

Avery found that even after many years of pain from breast surgery, healing is still possible:

> I had breast surgery twenty years ago, which left me with horrible nerve pain around both my nipples, so painful that I always had to cover them, even when taking a shower. Even a light touch would send shooting pains through my breasts. When I became pregnant, I was overjoyed, and also sad that I would never be able to breastfeed my baby.
>
> When he was born the nurse encouraged me to try. As I had predicted, the pain was excruciating. But a small voice in my head told me to keep trying. I took it one hour at a time. His latch was perfect, they said; he is so happy nursing, they said; he is gaining weight, they said; and meanwhile I was experiencing the worst pains of my life. Days turned into weeks, which turned into months. I honestly have no idea how I managed to push through

the pain all day and night, but a miracle happened. Gradually, my nerve damage seemed to miraculously start to heal. By month six, I barely had any pain and I was truly shocked. . . . A physician myself, I cannot explain this miracle scientifically. Anything is possible!

– *Avery, Colorado, United States*

Being in pain every time you nurse is really, *really* tough! Breastfeeding supporters are here to help – including finding alternative ways to feed your baby, if that's what you need to do.

If you've had surgery or procedures on your breasts or nipples, your baby's nappy output and weight will need to be closely monitored in the first couple of weeks. And it makes sense to get your milk production off to the strongest possible start.

"Milk Max" Tips

- Begin nursing or expressing as soon as possible after birth.
- Make sure your baby is deeply, comfortably attached at the breast (see Chapter 4).
- Nurse or express *at least* eight to twelve times in twenty-four hours.

If your baby needs extra milk, it can be given in ways that support your nursing relationship (see Chapter 18, Supplementing).

Trevor found that nursing became far more than just a method of feeding:

Before Jacob was born, I thought that I would try to breastfeed him because it would be good for him – it was the healthy choice. After I started nursing, it became a way of life and my best means of responding quickly to his signals and cries, to meeting his needs. Breastfeeding kept the hormones flowing and taught me how to look out for a baby who could do very little for himself. No matter how exhausted I was, how sleepy, how sore, how hungry, how thirsty, how badly I had to wee, no feeling I experienced seemed as important and urgent as satisfying my baby. I may be using a supplemental nursing system, but I have breastfeeding hormones. I am breastfeeding. And it has changed my life.

– *Trevor, Manitoba, Canada*

We've worked with many parents who've nursed after surgeries of all kinds – we'd love to support you, too.

Living with Low Milk Production

By far the most common cause of low milk production is a slow start with nursing or expressing. Not enough milk is removed from the breasts in the early days after birth, meaning that milk production never really achieves "lift off." That makes it sound simple…but we know that so often, it really isn't.

Helen had a perfect storm of difficulties:

> To recover from the anaesthetic and sudden onset of pre-eclampsia, I was left alone in a room for hours during which nobody told me anything about my babies. I assumed the worst. I wasn't allowed to hold them, and nobody thought to show them to me.
>
> The next challenge was that initially I wasn't producing any milk for some reason. The nurses' response to this was to give me a sucker-type syringe for me to pull out my sunken nipples. One nurse sold me a drink that was meant to help milk production. There ended the medical team's breastfeeding support! The twins were screaming with hunger. As the days wore on, my production kicked in, but I never had enough to fully feed both of them. Being so poor that I couldn't eat three square meals a day didn't help. I also never managed breastfeeding both at once and there was no support for that. I had this strong sense of guilt that I couldn't exclusively breastfeed.
>
> – Helen, from the UK, babies born in Ecuador

Beyond Breastfeeding Guilt

Helen describes feeling guilty – even though she faced barriers to breastfeeding that might have scared an Olympic hurdler. (Amazingly, she managed to nurse her twins for ten months.) Nobody can tell you how to feel when breastfeeding doesn't go the way you hoped, but it's worth thinking about the source of those feelings.

Guilt implies responsibility. You might also feel ashamed. Both of these emotions are based on the idea that you have done something wrong, that your breastfeeding difficulties were your fault. But the reality is that illness, healthcare systems, and many other factors are completely beyond our control. Some of these factors are under the control of other people. (Maybe they should be the ones feeling guilty!) Focusing only on individual choice misses a *huge* part of the picture.

If you feel you've let your baby down by not exclusively breastfeeding, remember that in your baby's eyes, you are the best beloved parent. He doesn't need you to be perfect – he won't grow up to be perfect, either.

So where does this leave guilt? We all want to do the very best for our babies and may feel a sense of personal failure if we can't. Disappointment and sadness often lurk just under the surface. Nursing our babies is the normal follow-on from pregnancy. At some level, if it doesn't happen, our bodies may react with grief – as if our babies had died – even though they're right there, healthy and happy. Mourning the nursing relationship you didn't have may be an important part of healing and recovery.

Sometimes, disappointment and sadness come out as envy of other people who seem to have it easier than we do. Marina saw this clearly:

> Every mother I saw breastfeeding I would congratulate and secretly envy. I even made a comment once that I felt sorry about; it was my pain speaking. I apologised immediately.
>
> – Marina, Madrid, Spain

Are you angry? Many of us have been taught not to express anger. But anger, targeted properly, is a normal and healthy response in some situations. If you've been treated unfairly because of who you are, or received poor care, or seen how a corporation makes money by undermining breastfeeding, anger might be an appropriate reaction. Many parents, healthcare professionals, and scientists are extremely concerned about barriers to breastfeeding. If you would like to use your anger to bring about change, you could consider making a complaint or supporting an advocacy organisation on this issue. You might prefer to find someone to talk to or express your feelings in writing or another art form. Putting your anger to use is healthier for you (and therefore your baby) than bottling it up.

Besides all these wider factors, some of us have physical limitations to how much milk we can produce, as Missy discovered:

> During my pregnancies there were no changes in my breasts. My breasts did not feel full before or after birth, and they did not increase in size. I did everything I could to bring up my supply, but all in vain. A few years later my mother-in-law told me she thought that I had insufficient glandular tissue.
>
> – Missy, United States

For more about physical causes of low milk production, see Chapter 18, Breast Tissue Insufficiency, Low Milk Supply, Weight Gain Worries.

While we know that exclusive breastfeeding is the ideal, *any* amount of your milk (or any human milk) your baby gets has great and irreplaceable value. Many parents, and sometimes even healthcare professionals, believe that formula is as good as human milk. But it simply isn't true. Formula is an adequate food for babies, and the only safe alternative for those who can't be fed on human milk. But it's an ultraprocessed product, marketed primarily to make profits for shareholders. Its ingredients vary according to the price of the raw components (when they get too expensive, manufacturers switch to cheaper alternatives). Human milk, on the other hand, is a living fluid, adapted over millennia specifically to feed, protect, and nurture human babies. It varies according to the baby's stage of development, time of day or night, and the needs of the baby's immune system. If someone invented a product that could do everything human milk does, they'd probably get several Nobel Prizes. Even a few drops of your milk go a very long way.

Whether or not you can produce all the milk your baby needs, you can nurse your baby if you want to – as Missy did:

> I do think that nursing and supplementing by bottle was worth it, because of the number of times I had to nurse a toddler out of a tantrum at Target or anywhere for that matter! Or in bed for a quick ten-minute bedtime. Or for the many times they come to me to snuggle during the day. I am sharing my story so that hopefully if you are like me and you can't make enough milk, you can see that there is still a benefit to nursing anyway. Even a little bit can make a difference in your connection and the baby's health.
>
> – Missy, United States

There are many options and tools for supporting your nursing relationship.

Leah began with formula and bottles, moved on to an at-breast supplementer, and with the help of medication, eventually nursed without any tools at all:

> I was expecting breastfeeding to be a new skill that I would need to master, but what I didn't expect was to have low supply. My son was born at full term and I started breastfeeding right away. By his third day, my milk still hadn't "come in," and I had a hungry, crying newborn on my hands. Being my first baby, I didn't know what to do and ended up giving him a bottle of formula. That was the beginning of close to three days of him not really wanting to breastfeed and only taking the bottle, until I could get in to see a lactation consultant through the local public health unit. The LC was very helpful, and immediately we started supplementing with a tube at the breast. Supplementing [and medications] ended up being our route to success. We went on to breastfeed for three years!
>
> – Leah, Ontario, Canada

"Technical support" is just part of what you need if you've got low milk production or other complex feeding challenges. Nursing always needs a support team. Nursing with complex challenges requires a more experienced one.

Marisela, who expressed for her son because of severe pain while nursing, found herself surrounded with support from family, friends, and a La Leche League community:

> I did not know the comforting effect of seeing other mums who were also going through similar situations to mine. My support network watched me suffer but never stopped encouraging me. My mum constantly told me not to give up; I will never forget that she was with me when Sandra [LLL Leader] visited us; she asked questions and made sure to record everything. My husband supported me in every crazy thing, taking me here and there to check my breastfeeding technique; he hugged me when he saw me cry many, many times. Plus my friends who were always supporting me, especially Bastian's mum, who told me something that I will never forget: "Follow your mummy instinct." Those words helped me to ground everything I learned and let me go as if I were on a slide.
>
> – Marisela, Mexico

Leah also found support at La Leche League:

> My local LLL group, and the mums and Leaders I met there, were a very important support for me. Talking about my challenges establishing breastfeeding helped other mums know that these challenges can be overcome with the right supports, and it also helped me heal from the experience.
>
> – Leah, Ontario, Canada

When your own breastfeeding journey is far from what you'd hoped for, being around others who seem to be nursing easily may be just too painful. But the range of parents and experiences in our groups might surprise you. Trevor describes his very first LLL meeting:

> After the introduction and an icebreaker, some people brought up specific problems they wanted help with. Soon enough, tears were streaming down the faces of a few parents. I saw that folks really do wait all month for the one day when they can vent, rage, grieve, learn, and celebrate about breastfeeding unreservedly in front of one another. . . . Following the structured part of the meeting, several women came up to me to say that they were amazed by my courage and determination to breastfeed. I left knowing that the work done in that church basement was essential.
>
> – Trevor, Manitoba, Canada

If you don't want or feel able to attend a meeting, you're warmly welcome to call a Leader or lurk in a social media group. Maybe you'll eventually feel comfortable to write a post or attend a virtual or in-person meeting. Or maybe you'll find the support you need elsewhere, from those who've got experience of challenges like yours. We'd love to be part of your network.

Babies with Special Needs

A baby born with a disability or medical problem, or who develops one later, needs the stimulation, comfort, and closeness that are part of breastfeeding even more than a healthy baby does. And – whether or not she's able to nurse – your milk supports her health and development like nothing else can. Parenting is *really* complicated when your child has complex medical issues. Nursing can be a haven of normality. Expressing your milk is the one thing that only *you* can do for your baby – even if professionals do much of your child's day-to-day care.

If you know in advance that your baby may have health complications, you might want to express colostrum during the last few weeks of your pregnancy, in case she needs extra milk quickly (see chapters 1 and 15).

Whatever the situation, there are almost always options for breastfeeding or providing human milk. You can find information and stories about breastfeeding babies with Down syndrome, cleft lip or palate, cystic fibrosis, and many other challenges at www.llli.org.

Fee (with the help of her friends) expressed milk for her daughter for two years:

> Willow suffered a brain injury at birth, which meant she didn't have many of the natural reflexes babies are usually born with. She had no suck, no swallow; she showed no interest in anything around her, let alone the breast. Willow spent her first five weeks of life in the neonatal and special care units. I didn't hold her until she was one week old, but I expressed for her from day one.
>
> Twelve incredible women pumped for Willow alongside me, regularly. I continued expressing for Willow beyond her first year; I was determined to get her to that magical two years. And I did. On the morning of her second birthday, Willow had that last breast milk, a 5 ml syringe of pure gold, magic milk, and I hung up my breast pump. It is almost certainly the hardest thing I've ever done, but something I am so proud of. If you're reading this and you are exclusively expressing for a poorly tube-fed baby, keep going. You *can* do this. I know how hard it is, but it really will be worth it.
>
> – Fee, UK

Kallyn's nursing journey took an unexpected turn when Liam became critically ill at seven months old:

> Following months of chronic infections, Liam was admitted to the local hospital with RSV and pneumonia. After a few days . . . he was airlifted to the nearest children's hospital, where he would remain in the intensive care unit for the next month of his life.
>
> He was no longer allowed oral feeds because he was now critically ill. A nasogastric tube was placed, and I went from an exclusively breastfeeding mother to an exclusively pumping mother overnight.
>
> He was able to gain enough coordination and strength to go on to breastfeed successfully. He was later diagnosed with 22q11.2 Deletion syndrome, a diagnosis that explained so many of the previous illnesses and

hardships that he faced. The medical appointments didn't slow, the hospital stays continued to happen, and we continued to nurse.
— *Kallyn, United States*

Emma's baby had kidney problems and eventually had to stop both nursing and drinking her milk:

Two days into our NICU experience, we were taken into a room and told about her kidney problems: they hadn't formed properly – there was no cure – she would need a transplant when she was big enough. In the meantime, her numbers were going in the wrong direction and there was a good chance she would need dialysis – very risky in such a tiny baby. Then they told me about potassium. She had too much potassium (regulating it is one of many jobs the kidneys have). The only way to reduce potassium is through diet – giving her a low-potassium special milk. To say I was devastated is an absolute understatement. Eighteen months on, I still can't talk about breastfeeding without crying. It was such a huge part of my bond and relationship with my toddler, I couldn't imagine not being able to feed my daughter at all.

My journey from then on was complicated. We were in hospital for eight weeks. I was allowed to do a little bit of breastfeeding under the supervision of an amazing speech and language team. But we had times when she wasn't allowed my milk at all. I kept pumping, but I'll never forget when they couldn't even add a few millilitres of my milk to her special recipe. I was sent home with all my bottles of breast milk that I had pumped for her. They didn't need it. I felt useless and crushed. Throughout her first six months her potassium improved, and we went to up to four breastfeeds a day, on top of her special milk that she was given through her feeding tube.

That was a special summer. I even experimented with tandem feeding with my toddler. However, then we had to stop again – it was too hard to measure and control the liquid she was having (which is essential for kidney disease). I could add 120 ml a day of my milk to her feed, but I found that so, so hard. Eventually I stopped pumping, and we had our last breastfeed. I still feel incredibly guilty that I couldn't continue – but my brain tells me how, considering her kidney disease, she really did get a decent amount.
— *Emma, London, UK*

Within our global LLL community, over more than sixty years, families have experienced pretty much every possible complication, illness, and disability. We might not always understand all the medical complexities you're dealing with, but we will always do our best to help you nurse or provide milk for your child – or stop doing so, if you need to.

Lactation After Loss

This section is for you if you've experienced the loss of a baby through miscarriage, stillbirth, or death shortly after birth, or the death of a breastfed child through illness or accident. We are so sorry this has happened to you. We've supported many bereaved families and are here for anything you need.

If you were already nursing or expressing, or were far enough through pregnancy that you're making milk, you will need to deal with your milk production.

If you're still nursing another child, you can continue. Expect some runny, maybe yellow, stools in the first few days – colostrum has a laxative effect. Over time, your milk production will settle down in line with the amount your child is taking.

Milk Production Immediately After Miscarriage or Birth

Our bodies start making milk from around sixteen weeks of pregnancy. Milk production is driven entirely by the hormones of pregnancy until a few days after birth. This means that if you have a miscarriage after about sixteen weeks, or if your baby is stillborn, or dies during or shortly after birth, your milk will increase as it usually would after birth.

If you are medically well yourself, you'll usually be discharged from the hospital before your milk increases. Your breasts are likely to become tender, swollen, and sore around two to three days or so after birth. Breast tissue can extend up into your armpits, so you might feel tenderness there, too. It can be quite a shock, even if you're expecting it. Cold packs, anti-inflammatory medication, and other remedies can help relieve the discomfort (see Chapter 18, Engorgement).

From this time on, milk is made only in response to milk being removed from your breasts. If you don't remove milk, your milk production will slow down and stop over a period of about two weeks.

This is your body working as it should in response to the loss of your baby.

Options for Dealing with Your Milk

Whatever stage of lactation you're in, you have several options for dealing with your milk production:

1. Physiological Suppression

Using your body's built-in brake to slow down and stop milk production gradually is called physiological suppression. This takes about two weeks if you've just had a miscarriage or given birth. If you've already started nursing or expressing, it takes longer. If your baby was older than about six weeks, it's likely to take about six weeks to completely wind down your milk production.

This is the approach Luisa took when her baby died at twenty-seven weeks of pregnancy after she became ill with Covid-19:

> My body was not yet prepared to let go. I had milk and I had enough of it. It was just heartbreaking that the child who should have got the milk was not there. So, I had to tell/teach my body to stop producing milk. I pumped the milk and then threw it away, which was hurtful. I know I could have kept the milk, but it would have reminded me every time that it was originally meant for someone else. The moment when the milk flow stopped entirely was difficult as well. It was a closure. I would have loved to breastfeed my daughter so much, but I couldn't. The positive thing I took from the whole situation was that I knew what my body could do.
>
> – Luisa, Switzerland

Here are some suggestions to help you through this process of physiological suppression:

- **When your breasts begin to feel uncomfortably full, remove just enough milk to feel comfortable again.** You may be worried that removing milk to ease your discomfort will only encourage more milk to be made, but this is the best way to stay comfortable and prevent mastitis (breast inflammation). The aim is to remove just enough milk to be comfortable but not enough to drain your breasts well. Using warm, wet cloths on the breast just before expressing may help milk flow more easily.

- At first, you may need to express several times a day, but over time **the milk will gradually subside** until the day comes when you no longer feel discomfort and don't need to remove any more milk.
- During this process, **your milk might leak** if you think about your baby, hear another baby cry, or hug someone. (You might find hugs uncomfortable if your breasts are very tender. Let family and friends know what you prefer.) Absorbent nursing pads may be helpful until your milk production decreases, and you might want to sleep on a towel or waterproof pad.
- Some bereaved parents find comfort in **collecting a small amount of milk as a keepsake of their baby,** to be made into a piece of jewellery. If this is an idea you'd like to explore, you can find providers online. Some families choose to do something else with the milk they collect, like bury it with their baby or put it somewhere else that has meaning for them.
- Use the measures described here and in Chapter 18, Engorgement, to ease swelling and discomfort while your milk production gradually winds down.

2. Milk Suppression

It used to be quite common to give powerful drugs to stop milk production. These days, medication is prescribed less often because some of the older drugs had dangerous side effects. But it's still an option after the death of a baby or child.

This was the way Verity chose to deal with her milk production when her daughter Marianne died of spinal muscular atrophy aged three months:

> I did hope to be able to donate breastmilk after she died, but emotionally it was too difficult to do, so one of the doctors prescribed me some tablets that would stop the breastmilk production. I started taking these a few days before she died, as I had enough stored milk for her; by then she was on a trickle comfort feed. The milk stopped the day before she died, but after she died I started leaking clear fluid from my breasts each time I cried. This lasted around a week – isn't the body amazing?
> – Verity, Oxfordshire, UK

To speed the process of milk reduction (but not as fast as powerful suppressant drugs), some mothers choose to use **herbs or over-the-**

counter medication. Talk to your healthcare provider or a breastfeeding specialist about herbs or medications that can decrease milk production, as well as any pain medication you need.

Breast binding has not been found to hurry the milk reduction process, but you may find a soft, supportive bra helps with comfort.

3. Milk Donation

Some bereaved mothers take great comfort from being able to give their milk away to other families with premature or sick babies, as Sam describes:

> That feeling of needing some good to come out of this awful situation was strong for me. I started to read up on what else I could do, particularly breastmilk donation. I had had a really positive and enjoyable lactation journey with my first child, so I knew roughly what to expect and I felt confident that my body could produce an impressive volume. This was important for me because at this stage in my pregnancy and grief, on some level, I felt like my body had let me down. So if it could perform this task for me (and the milk bank), then I saw that as the first step in rebuilding my trust in my physical self.
>
> I didn't know it at the time, but being a milk donor was a lifeline for me; it gave me a sense of daily purpose and eventually a sense of pride. It was my silver lining to a very, very dark cloud. Expressing milk for donation gave my day structure, regularity that otherwise would have been absent. My husband was brilliantly supportive of my decision to donate milk, and he was involved in the process, too – he would wash up and sterilise breast pumps, take the freezer temperature, and drive me to the milk bank to drop donations off. We were both still grieving and processing the babyless situation we were in, but the milk donation process gave us a way to feel connected to each other at a time when neither of us were ready to talk directly about what had just happened.
>
> I did enjoy the donation process, but at some point it felt right to stop. Expressing is a very physically and mentally demanding process, so as I felt more ready to rejoin the real world, I started to decrease the frequency and volumes of my expressing sessions until one day my donation journey came to a natural end. It was a bittersweet moment, but I am and will always be glad that I got to have that experience, and I just hope it helped a baby in need.
>
> – Sam, England

Milk banks are experienced in working with bereaved mothers to make the process of donation as stress-free as possible. You won't have to commit to donating a specific amount of milk and can stop whenever you want.

If you decide to keep your milk production going, you will need to express regularly, by hand or with a pump. The amount of milk you make will depend on how often you express. Any amount of milk is enormously valuable to the babies who receive it. Milk banks usually provide bottles for you to collect and freeze your milk at home before it's transported to the bank to be pasteurised. It's important to follow hygiene procedures carefully when expressing for a milk bank. You won't be able to donate your milk if you smoke or are taking certain medications.

Informal milk sharing is another option chosen by some families: donating milk directly to an individual baby rather than through a milk bank (see Chapter 18, Milk Sharing).

Expressing your milk has some health benefits for you, reducing your risk of some breast and ovarian cancers. It may also delay the return of your period.

Every bereaved mother feels different. It's important that you make the right choice for you. Milk bank staff, healthcare professionals, and breastfeeding supporters are all available to listen and help you work out what you want to do.

Luisa and her husband were supported by a midwife:

> [We worked with] a midwife who specialised in caring for parents after child loss. She was such a great person who helped us through the tough time. Looking back, skilled personnel, especially in such a situation, are a huge help for affected parents.
>
> – Luisa, Switzerland

Many families in the LLL community have lost a pregnancy or a child. If there is anything we can do to support you, at any stage, it would be our privilege.

Want to know more?

You can find extra resources for this chapter
at the "Art of Breastfeeding" tab at
www.llli.org.

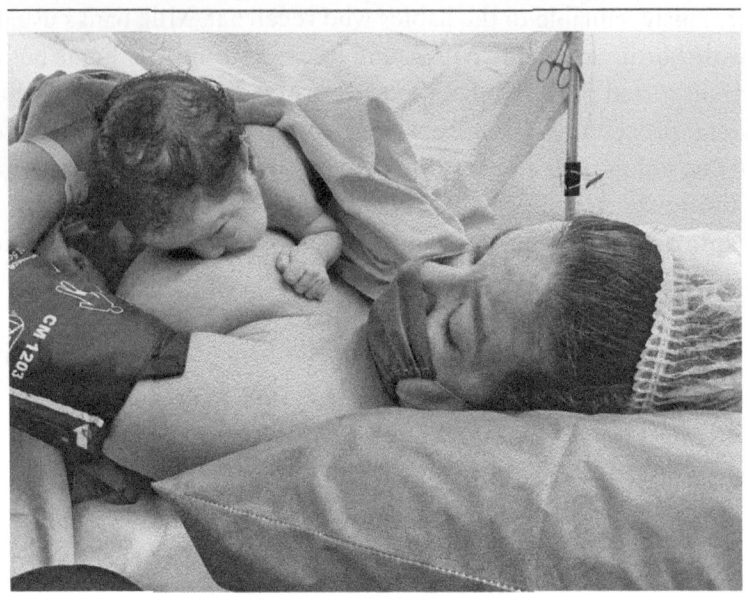

EIGHTEEN

A–Z "Tech Support" Tool Kit

Blebs (Milk Blisters)	508
Breast Lumps	509
Breast Tissue Insufficiency (Hypoplasia/IGT)	510
Colds and Minor Illnesses	512
Crying and Colic	513
Diet and Weight (Yours)	515
Dysphoric Milk Ejection Reflex (D-MER)	516
Engorgement (Full, Swollen Breasts)	517
Feeding in Emergencies	519
Hospitalisation or Surgery, Your Child's or Yours	522
Hypoglycaemia (Low Blood Sugar in Your Baby)	522
Hypothermia	524
Jaundice, or Hyperbilirubinaemia (Too Much Bilirubin)	524
Low Milk Supply	526
Mastitis and Blocked Ducts	530
Medications	533
Milk Sharing	535
Nipple Diversity	538
Nipple Shields	540
Nursing Strike (Breast Refusal)	543
Oversupply (Too Much Milk)	545
Postnatal Mood Disorders (Depression, Anxiety, OCD)	547
Reflux	551
Sore Nipples	553
Supplementing (Giving Extra Milk)	556
Tongue-Tie	562
Vasospasm	563
Weight Gain Worries	565
Yeast (Thrush/Candida Infections)	570

If you've used a computer or smartphone, you've probably run into a problem or two. What then? Well, you don't chuck the whole thing out the window. You might play around a little to see if there's a quick fix. You restart it. Maybe you check the manual or look online. If you can't fix it yourself, you contact tech support – a real person (not a bot!) who listens to your problem and talks you through possible solutions.

Sometimes, breastfeeding needs a little tech support, too. This chapter touches on some of the most common topics LLL Leaders are asked about, in alphabetical order. Some are very brief; others have more detail. There's much more to know! You'll see that for some topics we've put extra resources online.

Consider this chapter the first step. It isn't a real person; it's just a book. So, if the answer you're looking for isn't here (and isn't in the index at the back, either), find a breastfeeding supporter or breastfeeding-knowledgeable healthcare provider. And do it soon!

What if you have been to the relevant section of this chapter, followed the ideas, and things still aren't working? Maybe the issue wasn't quite what you thought, or you may have more than one issue happening. Or maybe your issue isn't covered here. Talking to a real person (and maybe more than one) is the best way to fix breastfeeding problems. The difference help makes can be dramatic.

Blebs (Milk Blisters)

A **bleb** is a little white or yellow spot on the tip of a nipple. It can hurt *a lot* (often described as stinging pain) during nursing. And sometimes a bleb blocks milk from coming out of part of the breast. If this happens, a section of the breast might be tender, sore, and warm. On light skin, you might see a red patch (see Mastitis and Blocked Ducts in this chapter).

When you get rid of a bleb, thickened milk behind it may come out as gritty granules or a tiny toothpaste-like ribbon. It may just disappear during a nursing (*harmlessly* into the baby). Once it's gone, any backed-up milk usually clears quickly.

The Backstory

There isn't much research on blebs yet, and no one knows for sure why they happen. Blebs may be more likely if the skin of your nipple has been damaged by your baby during nursing.

What You Can Do

Because we aren't even sure how blebs form, there are many possibilities for their treatment. If a bleb isn't causing any pain or other troublesome symptoms, you can just ignore it. It might last for weeks or months before mysteriously disappearing.

If a bleb is causing you discomfort, check with LLL websites, a breastfeeding helper, or your healthcare provider for current treatment suggestions. Make sure your baby is deeply attached at the breast to avoid further damaging the nipple. If a bleb comes back, you may need to repeat the treatment.

Want to know more?

You can find extra resources for this section at the "Art of Breastfeeding" tab, Chapter 18, at www.llli.org.

Breast Lumps

During breastfeeding, you can expect lumpy breasts, and you'll get to know your breasts better than ever before.

The Backstory

Most lumps get bigger and smaller as milk is made and removed. Lumps that come and go are not a concern. Lumps that *don't* change can sometimes result from surgery or injury to the breast. Most lumps in lactating breasts are benign (not cancer).

If your breast is lumpy *and sore*, see the section on Mastitis and Blocked Ducts in this chapter. Occasionally, an abscess (pocket of infected tissue) forms within the breast, usually as a complication of mastitis. This requires urgent medical treatment. Let your healthcare provider know if symptoms don't improve within two to three days of treatment for mastitis.

An uncommon type of breast lump is a **galactocele.** It forms when a milk duct traps milk in a pocket. It feels like a smooth, round, movable sac in the breast. The milk inside gradually thickens because it's unable to drain out. A galactocele can be diagnosed by ultrasound imaging of the breast, and can be treated, if necessary, by drawing fluid from it.

What You Can Do

Check with your healthcare provider if either of the following is true:

- You have a lump that doesn't change in size when you nurse or express.
- You notice changes on the skin of your breast (dimpling, or dipping inward).

If you have a family history of breast cancer, you can still have regular mammograms – they're safe for the nursing baby. The same is true of a needle or incisional biopsy. Continuing to breastfeed helps protect the health of your breasts as well as that of your baby. Nurse or express as thoroughly as you can before the scan, for your own comfort and to provide as unmilky a picture as possible.

If a galactocele isn't causing discomfort or getting in the way of nursing, you could just leave it alone. It can be drained with a needle, though it may refill. If you want to, you can have it surgically removed when you've finished nursing.

With any breast surgery, an incision that radiates from your nipple like the spoke on a wheel (rather than going around your nipple) causes the least damage. There's no need to wean for surgery. For more about breast procedures, see Chapter 17.

Breast Tissue Insufficiency (Hypoplasia/IGT)

While most breasts – whatever shape or size – work just fine, there are exceptions. **Hypoplastic** (*hypo* meaning less, *plastic* referring to growth) breasts have less milk-making tissue. However hard you try, it's just not possible for some breasts to produce a full milk supply. The term *insufficient glandular tissue (IGT)* is sometimes used to describe this situation when other potential causes of low milk production have been ruled out.

The Backstory

Hypoplastic breasts are different from small breasts. They may be tube-shaped rather than rounded, or have very little tissue on the underside. You may be able to put your whole hand on your chest between them. They may differ dramatically in size, and one or both areolae may be puffy. But this condition is not all about appearances. If your breasts look like this, you might be able to breastfeed just fine. And some people have more body fat or have had surgery (breast implants), which can mask the appearance of hypoplastic breasts. It's also possible to have one hypoplastic breast and one that's not.

Research on hypoplasia is still at an early stage; there are still more questions than answers. We know that previous cancer treatment and some genetic syndromes (like Poland syndrome) can cause it. Researchers have suggested other possibilities, too, some based on animal studies: chemical exposure when your mother was pregnant with you, obesity or an eating disorder during adolescence, insulin resistance, and more. We hope research will help us find more answers – and solutions.

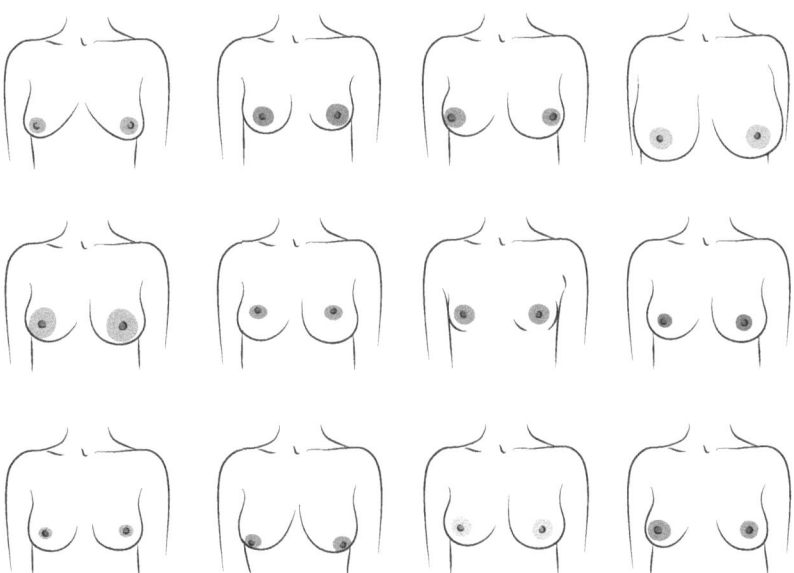

Breast variations: these breasts may or may not make enough milk

What You Can Do

If you sense something isn't right, or if your breasts match what we've described, talk to a breastfeeding supporter. They can help you make the most of your milk production and ensure your baby gets enough milk. It will be important to monitor your baby's nappies (wees and poos) and growth so any problems are noticed quickly. If your baby is unable to get all the milk he needs at the breast, your helper can support you to come up with a workable plan to keep him safely fed while protecting your nursing relationship. Feeding your baby might not be the way you hoped or imagined, but any amount of your milk is beneficial, and you can still nurture him at the breast or chest. You may have breast growth and more milk with each baby.

See also Low Milk Supply and Supplementing in this chapter.

Want to know more?

You can find extra resources for this section at the "Art of Breastfeeding" tab, Chapter 18, at www.llli.org.

Colds and Minor Illnesses

Sometimes you are unwell. Sometimes your baby is. Can you still breastfeed? Yes, almost always. For more about serious or long-lasting illnesses, see Chapter 17, Illnesses, and LLL websites.

The Backstory

You and your baby have been a unit since she was conceived. Not only does she live on your milk, she shares your immune system. By the time you know you're unwell, you've started passing on not only the illness but your immunities to your baby. If you stop breastfeeding when you're unwell – whatever the age of your child – you stop supporting her immune system when she needs it most.

And it works the other way around, too. If your baby picks up an illness that you haven't been exposed to yet, she passes those germs to you through nursing, and within the breast itself you begin making antibodies and passing them back to her, to help her recover.

What You Can Do

Bottom line: with *very few* exceptions, keep breastfeeding when either you or your baby is ill! The Centers for Disease Control and Prevention (United States) and the World Health Organization both have information on breastfeeding during specific illnesses. Most medications are safe while breastfeeding (see Medications in this chapter).

Illness in babies can come quickly, hit hard, and leave just as quickly. Nursing provides fluids and nutrition when your baby refuses other food and drinks or can't keep them down, and it provides excellent pain relief.

Here are suggestions for breastfeeding through minor illnesses:

Stuffy nose: try nursing out of doors or in a steamy bathroom. Upright positions can also help. Some parents use saline drops to flush their babies' noses, or you can get special "baby nasal aspirator" (snot sucker!) devices. If your baby really can't nurse, expressed milk can tide him over.

Vomiting and/or diarrhoea: if you have either of these, you might see a small dip in your milk production. Stay hydrated as best you can – your milk supply will bounce back as you recover. If your baby is vomiting or has diarrhoea, short, frequent feeds help keep him hydrated. If nursing triggers vomiting, you could try offering a freshly expressed breast to see if your baby can keep down smaller amounts of milk. If you're worried about either of you, contact your healthcare provider.

Crying and Colic

All over the world, most young babies cry. Starting a week or so after birth, crying builds during the first six weeks or so. It's typically most intense towards the end of the day. Some babies cry much more than others. Whatever the cause, most babies cry less after the first two months.

The Backstory

Colicky is the catch-all term for a healthy baby who cries hard at least three hours a day, several days a week. There are many possible causes of this behaviour:

- hunger (if your baby wants to nurse again, there's no problem in letting him; babies tend to cry less in cultures where they're kept close and can nurse whenever they like)

- an oversupply of milk or reflux (these have their own sections in this chapter) or food allergies
- bruising, tight muscles, or even broken bones from his position in utero or during birth
- a hair caught around a tiny body part, like a toe (ouch!)
- a nappy rash or other sore areas of skin
- an eye irritation
- a bladder or ear infection
- other illnesses

Many babies with colic never have an obvious cause.

A history of the mother having migraines or stress during pregnancy, premature birth, either parent being depressed, and domestic abuse are also factors researchers have linked to increased crying. And some babies are just more sensitive, intense, and hard to soothe (see Chapter 7). Sudden, intense crying that is not normal for your baby needs to be checked out with a healthcare provider right away.

What You Can Do

These ideas have been shown to help prevent crying and mellow unsettled babies:

- **Respond quickly to signals that your baby wants to nurse.** Try to do this before he gets worked up.
- **Keep him in contact with your body.** A sling or soft carrier frees up your hands.
- **Try rhythmic movement.** Walk, rock, sway, or dance with your baby.
- **Try a change of scenery,** like going outdoors or into a quiet, dark room.
- **Share the load.** It's hard to calm a crying baby if you're tense yourself. A different pair of familiar arms might help.

A few babies just cry, no matter what you try to do to calm them. Living with a baby who can't be comforted is *really* hard. You need support for yourself. If you're becoming overwhelmed or are worried you might harm your baby, reach out to family, friends, your healthcare provider, or a parent helpline. La Leche League Leaders and groups can offer solidarity, encouragement, and space to talk.

Want to know more?

You can find extra resources for this section at the "Art of Breastfeeding" tab, Chapter 18, at www.llli.org.

Diet and Weight (Yours)

Making milk takes fuel. This fuel comes from what we eat and from nutrients stored in our bodies.

You don't need to eat a perfect diet to make milk! Breastfeeding has worked just fine for thousands of years, through times of feast and famine, with every kind of food. Your baby is your body's first priority. If you're short of nutrients, you'll suffer before your baby does – and your health matters, too (not just because you make milk!).

The Backstory

Making milk for one baby requires about 500 kcal (2,100 kJ) of energy a day in the first year. You might only need to eat breakfast twice to more or less cover that. About 100 g (3 oz) of trail mix has that many calories. You don't need to have lunch twice or dinner twice. If you count calories, it might be helpful to know that you probably need to take in at least 1,800 kcal (7,500 kJ) a day to meet both your needs and your baby's. Regularly eating less than this may cause malnutrition, which over time can lead to reduced milk production.

Most of us gain fat in pregnancy and keep some of it for a while afterwards. This is our body's insurance plan against hard times. Our bodies expect to convert these reserves into milk in the months after birth.

What You Can Do

Many of us have enough reserves that we don't need to eat 500 kcal (2,100 kJ) extra. Health authorities often recommend aiming for a bit less: around 330 to 400 kcal (1,400 to 1,700 kJ) per day – so we gradually use up some reserves, too. It's considered safe to lose about 500 grams (1.1 pounds) of weight a week during breastfeeding. Losing weight much faster than this isn't recommended, because toxins stored in our fat get released into milk. For more about environmental contaminants, see Chapter 8.

If you're actively trying to lose weight, it's important to be aware that some kinds of food restriction might not be safe while you're making milk because you need energy faster than usual. Strict low-carbohydrate (keto) diets may be in this category. Check with a breastfeeding-knowledgeable healthcare provider, dietitian, or nutrition specialist for current advice, and see www.llli.org.

It's important to make sure you're getting the balance of food you and your baby need, especially in these situations:

- if you're nursing more than one child
- if you're avoiding certain foods, for instance, because of allergies
- if you have diabetes
- if you've previously had bariatric surgery

If you're vegetarian or vegan, be sure that you're getting enough vitamin B12, folate, zinc, and iron. Talk to your healthcare provider if you're concerned.

Dysphoric Milk Ejection Reflex (D-MER)

For some, nursing (or expressing) is accompanied by a wave of strong negative feelings just before the milk releases. For Rosie's story about this condition, see Chapter 6. These sensations, thought to be caused by hormones, have been named dysphoric milk ejection reflex, or D-MER for short. There are strategies that can help, including

- deep breathing and relaxation
- distraction
- drinking something cold when your milk releases
- vitamin supplements
- antidepressant medication

See LLL websites for further information, and contact a breastfeeding helper. We can support you through this – including weaning partially or fully if you need to (for more about weaning, see Chapter 16).

Want to know more?

You can find extra resources for this section at the "Art of Breastfeeding" tab, Chapter 18, at www.llli.org.

Engorgement (Full, Swollen Breasts)

Engorgement means extra fluid in body tissues. Engorged breasts feel heavy, full, hot, tender, or painful. Overfullness can make latching difficult. Without a well-nursing baby or some other means of frequent, effective milk removal, that heaviness and warmth can expand into tight, shiny breasts that are too full for milk to leave, the way a cold can leave you too stuffed up to blow your nose.

The Backstory

In the first three to five days after birth, blood flow to your breasts increases to get the "milk factory" running at full speed. Other fluids move through your body, too. As one mother put it, "After the birth, all that fluid that was in your ankles rushes up to your breasts to see what's going on." And if you've had intravenous fluids during labour and birth, some of the extra fluid pumped into your body goes to your breasts, exaggerating normal engorgement. Engorgement is often most noticeable around the third or fourth day, though you might not notice it at all or have engorgement that lasts longer or comes and goes over a few days.

Engorgement can also happen later on if your baby goes an unexpectedly long time between nursings. It may affect one or both breasts, depending on whether it was one or both that went unused for a while. This later engorgement is usually easy to relieve with nursing.

It's important to resolve engorgement as quickly as possible to avoid compounding the problem as more milk is made. It's like having a traffic jam in your breast – if everything gets really backed up, it's harder to get it flowing again. If engorgement is very severe, or lasts a long time, milk production reduces.

What You Can Do

- Keep your baby with you, and nurse as often as she's willing, beginning as soon as possible after birth.
- If your breast is too firm for your baby to latch easily, try **reverse pressure softening** to push fluids out of your breast and back into lymphatic circulation. Press steadily with the length of your index fingers on either side of your nipple's base, where your baby's upper and lower gums will be. Press firmly for about a minute, and immediately offer to nurse. Or press all the short-nailed fingertips of one hand around the base of your nipple to make five little dents. You can do this before every nursing session until the engorgement is gone.

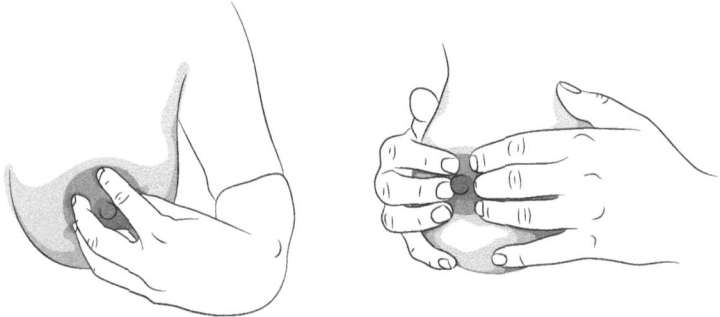

Reverse pressure softening: use finger tips or finger lengths to press fluid away from the nipple

- If your baby can't latch well, even with reverse pressure softening, **gentle hand expression or pumping** on a very low setting might help. (Pumping at a setting that's too high pulls more fluid into the area around the nipple, making things worse.)
- *Gentle* **breast massage** can help get rid of the extra fluids. Start with small circles near your shoulder to help you relax. Then make gentle strokes from your nipple to your shoulder or armpit, starting at different parts of the nipple each time. This is sometimes called lymphatic drainage.
- **Lie flat on your back** when you rest. Gravity will help drain fluids away from your breasts.
- **Nonsteroidal anti-inflammatory medication,** such as ibuprofen, helps reduce both pain and swelling. Talk to your healthcare provider if you can't take this or need something stronger.

- **Inflammation responds best to cold.** Wrap a bag of frozen peas, corn, or ice in a small towel and use it as a cold compress, alternating about twenty minutes on, about twenty minutes off as much as you like. Refreeze as needed. You could also use a chilled gel pack, a cloth wrung out in very cold water, or chilled green cabbage leaves (a traditional remedy that some find helpful).
- A **bath or shower** can help you relax (and help milk to flow) but try not to overheat your breasts. In the shower, let the water play over your back not your chest. And maybe have it a little cooler than usual.
- Occasionally, engorgement tips over into **mastitis** – runaway breast inflammation. If it's getting worse, or if you start to feel ill (like you have the flu), contact your healthcare provider, and see Mastitis and Blocked Ducts in this chapter.
- It's common to have **low mood** along with breast engorgement at any stage of nursing. Many of us have found ourselves weeping on the third or fourth day after birth, feeling we just can't cope. (When someone with a baby this age arrives at an LLL meeting, we quietly make sure the tissues are within reach.) Researchers are finding out more all the time about how inflammation anywhere in your body affects your brain and your emotions. As the swelling goes down, your mood will likely come up. Until then, you need plenty of loving care and support.

Feeding in Emergencies

If you live in an area where natural disasters are known to happen, you probably already have a plan for feeding your baby safely in an emergency.

But even if you don't, it's important to be prepared, in case of the following emergencies, which can happen anywhere:

- extreme weather events (which are becoming more common)
- needing to leave your home quickly, for example, because of fire or flooding
- failure of local power or water supplies

This section aims to give you key information to help keep your baby safe. The LLLI website has lots of information on feeding in emergencies, in multiple languages.

- **In an emergency, keep breastfeeding!** It's even more important than usual. Without breastfeeding, babies are at higher risk of infections and not getting enough fluids and nutrition. An emergency is not the time to switch to formula because it's very hard to prepare formula safely in emergency situations.
- **If you're breastfeeding and rely on expressing your milk, learn how to hand express.** This is a reliable backup in case of power cut or lack of clean water and facilities to clean a pump.
- **It's especially important to have an emergency preparedness plan if you're using formula.** Your national or regional government or health authority may provide information on what you need.

Cups are safer to use than bottles in an emergency because they are easier to clean properly. Bacteria on feeding equipment can make babies ill.

Breastfeeding Under Stress

Stress does not reduce milk production, though it can slow down your milk release. You will continue making milk even if you are not eating or drinking, or are ill.

Here are some suggestions for nursing while you are stressed:

- If you're in a very stressful situation and feel your milk is not flowing normally, **nurse your baby directly** if you can, rather than expressing. Milk usually flows more easily when nursing than when expressing, and nursing helps calm both you and your baby. Think about how breastfeeding and your milk are protecting your baby and helping her feel safe.
- Your milk might also flow more easily if you have **a private space to nurse in** – it's okay to ask for this if you need it. It can be hard to relax in an unfamiliar place, especially if you're surrounded by strangers. If there isn't a private space, you could use a scarf or blanket as a screen or sit in a corner and ask family members to sit between you and other people.
- **Don't panic.** It just isn't possible for milk production to suddenly stop unless you've taken medication to shut it down (or are pregnant). Your milk is still there – it will flow again.

- **Ask for help.** Find local LLL Leaders, helplines (in some communities), or online groups.

For more tips on encouraging milk release, see Chapter 15.

Making More Milk

If you're mixed feeding (both breastfeeding and using formula), you might be able to make more milk so you're less reliant on formula.

If you're already fully breastfeeding your own baby, it may be possible to make extra milk for another baby or child who needs feeding.

Key things to know:

- Putting a baby or child to your breast (or expressing your milk) more often signals your body to make more milk (see Low Milk Supply in this chapter).
- If your own baby is young and fed only on your milk, it's important to make sure he is fed first, before feeding another baby or child.
- If your own baby needs extra milk in an emergency situation, it may be safer for him to be breastfed by someone else than to be given formula (see Milk Sharing in this chapter).

Relactation

If you have stopped breastfeeding and want to bring back some milk production, you could relactate. You can do this by putting your baby or child to your breast or by expressing.

Here are some more tips about relactation:

- **The more recently you stopped breastfeeding,** and the more milk you were making at that point, the more likely it is that you'll be able to bring in a significant amount of milk (see Chapter 17, Relactation).
- Any amount of your milk will give your baby immune protection that no formula can provide.
- It's likely to take a few days or weeks to bring in your milk production, and you'll need support. **Your baby will need to be**

supplemented (given extra milk) during this process (see Supplementing in this chapter).

Want to know more?

You can find extra resources for this section at the "Art of Breastfeeding" tab, Chapter 18, at www.llli.org.

Hospitalisation or Surgery, Your Child's or Yours

When you or your baby, toddler, or child needs surgery or hospitalisation, planned or in an emergency, breastfeeding can almost always continue. Nursing helps your child feel safe and comforted, and recover faster. There are very few situations in which breastfeeding needs to be interrupted because of your own illness or surgery (see Medications in this chapter).

The Academy of Breastfeeding Medicine has a useful protocol (Supporting Breastfeeding During Maternal or Child Hospitalization) that strongly supports breastfeeding.

Contact an LLL Leader or see LLL websites for more information.

Hypoglycaemia (Low Blood Sugar in Your Baby)

Hypoglycaemia means "low blood sugar" (*hypo* means "less," *glycaemia* means "sugar"). It's normal for babies to have a drop in the level of sugar (energy) in their blood in the couple of hours after birth. Most babies don't need to have their blood sugar levels checked. However, in babies born early, or to diabetic mothers, or small or large for gestational age, blood sugar is more likely to drop low enough to cause problems and may need to be treated.

The Backstory

When you have diabetes in pregnancy, the amount of sugar in your blood is likely to be higher than normal. The baby gets used to this before birth, and after birth her blood sugar level can drop too low.

Babies who were born early, or very small or very large, may also have low blood sugar at first (being born very large often goes with diabetes). Bear in mind that large and small babies may also be just fine. However, symptoms of low blood sugar range from mild to serious, and hospitals usually have policies about testing blood sugar levels and protocols for when and how to treat babies with low blood sugar.

What You Can Do

The first and simplest thing you can do if there is concern about your baby's blood sugar level is to hold her skin-to-skin for as long as you like after birth. This can help raise her blood sugar or make it less likely to drop very low – whether or not she nurses.

The Academy of Breastfeeding Medicine has a useful protocol for hypoglycaemia (Guidelines for Glucose Monitoring and Treatment of Hypoglycaemia in Term and Late Preterm Neonates), which you can share with your doctors if needed. It says that:

- Breastfeeding within the first hour after birth is important.
- Babies with no risk factors or symptoms should not be tested.
- At-risk babies should be tested until their blood sugar is normal.
- There is no evidence that babies with low blood sugar who show no symptoms need to be treated.

If your baby does have symptoms of low blood sugar and needs treatment, there are several options:

- **Dextrose (sugar) gel** rubbed inside the baby's cheek works quickly and doesn't interfere with breastfeeding.
- If your baby needs **extra milk,** expressing by hand or pump will help you bring in plenty. If you're not able to express enough, donor breastmilk is the next best option (see Supplementing and Milk Sharing in this chapter, and Chapter 15 on expressing).

If you have diabetes of any kind (gestational, type 1, or type 2) – or you know you're likely to have an early, very small, or very large baby – it's helpful to plan with your healthcare provider for how your baby will be cared for if she does have low blood sugar. You might want to consider expressing and freezing some colostrum (early milk) in the last few weeks of pregnancy. This can be fed to your baby if she has low blood sugar after birth (see Chapter 15).

Hypothermia

Hypothermia means being too cold (*hypo* means "less," *thermia* means "heat"). This can be dangerous for babies.

The Backstory

Nothing has been found to warm a baby better than skin-to-skin contact with his mother. Nothing. Babies in warmers and incubators don't warm as thoroughly or hold their temperature as well.

What You Can Do

Keeping your baby with you, his skin against your skin, with a blanket over you both, is the best prevention for hypothermia. If your baby was born in a birthing pool or bath, he'll need to be dried off with a warm towel when he comes out of the water; wet babies lose heat faster. Premature babies (even if only a bit early) are more likely to get cold because they have less fat and aren't so good at managing their temperature yet. Kangaroo Care (spending as much time as possible skin-to-skin) is agreed to be the healthiest, happiest place for premature babies as soon as they're well enough to do it (see Chapter 17). Being snuggled toasty warm with you is also a good way to help prevent jaundice.

Jaundice, or Hyperbilirubinaemia (Too Much Bilirubin)

Babies can develop yellowed skin and eyes in the days following birth. The yellow colour is caused by a pigment called bilirubin (red bile) in the blood. A little jaundice is common; more than half of babies have it. In fact, it's thought that it might even be good for babies, protecting them from inflammation and infection. But too much can make a baby sleepy and not interested in eating. If levels get *really* high, bilirubin can even cause brain damage.

The Backstory

Before birth a baby needs extra red blood cells because she gets less oxygen through the placenta than she will via her lungs. After birth she doesn't need as many, so her body breaks down the extra red blood cells and bilirubin is formed in that process. Bilirubin leaves the body in poo, not wee, so milk (not water) intake is the most important way to prevent and resolve jaundice. The more milk the baby gets, the more she poos, and that helps get rid of the bilirubin.

Does jaundice need treatment? It depends. Here are some of the factors your healthcare providers will consider:

- Babies don't usually build up bilirubin from breaking down blood cells until they're two or three days old, so **the baby who has high bilirubin on her first day of life** is more likely to have something else going on and to need extra care.
- **Premature or sick babies** are at higher risk of building up too much bilirubin than healthy, full-term babies.
- Babies who have **ABO blood group incompatibility, an infection, a lot of bruising from birth,** or other issues, are more likely to get jaundice earlier and to need treatment.

Jaundice caused by not having enough poos tends to go away by about five days of age, as milk becomes more plentiful. Healthy, thriving babies sometimes have obviously yellow eyes, and yellowish or orangey skin for weeks or even a couple of months. Regardless of skin tone, pressing gently with your finger on the skin of the baby's forehead or nose will show a yellowish tinge if your baby has jaundice.

Jaundice that lasts past five days is sometimes called breastmilk jaundice. Breastfed babies are more likely to be jaundiced. If nursing is not going well, though, the baby may not get enough milk to clear the bilirubin and may need extra care.

What You Can Do

Giving your baby plenty of milk in the first few days helps keep bilirubin levels down. If she becomes jaundiced (the whites of her eyes start to look yellow), her bilirubin levels should be checked by a healthcare provider. Jaundice treatment has two parts:

1. **Food.** Keep your baby with you as much as possible so you can keep breastfeeding going strong. This is your first and best ally against jaundice. If she's away from you for treatment, or is very sleepy, your baby won't be nursing as frequently as she otherwise would. You can express your milk to protect your milk production (and give you plenty of milk to feed to your baby; see Chapter 15). Some healthcare providers may recommend supplementing with formula to bring down the bilirubin level faster. If you don't have enough milk of your own, adding formula to increase volume may lower bilirubin faster, but using formula in the early days involves some risks to the newborn gut. In some places, banked donor human milk may be an option (see Supplementing and Milk Sharing in this chapter).
2. **Light.** Some wavelengths of light can be safely absorbed by the baby's skin, changing bilirubin into a form that is excreted faster. Hospitals use phototherapy lights (bili-lights) to treat babies with higher levels of jaundice. Be prepared for some spinach-coloured poos as the extra bilirubin comes out.

Once your baby's jaundice levels have come down, and light therapy is finished, your previously sleepy baby may be unsettled for a while and want to nurse very often, making up for lost time.

Low Milk Supply

Sometimes a baby is not able to get all the milk he needs at the breast or chest. The good news: your nursing relationship doesn't depend on the amount of milk you can make! You may be able to increase your milk production, but however it turns out, any amount of your milk is beneficial – and your baby gets much more from nursing than just milk. When needed, extra milk can be given in ways that support your nursing relationship (see Supplementing in this chapter). For more about low milk supply, see Breast Tissue Insufficiency, Supplementing, and Weight Gain Worries in this chapter.

The Backstory

Worrying about not making enough milk is common (much more common than not actually making enough milk). In many parts of the world, more than half a century of formula-feeding – and advertising by formula companies – has undermined confidence that breastfeeding can work, and the know-how to help it work well. Many of us worry that we don't have enough milk even when we do. However, a few of us really *aren't* able to make all the milk our babies need, no matter how hard we try. No one knows exactly how many, but compared with previous generations, more of us find ourselves in this situation for many reasons, including that more of us are choosing to nurse our babies – which is a great reason!

These are *not* reliable signs of whether your baby is getting enough milk:

- your baby's feeding pattern (very often, or with long gaps)
- your baby's behaviour (how much he cries or fusses; whether he's happy to be put down between feeds)
- your baby's sleep pattern (waking every few minutes or sleeping for hours at a stretch)
- how your breasts feel (full or soft), and what they look like

These *are* reliable signs (the only ones!):

- your baby's weight
- your baby's pooey and wet nappies

For more detail on nappy output and growth at various ages, see chapters 5 to 7.

If you're concerned your baby might not be getting enough milk, work with your healthcare provider to monitor his growth and find breastfeeding support quickly.

If your baby really isn't getting enough milk, it's important to figure out if he's not taking enough milk because you're not making enough. Or are you not making enough because he's not taking enough? Or is he taking plenty but not using it well? These are three completely different issues that your breastfeeding support person and healthcare provider can help you figure out.

Reasons why your baby might have trouble taking enough milk include

- the way he's held and attaches at the breast
- not feeding often enough, or long enough
- being born prematurely

- having a tongue-tie or other "body" problems
- being jaundiced or sick; for example, having an infection

Reasons why your baby might be taking enough milk but not using it well include

- food allergy
- heart problems (such as a hole in the heart)
- some other illness that affects digestion or uses extra energy

Reasons why you may be having trouble making enough milk include

- hormonal issues
  - retained fragments of placenta
  - thyroid problems (which can affect milk production or release)
  - polycystic ovary syndrome (PCOS)
  - hormone treatments (oestrogen or testosterone)
- structural issues
  - breast hypoplasia (see Breast Tissue Insufficiency in this chapter)
  - previous nipple or breast surgeries and procedures (see Chapter 17)

Evidence suggests diabetes, obesity, and other metabolic health issues may affect milk production, though of course, many heavier mothers make milk just fine.

If you have a physical limit on how much milk you can make, you've probably had a low supply from the start, and the usual ways to increase milk production (see the next section) may not have much effect. It can take some detective work to figure out what's causing the problem. Fortunately, researchers are looking at the underlying causes of low milk production now, so please reach out to your breastfeeding helper for the latest information.

What You Can Do

By far the most common cause of low milk supply is not enough milk being removed from the breasts in the early days after birth. Whether or not you've worked out the likely cause, if you suspect milk production is low, it makes sense to take steps to increase it by removing milk more often. The earlier you act, the better the results are likely to be. You can start with the following steps:

- Check that your baby is as **efficient** as possible at the breast.
- Offer each breast **as often as your baby will take it** (it can be more than two per feed!).
- **Compress** the breast with your hands to help your baby get more milk when nursing, and **switch sides** when she stops actively feeding (when she's just doing light, fluttery sucks and not much swallowing – see Chapter 4).
- If this doesn't do the trick, **express your milk as often as possible** (see Chapter 15).

You might have heard about **galactagogues,** the medical term for a food, herb, or medication that can increase milk production. Some of these have been used for centuries. Work with a breastfeeding supporter and your healthcare provider if you want to give any of them a try. You will also need to nurse or express frequently for these to work. There are also some anti-galactagogues, which can reduce milk production (see Medications in this chapter). A breastfeeding supporter can help you check that none of these is likely to be causing the problem.

There's much, much more to know! Working on milk supply issues can be hard. It's time-consuming, and you might feel a mixture of emotions, including frustration, disappointment, and wondering whether it's worth it. It can be helpful to connect with others who have been through the same thing. We've supported thousands of families to find a nursing relationship that works well for them, even if it doesn't look like what they had imagined. We're here for you, too. And one more thing – many of us who have had problems making enough milk for our first baby make more for the next baby, and any after that as well.

Want to know more?

You can find extra resources for this section
at the "Art of Breastfeeding" tab, Chapter 18, at
www.llli.org.

Mastitis and Blocked Ducts

Maybe you discover a tender or painful area in your breast. It might feel lumpy or warm to touch, and if you've got lighter skin, it might look pink or red. This is commonly called a blocked duct. Maybe you're running a slight fever, or you're beginning to feel flu-like aches and chills. These are all signs of mastitis.

Mastitis (inflammation of the breast) can come and go like a whirlwind over a couple of days. But it can last for longer; and if it's not dealt with effectively, mastitis can keep coming back – or even make you severely ill. Uncommon but serious complications of poorly treated mastitis are **abscess** (a collection of pus in the breast, requiring drainage) and **sepsis,** a life-threatening whole-body response to infection. It's important to know the signs of mastitis and the basics of treating it. Our understanding of mastitis – and how to deal with it – has changed quite a bit recently. Medical advice may change further as more research is done; check with your healthcare provider and breastfeeding supporter for current recommendations.

The Backstory

Blocked ducts and mastitis are now recognised as being on a mastitis spectrum of interrelated conditions. They have one thing in common: inflammation in the breast. Inflammation happens when the body senses a threat, such as pressure, damage, or infection, and sends protective cells to control or fight it. This process causes the symptoms you experience.

Possible causes of mastitis include the following:

- **Not enough milk being removed.** Maybe because of widely spaced feedings, or the baby not nursing efficiently, milk can build up in the breast, increasing pressure and triggering swelling. Overusing a breast pump or milk collection device can cause you to make a lot more milk than you need.
- **Nipple damage.** Usually caused by a baby who's not latching well, or an older baby biting, nipple damage can let in bacteria.
- **Breast injury.** Your breast could have been injured by **trauma** (a blow to the breast) or **pressure** (from wearing an underwire or too-tight bra, bag strap, seatbelt, baby carrier, or something else in contact with your breast). You might also be more prone to

mastitis if you've had breast surgery, such as implants, which increase pressure in the breast.
- **Stress.** Extra stress (including being unusually tired, travelling, or hosting guests) can put your immune system under extra strain and make mastitis more likely.

What You Can Do

- **Make sure your baby is attached deeply and nursing effectively.** If you're not sure, a breastfeeding supporter can assist you.
- **Check for blebs.** These tiny white or yellow dots on the tip of the nipple can block milk coming out, causing mastitis symptoms (see Blebs in this chapter).
- **Continue nursing or expressing.** You don't need to try to remove every drop of milk. Doing this can even make things worse by increasing supply and pressure within the breast. Be guided by how often your baby wants to nurse and what helps your breast feel most comfortable. Milk can taste saltier during mastitis, and some babies refuse it. If you still feel very full after nursing, or if your baby doesn't want to (or can't) nurse, gently express just enough milk to soften the breast.
- **Rest.** As the saying goes: don't stand if you can sit, sit if you can lie down, or stay awake if you can sleep! You're ill – go to bed with your baby if you can. Ask for all the help you can get until you're fully recovered.

Is My Milk Safe for My Baby?

Almost always – and keeping it flowing will protect the health of your breast. If you have infective mastitis, and the infection is an unusual one, or very severe, *and* your baby is premature or sick, you might occasionally need to pause giving your milk until antibiotic treatment has started. But this is rare. Check with your healthcare provider if you're concerned.

I'm Nursing (or Expressing), but the Milk Isn't Coming Out – Help!

If your milk doesn't flow easily, it's probably because inflammation in your breast is acting like a traffic jam. Anti-inflammatory measures (see the next section) used twenty to thirty minutes before nursing (or expressing) may help. Don't be rough with the breast to force milk out; this can make swelling worse (and it really hurts!). Any temporary drop in milk production during mastitis usually sorts itself out once the breast is back to normal.

What Else Can You Do?

These are further things you can try to relieve your mastitis:

- **Nonsteroidal anti-inflammatory medications,** like ibuprofen, can relieve both pain and inflammation. Your healthcare provider may be able to suggest alternatives if you can't take them, or stronger medication if you need it.
- **Cold** can help ease swelling in the breast, just like it does in other areas of your body. It probably won't get rid of the mastitis on its own, but it may feel good. You could use cold gel packs, washcloths soaked in cold water and wrung out, or a bag of frozen vegetables or crushed ice wrapped in a towel (be careful not to burn your skin with cold).
- If cold sounds unpleasant (as it might if you're shivery), or your community's practice is to avoid cold in the period after birth, you could try **warm** compresses to help milk flow, or for comfort between feeds. A warm bath might feel good, too. Don't use heat for too long, though, as it can make swelling worse.
- If you feel more comfortable with a **bra,** a well-fitted, supportive one might help. If you feel better without one, that's fine, too.
- **Massaging and moving the breast** can sometimes be helpful. The pressure should be *very* gentle (be guided by what feels good) and done by hand (avoid electric massage devices). Massaging an inflamed area can cause it to become more inflamed, so it may be soothing to apply a cold compress or ice afterwards.
- **Lymphatic drainage,** described in the Engorgement section of this chapter, may be helpful.
- You might like to try some **different feeding positions** from your usual. There may be areas of the breast that don't get drained so well if you always stick to one or two positions. Some people find it helps to lay their baby down on her back on a flat surface and, kneeling above her, dangle the breast into her mouth. This position swings the breast away from the rib cage (which might

especially help if the sore area is under the breast) and gives you a full circle of angles to try!
- There's some evidence that probiotics, soy lecithin, and therapeutic ultrasound might have beneficial effects on mastitis. But it's too early to be sure. We hope there will be more high-quality research during the lifetime of this book. Ask your healthcare provider for up-to-date advice.

When Do I Need to Get Medical Help?
If you're not getting worse, you can treat yourself for twenty-four hours. If nothing has changed, or you're starting to feel better, try another twenty-four hours. After forty-eight hours, if you're still not improving, or you're getting worse, continue with the same measures *and* talk to your healthcare provider.

Get medical help right away if

- you see any pus
- you have a fever (more than 100.4°F/38°C)
- you feel much worse
- you see darker streaks (on dark skin) or reddish streaks (on light skin)

Your provider may prescribe antibiotics. Most people start feeling better within a day or two of starting them. Keep up the self-help measures just listed alongside the antibiotics.

If you're not feeling better by the third day of antibiotics, let your healthcare provider know. And be sure to take your whole course of medication, even if you feel better. If you stop too soon, the mastitis is more likely to come back. If you're not feeling completely better by the time you've finished the medication, contact your provider to see if you might need a longer course, or a different medication.

If you keep getting mastitis, an LLL Leader or other breastfeeding supporter can help you figure out any underlying breastfeeding issues. Mastitis is horrible – we hope you feel better soon.

Medications

We know to be careful about medications during pregnancy, but what happens after your baby is born? There are very few medications that are unsafe to take during breastfeeding. These are mostly very toxic ones, like chemotherapy drugs, plus a few that suppress milk production. However, if you read the package insert that comes with many medications, it might tell you that it's not safe to take during pregnancy or breastfeeding. What's going on?

The Backstory

Taking a medication before your baby is born can be risky because the baby is growing arms, legs, internal organs, and brain. Drugs that are fine for fully grown adults can affect this development in harmful ways. After birth, like in adults, your baby's liver is responsible for eliminating most medications from his blood. However, his liver is not fully mature at first and, of course, is smaller than yours. Not all medications are absorbed the same way, so the decision about whether to take a medication depends on many factors.

So how can you know what's safe and what isn't? A few drugs concentrate in breastmilk, while many don't get into milk at all, or appear only in tiny amounts. In some cases, the amount of the medication that gets into the milk depends on your genetics. Drug companies usually try to be supercautious, often suggesting you don't use their drugs during breastfeeding at all. But that's not the whole story. You will also want to consider these factors:

- **The risks to your baby of not being breastfed.** There is no risk-free substitute for breastfeeding.
- **The risks to you of weaning, especially if you don't want to.** This may be particularly important if you take medication for a mood disorder, such as depression or anxiety (see Postnatal Mood Disorders in this chapter) that can be made worse by weaning. Almost all mood medications (and some medications for ADHD) can be taken while breastfeeding. To be told you must choose between medication and nursing when you're already depressed or anxious puts you in a terrible dilemma. It's almost never necessary.
- The risks **of not taking a medication you really need.**
- And **what your nursing relationship means** to both of you.

A small theoretical risk from a medication might be outweighed by the potential costs of pausing or stopping breastfeeding.

What You Can Do

Fortunately, many drugs have been well studied, and good information is available to tell us how much of a drug is likely to get into breastmilk and what effect, if any, it might have on babies. Healthcare providers may not be familiar with resources about medications and breastfeeding. If you're told you must stop nursing to take a medication you need, or aren't sure about the safety of a medication you plan to take, check with a breastfeeding supporter or breastfeeding-knowledgeable pharmacist.

Want to know more?

You can find extra resources for this section at the "Art of Breastfeeding" tab, Chapter 18, at www.llli.org, to help you and your healthcare provider make an informed decision.

Milk Sharing

Sharing milk with other people's babies who need it is an ancient practice that's becoming more widespread. If you're considering milk sharing, either as a donor or as a recipient, for your baby, it's important to be aware of the potential risks and ways to minimise them.

Please note that LLL Leaders are not able to link milk donors with families needing milk.

The Backstory

Milk sharing was common before commercial infant formula was widely available. If a mother didn't have enough milk for her baby, or was unavailable for some reason, another mother would nurse the baby. Milk sharing might be done occasionally, by family or friends, or it might be a formal arrangement for the complete feeding of the child (known as wet nursing). In some parts of the world, wet nursing has a long and painful history of being imposed on enslaved and underprivileged women. In other places, wet nursing was a well-paid and respectable profession.

Formula is now widely available and accepted, but it's not the only option for babies needing more milk. Shared nursing is still practised in many places, especially among close family (see Chapter 5, Traditional Supplementation Methods). Technology has expanded the options: breast pumps make it possible to use milk expressed by someone else without them nursing your baby directly.

Some countries have systems of registered **milk banks,** with rules to make sure the milk is safe. Usually, milk goes first to premature or sick babies in hospitals. Some milk banks are also able to supply milk for babies at home. But milk banks aren't available everywhere. Many milk banks closed in the 1980s because people were concerned about HIV being passed on through milk. Fortunately, pasteurisation (a special heat treatment) is now proven to completely inactivate the HIV virus and many more, including Covid-19, in milk.

Most majority Muslim countries (though not all – Iran launched its first milk bank in 2016) have avoided milk banking because of beliefs about "milk kinship" between children who have been fed by the same woman. Wet nursing, which makes milk kinship bonds clear to everyone involved, may be a more acceptable alternative.

Thanks to research and easy access to information, we understand more than ever the importance of human milk for babies. It's not surprising that families in need of extra milk are turning to other parents to share milk with them. This may just mean that someone close to the family nurses, or expresses for, a baby in need. But the internet has widened the possibilities. Milk-sharing websites and social media groups enable sharing on a wider scale.

What You Can Do

It's important to be aware of the main risks involved in informal milk sharing:

- passing on diseases
- exposing your baby to medications, illegal drugs, or other substances
- being given something else instead of, or mixed with, human milk

Healthcare professionals are often reluctant even to mention milk sharing as an option because of these risks. Yet health professionals advise parents every day on how to use formula as safely as possible, even though formula has more risks.

As a parent, you have the responsibility to make sure your baby's food is safe. Our role is to provide information to help you make the best possible choice in your situation, and to carry it through safely.

Here are some safety tips for using milk that is informally shared (not obtained via a milk bank):

- **Know exactly where the milk comes from.** Getting to know the donor is much safer than sourcing milk anonymously. It helps if you have a personal connection, or if your donor is a part of your community.
- **Using freely donated milk is safer than buying it.** People are more likely to lie about medical history or to add something to the milk to increase the amount if they are getting money for it.
- **Get a full medical history.** Some of these things might not be easy to ask about, but they are important to protect your baby from: illnesses, medications, smoking, illegal drug use, and any risky behaviours in a sexual partner. You can find detailed questions to ask in the Academy of Breastfeeding Medicine's "Position Statement on Informal Breast Milk Sharing for the Term Healthy Infant."
- **Consider heat-treating milk at home.** Heat-treating inactivates viruses while protecting the nutrients and most of the immune factors in breastmilk. No special equipment is needed; you just have to be able to boil water. It's important to follow your chosen method closely. You can find one method in the Academy of Breastfeeding Medicine's "Position Statement on Informal Breastmilk Sharing."

The Academy of Breastfeeding Medicine's protocol "Human Milk Storage Information for Home Use for Full-Term Infants" has useful information on cleaning hands and equipment and storing, transporting, freezing, defrosting, and warming shared milk.

Having your milk donor nurse your baby directly is the safest form of milk sharing if you're confident they are healthy. With direct nursing there is no risk of milk getting contaminated between the donor and the baby. Where possible, direct breastfeeding has other benefits for babies, too (see Chapter 17, Exclusive Pumping).

Thinking of donating milk? You'll first want to be sure you will have plenty for your own baby. If you increase your milk production to donate, it can be a bit frustrating if the milk flows faster than your baby likes, or if your breasts are very full between feedings. You might need to have a regular plan to express. You'll require fridge or freezer space to store the milk, plus suitable containers (see Chapter 15). Some milk sharing networks suggest having a written agreement to make clear who is covering expenses and to protect yourself against any legal issues.

Nipple Diversity

Nipples come in different shapes and sizes but still work just fine for breastfeeding. Nipples are like rubber bands that can stretch and then relax back to their original size. But, like rubber bands, some are stretchier than others.

The Backstory

Most babies can give you a bruise by just sucking on your neck; they don't need an ideal nipple in order to latch, just a little matching of parts. Some babies do find it harder to latch on if your nipples are flat, inverted, or very large.

What You Can Do

Flat nipples are really just short-stemmed. Your baby will find them by their texture, taste, smell, and seeking the point on your breast's contour where she expects a nipple to be. You can rub or fiddle with short nipples to make them more prominent, or use your finger to push up

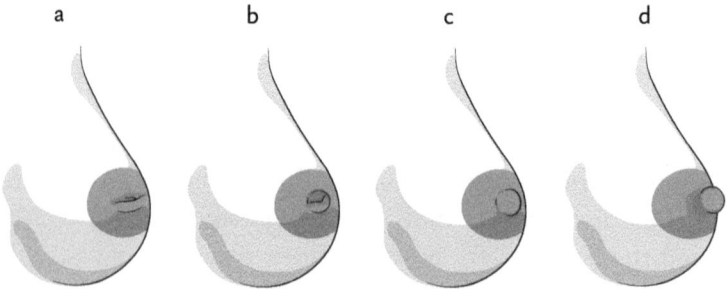

Nipple variations: (a) inverted, (b) slightly inverted, (c) flat, (d) protruding

into the breast from underneath and help push your nipple out further (this is called a nipple nudge). You might find using your hand to make a breast "sandwich" or "taco" helpful as well. For more tips on latching and attaching, see Chapter 4.

While both you and your baby are learning, it may help to avoid artificial teats (bottles and dummies). Many babies can switch easily between them and the breast; however, if you've got flat nipples, it may be harder for her to transition, at least until your baby is nursing well. Once she has got used to the super-stimulation of a large, firm artificial teat, she may find it harder to recognise your nipple. If your baby needs extra milk, there are other options (see Supplementing in this chapter).

Some nipples aren't really short or flat; they just seem that way if you're engorged (see Engorgement in this chapter).

Inverted nipples tuck in instead of sticking out. If you have inverted nipples, you can try nursing after first gently pressing around your nipple with your fingers until it comes out. Some nipples look inverted but will pop out nicely if you do this. Some inverted nipples get more exposed during pregnancy, and there are commercial devices that help pull the nipple out. It may be wise to wait until your baby is born to see if you need to use them. Pumping briefly before nursing may also help.

Over time, just as a rubber band becomes more stretched out and doesn't snap all the way back, some nipples stretch out and stop being inverted. As adhesions (bands of tissue holding the nipple in) stretch or break, you may be a little sore. Skin can also get chapped if the nipple tucks itself away while it's still damp. After nursing or expressing, it may be helpful to quickly pat it dry or hold it open until it dries.

If your nipple won't come out at all, breastfeeding may be more difficult. If your baby *will* latch and suckle, the nipple should work just fine; the problem tends to be that the baby doesn't recognise the nipple and gets frustrated trying to find it.

Here are a few of the many options to try if your baby struggles to latch:

- Some babies can feed well with a **nipple shield.** If this works for you, it may be a good option for as long as you need it. (See the next section.)
- If you've got only one inverted nipple, you could **express** on that side and nurse on the other.

- You could **let the inverted-nipple side dry up.** Your functioning side might make enough milk for your baby all by itself. If not, you could fill the gap with donor milk or formula (see Supplementing in this chapter).

Other nipple shapes are common. If your nipple tip is oval instead of round, try having your baby take the longer dimension from corner to corner in her mouth.

Some of us have very **large nipples.** If your baby's mouth is just too small for your nipples at first, she'll grow into them. You can express your milk for her. It won't take long before she's big enough to manage. As one LLL Leader pointed out, "Right now, we need to keep your milk supply up and keep your baby fed. We can sort out the utensils later." For tips on keeping your milk supply high, see Chapter 4, The Three Keeps, and Chapter 15. Whether or not your baby can nurse directly, we can help you figure out something that works.

Nipple Shields

A nipple shield is a thin piece of material, usually silicone, that looks something like a wide-brimmed hat that sits over your nipple during nursing. Shields can be useful in a number of situations:

- **helping premature or very small babies** who don't have a lot of strength. The shield stays put when the baby pauses, so less energy goes into holding everything in place.
- helping a baby transition from **bottle teats** to nursing.
- helping a baby latch on to a **flat or inverted nipple.**
- helping parents who have **sensory issues** or have experienced **sexual trauma** and may find that a shield helps them tolerate the sensations of nursing.

A nipple shield is often suggested as a solution for **nipple pain.** We've seen this work well for some people, though the evidence is not as good as for the uses already mentioned, and it can even make things worse. There may be other things that help more (see Sore Nipples in this chapter and Chapter 4).

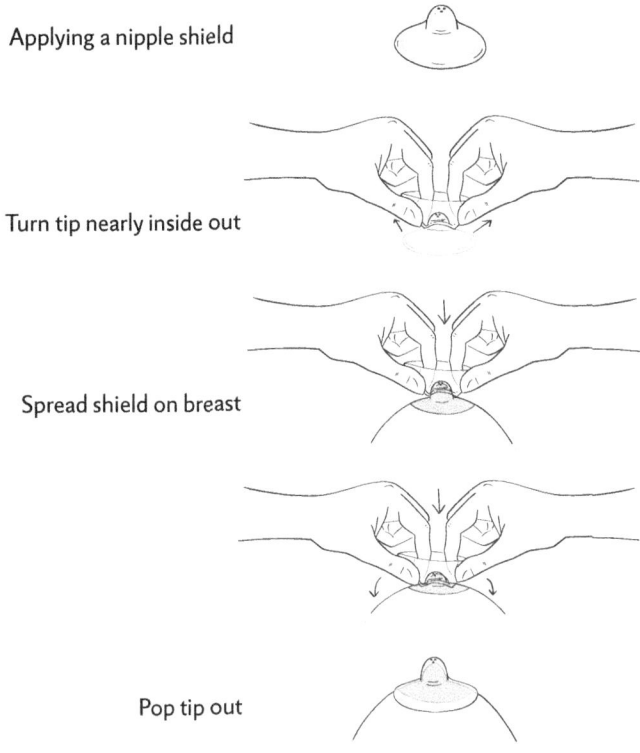

Applying a nipple shield

Turn tip nearly inside out

Spread shield on breast

Pop tip out

The Backstory

Nipple shields aren't "one size fits all." If possible, try a few to see what style and size works best for you. Even better, work with a breastfeeding supporter who's experienced in using them.

Here are some tips for applying a shield:

- A shield may stay on better if it's wet when you put it on.
- Turn it almost inside out.
- Put the end of your nipple against the inside of the tip.
- Push the rim back down into place and wiggle the nipple section to pop it out. Your nipple will be pulled into the shield a bit.
- It can be helpful to hand express a few drops of milk into the shield before latching your baby so he gets an instant reward as soon as he sucks.
- If your shield has a cut-out section, you can experiment to see if your baby prefers it by his nose, chin, or cheek.

Breastfeeding supporters are sometimes cautious about shields because they're aware of the problems with earlier shields. These were made of rubber and so thick that the breast didn't get much stimulation through the shield. Milk production tended to suffer unless the mother also expressed. The newer, thin silicone shields allow much better stimulation of the breast. If a baby can nurse effectively with a shield, you might not need to express at all. You'll know things are going well if you hear or notice plenty of swallowing and your breast is softer after nursing. Keep an eye on your baby's nappies and weight to make sure he gets enough milk.

Babies sometimes remove milk poorly with a nipple shield for the same reasons they can't nurse well: because of shallow latch or a tongue-tie, for instance, or because they're premature and low on energy. While working on the feeding issues – or just waiting for your preemie to get bigger and stronger – you may need to express as well to keep up milk production (see Supplementing in this chapter).

Ideas for Weaning from Nipple Shields

Nipple shields can be useful aids, like reading glasses or crutches. While you need them, if they're working well, there's no need to rush to stop using them. There may come a point, though, where you'd be glad to do without them but your baby isn't keen to give them up. What can you do?

- **Try removing the shield after the baby is fed,** when he is dozing and still contentedly sucking.
- **Try removing the shield in the middle of a nursing session.** Pick a calm moment when your baby's stopped actively sucking. If he starts to get upset, put the shield back and try again later. With an older baby you may need to wait a day or two between tries.
- **Try rinsing your nipple and areola before offering the breast.** A baby who's used to the bland taste of a silicone shield may at first be bothered by the taste of your skin. Or coat your nipple and areola with your milk to make it more enticing.

Sometimes, something just... changes. Often, the first shield-free feed comes as a surprise. The shield falls off and the dog steals it. Or you're away from home and realise you forgot to bring it. And suddenly, your baby is ready. Most babies who need shields will eventually nurse without them. And if you end up continuing to nurse with shields? They might be a bit of a nuisance, but you're *nursing*!

Nursing Strike (Breast Refusal)

Sometimes a baby who's been nursing happily for months suddenly starts refusing. This is different from when a baby is ready to wean because it happens so abruptly. She's clearly unhappy but still unwilling to nurse. This is often called a **nursing strike,** or breast refusal, and it's most common around eight to ten months. If your younger, not-yet-on-solids baby suddenly stops nursing, contact your healthcare provider and find breastfeeding support.

The Backstory

The cause of a nursing strike can be physical — a stuffy nose or sore mouth, throat, or ear, for instance — or emotional. Some possibilities include the following:

- **A loud noise** (maybe your reaction when your baby bit you!) could have startled her while she was nursing.
- **A dip in your milk supply** can happen during your menstrual cycle or a new pregnancy (along with a change in milk taste). Or milk supply can gradually drift downward if you're nursing less, perhaps because you're separated from your baby. Many babies don't mind a small decrease in supply, but some get frustrated with the breast if the milk drops below the satisfaction zone, especially if they can get milk another way, from a bottle or cup.
- **An oversupply of milk** can frustrate a baby who wants to sleep or just wants comfort.
- **Family stress,** such as that caused by a new job, move, illness, separation, or bereavement, can lead to a nursing strike.

Now you have a baby who has lost her main food source and her biggest comfort, yet she turns away whenever you offer. Some babies on strike will nurse at night or during naps. Some won't nurse at all. It's a tough time for you both. It's normal to feel shocked, and sad. While it's worth trying to figure out what happened, sometimes you'll never know the cause.

What You Can Do

Don't be too quick to give other drinks and foods to make up for the milk your baby's missing. She's probably a sturdy little gal by now and may just need a bit of time. Do hand express or pump your milk while the strike lasts to keep your breasts comfortable. Keeping your milk supply high isn't so urgent as your baby gets older; unlike during the early weeks of nursing, production with an older baby goes down only very slowly, even if the baby nurses less.

If the strike continues for more than a day, you could offer your expressed milk in a cup. It might be a good idea to avoid bottles if you can, so that your baby's sucking urge will also encourage her towards nursing.

Try these time-honoured approaches to resolving a nursing strike:

- Nurse your baby in her sleep. This is probably the most commonly helpful suggestion.
- Sing or rock her skin-to-skin.
- Nurse somewhere different – walking around, outdoors, or in a warm bath.
- Spend time around other nursing babies and children.
- Try new positions – sitting facing you, for instance; or put her up against your shoulder and slide her down.
- Do a dance or baby bounce – starting small but getting bouncier and bouncier – while holding her in a nursing position. (Stop if she doesn't like it.) You could also try sitting on an exercise ball.
- And here's a wild one that worked for one mother: sit in an office chair holding the baby in your lap near but not at your breast. Have someone spin the chair (not too fast) until you're a little dizzy and then offer your breast. Sometimes being a little disoriented lets our instincts rise to the surface!

If nothing is working, try *not* trying for a day or so to let the tensions (whatever they are) cool. Then keep your shirt up and your breast available but don't push the issue. Almost all nursing strikes end happily, but they don't all end quickly. It may be helpful to talk to a breastfeeding supporter or connect with others who've been through a nursing strike. Having someone to talk to about your own feelings can give your child space to work out hers.

Oversupply (Too Much Milk)

At first, you're happy: your breasts work! You're making milk! You can hear your baby gulping. But then you notice that he pulls off, spluttering, and your milk sprays like a fire hose. Soon he gets fussy about feeding. He may nurse a bit, let go, nurse some more, squirm and grumble and let go, then start all over again. He rarely falls asleep on the breast. He might spit up frequently or need a lot of burping. He might cry if you try to switch sides. His poos might have started out yellow, but over time they turn green or may look frothy and mucousy. You might even see streaks of blood in his poo. Nursing feels like a real struggle, though your baby's probably gaining weight fast. And your breasts still feel uncomfortably full after nursing; you might leak a lot longer than your friends did, plus you may keep getting mastitis. What's going on?

It sounds like you have an **overabundant milk supply** (oversupply – also known as hyperlactation). Other people might assume that's a good thing, but as you're discovering, it can be a big nuisance. We tend to have more milk with each baby, so oversupply is more likely with every baby after the first. The good news: it's almost always fixable.

The Backstory

Part of the problem with oversupply is just plain mechanics. You have a lot of milk, and it can come out *fast*. It's hard for your baby to keep up with the flow.

Then there's the digestion part. When there is a *lot* of milk, it can rush through the baby faster than he can easily digest it. Your baby has a gas factory going on in there, and it *hurts* (search "lactose overload" on LLL websites for a fuller explanation). If your baby has other symptoms, such as a rash, eczema, stuffy nose, or wheezing, there may be more going on than just oversupply; talk to your healthcare provider to rule out food sensitivity.

What You Can Do

It may be that all you need to do is help your baby manage the flow until he grows a bit or gets used to it:

- **Make sure he's got a big mouthful of breast.** When he's deeply latched, he's best able to control the flow of milk in his mouth (see Chapter 4).

Caution! Sometimes a baby *looks* like he's struggling with fast milk flow when actually he has sucking or swallowing issues and can't cope with a *normal* flow. This baby is likely to be newborn, premature, or small-for-dates, or may have other feeding issues, such as tongue-tie. He may be growing more slowly than expected. Don't do anything that might reduce your milk production until you've found breastfeeding support.

- **Shift positions.** Try laid-back positions (see Chapter 4). Leaning back turns your fast flow into a fountain, which may be enough. Or try sitting up but hugging your baby's back and shoulders more closely, tipping his head back a bit more and giving the milk a straighter shot down his throat. Or try nursing lying down, which some oversupply babies prefer.
- **Let him come off the breast** when the milk releases for the first time. Have a cloth handy, to catch the spray! The second milk release and the ones after that are usually smaller and easier to manage (but do let your baby come off whenever he needs to).
- **Use your hands to trigger just one milk release** before he comes to the breast. Do this only when you really need to – like when you've got a few hours of built-up milk.
- **Nurse more often.** This will keep your milk from building up so much.
- **Nurse when your baby is sleepy.** Feeds may be calmer this way.

If, after trying several of these ideas, your baby is still not coping (but is growing fast), you may need to tell your breasts to calm down. Basically, you'd aim to use each breast less often during each twenty-four-hour period, signalling it to slow down milk production. This may mean nursing on one breast per feed or for several hours in a row.

You might be advised to express milk before you nurse, so the baby doesn't have so much to deal with. That encourages your breasts to make even more milk, though, making the problem worse.

Search "Oversupply" on LLL websites for tips, or work with a breastfeeding supporter. Keep an eye on your baby's growth to make sure you don't overdo it!

Postnatal Mood Disorders (Depression, Anxiety, OCD)

Postnatal mood disorders are very common, and sometimes breastfeeding can actually help. If you need medication, breastfeeding can almost always continue.

Depression

Depression that hits after the birth of your baby, known as postnatal depression (PND), lasts longer than the common, very short-term baby blues, which often occur around the fourth day after birth.

The Backstory
The term *postnatal depression* describes low mood that starts at any time in your baby's first year (though it most often begins by about ten weeks after birth) and lasts at least a couple of weeks. Globally, about one in five new mothers experience it. There's quite a range among countries, however. Many reasons may account for these differences, including how postnatal depression is diagnosed and reported, as well as how pregnant women and new parents are cared for in different cultures.

You're more likely to experience depression or other mood disorders after birth if you've had one or more of these experiences:

- You've had depression or other mental health issues before.
- You've experienced recent trauma, such as domestic abuse or sexual violence.
- You experienced abuse or neglect as a child.
- You're parenting alone and have no one to help.
- Your birth was difficult.
- You've been separated from your baby.
- Your baby had to stay in hospital.
- Breastfeeding isn't going well.
- You're having trouble sleeping (even when your baby does) and so are extremely tired.
- You're living with basic survival stresses: poverty, poor housing, homelessness, being a refugee.

Low mood can sometimes be caused by hormonal imbalances, such as underactive thyroid (hypothyroidism), which is not as common as once thought but is worth investigating if you had diabetes while you were pregnant or you're very tired all the time. Other symptoms of underactive thyroid include sensitivity to cold, constipation, dry skin, hair loss, and muscle weakness. It's very treatable. Talk to your healthcare provider if you notice any of these symptoms. If you already know you've got thyroid issues, you might need to be tested more often than usual as things settle down after birth. Medications for hypothyroidism are safe for your baby.

Aside from physical causes, postnatal depression is more common in societies where new families are not well supported by extended family or community. Fathers and other partners can also experience it, so it's clearly not just about what's going on in the postbirth body.

Anxiety

Anxiety is a separate condition that can happen either with postnatal depression or on its own. Anxiety is a sense of worry, fear, or dread. Some anxiety during pregnancy, childbirth, and early parenthood is normal; it keeps us attentive to protect our babies. But it can get out of control. Almost constant or overwhelming anxiety, sometimes diagnosed as general anxiety disorder, can rob you of your joy and make life very hard.

Anxiety sometimes develops a particular focus, such as one of these:

- **phobias:** fear of specific things, such as germs
- **social anxiety:** fear of being with other people
- **agoraphobia:** fear of being outside or in public places
- **panic disorder:** suddenly feeling terrified, as if you might die

Obsessive-Compulsive Disorder (OCD)

Untreated postnatal anxiety can sometimes lead to obsessive-compulsive behaviours, which might be diagnosed as obsessive-compulsive disorder (OCD). Obsessions are thoughts that keep coming back even when you don't want them to. Compulsions are actions performed repeatedly to cope with and reduce fears; examples are washing your hands unusually often or checking that doors are locked. Obsessive-compulsive disorder is exhausting, and it can dominate your life. If you've had OCD before, like other disorders it can start up again after you've had a baby.

Some mothers become afraid that their babies might be harmed – or that they might harm their babies. They engage in endless rituals (compulsions) to keep their babies safe. And they're frightened that if anyone finds out about these thoughts, they might take the baby away. If you have these types of thoughts, it's important to find someone you can talk to. Antidepressants can also help. There are tragic situations where mothers do harm their babies. *But there is a big difference between this and OCD.* Mothers are more likely to harm their babies when they have **postnatal psychosis (PPP),** a rare but serious condition during which they break with reality. While they're in the psychotic state, they may believe that they really do need to harm themselves or their babies. You can read a bit more about postnatal psychosis in Chapter 6. In contrast, people with OCD feel horrible about their thoughts and go to great lengths to keep their babies safe.

What You Can Do

If you have depression, anxiety, or obsessive-compulsive disorder, it's easy to feel there's nothing you can do about it. It's common to feel that it's shameful to talk about it, that no one could understand or help, or even that you brought it on yourself and don't deserve to get better. These thoughts are your mood disorder talking – they aren't true. You need, and deserve, help.

It might be easier for people close to you to see what's going on than it is for you. If you're reading this because you're worried about your partner or someone else you care about, talk to them about what you notice and why you feel concerned. Reassure them that you will support them to find help and through whatever happens after that. When we're having a tough time, we need our loved ones alongside us more than ever.

Medical Emergency

If your partner or loved one who has just given birth is becoming disconnected from reality, *please don't wait.* Get medical help right away.

We know that reaching out for help might be the hardest thing you've ever done. But it can be the first small step on your road to recovery. If your depression or anxiety is mild, enlisting the support of your partner, family, or friends and starting one or more supportive practices (such as exercise, meditation, mindfulness, or light therapy) may be all you need to do. Reach out to safe people and let them know how hard you're finding life right now. If you need more help than they can give, talk to a healthcare provider you trust.

Fortunately, there are many treatments for overcoming mood disorders. They're similar for all of them (although medications may be different). Most anti-anxiety and antidepressant medications are compatible with breastfeeding. If you're ever told that you need to pause or stop nursing because you have to take medication for your mood, check out the Medications section of this chapter and get a second opinion. There are also non-medication treatments, including

- cognitive-behavioural therapy (CBT)
- interpersonal psychotherapy
- eye movement desensitization and reprocessing (EMDR) therapy for post-traumatic stress disorder (see Chapter 3)
- acupuncture

Sometimes, a combination of talking therapy and medication helps more than either approach alone.

Continuing to breastfeed helps both you and your baby. Breastfeeding hormones help reduce your feelings of stress, anxiety, and hopelessness. Your presence and touch provide emotional connection and security for your baby even if you don't feel it. If breastfeeding challenges are making your depression or anxiety worse, help from an LLL Leader or another breastfeeding helper is only a text, click, call, or visit away. If you want to stop nursing or expressing, of course we can help with that, too. It's usually safest to wean gradually, to let your hormones adjust (see Chapter 16).

If you feel up to connecting with an LLL group (or any other group for new parents), we guarantee that you won't be the only person there who's struggled with mental health. We'd love to be part of your support network.

Want to know more?

You can find extra resources for this section in the "Art of Breastfeeding" tab, Chapter 18, at www.llli.org.

Reflux

Does your baby do any of these things?

- arch her back when nursing
- pull on and off the breast as if she wants to nurse but for some reason can't
- swallow frequently *between* feedings
- fuss in a car seat or when lying flat
- drool, have noisy breathing, or have a stuffed-up nose most of the time

She may have reflux. The problem is, some of these symptoms may be normal baby behaviour, too, so it can be hard to figure out whether there really is a problem and what, if anything, you need to do about it.

The Backstory

Gastroesophageal reflux occurs when the connection between the stomach and oesophagus (the tube connecting your mouth and your stomach) opens or does not close completely and stomach contents rise into the oesophagus. People have minor reflux many times a day, babies more often than adults. Not all reflux is noticeable, and not all reflux makes us uncomfortable.

Reflux is a spectrum. At the mild end, a baby might vomit a bit (or even a lot) but it doesn't bother him. He feeds well and grows normally. As a wise doctor put it, this kind of vomiting is a laundry problem, not a medical one! At the severe end, reflux interferes with feeding, growing, and even breathing, and it can be extremely painful. This severe reflux – known as gastroesophageal reflux *disease* (GORD) – is more common in babies who were born prematurely or who have other health issues. These babies may need medication or even (in rare cases) surgery.

And then there are all the healthy but refluxy babies in the middle. They might bring up milk or look like they're working hard not to (known as "silent reflux"). And they seem bothered by it to some extent.

What You Can Do

- **Rule out other feeding or health issues.** Oversupply (too much milk), not enough milk, tongue-tie, and allergies can look like reflux or make reflux symptoms worse. If reflux comes on very suddenly, is very severe (projectile vomiting), and your baby seems unwell, get medical help right away.
- **Offer to nurse frequently.** Nursing is soothing for uncomfortable babies. Feeding little and often minimises the pressure from a very full stomach and helps your baby with digestion.
- **Keep your baby close.** A sling or soft carrier can be hugely helpful during the day. Being upright after feedings may help him keep milk down, and carrying helps keep him calm. A cloth or towel between you and the baby can catch any spit-up.
- **Avoid putting pressure on his stomach.** Your baby might be more comfortable, for now, in an all-in-one sleep suit rather than those cute little jeans, and in a sling rather than a car seat.
- **Stop or reduce smoking and consuming diet drinks.** Secondhand smoke (passive smoking) is known to cause or worsen reflux in babies, and there's some evidence that artificially sweetened beverages might do the same.

The opening from the stomach to the oesophagus is usually on the right side, so anything that puts the right side higher than the left side may keep your baby's stomach contents down better. Here are some ways you can help:

- During nappy changes, instead of bending your baby in half to wipe his bottom, try rolling him onto his left side.
- Try the Magic Baby Hold (see Chapter 6).
- If your baby sleeps badly flat on his back (recommended for safer sleep), discuss options with your healthcare provider. For more on sleep safety, see Chapter 12.

Almost all babies grow out of reflux by their first birthday, with many families finding that the symptoms improve after four or five months. If your baby can feed and grow well, carrying mop-up washcloths and spare clothes might be all you need to do. Get support from people who understand what you're going through. La Leche League groups can be a good place to start. If your baby is really struggling, and you feel like you're just not coping, talk to your healthcare provider. You, as well as your baby, need support. There are treatment options for babies who really need them.

Sore Nipples

You've probably heard a few stories about nipple pain. Some people have horror stories about cracked, bleeding nipples. Others warn you that breastfeeding hurts until your nipples "toughen up." Some say nursing should never hurt at all, and if it does, you're "doing it wrong." So where does this leave you, if you're sore?

Research has found that nipple pain affects many, maybe even most of us in the early days after birth. Nipple soreness is a common reason for stopping breastfeeding before you'd planned to. But we also know that when the baby's latch is deeper, the pain is less. Getting an effective latch right from the beginning can make a big difference. In most cases, nipple pain improves significantly by seven to ten days after birth as the two of you figure out how to nurse comfortably. That might give you some hope!

The Backstory

Most often, sore nipples happen when a baby doesn't take quite a big enough mouthful of breast. If this is happening, you'll probably see a change in the appearance of your nipple when she lets go – it may have a paler stripe across the top, look creased, or have one side flattened (like the tip of a new lipstick). The skin might start to break down, or crack.

- **The way the baby is being held** might be making it hard for her to open wide and take a big mouthful. This is the most common reason for nipple pain, and it's usually very fixable.
- **Medications** given in labour or at birth can affect the baby at first, making it harder for her to use all her reflexes to feed well.

- **Engorgement** (a very full, swollen breast) can make the breast too firm for the baby to get a deep mouthful (see Engorgement in this chapter).
- **A very small baby** (born prematurely or small-for-dates) and/or **very large nipples** can be a challenge. A little extra time may be needed before everything fits easily (see Nipple Diversity in this chapter).
- Occasionally, a baby has **physical challenges,** such as tongue-tie, making it impossible to get a deep latch (see Tongue-Tie in this chapter).

If you get pain only during the first few seconds after your baby latches, which quickly fades to little or nothing, it's usually a sign you've had nipple damage that's now healing. The pain occurs as the baby stretches out the damaged nipple to the back of her mouth at the start of the feed. Ouch! As long as it doesn't keep getting damaged, your nipple will soon heal.

Here are some other causes of sore nipples:

- **Nipple tenderness** caused by hormones is common in the first couple of weeks after birth, even if nursing is comfortable. You might feel like you can't stand anything, even clothing, touching your breasts. The only real fix is time, though pain medication, distraction, and deep breathing (like you might have learned for labour) can also help.
- You might find you have nipple tenderness for a day or two during your **menstrual cycle.**
- Sore nipples can also be an early sign of **pregnancy.** For more about breastfeeding while pregnant, see Chapter 16.
- **Blebs, vasospasm, tongue-tie, and yeast (thrush) infection** can also cause sore nipples – each of these has its own section in this chapter.
- Less common causes for sore nipples include skin conditions like **eczema, or skin reactions** to creams, ointments, or feeding tools (pump flanges, nipple shields, etc.).

What You Can Do

Nipple pain accompanied by nipple damage or compression of the nipple in the baby's mouth is always a sign that something needs attention.

- **Don't forget pain medication if you need it!** There are many options that are safe for your nursing baby (see Medications in this chapter).
- Research suggests that **using laid-back nursing positions** can help a lot (see Chapter 4 for all aspects of latching and attaching).
- **Don't be afraid to experiment.** A tiny adjustment here or there can make a big difference to your comfort (and your baby's efficiency). You might not need to take her off the breast every time – try cuddling her shoulders and bottom a fraction closer while letting her head tip back a little more. If that's still uncomfortable, you might need to take her off and try again.
- **Face-to-face help from a breastfeeding supporter** (in person or via video call) can make a big difference. You might want to do this more than once or see more than one person. Progress towards comfortable feeding often involves lots of baby steps.
- If things aren't improving, even with plenty of help, you might want to **talk to a breastfeeding specialist** about the possibility of tongue-tie.

Wound Care

Many treatments have been offered for sore nipples – purified lanolin, all-purpose nipple ointment, and hydrogel dressing, for example – but the research suggests none of those make a significant difference when it comes to relieving pain. If you find one or more of these treatments helpful for you, though, they're unlikely to cause any harm. There is some evidence that silver cups (worn over your nipples between feeds) may aid healing. Silver is widely used for treating wounds on other parts of the body.

A traditional remedy that some people find helpful is to hand express some milk and let it dry on your nipples. If you're going to rub anything on your nipples, wash your hands first! Some doctors also suggest washing wounded nipples once a day with a mild soap to prevent infection. If you see any crustiness, yellow ooze, swelling, or change in colour or shape, check with your healthcare provider to see if you need further treatment.

Nipple shields are sometimes suggested, to protect the nipple while it's healing (see Nipple Shields in this chapter). They're not ideal for sore nipples, though, the main problem being that they can mask, rather than fix, the underlying issue. If your nipples are so sore that you can't tolerate the baby feeding on your bare breast, a shield might give temporary relief, but it's probably even more helpful to find a breastfeeding supporter to help you work on getting a deeper, more comfortable latch.

Another option is to take a break and express your milk while your nipples heal. You could do this for a few days or just on a feed-by-feed basis. As long as your milk is flowing, and your baby is fed, you have plenty of time to work on breastfeeding. For more on how to keep things going while your baby's not directly nursing, see Chapter 4, The Three Keeps.

Many of us have had a painful beginning to our nursing relationship. Usually it lasts only a few days, sometimes a few weeks, occasionally longer. It almost always gets better with time, practice, and the baby growing. Working with one or more breastfeeding supporters can often help you get comfortable faster. Encouragement from others who have been through it is often the very best thing to help you keep going at times when you're wondering if it's worth it. You don't need to put up with nipple pain, and there are lots of people who can support you.

Supplementing (Giving Extra Milk)

Supplementing (giving extra milk) can be both emotional and confusing. Does your baby really need it? If so, what should you give, when, and how much? Will it undermine breastfeeding? Will you be able to stop doing it? As with causes of low milk supply, we know a lot more than we used to. We at LLL can support you to supplement in a way that protects your long-term nursing relationship.

The Backstory

Before you give your baby extra milk, be sure he really needs it. Giving unnecessary supplements can decrease your milk production; your baby may fill up on the supplement and take less milk at the breast. But if he truly isn't getting enough milk, he'll need that supplement, plus the milk he gets from you, to grow the way he should. While you're trying to fix any breastfeeding problem, it's vital to make sure your baby is getting enough milk. Babies breastfeed better when they're calm and not frantically hungry. Premature, small-for-dates, or sick babies, and those who have been getting less milk than they really need for a while, often need extra milk to give them enough energy to nurse. In these cases the supplement can actually be helpful in solving your breastfeeding issues.

What You Can Do

Work closely with a breastfeeding supporter and your healthcare provider. They can help you figure out whether supplements are necessary and if so, how to use them in a way that supports breastfeeding, including reducing them if it's safe to do so.

What Supplement?
When it comes to supplements, there is more than one option:

- **Your own expressed milk.** Your milk is tailor-made for your baby, and expressing it protects your milk production.
- **Human milk from another source.** If you don't have enough expressed milk of your own, donor milk is the next best option. See Milk Sharing in this chapter.
- **Formula.** Unless your baby is allergic to cow's milk, a standard first-stage infant formula is usually appropriate for babies up to twelve months old. "Follow-on" milks are not necessary. All formula manufacturers must adhere to the same rules about nutritional content. The extra health benefits claimed by more expensive brands aren't backed up by good evidence (if they were, all brands would have to put them in). Always make up powdered formula with the exact amounts of powder and water specified. Check with your healthcare provider if you're not sure how to use it. For more about using formula, see Weight Gain Worries in this chapter.

How Much?
Only your baby knows the answer! Let's look at three different babies:

- The first baby has recently **begun to seem fussy and extra hungry** since he started sleeping for longer stretches at night or since you started packing for a move. What supplement does he need? Probably just some extra nursing, because things are basically going well and you've hit a small dip.
- The second baby has **begun to grow more slowly.** The supplement he needs may just be the extra that you express while you get a

minor nursing problem sorted out. He'll probably soon start refusing some of what you've expressed, and you can begin phasing out the extra. Often you never find out exactly what the problem was, but a little expressing takes care of it for good.

- The third baby's **weight gain is faltering** (much slower than expected). He'll need more in terms of supplementation. You'll probably be expressing to build your supply but also giving your baby extra supplements. At first, he might not take much. You might even wonder whether he needs it, despite what the scale says. But then he might start to act like milk might go out of fashion, demanding large amounts. His stomach had become accustomed to smaller volumes, and it can take a few days for his appetite to start working properly.

Your baby may need to gain weight extra-fast to catch up. If he's fallen behind and *then* starts growing at his normal rate, he'll stay as far behind as he was. He needs to grow faster than normal for a while to catch up, and that takes more food than normal. Once he catches up, his appetite will settle down, but until then, expect a steeper-than-average line on his growth chart and a very hungry baby! When he's growing well, you can trust him to show you how much he needs. Paced bottle-feeding or another careful feeding method allows him to stop when he's had enough.

When?
People often suggest nursing the baby first and then "topping up" with the supplement. But this order can be unhelpful because the baby may come to associate nursing with hunger and frustration. You could try offering the supplement *before* nursing or between sides. As often as you can, *finish feeds at the breast.* This helps the baby associate the breast with satisfaction. Depending on how much supplement your baby needs, you might not have to supplement at every feed. Some families find that they can supplement during the day, for example, but just nurse at night. The key is to make sure your baby gets enough total milk in every twenty-four-hour period. When you provide it is entirely up to you.

What With?
The best supplementation device for you is the one you and your baby feel most comfortable with.

- **A nursing supplementer** (or "lactation aid") enables you to feed expressed milk or formula at the breast while your baby nurses. It consists of a tube with one end in a container of milk and the other held or taped on your breast, next to your nipple. As she nurses, your baby draws milk from the container. Using a supplementer has several advantages: you can supplement while you nurse, your milk production gets stimulated, you might not even need to express or use bottles. But your baby has to be able to nurse reasonably well to use one. Talk to your breastfeeding supporter about whether a nursing supplementer might be suitable in your situation.
- **Finger feeding** is a different way to use a tube. One end of the tube is placed in a bottle of milk. The other end is placed on your finger. The baby sucks on your finger to draw milk down the tube. The sucking action is a bit more like breastfeeding than bottle-feeding is, and the baby gets the familiar feel and taste of skin. If you're interested in trying this, contact a breastfeeding supporter.
- **Cups** are commonly used to supplement premature babies, especially in places where bottles are unsafe (you need good hygiene as well as reliable water and power supplies to use bottles safely). There is some evidence that for premature babies, using cups rather than bottles increases the odds of successful breastfeeding. If you'd prefer to avoid bottles, cups may be an option to consider; they can be used to supplement at any stage. Special baby-feeding cups are available – some have spouts, like the paladai, from India – but any small, clean cup can work. Cups are messier than bottles, though – it takes more skill and practice to cup-feed without spillage, and of course you can't carry milk around in them.
- **Baby feeding bottles** are convenient, socially acceptable in most places, and easy to use once you get the hang of them. It's easy to overfeed a baby with a bottle, though – babies love to suck, and if a bottle teat is what's on offer, they may keep on sucking even after they've had enough milk. And it's easy to override the baby's signals that she has had enough. Read on for tips on how to use bottles well.

Paced Bottle-Feeding

With paced bottle-feeding, your baby gets to eat at the speed she wants, stopping when she needs a break or has had enough. Here's how to do it:

- Your baby is **sitting upright,** *not* lying in your arms.
- **The bottle is fairly flat,** *not* angled steeply down (except right at the end of the feed, if *she* wants the last bit from the bottle). Many parents worry that if there's air in the bottle teat, the baby will swallow it and be gassy and upset. In reality, it's more of a problem for babies to be fed too fast. There has to be milk in the tip of the teat, but the whole teat *doesn't* need to be full of milk the whole time.
- **You're paying attention to your baby** throughout the feed. If she starts to look stressed (wide, alarmed eyes and "starfish" fingers, fidgeting, trying to turn away) give her a break by lowering the bottle so the milk is not flowing or removing it until she's calm and asks for more.

Check out paced bottle-feeding videos online to see the process in action. See Weight Gain Worries in this chapter for more on how to avoid overfeeding.

There's no kind of bottle or teat that's more like breastfeeding or works well for all babies (despite what advertisements claim). In general, start with a slow-flow nipple and change it to a faster one only if your baby is obviously frustrated. Flow rates are not standardised; one brand's slow might be the same as another brand's medium, or even fast. You may need to try a few to find one your baby prefers. And remember that pacing is key, no matter what kind of bottle or teat you use.

Side-Lying Bottle-Feeding

If your baby is premature, newborn (in the first month or so), or has health issues that decrease her muscle tone (making her a bit floppy), this alternative way of using a bottle might work better than upright paced feeding.

- Sit upright in a chair, with your knees slightly higher than your hips – if necessary, prop up your feet.
- Put a firm pillow on your lap (short end towards you if it's a rectangular pillow).
- Lie your baby on her side on the pillow, feet pointing towards you, facing the hand you want to hold the bottle in. Hold the bottle parallel to the floor.

If the milk is coming too fast, it will drip harmlessly out of the side of her mouth rather than down her throat (you might want to put a towel underneath her!). Again, watch your baby carefully so she can speed up, pause, and stop when she needs to.

When and How to Stop?
Often supplementing can be a short-term bridge to full breastfeeding. It's important to monitor your baby's weight while you're working towards reducing supplements. You've got the right amount of supplement when your baby is growing steadily, her growth curve tracking one of the lines on the growth chart, usually not far below where she started at birth.

Reduce the amount of supplement gradually, weighing your baby regularly to make sure she's still growing well. (Once a week is often about right to start with.) If she is, try reducing the supplement a bit more. You can weigh less often once she's got a solid track record of growth.

If her growth curve starts dropping, go back a step. It's tempting to rush it, but it pays to be patient and careful while you make this transition. It's a bit like crossing a rope bridge you're not totally certain will hold your weight. You don't run straight into the middle – you take one step at a time, ready to jump backward if it starts to give way!

Longer-Term Supplementing
Whether or not you can reduce and stop using supplements depends on your reason for needing them. If you have an underlying reason for low milk production (see Low Milk Supply in this chapter), you might need to use them until your baby is eating family foods or through the first year. A nursing supplementer can help you to enjoy nursing your baby regardless of how much milk you're producing. It's possible to

use a supplementer part-time, say, at home, while using bottles when out and about.

Once your baby is eating family foods as well, she may eventually be able to get the extra calories she needs from other foods instead of milk supplements. Many of us who needed to supplement with formula in the early months find that eventually we can just nurse alongside solids. We can relax into the later months and years of breastfeeding, leaving behind our early worries about milk production. Breastfeeding is not an all-or-nothing process. Every drop of your milk your baby gets is a gift.

Want to know more?

You can find extra resources for this section at the "Art of Breastfeeding" tab, Chapter 18, at www.llli.org.

Tongue-Tie

You've been trying hard to help your baby latch deeply, maybe with lots of help, but it's still not working. Your nipples are very sore, and look flattened or pinched when he lets go. You might feel a sensation like hammering or sandpapering during nursing. Your baby's weight gain may also be slow, and feeds may be frustrating as he frequently stops and starts, slips off the breast, or falls asleep. He might even refuse to nurse altogether. It's possible that your baby has a tongue-tie.

If you or your breastfeeding supporters suspect this might be the case, you will need to see a tongue-tie specialist (this might be a

Tongue Variations

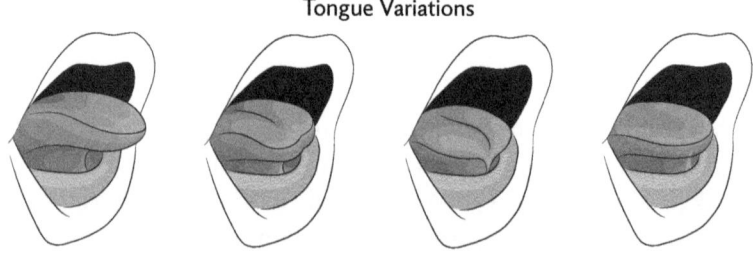

Some tongue variations may affect breastfeeding. What the tongue *looks like*, though, is not as important as *how it works*.

doctor or, in some places, a midwife, dentist, or other healthcare provider) for an assessment, diagnosis, and plan for treatment. See LLL websites or talk to a breastfeeding supporter for more information. We can support you through the process.

Want to know more?

You can find extra resources for this section at the "Art of Breastfeeding" tab, Chapter 18, at www.llli.org.

Vasospasm

A nipple **vasospasm** happens when the tiny blood vessels inside the nipple contract so tightly that blood is forced out of the nipple, turning the tip paler. This colour change is known as blanching (whitening). When the spasm relaxes and the blood flows back, on dark skin tones the nipple returns to its usual colour. On light skin tones, the nipple might turn bluish or purple to bright red before going back to its usual colour.

It can be painful when the blood returns, because those tiny blood vessels also supply the nerves. Like the "pins and needles" discomfort you get when you sit or sleep on part of your body, there can be a delay in the sensation returning. You may feel stinging or burning following a feed, or pain that shoots deep into the breast. You might feel it in one nipple but not the other. It can last several minutes and can also occur between feeds. It may be misdiagnosed as a yeast infection.

The Backstory

Vasospasms usually occur because of nipple trauma – a nipple's way of saying, "Ow!" It's also fairly common if you've had breast or nipple surgery, possibly as a result of nerve or tissue damage. Some drugs, including nicotine and caffeine, can contribute to vasospasm.

The medical condition Raynaud's phenomenon, a disorder of the small blood vessels in the skin, also causes vasospasms. It's more common in women than men, and it tends to run in families. If you have true Raynaud's, you'll typically be very sensitive to cold. Your hands and feet, maybe your nose and ears, will tingle and burn when you get cold. Your nipple vasospasms might be triggered by cold, too. If you had these symptoms before having your baby and are now having vasospasms in your nipples, consult with your healthcare provider about treatment options.

Most cases of nipple vasospasm, though, are caused not by Raynaud's, but by the baby compressing the nipple during a feeding. It might look squashed (misshapen, maybe with a stripe across the tip) when your baby lets go. This is most often because she didn't get quite a big enough mouthful. A baby might also "clamp down" on the nipple if the position she's in feels unstable or if she has a tongue-tie (see previous section).

What You Can Do

Vasospasms caused by shallow latch usually resolve once the cause is addressed (see Sore Nipples in this chapter and Chapter 4). In the meantime, to ease a spasm, you can try getting blood back into the nipple by squeezing it at the base (this might even stop the pain immediately). It can also feel good to massage your nipple. It looks a bit like hand expressing, but instead of trying to get milk *out*, you're gently easing blood back *in*, from breast to nipple. This might feel more comfortable if you use a little edible oil (such as olive oil) on your fingers.

Warmth can help prevent vasospasms caused by Raynaud's or ease vasospasm caused by compression in the baby's mouth. To keep your breast warm, here are some things you could try:

- Wear an undershirt or extra layer.
- Keep your home (or at least the room you're nursing in) a little warmer if possible.
- Get woollen breast pads – a fine wool-silk mix – popular in some cold countries. If you like them, you could even get two pairs and double up!
- Cup the nipple with your warm hand.
- As soon as your baby comes off the breast, hold a hot water bottle against the nipple, or use a wheat bag, cherry pit pillow, or sock filled with rice and sewn or tied shut. Microwaved on high for about a minute, any of these will hold a gentle heat for quite a while.

We know how miserable vasospasms can be, and we're here to help.

Weight Gain Worries

Weight gain is one way to monitor how things are going with your baby's feeding and overall health. Parents often worry that their babies aren't gaining enough weight or are gaining it too fast.

The Backstory

Healthy babies can gain weight at very different rates. Boys tend to grow faster than girls. Babies with tall biological relatives tend to grow faster than those whose family members are petite. Sometimes everyone forgets to look at the baby and his family as well as the numbers. And sometimes there really is a problem, and the scale can alert you.

The 2006 World Health Organization growth charts and more recent Intergrowth-21st charts for premature babies are reliable tools that show whether a baby's growth is within the (wide) range of normal. An unusual growth pattern is a good reason to check how feeding is going – and to get a medical checkup, since this kind of pattern can be an early sign of illness.

What You Can Do

Part 1: The Slow-Growing Baby

If your healthcare provider says your baby's weight gain is too low, a good first step is to confirm the numbers. Since scales can vary, try to have your baby weighed on the same scale each time, naked or wearing the same or similar clothes. Avoid weighing a full baby one time and a hungry baby the next. It's also helpful to weigh your baby at the same time of day; babies' weights fluctuate throughout the day, just as ours do. Once you've got accurate weight information, take a close look at your baby and ask these questions:

- **Does she look plump and rounded?** Slow-gaining babies who are doing well usually have rounded cheeks, plump thighs, creases around their wrists and ankles, etc. If she was premature or born small-for-dates, it may take her a few weeks to get that chubby baby look.

- **Does she relax after feedings (hands open, arms limp) and stay content for at least a few minutes?**
- **Is she doing the things your healthcare provider expects a baby of her age to do?**
- **Is she energetic?**
- **Are you seeing enough pooey nappies?** For what to expect at each stage, see chapters 5, 6, and 7.

If your baby is nursing as often as she wants, including plenty of "conversational" nursings; seems plump, healthy, active, cheerful, and developmentally on target; but still is gaining slowly, what should you do?

Ideally, you should have her checked over by a healthcare provider. Rarely, slow growth can be a sign of an underlying health issue, so it's important to rule this out. Babies who look healthy and thriving usually are! With everything else looking good, this may simply be your baby's normal growth pattern.

It's different if your baby is not only growing slowly but is also miserable or low in energy. In this case, consulting with your healthcare provider is vital and so is finding breastfeeding support, fast. You'll need a plan to keep your baby safely fed while you figure out what's going on.

These are the steps to increase weight gain for a well but slow-growing baby:

1. Make sure your baby is nursing as **effectively** as possible.
2. Make sure she **nurses as often as she's willing** (at least ten times in twenty-four hours) and **takes as many breasts as she will take each time** (it can be more than two!). You can use your hands to compress your breast while she nurses to help her get more milk.
3. If this doesn't do the trick, **add in some expressed milk,** increasing the amount until she's growing well. This may mean limiting the time she spends nursing to free up enough time to express (see Low Milk Supply in this chapter and Chapter 15).
4. If you can't express enough milk, **donor milk or formula** can fill the gap (see Supplementing in this chapter).

You may need to discuss with your baby's healthcare provider whether it's more important for your baby to grow faster or to benefit as much as possible from the protection and brain development she gets from human milk. If your baby is not able to take larger volumes of milk (e.g., because she's premature), supplementing with extra cream skimmed from expressed milk may be an option to consider.

Babies who are fed better, feed better. Supplements can be given in ways that support your nursing relationship. There is no reason why you shouldn't continue to enjoy nursing your baby as long as you both want, whether or not you need to supplement.

OLDER BABIES

If your very slow-growing baby is older than four months (but not before) and you don't have enough expressed milk to get her growing well, you could discuss with your healthcare provider whether it would be better to offer high-calorie family foods a little early, instead of formula. If your baby is already eating family foods, work with your healthcare provider to make sure she gets the nutrition she needs. It's possible to fill up a baby on low-calorie foods so that growth slows down even if she seems to eat quite a bit.

Some babies need more active encouragement and help with eating than others (see Chapter 13).

Part 2: The Very Fast-Growing Baby or Child

Maybe your concerns are in the other direction. Earlier editions of this book barely mentioned childhood overweight and obesity, but it's become such a widespread issue that we need to do it justice here. In the four decades up to 2016, it's estimated that the number of children in the world living with overweight or obesity increased tenfold, and in some areas it is still increasing.

We understand that the relationship between weight and health is not simple. Being a particular size is not a guarantee of good health (or ill health). Many larger people are fit and healthy. However, we do know that higher weight-to-height ratios are associated with higher risk of some health problems. Baby and childhood overweight and obesity tend to track through into adulthood – and the longer a person lives with overweight or obesity, the greater the potential cost to their health.

Evidence is mounting that ultraprocessed foods, including formula, increase the risk of overweight and obesity. But this is complicated, because size depends on so many factors beyond what we eat.

At highest risk of overweight are formula-fed children of mothers with overweight. Any amount of breastfeeding seems to help, with breastfeeding for longer, and exclusive breastfeeding, probably providing stronger protection. Children who are not breastfed grow differently from those who are. They tend to gain more slowly than breastfed babies in the first two or three months. After that, weight gain for breastfed babies slows down but it stays higher for formula-fed babies. Breastfed babies are leaner by twelve months. Very fast weight gain throughout the first year increases the likelihood of overweight later on.

Researchers are still in the early stages of finding out exactly how early feeding contributes to children's long-term growth and health. Scientists have discovered hormones in human milk that seem to help regulate appetite and energy use. We are far from understanding how all these "bioactive" components of human milk work, but we do know, for example, that insulin levels are very different in babies who are not breastfed.

We are also learning that the milk of mothers living with overweight or obesity has some differences from the milk of lower-weight mothers, possibly increasing the risk of overweight for their babies. Your own milk is still by *far* the best food for your baby, whatever your shape and size. Formula-feeding has many more risks besides overweight and obesity. But it does seem that the tendency towards overweight can be passed on to our children in many ways: through genetics, during pregnancy, and potentially through milk, as well as at mealtimes.

So, if you want to maximise the chances of your child having a healthy weight, what can you do? Here's what research tells us. Some of these factors will of course be beyond your control:

- **Aim for a healthy weight gain in pregnancy.** Your healthcare provider can make recommendations based on your pre-pregnancy weight.
- **Avoid or minimise smoking** in pregnancy, and after your baby is born. The reasons aren't fully understood, but smoking is associated with increased risk of overweight.
- **Aim to give birth vaginally** if you can. Babies born by caesarean have a higher risk of overweight, possibly because of differences in their microbiome (gut bacteria).
- **Breastfeed your baby** according to World Health Organization recommendations – exclusively for six months, continuing until two years or beyond.

- **Nurse responsively, according to your baby's appetite.** There's no benefit to restricting breastfeeding in any way, even if your baby becomes "pleasingly plump" (see Chapter 7).
- **Nurse directly,** as far as possible. Feeding expressed milk by bottle increases risk of overweight; the risk is somewhere between direct breastfeeding and using formula. Babies tend to take more milk by bottle than they do at the breast, even if it's your (or someone else's) milk in the bottle.
- If using a bottle, pay careful attention while feeding, and **let your baby show you when she's finished drinking.** Don't encourage her to take a bit more or to finish the bottle. If she wants more, offer it – again watching for signs that she wants to stop. Healthy babies are good at regulating their own appetite.
- **Avoid using large bottles** (bigger than 180 ml, 6 ounces).
- If you need to use formula, consider choosing one with a lower protein content. **Standard (high)-protein formulas increase the risk of overweight.**
- **Make up powdered formula carefully,** according to the instructions. Measurements on feeding bottles may not be accurate (especially the kind with bag liners). Consider weighing the water and powder on accurate scales to check.
- **Wait to introduce family foods** until around six months, when your baby shows clear signs of readiness. If she was born prematurely, or has food allergies, consult with your healthcare provider about the timing of introducing family foods.
- When you start family foods, let your baby feed herself. She can pick up pieces of food or hold a larger piece and gnaw on it. **Spoon feeding increases the risk of overfeeding.**
- **Inform yourself about healthy foods and portion sizes. As much as you can, offer your baby real food.** Babies and toddlers don't need artificially sweetened foods, and it's best to keep ultraprocessed foods to a minimum. "Juice drinks," and semi-liquid food served in pouches are usually full of processed sugars even if they're marketed as healthy. For more about family foods and healthy eating, see Chapter 13. For more about drinks for babies and toddlers, see Chapter 10.

Want to know more?

You can find extra resources for this section at the "Art of Breastfeeding" tab, Chapter 18, at www.llli.org.

Yeast (Thrush/Candida Infections)

If you have a thrush infection (caused by Candida – a kind of yeast) on your breast, breastfeeding usually hurts. A lot! Your nipples might be shiny looking, sometimes with flaking skin, regardless of skin tone. Lighter skin tones might look pinker than usual. You might feel an intense burning, itching, shooting, or stabbing pain in *both* breasts, especially after or between feeds. Your baby may have a yeast overgrowth in his mouth, too, making him a miserable nurser.

If you think you or your baby might have a yeast infection, contact your healthcare provider and reach out to a breastfeeding supporter for up-to-date information.

Want to know more?

You can find extra resources for this section at the "Art of Breastfeeding" tab, Chapter 18, at www.llli.org.

ACKNOWLEDGEMENTS

The writing team for *The Art of Breastfeeding* is grateful for the generosity of all who participated in bringing this ninth edition to life.

Thank you, La Leche League International, for the honour of joining the decades-long roll of writers of this book. The title might be new, but the message is timeless.

Warm thanks to Lydia de Raad, GG Williams, Zion Tankard, and the LLLI Board of Directors for their encouragement, enthusiasm, responsiveness, and support.

At the heart of this book are the hundreds of stories shared with us by families all around the world, who wrote beautifully about their experiences. Thank you. We laughed, cried, and were amazed as we read them. Nursing or providing milk for your baby truly transcends culture and countries.

Many stories were translated into English from other languages. Thanks go to all who worked on translations: Hiroko Hongo and Shoko Jin (Japanese), Veronique Lesoinne (French), Lydia de Raad (German), GG Williams (Italian), Vicky Bazoula Papadaki (Greek), and Carolyn Driver Burgess (Chinese).

Several published authors shared parts of their work or wrote new material for us: Aurelia Dávila Pratt (author of *A Brown Girl's Epiphany: Reclaim Your Intuition and Step into Your Power*), BJ Woodstein (author of *We're Here! A Practical Guide to Becoming an LGBTQ+ Parent*), and Trevor McDonald (author of *Where's the Mother? Stories from a Transgender Dad*).

Special appreciation to Edna Kelly, longtime LLL Leader, who donated the use of her lovely beach house so the writing team could meet and work together in person.

Reviewers were crucial in ensuring that information was correct, up-to-date, and relevant to our readers. Appreciation for their time and expertise goes to the following, and others who have chosen to be anonymous:

Helen Gray, LLL Leader and member of LLLI group on Infant Feeding in Emergencies. She's from the UK. She reviewed Chapter 18, Feeding in Emergencies.

Meg Harcourt, LLL Leader, special needs and Forest School teacher, and gardener. She's from the UK. She reviewed Chapter 13, Feeding a Family on a Budget.

Hiroko Hongo, co-chair of the Action, Networking, and Advocacy Committee; LLLI chair of the Infant Young Child Feeding Support Network in Japan; and member of the Infant Feeding in Emergencies Core Group. She's from Japan. She reviewed Chapter 18, Feeding in Emergencies.

Claire Inness, LLL member and scientific director. She's from the UK. She reviewed part of Chapter 18.

Kathy Kendall-Tackett, IBCLC. She has a PhD in psychology and is from the United States. She reviewed chapter 18, Postnatal Mood Disorders.

Louise Perkins, consultant midwife and specialist in tokophobia (fear of birth). She's from the UK. She reviewed Chapter 3.

Justice Reilly, LLL Leader, IBCLC, and breast surgeon. She's from the UK. She reviewed language on skin tone in Chapter 18.

Faith Wilson, RN, IBCLC, and mum of a baby who was in the NICU. She's from the United States. She reviewed pumping in chapters 14, 15, and 17.

Kerry Young, clinical psychologist and trauma specialist. She's from the UK. She reviewed birth, PTSD (Chapter 3).

Appreciation to Brigitte Sparnaaij, Jessica de Jong, and Laura Surentu for their illustrations. We are delighted to include photos submitted by mothers and parents from around the world, which reflect a range of feeding experiences. With thanks to Sophia Koutsou, the mothers of Liga de La Leche Republica Dominicana, Breea Seward, Itzul Bayardo, Anna Swisher, Nikoesi Lisane, Kim Moreau, Jennifer Hanratty, Paola Prince, Rhiannon Cooper, Justine Fieth, Pirat Aurélie, Laura Merryweather, Aylin Ebe Gaziantep, and Sandra Diosdado.

We thank Sara Weiss and Sydney Collins, our editors at Ballantine Books, for all their work. Amber Salik did a superb job as an authenticity reader, and we are very grateful for her insights. We appreciate the encouragement and support of our agent, Maura Kye-Casella of Don Congdon Associates. Warm thanks also to LLLI's agent, Stephanie Rostan of Levine, Greenberg, Rostan Literary Agency.

We are grateful for many contributors and reviewers named in the previous edition – their wisdom and expertise continue to resonate in this new book.

And finally, dear reader, we hope you will find useful ideas and strategies to help you meet your breastfeeding goals. And that you will know that, whatever your story, you are not alone, and there is a place in La Leche League for you.

From Bibiana Moreno Carranza

My deepest thanks to the greatest teachers in my life, my children, Ferran and Pol. None of what I have achieved today would have happened had it not been for your teachings. And, of course, without you, I would never have envisaged myself on this path of helping to improve the world through breastfeeding. To Mario, for always trusting me and supporting me in my madness. To my parents, whose tireless effort, support, and love made me the person I am. To my sister, for teaching me that growth comes when you step out of your comfort zone. To all my family and friends, comrades in this journey of life, infinite thanks for allowing me to share a little bit of me with you!

Undoubtedly, a big thank-you to all the people who contributed their stories, as they are the basis of this book. Also to all my LLL colleagues who accompany me on this journey of giving and contributing to a better world.

And, of course, to my dear Anna, Jayne, and Teresa, partners in this work, from whom I have learned so much that words cannot tell. Our Zoom meetings – full of stories, anecdotes, laughs, warmth, and acceptance – were real oxytocin rushes. It has been an honour to work with you.

From Jayne Joyce

La Leche League taught me how much I need other women, and that has never been truer than while writing this book. Thank you, dearest Anna, Bibiana, and Teresa – you are the best team I could have wished for. I can't wait to hug you in person.

For over twenty years, my co-Leaders have been the sisters I never had. I am continually grateful to you, and to the families of LLL Oxfordshire and LLLGB, who have taught me more about the art of breastfeeding than any book could.

Thank you to my family, for your tolerance, encouragement, distraction, and baking. I love you.

My work on this book is dedicated to the memory of my best friend, Dr. Ruth Graham (1969–2021), who first put the book in my hands, and told me I needed to find out about breastfeeding. I've never stopped.

And to the memory of Neve Tammam (2012–2023), much-loved daughter of my former co-Leader Emily and her husband, Jonathan, and sister of Maya, Orli, and Libi. Your ripples will keep on spreading.

From Teresa Pitman

First, I would like to acknowledge Stephen Douglas, who helped us find mothers in Sierra Leone who were willing to share their breastfeeding experiences. Stephen was my longtime friend and an excellent journalist and photographer.

His death in December 2023 was tragic, and it saddens me to realise that this book will be the last time we work together. You are missed, Stephen!

My baby sister, Lotus, who died of cancer in October 2022, is also deeply missed. Lotus breastfed her two children, Soren and Raven, and claimed that nursing was pretty easy for her because she had seen me and my sister breastfeeding. (She lived with me for a year, so she had lots of opportunities to see a baby at the breast!)

The support I have had from my La Leche League friends and colleagues, and from my family (which has grown to include not just my four children and their spouses but a total of ten amazing grandchildren) continues to be what keeps me going.

I am the only one of the four of us writers who worked on the previous edition, a book I was very proud to have been involved with, and it's been exciting to see the new research on birth, breastfeeding, and sleep added, as well as the stories from around the world. But for me, getting to know Anna, Jayne, and Bibi has been the biggest joy – and I love the different perspectives that each of them brings to this book. I hope you will love it, too.

From Anna Swisher

La Leche League changed my life's calling, and I am so grateful. The warmth, acceptance, and belonging given in meetings and by all the Leaders and mothers over the years have helped me to "learn a loving way of life," as one LLL book calls it. The friendships, understanding, and support can be lifelong, and make life sweeter and richer. La Leche League's loving concepts continue long after our children have grown up, and to see them passed to the next generation fills my heart with deep gratitude. The invitation to participate in the writing of this edition is still an unbelievable honour.

Heartfelt thanks and love to my family and friends, who understood that writing really is work and supported me with love, encouragement, and lots of coffee.

I am deeply grateful for the friendships that Bibiana, Teresa, Jayne, and I have developed over the past two-plus years as we worked together closely across four countries and four time zones. Our Zoom calls became our own LLL group of sorts, where we hashed out topics, shared personal joys and griefs, and collaborated on different platforms. Each of these wise, brilliant Leaders brought different skills and talents to the process, and I learned so much! We are truly sisters of the heart, and I am so thankful and humbled to have worked together.

NOTES

Chapter 1: Preparing

4. **Today, most expectant mothers choose breastfeeding**
   UNICEF. 2023. "Global Breastfeeding Scorecard 2023." www.unicef.org/media/150586/file/Global%20breastfeeding%20scorecard%202023.pdf.

5. **diabetes of any kind**
   Stuebe, A. M. 2015. "Does Breastfeeding Prevent the Metabolic Syndrome, or Does the Metabolic Syndrome Prevent Breastfeeding?" *Semin Perinatol* 39 (4): 290–95.

5. **The last few weeks of pregnancy may be a good time to learn how to express milk**
   Foudil-Bey, I., et al. 2021. "Evaluating Antenatal Breastmilk Expression Outcomes: A Scoping Review." *Int Breastfeed J* 16 (1): 25.
   Juntereal, N. A., and D. L. Spatz. 2021. "Integrative Review of Antenatal Milk Expression and Mother-Infant Outcomes During the First 2 Weeks After Birth." *J Obstet Gynecol Neonatal* 50 (6): 659–68.

6. **Just as pregnancy causes changes in your breasts and uterus**
   Hoekzema, E., et al. 2017. "Pregnancy Leads to Long-Lasting Changes in Human Brain Structure." *Nat Neurosci* 20 (2): 287–96.

7. **There is almost nothing you can do for your child in her whole life**
   Pérez-Escamilla, R., et al. 2023. "Breastfeeding: Crucially Important, but Increasingly Challenged in a Market-Driven World." *Lancet* 401 (10375): 472–85.

9. **the deaths of 823,000 babies would be prevented**
   Victora, C. G., et al. 2016. "Breastfeeding in the 21st Century: Epidemiology, Mechanisms, and Lifelong Effect." *Lancet* 387 (10017): 475–90.

9. **Formula-feeding increases the burden**
   Andresen, E. C., et al. 2022. "Environmental Impact of Feeding with Infant Formula in Comparison with Breastfeeding." *Int J Environ Res Public Health* 19 (11): 6397.

9. **A baby who is not breastfed averages several points**
   Horta, B. L., et al. 2015. "Breastfeeding and Intelligence: A Systematic Review and Meta-Analysis." *Acta Paediatr* 104 (467): 14–19.

9. **Have you seen the list of components in human milk**
Kim, S. Y., and D. Y. Yi. 2020. "Components of Human Breast Milk: From Macronutrient to Microbiome and MicroRNA." *Clin Exp Pediatr* 63 (8): 301–9.
9. **"If breastfeeding did not already exist"**
Hansen, K. 2016. "Breastfeeding: A Smart Investment in People and in Economies." *Lancet* 387 (10017): 416.
15. **"Pain is the body's way of guiding us"**
Smillie, C. 2024. Email correspondence. April 26, 2024.

Chapter 2: Connecting

22. **"I don't think one parent"**
Morrison, T. Quoted in Stadlen, N. 2020. *What Mothers Learn: Without Being Taught.* London: Piatkus.
26. **As shared nursing, wet nursing, and donor milk**
Baumgartel, K. L., et al. 2016. "From Royal Wet Nurses to Facebook: The Evolution of Breastmilk Sharing." *Breastfeed Rev* 24 (3): 25–32.
Kullmann, K. C., et al. 2022. "Human Milk Sharing in the United States: A Scoping Review." *Breastfeed Med* 17 (9): 723–35.
26. **milk is tailored to the exact age and stage of your baby**
Toscano, M., et al. 2017. "Role of the Human Breast Milk-Associated Microbiota on the Newborns' Immune System: A Mini Review." *Front Microbiol* 8: 2100.
26. **This triggers the production of targeted antibodies**
Bode, L., et al. 2014. "It's Alive: Microbes and Cells in Human Milk and Their Potential Benefits to Mother and Infant." *Advances in Nutrition* 5 (5): 571–73.
Breakey, A. A., et al. 2015. "Illness in Breastfeeding Infants Relates to Concentration of Lactoferrin and Secretory Immunoglobulin A in Mother's Milk." *Evol Med Public Health* 1: 21–31.
Lyons, K. E., et al. 2020. "Breast Milk, a Source of Beneficial Microbes and Associated Benefits for Infant Health." *Nutrients* 12 (4): 1039.
27. **The World Health Organization estimates that almost one in three women**
World Health Organization. 2021. "Violence Against Women." March 9. www.who.int/news-room/fact-sheets/detail/violence-against-women.
27. **The American College of Obstetricians and Gynecologists says that one in six**
American College of Obstetricians and Gynecologists (ACOG). 2012. "Intimate Partner Violence." February. www.acog.org/clinical/clinical-guidance/committee-opinion/articles/2012/02/intimate-partner-violence.
29. **Babywearing – carrying a baby in a sling or soft carrier**
Little, E. E., et al. 2019. "Culture, Carrying, and Communication: Beliefs and Behavior Associated with Babywearing." *Infant Behav Dev* 57: 101320.
Olsson, E., et al. 2017. "Skin-to-Skin Contact Facilitates More Equal Parenthood – A Qualitative Study from Fathers' Perspective." *J Pediatr Nurs* 34 (May–June): e2–e9.
29. **About one in five women worldwide experiences depression**
Wang, Z., et al. 2021. "Mapping Global Prevalence of Depression Among Postpartum Women." *Transl Psychiatry* 11 (1): 543.

Chapter 3: Birth!

43. **one of the best ways to improve your labour and birth experience**
Acquaye, S. N., and D. L. Spatz. 2021. "An Integrative Review: The Role of the Doula in Breastfeeding Initiation and Duration." *J Perinat Educ* 30 (1): 29–47.
Bohren, M. A., et al. 2017. "Continuous Support for Women During Childbirth." *Cochrane Database Sys Rev* no. 7. July 6. CD003766.
Ramey-Collier, K., et al. 2023. "Doula Care: A Review of Outcomes and Impact on Birth Experience." *Obstet Gynecol Surv* 78 (2): 124–27.

44. **A birth supporter can help advocate for your needs**
Horton, C., and S. Hall. 2020. "Enhanced Doula Support to Improve Pregnancy Outcomes Among African American Women with Disabilities." *J Perinat Educ* 29 (4): 188–96.
McGarry, A., et al. 2016. "How Do Women with an Intellectual Disability Experience the Support of a Doula During Their Pregnancy, Childbirth, and After the Birth of Their Child?" *J Appl Res Intellect Disabil* 29 (1): 21–33.
Ross, L. E., et al. 2006. "Service Use and Gaps in Services for Lesbian and Bisexual Women During Donor Insemination, Pregnancy, and the Postpartum Period." *J Obstet Gynaecol Can* 28 (6): 505–11.

44. **countries where there is a large gap**
Dawson, P., et al. 2022. "Social Determinants and Inequitable Maternal and Perinatal Outcomes in Aotearoa New Zealand." *Women's Health (London)* 18: 17455065221075913.
Hill, Latoya, Samantha Artiga, and Usha Ranji. 2022. "Racial Disparities in Maternal and Infant Health: Current Status and Efforts to Address Them." Kaiser Family Foundation, November 1. www.kff.org/racial-equity-and-health-policy/issue-brief/racial-disparities-in-maternal-and-infant-health-current-status-and-efforts-to-address-them.
MBRRACE-UK. 2023. "Mothers and Babies: Reducing Risk Through Audits and Confidential Enquiries Across the UK." National Perinatal Epidemiology Unit, Oxford Population Health. Updated December 14. www.npeu.ox.ac.uk/mbrrace-uk.

46. **Ten Steps to Successful Breastfeeding**
World Health Organization. 2019. "Ten Steps to Successful Breastfeeding." December 23. www.who.int/multi-media/details/ten-steps-to-successful-breastfeeding.

46. **Baby-Friendly accreditation**
World Health Organization. 2018. *Implementation Guidance: Protecting, Promoting, and Supporting Breastfeeding in Facilities Providing Maternity and Newborn Services – The Revised Baby-Friendly Hospital Initiative*. Geneva: World Health Organization.
World Health Organization. 2017. *National Implementation of the Baby-Friendly Hospital Initiative, 2017*. Geneva: World Health Organization.

47. **Many give excellent care for uncomplicated pregnancies**
Aubrey-Bassler, K., et al. 2015. "Outcomes of Deliveries by Family Physicians or Obstetricians: A Population-Based Cohort Study Using an Instrumental Variable *CMAJ* 187 (15): 1125–32.

48. **home birth is just as safe as hospital birth for low-risk**
Hutton, E. K., et al. 2019. "Perinatal or Neonatal Mortality Among Women Who Intend at the Onset of Labour to Give Birth at Home Compared to Women of Low Obstetrical Risk Who Intend to Give Birth in Hospital: A

Systematic Review and Meta-Analyses." *E Clinical Medicine* 14: 59–70.

Scarf, V. L., et al. 2018. "Maternal and Perinatal Outcomes by Planned Place of Birth Among Women with Low-Risk Pregnancies in High-Income Countries: A Systematic Review and Meta-Analysis." *Midwifery* 62: 240–55.

48. **the hospital environment is what causes**

Akyıldız, D., et al. 2021. "Effects of Obstetric Interventions During Labor on Birth Process and Newborn Health." *Florence Nightingale J Nurs* 29 (1): 9–21.

Devane, D., et al. 2017. "Cardiotocography versus Intermittent Auscultation of Fetal Heart on Admission to Labour Ward for Assessment of Fetal Wellbeing." *Cochrane Database Sys Rev* 1 (1): CD005122.

50. **birth at home, which helps**

Quigley, C., et al. 2016. "Association Between Home Birth and Breastfeeding Outcomes: A Cross-Sectional Study in 28,125 Mother-Infant Pairs from Ireland and the UK." *BMJ Open* 6 (8): e010551.

53. **Vaginal exams can increase the risk of infection**

Gluck, O., et al. 2020. "The Correlation Between the Number of Vaginal Examinations During Active Labor and Febrile Morbidity, a Retrospective Cohort Study." *BMC Pregnancy Childbirth* 20 (1): 246.

53. **It's safe for babies to be born underwater**

Burns, E., et al. 2022. "Systematic Review and Meta-Analysis to Examine Intrapartum Interventions, and Maternal and Neonatal Outcomes Following Immersion in Water During Labour and Waterbirth." *BMJ Open* 12 (7): e056517. Erratum in *BMJ Open* 2022; 12 (9): e056517corr1.

Neiman, E., et al. 2020. "Outcomes of Waterbirth in a US Hospital-Based Midwifery Practice: A Retrospective Cohort Study of Water Immersion During Labor and Birth." *J Midwifery Womens Health* 65 (2): 216–23.

54. **abundant research to support the importance of skin-to-skin**

Moore, E. R., et al. 2016. "Early Skin-to-Skin Contact for Mothers and Their Healthy Newborn Infants." *Cochrane Database Syst Rev* 11 (11): CD003519.

Widström, A. M., et al. 2019. "Skin-to-Skin Contact the First Hour After Birth, Underlying Implications and Clinical Practice." *Acta Paediatr* 108 (7): 1192–1204.

55. **helps protect you from excessive bleeding**

Ruiz, M. T., et al. 2023. "Skin-to-Skin Contact in the Third Stage of Labor and Postpartum Hemorrhage Prevention: A Scoping Review." *Matern Child Health J* 27 (4): 582–96.

56. **induction of labour**

Little, S. E. 2017. "Elective Induction of Labor: What Is the Impact?" *Obstet Gynecol Clin North Am* 44 (4): 601–14.

56. **increase the need for pain medication**

Komatsu, R., et al. 2018. "Prediction of Outliers in Pain, Analgesia Requirement, and Recovery of Function after Childbirth: A Prospective Observational Cohort Study." *Br J Anaesth* 121 (2): 417–26.

57. **risk of infection increases**

Ray, A., and S. Ray. 2014. "Antibiotics prior to Amniotomy for Reducing Infectious Morbidity in Mother and Infant." *Cochrane Database Syst Rev* (10): CD010626.

57. **can cause more breast engorgement**

Kujawa-Myles, S., et al. 2015. "Maternal Intravenous Fluids and Postpartum Breast Changes: A Pilot Observational Study." *Int Breastfeed J* 10: 18.

57. **Added fluids also increase your baby's weight**
Chantry, C. J., et al. 2011. "Excess Weight Loss in First-Born Breastfed Newborns Relates to Maternal Intrapartum Fluid Balance." *Pediatrics* 127 (1): e171–79.
Kelly, N. M., et al. 2020. "Neonatal Weight Loss and Gain Patterns in Caesarean Section Born Infants: Integrative Systematic Review." *Matern Child Nutr* 16 (2): e12914.

57. **researchers have suggested calculating the baby's weight**
Noel-Weiss, J., et al. 2011. "An Observational Study of Associations Among Maternal Fluids During Parturition, Neonatal Output, and Breastfed Newborn Weight Loss." *Int Breastfeed J* 6: 9.

57. **Sixty percent of those giving birth in the United States**
Halliday, L., et al. 2022. "Epidural Analgesia in Labor: A Narrative Review." *Int J Gynaecol Obstet* 159 (2): 356–64.

57. **babies are more likely to be in less desirable positions for birth**
Menichini, D., et al. 2022. "Fetal Head Malposition and Epidural Analgesia in Labor: A Case-Control Study." *J Matern Fetal Neonatal Med* 35 (25): 5691–96.

58. **find the breast, latch, and suck effectively**
French, C. A., et al. 2016. "Labor Epidural Analgesia and Breastfeeding: A Systematic Review." *J Hum Lact* 32 (3): 507–20.
Lee, A. I., et al. 2017. "Epidural Labor Analgesia-Fentanyl Dose and Breastfeeding Success: A Randomized Clinical Trial." *Anesthesiology* 127 (4): 614–24.

58. **especially after higher doses of anaesthetic**
Beilin, Y., et al. 2005. "Effect of Labor Epidural Analgesia with and without Fentanyl on Infant Breast-Feeding: A Prospective, Randomized, Double-Blind Study." *Anesthesiology* 103 (6): 1211–17.

58. **good amount of iron stored up if the umbilical cord**
World Health Organization. 2014. *Guideline: Delayed Umbilical Cord Clamping for Improved Maternal and Infant Health and Nutrition Outcomes.* Geneva: World Health Organization.
Zhao, Y., et al. 2019. "Effects of Delayed Cord Clamping on Infants After Neonatal Period: A Systematic Review and Meta-Analysis." *Int J Nurs Stud* 92: 97–108.

58. **The majority of the babies in some countries are born**
Haggar, F., and K. Einarsdóttir. 2021. "Trends in Cesarean Birth Rates in Iceland over a 19-Year Period." *Birth* 48 (1): 36–43.
Rudey, E. L., et al. 2020. "Cesarean Section Rates in Brazil: Trend Analysis using the Robson Classification System." *Medicine (Baltimore)* 99 (17): e19880.
World Health Organization. 2021. "Caesarean Section Rates Continue to Rise, amid Growing Inequalities in Access." June 16. www.who.int/news/item/16-06-2021-caesarean-section-rates-continue-to-rise-amid-growing-inequalities-in-access.

59. **caesarean birth may have potential long-term health effects**
Chiavarini, M., et al. 2023. "Overweight and Obesity in Adult Birth by Cesarean Section: A Systematic Review with Meta-Analysis." *J Public Health Manag Pract* 29 (2): 128–41.
Papandreou, D., et al. 2023. "Relation of Maternal Pre-Pregnancy Factors and Childhood Asthma: A Cross-Sectional Survey in Pre-School Children Aged 2–5 Years Old." *Medicina (Kaunas)* 59 (1): 179.

Sandall, J., et al. 2018. "Short-Term and Long-Term Effects of Caesarean Section on the Health of Women and Children." *Lancet* 392 (10155): 1349–57.

59. **All of us have microbes (bacteria, etc.) living**
Kennedy, K. M., et al. 2023. "Questioning the Fetal Microbiome Illustrates Pitfalls of Low-Biomass Microbial Studies." *Nature* 613 (7945): 639–49.

59. **Babies born by C-section, though, grow a gut microbiome different**
Fouhy, F., et al. 2019. "Perinatal Factors Affect the Gut Microbiota up to Four Years After Birth." *Nat Commun* 10: 1517.
Korpela, K. 2021. "Impact of Delivery Mode on Infant Gut Microbiota." *Ann Nutr Metab* 30: 1–9.
Romano-Keeler, J., and J. Sun. 2022. "The First 1000 Days: Assembly of the Neonatal Microbiome and Its Impact on Health Outcomes." *Newborn (Clarksville)* 1 (2): 219–26.

59. **swabbing the baby's mouth, nose, and skin**
Dominguez-Bello, M. G., et al. 2016. "Partial Restoration of the Microbiota of Cesarean-Born Infants via Vaginal Microbial Transfer." *Nat Med* 22 (3): 250–53.
Kelly, J. C., et al. 2021. "Vaginal Seeding After Cesarean Birth: Can We Build a Better Infant Microbiome?" *Med (NY)* 2 (8): 889–91.
Song, S. J., et al. 2021. "Naturalization of the Microbiota Developmental Trajectory of Cesarean-Born Neonates After Vaginal Seeding." *Med (NY)* 2 (8): 951–64.e5.

60. **Nurse your baby in the operating room**
Stevens, J., et al. 2014. "Immediate or Early Skin-to-Skin Contact After a Caesarean Section: A Review of the Literature." *Matern Child Nutr* 10 (4): 456–73.

61. **the temperature on each breast rises and falls**
Ludington-Hoe, S. M., et al. 2006. "Breast and Infant Temperatures with Twins During Shared Kangaroo Care." *J Obstet Gynecol Neonatal Nurs* 35 (2): 223–31.

61. **stress hormones are much higher in babies**
Ionio, C., et al. 2021. "Parent-Infant Skin-to-Skin Contact and Stress Regulation: A Systematic Review of the Literature." *Int J Environ Res Public Health* 18 (9): 4695.

61. **Skin-to-skin contact after birth helps you**
Guala, A., et al. 2017. "Skin-to-Skin Contact in Cesarean Birth and Duration of Breastfeeding: A Cohort Study." *Scientific World Journal* 2017: 1940756.
Juan, J., et al. 2022. "Association Between Skin-to-Skin Contact Duration After Caesarean Section and Breastfeeding Outcomes." *Children (Basel)* 9 (11): 1742.
Sheedy, G. M., et al. 2022. "Exploring Outcomes for Women and Neonates Having Skin-to-Skin Contact During Caesarean Birth: A Quasi-Experimental Design and Qualitative Study." *Women Birth* 35 (6): e530–e538.
Stevens, J., et al. 2019. "Skin-to-Skin Contact and What Women Want in the First Hours After a Caesarean Section." *Midwifery* 74: 140–46.

63. **the next best place for your baby**
Ayala, A., et al. 2021. "Newborn Infants Who Received Skin-to-Skin Contact with Fathers After Caesarean Sections Showed Stable Physiological Patterns." *Acta Paediatr* 110 (5): 1461–67.

66. **birth is complicated by past traumas**
Simkin, P., and P. Klaus. 2004. *When Survivors Give Birth: Understanding and Healing the Effects of Early Sexual Abuse on Childbearing Women.* Seattle: Classic Day Publishing.

67. **effective treatments for PTSD**
Bisson, J. I., and M. Olff. 2021. "Prevention and Treatment of PTSD: The Current Evidence Base." *Eur J Psychotraumatol* 12 (1): 1824381.
De Bruijn, L., et al. 2020. "Treatment of Posttraumatic Stress Disorder following Childbirth." *J Psychosom Obstet Gynaecol* 41 (1): 5–14.
Watkins, L. E., et al. 2018. "Treating PTSD: A Review of Evidence-Based Psychotherapy Interventions." *Front Behav Neurosci* 12: 258.

Chapter 4: Latching and Attaching

71. **Ideally, your baby will be in your arms**
Brimdyr, K., et al. 2018. "An Implementation Algorithm to Improve Skin-to-Skin Practice in the First Hour After Birth." *Matern Child Nutr* 14 (2): e12571.
Brimdyr, K., et al. 2020. "The Nine Stages of Skin-to-Skin: Practical Guidelines and Insights from Four Countries." *Matern Child Nutr* 16 (4): e13042.
Widström, A. M., et al. 2019. "Skin-to-Skin Contact the First Hour After Birth, Underlying Implications and Clinical Practice." *Acta Paediatr* 108 (7): 1192–1204.

73. **Leaning back and nursing baby-on-top**
Milinco, M. V., et al. 2020. "Effectiveness of Biological Nurturing on Early Breastfeeding Problems: A Randomized Controlled Trial." *Int Breastfeed J* 15 (1): 21.
Wang, Z., et al. 2021. "The Effectiveness of the Laid-Back Position on Lactation-Related Nipple Problems and Comfort: A Meta-Analysis." *BMC Pregnancy Childbirth* 21 (1): 248.

74. **Lying completely flat, face down on your body**
Association of Women's Health, Obstetric, and Neonatal Nurses. 2020. "Sudden Unexpected Postnatal Collapse in Healthy Term Newborns: AWHONN Practice Brief Number 8." *Nurs Womens Health* 24 (4): 300–302.
Ludington-Hoe, S. M., and Addison, C. 2024. "Sudden Unexpected Postnatal Collapse: Review and Management." *Neonatal Netw* 43 (2): 76–91.

92. **Your baby's bare skin against yours**
Chi Luong, K., et al. 2016. "Newly Born Low Birthweight Infants Stabilise Better in Skin-to-Skin Contact Than When Separated from Their Mothers: A Randomised Controlled Trial." *Acta Paediatr* 105 (4): 381–90.
Linnér, A., et al. 2022. "Immediate Skin-to-Skin Contact May Have Beneficial Effects on the Cardiorespiratory Stabilisation in Very Preterm Infants." *Acta Paediatr* 111 (8): 1507–14.

Chapter 5: The First Few Days: Hello Baby . . .

98. **Yes, there are very good reasons to breastfeed exclusively**
Kramer, M. S., and R. Kakuma. 2012. "Optimal Duration of Exclusive Breastfeeding." *Cochrane Database Syst Rev* 2012 (8): CD003517.
Quigley, M. A., et al. 2016. "Exclusive Breastfeeding Duration and Infant Infection." *Eur J Clin Nutr* 70 (12): 1420–27.

99. **Colostrum is the very concentrated milk**
Academy of Breastfeeding Medicine. 2017. "Clinical Protocol #3: Supplementary Feedings in the Healthy Term Breastfed Neonate, Revised 2017." *Breastfeed Med* 12: 188–98.

99. **Your milk production won't be affected**
Aumeistere, L., et al. 2019. "Impact of Maternal Diet on Human Milk Composition Among Lactating Women in Latvia." *Medicina (Kaunas)* 55 (5): 173.
Innis, S. M. 2014. "Impact of Maternal Diet on Human Milk Composition and Neurological Development of Infants." *Am J Clin Nutr* (99) 3: 734S–741S.

100. **And every baby has a unique, inborn temperament**
Planalp, E. M., and H. H. Goldsmith. 2020. "Observed Profiles of Infant Temperament: Stability, Heritability, and Associations with Parenting." *Child Dev* 91 (3): e563–e580.
Takegata, M., et al. 2021. "Prenatal and Intrapartum Factors associated with Infant Temperament: A Systematic Review." *Front Psychiatry* 12: 609020.

100. **You can't sleep**
Stremler, R., et al. 2020. "Self-Reported Sleep Quality and Actigraphic Measures of Sleep in New Mothers and the Relationship to Postpartum Depressive Symptoms." *Behav Sleep Med* 18 (3): 396–405.

101. **Swelling is usually due to normal hormonal changes**
Kujawa-Myles, S., et al. 2015. "Maternal Intravenous Fluids and Postpartum Breast Changes: A Pilot Observational Study." *Int Breastfeed J* 10: 18.

104. **Blue light, from a phone or TV screen**
Silvani, M. I., et al. 2022. "The Influence of Blue Light on Sleep, Performance, and Wellbeing in Young Adults: A Systematic Review." *Front Physiol* 13: 943108.
Tähkämö, L., et al. 2019. "Systematic Review of Light Exposure Impact on Human Circadian Rhythm." *Chronobiol Int* 36 (2): 151–70.

104. **the closest thing to magic we have**
Bigelow, A. E., and M. Power. 2020. "Mother-Infant Skin-to-Skin Contact: Short- and Long-Term Effects for Mothers and Their Children Born Full-Term." *Front Psychol* 11: 1921.
Gupta, N., et al. 2021. "Systematic Review Confirmed the Benefits of Early Skin-to-Skin Contact but Highlighted Lack of Studies on Very and Extremely Preterm Infants." *Acta Paediatr* 110 (8): 2310–15.
Moore, E. R., et al. 2016. "Early Skin-to-Skin Contact for Mothers and Their Healthy Newborn Infants." *Cochrane Database Syst Rev* 11 (11): CD003519.
Widström, A. M., et al. 2019. "Skin-to-Skin Contact the First Hour After Birth, Underlying Implications and Clinical Practice." *Acta Paediatr* 108 (7): 1192–1204.

105. **is likely to happen a little later**
Caparros-Gonzalez, R. A., et al. 2019. "Maternal and Neonatal Hair Cortisol Levels and Psychological Stress Are Associated with Onset of Secretory Activation of Human Milk Production." *Adv Neonatal Care* 19 (6): E11–E20.
Mullen, A. J., et al. 2022. "Associations of Metabolic and Obstetric Risk Parameters with Timing of Lactogenesis II." *Nutrients* 14 (4): 876.
Preusting, I., et al. 2017. "Obesity as a Predictor of Delayed Lactogenesis II." *J Hum Lact* 33 (4): 684–91.
Suwaydi, M. A., et al. 2022. "Delayed Secretory Activation and Low Milk Production in Women with Gestational Diabetes: A Case Series." *BMC Pregnancy Childbirth* 22 (1): 350.

105. **it's milk removal that tells your breasts**
Lian, W., et al. 2022. "Determinants of Delayed Onset of Lactogenesis II Among Women Who Delivered via Cesarean Section at a Tertiary

105. **Feeding fewer times than this**
Kent, J. C., et al. 2016. "Breastmilk Production in the First 4 Weeks After Birth of Term Infants." *Nutrients* 8 (12): 756.

107. **How long a baby nurses**
Dienelt, K., et al. 2020. "An Investigation into the Use of Infant Feeding Tracker Apps by Breastfeeding Mothers." *Health Informatics J* 26 (3): 1672–83.
Harris, D. L., et al. 2022. "Feeding Patterns of Healthy Term Newborns in the First 5 Days – The Glucose in Well Babies Study (GLOW)." *J Hum Lact* 38 (4): 661–69.

107. **Some babies always take two sides**
Kent, J. C., et al. 2006. "Volume and Frequency of Breastfeedings and Fat Content of Breast Milk Throughout the Day." *Pediatrics* 117 (3): e387–e395.

109. **"Enable mothers and their infants"**
World Health Organization. 2019. "Ten Steps to Successful Breastfeeding." December 23. www.who.int/multi-media/details/ten-steps-to-successful-breastfeeding.

110. **It's also riskier for a premature baby**
Baby Sleep Info Source. n.d. "SIDS and Safety." BASIS. www.basisonline.org.uk/sids-and-safety.
Moon, R. Y., et al. 2022. "Evidence Base for 2022 Updated Recommendations for a Safe Infant Sleeping Environment to Reduce the Risk of Sleep-Related Infant Deaths." *Pediatrics* 150 (1): e2022057991.

111. **"Do not provide breastfed newborns"**
World Health Organization. 2019. "Ten Steps to Successful Breastfeeding." December 23. www.who.int/multi-media/details/ten-steps-to-successful-breastfeeding.

112. **unethical marketing, misinformation, and cultural expectations**
Pérez-Escamilla, R., et al. 2023. "Breastfeeding: Crucially Important, but Increasingly Challenged in a Market-Driven World." *Lancet* 401 (10375): 472–85.
Rollins, N., et al. 2023. "Marketing of Commercial Milk Formula: A System to Capture Parents, Communities, Science, and Policy." *Lancet* 401 (10375): 486–502.

112. **babies are often given formula in hospitals for reasons**
Biggs, K. V., et al. 2018. "Formula Milk Supplementation on the Postnatal Ward: A Cross-Sectional Analytical Study." *Nutrients* 10 (5): 608.

113. **Parents . . . may ask for formula**
Doherty, T., et al. 2023. "Stemming Commercial Milk Formula Marketing: Now Is the Time for Radical Transformation to Build Resilience for Breastfeeding." *Lancet* 401 (10375): 415–18.

113. **if formula is used carefully and sparingly**
Azad, M. B., et al. 2018. "Infant Feeding and Weight Gain: Separating Breast Milk from Breastfeeding and Formula from Food." *Pediatrics* 142 (4): e20181092.
Flaherman, V. J., et al. 2019. "Effect of Early Limited Formula on Breastfeeding Duration in the First Year of Life: A Randomized Clinical Trial." *JAMA Pediatr* 173 (8): 729–35.

116. **If you had a lot of IV fluids during labour**
Chantry, C. J., et al. 2011. "Excess Weight Loss in First-Born Breastfed Newborns Relates to Maternal Intrapartum Fluid Balance." *Pediatrics* 127 (1): e171–e179.

116. **Some research has suggested that weight loss be calculated**
Noel-Weiss, J., et al. 2011. "An Observational Study of Associations Among Maternal Fluids During Parturition, Neonatal Output, and Breastfed Newborn Weight Loss." *International Breastfeed J* 6: 9.

120. **healthy human babies sleep when they need**
Galland, B. C., et al. 2012. "Normal Sleep Patterns in Infants and Children: A Systematic Review of Observational Studies." *Sleep Medicine Rev* 16 (3): 213–22.
Kent, J. C., et al. 2006. "Volume and Frequency of Breastfeedings and Fat Content of Breast Milk Throughout the Day." *Pediatrics* 117 (3): e387–e395.

121. **Swaddling has been practised in many cultures**
Dixley, A., and H. L. Ball. 2022. "The Effect of Swaddling on Infant Sleep and Arousal: A Systematic Review and Narrative Synthesis." *Front Pediatr* 10: 1000180.
Dixley, A., and H. L. Ball. 2023. "The Impact of Swaddling upon Breastfeeding: A Critical Review." *Am J Hum Biol* 35 (6): e23878.
Nelson, A. M. 2017. "Risks and Benefits of Swaddling Healthy Infants: An Integrative Review." *Am J Matern Child Nurs* 42 (4): 216–25.
Pease, A. S., et al. 2016. "Swaddling and the Risk of Sudden Infant Death Syndrome: A Meta-Analysis." *Pediatrics* 137 (6): e20153275.
Ulziibat, M., et al. 2021. "Traditional Mongolian Swaddling and Developmental Dysplasia of the Hip: A Randomized Controlled Trial." *BMC Pediatrics* 21 (1): 450.
Van Sleuwen, B. E., et al. 2007. "Swaddling: A Systematic Review." *Pediatrics* 120 (4): e1097–e1106.

122. **some level of tenderness, soreness, or pain**
Dennis, C. L., et al. 2014. "Interventions for Treating Painful Nipples Among Breastfeeding Women." *Cochrane Database Syst Rev* (12): CD007366.
Douglas, P. 2022. "Re-Thinking Lactation-Related Nipple Pain and Damage." *Women's Health (Lond)* 18: 17455057221087865.
Kent, J. C., et al. 2015. "Nipple Pain in Breastfeeding Mothers: Incidence, Causes, and Treatments." *Int J Environ Res Public Health* 12 (10): 12247–63.
Puapornpong, P., et al. 2017. "Nipple Pain Incidence, the Predisposing Factors, the Recovery Period After Care Management, and the Exclusive Breastfeeding Outcome." *Breastfeed Medicine* 12: 169–73.

124. **can't tell for sure how much milk a baby is getting**
Perrella, S. L., et al. 2020. "Estimates of Preterm Infants' Breastfeeding Transfer Volumes Are Not Reliably Accurate." *Adv Neonatal Care* 20 (5): E93–E99.

Chapter 6: Four to Fourteen Days: Milk!

136. **Rarely, babies may not poo or wee enough**
National Institute of Diabetes and Digestive and Kidney Diseases. 2013. "Urine Blockage in Newborns." NIH Publication No. 13-5630. September. www.urologic.niddk.nih.gov.

139. **The more milk removed during these early**

Geddes, D. T., et al. 2021. "25 Years of Research in Human Lactation: From Discovery to Translation." *Nutrients* 13 (9): 3071.

Huang, S. K., and M. H. Chih. 2020. "Increased Breastfeeding Frequency Enhances Milk Production and Infant Weight Gain: Correlation with the Basal Maternal Prolactin Level." *Breastfeed Med* 15 (10): 639–45.

139. **The process starts fresh for each baby**
Zuppa, A. A., et al. 1988. "Relationship Between Maternal Parity, Basal Prolactin Levels, and Neonatal Breast Milk Intake." *Biol Neonate* 53 (3): 144–47.

141. **most mothers who have given birth**
World Health Organization. 2023. "Infant and Young Child Feeding." December 20. www.who.int/news-room/fact-sheets/detail/infant-and-young-child-feeding.

141. **"Breastmilk is the ideal food"**
World Health Organization. n.d. "Breastfeeding." www.who.int/health-topics/breastfeeding#tab=tab_1.

146. **Many babies are still very wakeful**
Baby Sleep Info Source. n.d. "Normal Sleep Development." BASIS. www.basisonline.org.uk/normal-sleep-development.

149. **the taste and smell of your milk**
Lan, H. Y., et al. 2021. "Breastmilk as a Multisensory Intervention for Relieving Pain During Newborn Screening Procedures: A Randomized Control Trial." *Int J Environ Res Public Health* 18 (24): 13023.

156. **your breasts *make* only one kind of milk**
Kent, J. C., et al. 2006. "Volume and Frequency of Breastfeedings and Fat Content of Breast Milk Throughout the Day." *Pediatrics* 117 (3): e387–e395.

160. **when mothers want to breastfeed**
Jaafar, S. H., et al. 2016. "Effect of Restricted Pacifier Use in Breastfeeding Term Infants for Increasing Duration of Breastfeeding." *Cochrane Database Syst Rev* 8: CD007202.

Tolppola, O., et al. 2022. "Pacifier Use and Breastfeeding in Term and Preterm Newborns – A Systematic Review and Meta-Analysis." *Eur J Pediatr* 181 (9): 3421–28.

160. **if the baby usually uses a dummy**
Moon, R. Y., et al. 2022. "Sleep-Related Infant Deaths: Updated 2022 Recommendations for Reducing Infant Deaths in the Sleep Environment." *Pediatrics* 150 (1): e2022057990.

160. **Using a dummy can affect the development**
Schmid, K., et al. 2018. "The Effect of Pacifier Sucking on Orofacial Structures: A Systematic Literature Review." *Progress in Orthodontics* 19 (1): 8.

160. **Orthodontists and dentists tend to warn against**
American Dental Association. n.d. "Thumbsucking." MouthHealthy. www.mouthhealthy.org/all-topics-a-z/thumbsucking.

British Orthodontic Society. 2019. "Dummy and Thumb-Sucking Habits." www.bos.org.uk/wp-content/uploads/2022/03/British-Orthodontic-Society-DigitsMarch2019.pdf.

160. **overuse of dummies during the daytime may slow**
Strutt, C., et al. 2021. "Does the Duration and Frequency of Dummy (Pacifier) Use Affect the Development of Speech?" *Int J Lang Commun Disord* 56 (3): 512–27.

160. **dummy use may be linked to increased ear infections**
Niemelä, M., et al. 2000. "Pacifier as a Risk Factor for Acute Otitis Media: A Randomized, Controlled Trial of Parental Counseling." *Pediatrics* 106 (3): 483–88.

Chapter 7: Two to Six Weeks: Finding Your Way

168. **Many communities once supported new mothers**
Astbury, L. 2017. "Being Well, Looking Ill: Childbirth and the Return to Health in Seventeenth-Century England." *Soc Hist Med* 30 (3): 500–519.
171. **Some breasts simply can't store a lot of milk**
Kent, J. C., et al. 1999. "Breast Volume and Milk Production During Extended Lactation in Women." *Exp Physiol* 84 (2): 435–47.
173. **"Support mothers to recognise"**
World Health Organization. 2019. "Ten Steps to Successful Breastfeeding." December 23. www.who.int/multi-media/details/ten-steps-to-successful-breastfeeding.
174. **No one counts or times feedings**
Konner, M. 1978. "Nursing Frequency and Birth Spacing in Kung Hunter-Gatherers." *IPPF Med Bull* 15 (2): 1–3.
174. **A roly-poly, exclusively breastfed baby**
Horta, B. L., et al. 2023. "Systematic Review and Meta-Analysis of Breastfeeding and Later Overweight or Obesity Expands on Previous Study for World Health Organization." *Acta Paediatr* 112 (1): 34–41.
175. **Breastfed babies tend to grow fast in the early months**
Bell, K. A., et al. 2017. "Associations of Infant Feeding with Trajectories of Body Composition and Growth." *Am J Clin Nutr* 106106 (2): 491–98.
175. **It's easy to overfeed a baby**
Anderson, C. E., et al. 2020. "Potential Overfeeding Among Formula Fed Special Supplemental Nutrition Program for Women, Infants and Children Participants and Associated Factors." *Pediatr Obes* 15 (12): e12687.
Golen, R. B., and A. K. Ventura. 2015. "Mindless Feeding: Is Maternal Distraction During Bottle-Feeding Associated with Overfeeding?" *Appetite* 91: 385–92.
175. **"Responsive breastfeeding involves"**
The Baby Friendly Initiative. 2016. "Responsive Feeding: Supporting Close and Loving Relationships." UNICEF UK, October. www.unicef.org.uk/babyfriendly/wp-content/uploads/sites/2/2017/12/Responsive-Feeding-Infosheet-Unicef-UK-Baby-Friendly-Initiative.pdf.
176. **some books *did* advise mothers**
Hardyment, C. 2007. *Dream Babies: Childrearing Advice from John Locke to Gina Ford*. London: Frances Lincoln.
176. **starved of interaction end up**
Brauer, J., et al. 2016. "Frequency of Maternal Touch Predicts Resting Activity and Connectivity of the Developing Social Brain." *Cereb Cortex* 26 (8): 3544–52.
Maitre, N. L., et al. 2017. "The Dual Nature of Early-Life Experience on Somatosensory Processing in the Human Infant Brain." *Curr Biol* 27 (7): 1048–54.
Ulmer, Y. A., et al. 2021. "Synchronous Caregiving from Birth to Adulthood

Tunes Humans' Social Brain." *Proc Nat Acad Sci USA* 118 (14): e2012900118.

176. **"fertilizer for the brain"**
The Baby Friendly Initiative. 2023. "Building a Happy Baby: A Guide for Parents." UNICEF UK, July. www.unicef.org.uk/babyfriendly/wp-content/uploads/sites/2/2018/04/happybaby_leaflet_web.pdf.

180. **an average of 750 to 800 ml**
Kent, J. C., et al. 2006. "Volume and Frequency of Breastfeedings and Fat Content of Breast Milk Throughout the Day." *Pediatrics* 117 (3): e387–e395.

182. **hormonal contraception**
Academy of Breastfeeding Medicine. 2015. "ABM Clinical Protocol #13: Contraception During Breastfeeding, Revised 2015." *Breastfeed Med* 10 (1): 3–12.

186. **feed more like earlier preemies**
Jónsdóttir, R. B., et al. 2020. "Breastfeeding Progression in Late Preterm Infants from Birth to One Month." *Matern Child Nutr* 16 (1): e12893.
Keir, A., et al. 2022. "Breastfeeding Outcomes in Late Preterm Infants: A Multi-Centre Prospective Cohort Study." *PLoS One* 17 (8): e0272583.

190. **make babies happier and more settled**
Pérez-Escamilla, R., et al. 2023. "Breastfeeding: Crucially Important, but Increasingly Challenged in a Market-Driven World." *Lancet* 401 (10375): 472–85.

190. **not mention their known risks**
Rollins, N., et al. 2023. "Marketing of Commercial Milk Formula: A System to Capture Parents, Communities, Science, and Policy." *Lancet* 401 (10375): 486–502.

190. **He relies on caretaking adults**
Abraham, E., et al. 2016. "Network Integrity of the Parental Brain in Infancy Supports the Development of Children's Social Competencies." *Soc Cogn Affect Neurosci* 11 (11): 1707–18.

190. **The more babies are held**
Norholt, H. 2020. "Revisiting the Roots of Attachment: A Review of the Biological and Psychological Effects of Maternal Skin-to-Skin Contact and Carrying of Full-Term Infants." *Infant Behav Dev* 60: 101441.

190. **parents and others instinctively pick up, hold, and soothe**
Bornstein, M. H., et al. 2017. "Neurobiology of Culturally Common Maternal Responses to Infant Cry." *Proc Nat Acad Sci USA* 114 (45): E9465–E9473.
Zeifman, D. M., and I. St. James-Roberts. 2017. "Parenting the Crying Infant." *Current Opinion in Psychology* 15: 149–54.

191. **Relaxed, well-loved babies have the best chance**
Winston, R., and R. Chicot. 2016. "The Importance of Early Bonding on the Long-Term Mental Health and Resilience of Children." *London J Prim Care (Abingdon)* 8 (1): 12–14.

191. **adults who know how to make loving relationships**
Schmoeger, M., et al. 2018. "Maternal Bonding Behavior, Adult Intimate Relationship, and Quality of Life." *Neuropsychiatry* 32 (1): 26–32.

198. **exclusively breastfeeding mothers get the most sleep**
Doan, T., et al. 2007. "Breast-Feeding Increases Sleep Duration of New Parents." *J Perinat Neonatal Nurs* 21 (3): 200–206.
Zimmerman, D., et al. 2023. "Academy of Breastfeeding Medicine Clinical Protocol #37: Physiological Infant Care – Managing Nighttime Breastfeeding in Young Infants." *Breastfeed Med* 18 (3): 159–68.

200. **fight-or-flight response to stress**
Taylor, S. E. 2006. "Tend and Befriend: Biobehavioral Bases of Affiliation under Stress." *Curr Dir Psych Sci* 15 (6): 273–77.

Chapter 8: Six Weeks to Four Months: Hitting Your Stride

207. **your baby is probably crying less**
Wolke, D., et al. 2017. "Systematic Review and Meta-Analysis: Fussing and Crying Durations and Prevalence of Colic in Infants." *J Pediatr* 185: 55–61.e4.
208. **most babies tend to take fewer and shorter nursings**
Kent, J. C., et al. 2013. "Longitudinal Changes in Breastfeeding Patterns from 1 to 6 Months of Lactation." *Breastfeed Med* 8 (4): 401–7.
209. **very common for babies to wake more often**
Academy of Breastfeeding Medicine. 2023. "ABM Clinical Protocol #37: Physiological Infant Care-Managing Nighttime Breastfeeding in Young Infants." *Breastfeed Med* 18 (3): 159–68.
Rudzik, A.E.F., and H. L. Ball. 2021. "Biologically Normal Sleep in the Mother-Infant Dyad." *Am J Hum Biol* 33 (5): e23589.
210. **The risk of SIDS is highest between about two and four months**
Cowgill, B. 2020. "Back to the Breast: An Historical Overview of the Perceived Connections Between Sudden Infant Death Syndrome and Breastfeeding." *J Hum Lact* 36 (2): 310–17.
Jullien, S. 2021. "Sudden Infant Death Syndrome Prevention." *BMC Pediatrics* 21 (Suppl 1): 320.
Thompson, J.M.D., et al. 2017. "Duration of Breastfeeding and Risk of SIDS: An Individual Participant Data Meta-Analysis." *Pediatrics* 140 (5): e20171324.
211. **learning to coordinate the muscles required for pooing**
Kramer, E. A., et al. 2015. "Defecation Patterns in Infants: A Prospective Cohort Study." *Arch Dis Child* 100 (6): 533–36.
212. **health agencies don't recommend numbing ointments for babies**
U.S. Food and Drug Administration (FDA). 2018. "Safely Soothing Teething Pain and Sensory Needs in Babies and Older Children." May 23. www.fda.gov/consumers/consumer-updates/safely-soothing-teething-pain-and-sensory-needs-babies-and-older-children.
212. **no significant difference in the volume**
Bane, S. M. 2015. "Postpartum Exercise and Lactation." *Clin Obstet Gynecol* 58 (4): 885–92.
Campos, M.D.S.B., et al. 2021. "Position Statement on Exercise During Pregnancy and the Post-Partum Period – 2021." *Arq Bras Cardiol* 117 (1): 160–80.
214. *far* **more environmental contaminants**
Gardener, H., et al. 2019. "Lead and Cadmium Contamination in a Large Sample of United States Infant Formulas and Baby Foods." *Sci Total Environ* 651 (Pt 1): 822–27.
Lehmann, G. M., et al. 2018. "Environmental Chemicals in Breast Milk and Formula: Exposure and Risk Assessment Implications." *Environ Health Perspect* 126 (9): 96001.
Pereira, B.F.M., et al. 2020. "Occurrence, Sources, and Pathways of Chemical Contaminants in Infant Formulas." *Compr Rev Food Sci Food Saf* 19: 1378–96.

214. **Breastfeeding builds your baby's immune system**
Donald, K., et al. 2022. "Secretory IgA: Linking Microbes, Maternal Health, and Infant Health Through Human Milk." *Cell Host Microbe* 30 (5): 650–59.

215. **low vitamin D may put us at higher risk**
Academy of Breastfeeding Medicine. 2018. "ABM Clinical Protocol #29: Iron, Zinc, and Vitamin D Supplementation During Breastfeeding." *Breastfeed Med* 13 (6): 398–404. Erratum in: *Breastfeed Med* 2018; 13 (9): 639. Erratum in: *Breastfeed Med* 2020; 15 (7): 481.
Creo, A. L., et al. 2017. "Nutritional Rickets Around the World: An Update." *Paediatr Int Child Health* 37 (2): 84–98.
National Health Service. 2020. "Vitamin D." August 3. www.nhs.uk/conditions/vitamins-and-minerals/vitamin-d.
Wang, H., et al. 2017. "Vitamin D and Chronic Diseases." *Aging Dis* 8 (3): 346–53.

215. **buildup of calcium in your blood**
Marcinowska-Suchowierska, E., et al. 2018. "Vitamin D Toxicity – A Clinical Perspective." *Front Endocrinol (Lausanne)* 9: 550.

216. **five to thirty minutes of sun exposure**
Office of Dietary Supplements. 2023. "Vitamin D: Fact Sheet for Health Professionals." National Institutes of Health, September 18. https://ods.od.nih.gov/factsheets/VitaminD-HealthProfessional.

216. **If you follow a vegan diet**
Office of Dietary Supplements. 2024. "Vitamin B12 Fact Sheet for Health Professionals." National Institutes of Health, February 27. https://ods.od.nih.gov/factsheets/Vitaminb12-HealthProfessional.

217. **normal and temporary stage**
Gizlenti, S., and T. R. Ekmekci. 2014. "The Changes in the Hair Cycle During Gestation and the Post-Partum Period." *J Eur Acad Dermatol Venereol* 28 (7): 878–81.

221. **hefty portion of their calories at night**
Geddes, D. T., et al. 2021. "25 Years of Research in Human Lactation: From Discovery to Translation." *Nutrients* 13 (9): 3071.

227. **time line for re-establishing any form of sex**
Labbok, M. H. 2015. "Postpartum Sexuality and the Lactational Amenorrhea Method for Contraception." *Clin Obstet Gynecol* 58 (4): 915–27.

230. **Partners can also experience depression**
Bruno, A., et al. 2020. "When Fathers Begin to Falter: A Comprehensive Review on Paternal Perinatal Depression." *Int J Environ Res Public Health* 17 (4): 1139.
Dhillon, H. S., et al. 2022. "Paternal Depression: 'The Silent Pandemic.'" *Ind Psychiatry* 31 (2): 350–53.

231. **The World Health Organization found a pregnancy rate**
World Health Organization. 2023. "Family Planning/Contraception Methods." September 5. www.who.int/news-room/fact-sheets/detail/family-planning-contraception.

232. **oestrogen-containing hormonal contraceptives**
Bryant, A. G., et al. 2019. "The Lactational Effects of Contraceptive Hormones: An Evaluation (LECHE) Study." *Contraception* 100 (1): 48–53.
Sridhar, A., and J. Salcedo. 2017. "Optimizing Maternal and Neonatal Outcomes with Postpartum Contraception: Impact on Breastfeeding and Birth Spacing." *Matern Health Neonatol Perinatol* 3: 1.

232. **mothers also report decreased milk production**
Academy of Breastfeeding Medicine. 2015. "ABM Clinical Protocol #13: Contraception During Breastfeeding, Revised 2015." *Breastfeed Med* 10 (1): 3–12.

Chapter 9: Four to Nine Months: In the Zone

238. **Your baby is more efficient now**
Kent, J. C., et al. 2013. "Longitudinal Changes in Breastfeeding Patterns from 1 to 6 Months of Lactation." *Breastfeed Med* 8 (4): 401–7.

243. **normal and healthy for a baby this age to nurse frequently**
Barry, E. S. 2021. "Sleep Consolidation, Sleep Problems, and Co-Sleeping: Rethinking Normal Infant Sleep as Species-Typical." *J Genet Psychol* 182 (4): 183–204.
Pennestri, M. H., et al. 2020. "Sleeping Through the Night or Through the Nights?" *Sleep Med* 76: 98–103.

244. **WHO charts are based on a large group**
De Onis, M., et al. 2009. "Les standards de croissance de l'Organisation mondiale de la santé pour les nourrissons et les jeunes enfants" [WHO growth standards for infants and young children]. *Arch Pediatr* 16 (1): 47–53.

244. **starting hormonal contraception**
Academy of Breastfeeding Medicine. 2015. "ABM Clinical Protocol #13: Contraception During Breastfeeding, Revised 2015." *Breastfeed Med* 10 (1): 3–12.

246. **Many people have a built-in preference**
Montaruli, A., et al. 2021. "Biological Rhythm and Chronotype: New Perspectives in Health." *Biomolecules* 11 (4): 487.

247. **Exclusively breastfed babies can get all the fluid they need**
World Health Organization. 2023. "Infant and Young Child Feeding." December 20. www.who.int/news-room/fact-sheets/detail/infant-and-young-child-feeding.

248. **not using any topical teething medications**
U.S. Food and Drug Administration. 2018. "Safely Soothing Teething Pain and Sensory Needs in Babies and Older Children." May 23. www.fda.gov/consumers/consumer-updates/safely-soothing-teething-pain-and-sensory-needs-babies-and-older-children.

251. **Will Night Nursing Cause Tooth Decay?**
Anil, S., and P. S. Anand. 2017. "Early Childhood Caries: Prevalence, Risk Factors, and Prevention." *Front Pediatr* 5: 157.
Branger, B., et al. 2019. "Breastfeeding and Early Childhood Caries. Review of the Literature, Recommendations, and Prevention." *Arch Pediatr* 26 (8): 497–503. Erratum in *Arch Pediatr* 2020; 27 (3): 172.
Kharouba, J., et al. 2023. "Knowledge of Breastfeeding Mothers Regarding Caries Prevention in Toddlers." *Children (Basel)* 10 (1): 136.

254. **Am I Still Protected Against Pregnancy?**
Labbok, M. H., et al. 1994. "The Lactational Amenorrhea Method (LAM): A Postpartum Introductory Family Planning Method with Policy and Program Implications." *Adv Contracept* 10 (2): 93–109.
Van der Wijden, C., and C. Manion. 2015. "Lactational Amenorrhoea Method for Family Planning." *Cochrane Database Syst Rev* (10): CD001329.

Chapter 10: Nine to Eighteen Months: On the Move

264. **Your baby is still getting many of her essential nutrients**
Czosnykowska-Łukacka, M., et al. 2018. "Breast Milk Macronutrient Components in Prolonged Lactation." *Nutrients* 10 (12): 1893.
Scott, J., et al. 2016. "A Comparison by Milk Feeding Method of the Nutrient Intake of a Cohort of Australian Toddlers." *Nutrients* 8 (8): 501.

264. **Your milk is adapting to her changing needs**
Perrin, M. T., et al. 2017. "A Longitudinal Study of Human Milk Composition in the Second Year Postpartum: Implications for Human Milk Banking." *Maternal Child Nutrition* 13 (1): e12239.

265. **can negatively affect your child's health**
Guo, L., et al. 2023. "Association of Ultra-Processed Foods Consumption with Risk of Cardio-Cerebrovascular Disease: A Systematic Review and Meta-Analysis of Cohort Studies." *Nutr Metab Cardiovasc Dis* 33 (11): 2076–88.
Pagliai, G., et al. 2021. "Consumption of Ultra-Processed Foods and Health Status: A Systematic Review and Meta-Analysis." *Br J Nutr* 125 (3): 308–18.

265. **different textures, shapes, and sizes**
Westland, S., and H. Crawley. 2018. "Fruit and Vegetable Based Purées in Pouches for Infants and Young Children. First Steps Nutrition Trust." www.firststepsnutrition.org/composition-of-food-marketed-for-children-1?rq=Fruit%20and%20Vegetable%20Based%20.

265. **Formula is heavily marketed**
Rollins, N., et al. 2023. "Marketing of Commercial Milk Formula: A System to Capture Parents, Communities, Science, and Policy." *Lancet* 401 (10375): 486–502.
Romo-Palafox, M. J., et al. 2020. "Infant Formula and Toddler Milk Marketing and Caregiver's Provision to Young Children." *Maternal Child Nutrition* 16 (3): e12962.
Vilar-Compte, M., et al. 2022. "Follow-up and Growing-up Formula Promotion Among Mexican Pregnant Women and Mothers of Children under 18 Months Old." *Maternal Child Nutrition* 18 (Suppl 3): e13337.

266. ***none* of these "follow-up" or "growing up" formulas are necessary**
World Health Organization. 2017. *Guidance on Ending the Inappropriate Promotion of Foods for Infants and Young Children: Implementation Manual.* Geneva: World Health Organization.

266. **Humans in some parts of the world began taking milk**
Gerbault, P., et al. 2013. "How Long Have Adult Humans Been Consuming Milk?" *IUBMB Life* 65 (12): 983–90.

266. **most adults lose the ability to digest milk**
Storhaug, C. L., et al. 2017. "Country, Regional, and Global Estimates for Lactose Malabsorption in Adults: A Systematic Review and Meta-Analysis." *Lancet Gastroenterol Hepatol* 2 (10): 738–46.

266. **If you want to give your baby juice**
Heyman, M. B., and S. A. Abrams. 2017. "Fruit Juice in Infants, Children, and Adolescents: Current Recommendations." *Pediatrics* 139 (6): e20170967.

266. **Sweetened "fruit drinks" aimed at babies**
Fleming-Milici, F., et al. 2022. "Marketing of Sugar-Sweetened Children's Drinks and Parents' Misperceptions About Benefits for Young Children."

Maternal Child Nutrition 18 (3): e13338.
267. **World Health Organization growth charts reflect**
World Health Organization. 2022. "Infant Growth Patterns on the WHO and CDC Growth Charts." www.cdc.gov/nccdphp/dnpao/growthcharts/who/using/growth_patterns.htm.

Chapter 11: Nursing Toddlers and Beyond: Moving On

284. **the normal time frame for ending breastfeeding**
Chinique de Armas, Y., et al. 2022. "Tracking Breastfeeding and Weaning Practices in Ancient Populations by Combining Carbon, Nitrogen, and Oxygen Stable Isotopes from Multiple Non-Adult Tissues." *PloS One* 17 (2): e0262435.
Dettwyler, K. A., 2004. "When to Wean: Biological Versus Cultural Perspectives." *Clin Obstet Gynecol* 47 (3): 712–23.
285. **breastfeeding promotes normal development of the jaw and palate**
Abate, A., et al. 2020. "Relationship Between Breastfeeding and Malocclusion: A Systematic Review of the Literature." *Nutrients* 12 (12): 3688.
285. **Human milk promotes brain growth**
Brown Belfort, M. 2017. "The Science of Breastfeeding and Brain Development." *Breastfeed Med* 12 (8): 459–61.
285. **immune factors in your milk**
Czosnykowska-Łukacka, M., et al. 2020. "Changes in Human Milk Immunoglobulin Profile During Prolonged Lactation." *Front Pediatr* 8: 428.
286. **"Children should continue to be breastfed"**
Alliance for Transforming the Lives of Children. 1990. "The Innocenti Declaration." https://atlc.org/Resources/innocenti_declaration.php.

Chapter 12: Sleeping Like a Baby

304. **formula advertising plays into parents' concerns**
Rollins, N., et al. 2023. "Marketing of Commercial Milk Formula: A System to Capture Parents, Communities, Science, and Policy." *Lancet* 401 (10375): 486–502.
304. **babies around the world have behaved**
Tomori, C. 2017. "Breastsleeping in Four Cultures: Comparative Analysis of a Biocultural Body Technique." In *Breastfeeding: New Anthropological Approaches*, ed. C. Tomori, A.E.L. Palmquist, and E. A. Quinn, 55–68. Abingdon, England, and New York: Routledge.
305. **What's Normal for Babies When It Comes to Sleep?**
Galland, B. C., et al. 2014. "Children's Sleep Patterns from 0 to 9 Years: Australian Population Longitudinal Study." *Arch Dis Child* 99 (2): 119–25.
Galland, B. C., et al. 2012. "Normal Sleep Patterns in Infants and Children: A Systematic Review of Observational Studies." *Sleep Med Rev* 16 (3): 213–22.
306. **his heart rate, breathing, and temperature are less stable**
Moore, E. R., et al. 2016. "Early Skin-to-Skin Contact for Mothers and Their Healthy Newborn Infants." *Cochrane Database Syst Rev* 11 (11): CD003519.

306. **His stress level increases**
Middlemiss, W., et al. 2012. "Asynchrony of Mother-Infant Hypothalamic-Pituitary-Adrenal Axis Activity following Extinction of Infant Crying Responses Induced During the Transition to Sleep." *Early Hum Dev* 88 (4): 227–32.

308. **loving interaction with caregivers is vital**
Baddock, S. A., et al. 2019. "The Influence of Bed-Sharing on Infant Physiology, Breastfeeding, and Behaviour: A Systematic Review." *Sleep Med Rev* 43: 106–17.
Bigelow, A. E., and L. R. Williams. 2020. "To Have and to Hold: Effects of Physical Contact on Infants and Their Caregivers." *Infant Behav Dev* 61: 101494.
Ilyka, D., et al. 2021. "Infant Social Interactions and Brain Development: A Systematic Review." *Neurosci Biobehav Rev* 130: 448–69.

309. **Your milk varies in composition**
Italianer, M. F., et al. 2020. "Circadian Variation in Human Milk Composition, A Systematic Review." *Nutrients* 12 (8): 2328.
Qin, Y., et al. 2019. "Variations in Melatonin Levels in Preterm and Term Human Breast Milk During the First Month After Delivery." *Sci Rep* 9 (1): 17984.

309. **If you sleep with your baby**
Ball, H. L., et al. 2016. "Bed-Sharing by Breastfeeding Mothers: Who Bed-Shares and What Is the Relationship with Breastfeeding Duration?" *Acta Paediatr* 105 (6): 628–34.
Bovbjerg, M. L., et al. 2018. "Women Who Bedshare More Frequently at 14 Weeks Postpartum Subsequently Report Longer Durations of Breastfeeding." *J Midwifery Womens Health* 63 (4): 418–24.
Little, E. E., et al. 2018. "Mother-Infant Physical Contact Predicts Responsive Feeding Among U.S. Breastfeeding Mothers." *Nutrients* 10 (9): 1251.

309. **babies randomly assigned to sleep**
Ball, H. L., et al. 2006. "Randomised Trial of Infant Sleep Location on the Postnatal Ward." *Arch Dis Child* 91 (12): 1005–10.

309. **if you bed-share with your baby**
Doan, T., et al. 2014. "Nighttime Breastfeeding Behavior Is Associated with More Nocturnal Sleep Among First-Time Mothers at One Month Postpartum." *J Clin Sleep Med* 10 (3): 313–19.
Rudzik, A.E.F., and H. L. Ball. 2021. "Biologically Normal Sleep in the Mother-Infant Dyad." *Am J Hum Biol* 33 (5): e23589.
Srimoragot, M., et al. 2022. "Infant Feeding Type and Maternal Sleep During the Postpartum Period: A Systematic Review and Meta-Analysis." *J Sleep Res* 32 (2): e13625.

310. **It takes both of you more time to settle**
Mosko, S., et al. 1997. "Maternal Sleep and Arousals During Bedsharing with Infants." *Sleep* 20 (2): 142–50.

310. **think twice about whether sleep tracker apps**
Ball, H. L., and A. A. Keegan. 2022. "Digital Health Tools to Support Parents with Parent-Infant Sleep and Mental Well-Being." *NPJ Digit Med* 5 (1): 185.

311. **night feedings are especially important for overall milk supply**
O'Shea, K. J., et al. 2022. "The Impact of Reducing the Frequency of Night Feeding on Infant BMI." *Pediatr Res* 91 (1): 254–60.

312. **It can also trigger your period**
Labbok, M. H., et al. 1997. "Multicenter Study of the Lactational Amenorrhea Method (LAM): I. Efficacy, Duration, and Implications for Clinical Application." *Contraception* 55 (6): 327–36.

313. **Room-Sharing with Your Baby**
Carpenter, R. G., et al. 2004. "Sudden Unexplained Infant Death in 20 Regions in Europe: Case Control Study." *Lancet* 363 (9404): 185–91.

314. **Babies who are formula-fed**
Hauck, F. R., et al. 2011. "Breastfeeding and Reduced Risk of Sudden Infant Death Syndrome: A Meta-Analysis." *Pediatrics* 128 (1): 103–10.

314. **a formula-feeding mother who sleeps with her baby**
Volpe, L. E., et al. 2013. "Nighttime Parenting Strategies and Sleep-Related Risks to Infants." *Soc Sci Med* 79: 92–100.

314. **Researchers tickled both breastfed and formula-fed babies**
Horne, R. S., et al. 2004. "Comparison of Evoked Arousability in Breast and Formula Fed Infants." *Arch Dis Child* 89 (1): 22–25.

316. **families that immigrated from South Asian countries**
Ball, H. L., et al. 2012. "Infant Care Practices Related to Sudden Infant Death Syndrome in South Asian and White British Families in the UK." *Paediatr Perinat Epidemiol* 26 (1): 3–12.

316. **Non-smoking**
Mileva-Seitz, V. R., et al. 2017. "Parent-Child Bed-Sharing: The Good, the Bad, and the Burden of Evidence." *Sleep Med Rev* 32: 4–27.

316. **Being sober**
Mileva-Seitz, V. R., et al. 2017. "Parent-Child Bed-Sharing: The Good, the Bad, and the Burden of Evidence." *Sleep Med Rev* 32: 4–27.

318. **An Australian study found**
Cunningham, H. M., et al. 2018. "Bed-Sharing in the First 8 Weeks of Life: An Australian Study." *Matern Child Health J* 22 (4): 556–64.

320. **Is It Safer for My Baby to Go to Sleep with a Dummy?**
Alm, B., et al. 2016. "Breastfeeding and Dummy Use Have a Protective Effect on Sudden Infant Death Syndrome." *Acta Paediatr* 105 (1): 31–38.
Psaila, K., et al. 2017. "Infant Pacifiers for Reduction in Risk of Sudden Infant Death Syndrome." *Cochrane Database Syst Rev* 4 (4): CD011147.

324. **Some evidence suggests the mother's health**
Blum, J., et al. 2022. "Temporal Development of the Infant Oral Microbiome." *Crit Rev Microbiol* 48 (6): 730–42.

325. **Avoid the blue light**
Figueiro, M. G. 2017. "Disruption of Circadian Rhythms by Light During Day and Night." *Curr Sleep Med Rep* 3 (2): 76–84.
Fisk, A. S., et al. 2018. "Light and Cognition: Roles for Circadian Rhythms, Sleep, and Arousal." *Front Neurol* 9: 56.

325. **Phones can steal sleep**
Heo, J. Y., et al. 2017. "Effects of Smartphone Use with and without Blue Light at Night in Healthy Adults: A Randomized, Double-Blind, Cross-Over, Placebo-Controlled Comparison." *J Psychiatr Res* 87: 61–70.

328. **Get outside for at least an hour**
Bathory, E., and S. Tomopoulos. 2017. "Sleep Regulation, Physiology and Development, Sleep Duration and Patterns, and Sleep Hygiene in Infants,

Toddlers, and Preschool-Age Children." *Curr Prob Pediatric Adolescent Health Care* 47 (2): 29–42.

328. **If you're using a white noise app**
Hong, S. A., et al. 2021. "Hazardous Sound Outputs of White Noise Devices Intended for Infants." *Int J Pediatr Otorhinolaryngol* 146: 110757.

329. **a rather lengthy middle-of-the-night period of wakefulness**
Ekirch, A. R. 2016. "Segmented Sleep in Preindustrial Societies." *Sleep* 39 (3): 715–16.

330. **Sleep training can work**
Hohman, E. E., et al. 2022. "Effect of the INSIGHT Firstborn Parenting Intervention on Secondborn Sleep." *Pediatrics* 150 (1): e2021055244.

330. **babies who are sleep-trained**
Hall, W. A., et al. 2015. "A Randomized Controlled Trial of an Intervention for Infants' Behavioral Sleep Problems." *BMC Pediatrics* 15: 181.

331. **stress levels may still be high**
Middlemiss, W., et al. 2012. "Asynchrony of Mother-Infant Hypothalamic-Pituitary-Adrenal Axis Activity following Extinction of Infant Crying Responses Induced During the Transition to Sleep." *Early Hum Dev* 88 (4): 227–32.

331. **sleep training doesn't make any difference**
Cassels, T., and J. G. Rozier. 2022. "The Effectiveness of Sleep Training: Fact or Fiction?" *Clinical Lactation* 13 (2): 65–76.

331. **classic sleep training, such as cry-it-out**
D'Souza, L., and T. Cassels. 2023. "Contextual Considerations in Infant Sleep: Offering Alternative Interventions to Families." *Sleep Health* 9 (5): 618–25.

331. **adding solid foods doesn't help babies sleep more**
Messayke, S., et al. 2021. "Infant Feeding Practices and Sleep at 1 Year of Age in the Nationwide ELFE Cohort." *Matern Child Nutr* 17 (1): e13072.

331. **Starting family foods early increases**
Ong, Y. Y., et al. 2023. "Timing of Introduction of Complementary Foods, Breastfeeding, and Child Cardiometabolic Risk: A Prospective Multiethnic Asian Cohort Study." *Am J Clin Nutr* 117 (1): 83–92.
Woo Baidal, J. A., et al. 2016. "Risk Factors for Childhood Obesity in the First 1,000 Days: A Systematic Review." *Am J Prev Med* 50 (6): 761–79.

Chapter 13: Beginning Family Foods

337. **Doctors sought solutions to this man-made problem**
Rollins, N., et al. 2023. "Marketing of Commercial Milk Formula: A System to Capture Parents, Communities, Science, and Policy." *Lancet* 401 (10375): 486–502.
Baker, P., et al. 2023. "The Political Economy of Infant and Young Child Feeding: Confronting Corporate Power, Overcoming Structural Barriers, and Accelerating Progress." *Lancet* 401 (10375): 503–24.

338. **early introduction of solids**
Rippey, P.L.F., et al. 2020. "Health Impacts of Early Complementary Food Introduction Between Formula-Fed and Breastfed Infants." *J Pediatr Gastroenterol Nutr* 70 (3): 375–80.

338. **"Infants should be exclusively breastfed"**
World Health Organization. 2023. "Exclusive Breastfeeding for Optimal

Growth, Development, and Health of Infants." August 9. www.who.int
/tools/elena/interventions/exclusive-breastfeeding.

338. **Maybe you're wondering**
Messayke, S., et al. 2021. "Infant Feeding Practices and Sleep at 1 Year of Age in the Nationwide ELFE Cohort." *Matern Child Nutr* 17 (1): e13072.

339. **your time frame may be different**
Baldassarre, M. E., et al. 2022. "Complementary Feeding in Preterm Infants: A Position Paper by Italian Neonatal, Paediatric, and Paediatric Gastroenterology Joint Societies." *Ital J Pediatr* 48 (1): 143.
Gómez-Martín, M., et al. 2021. "Longitudinal Study Depicting Differences in Complementary Feeding and Anthropometric Parameters in Late Preterm Infants up to 2 Years of Age." *Nutrients* 13 (3): 982.

342. **formula-fed babies don't accept**
Forestell, C., et al. 2017. "Flavor Perception and Preference Development in Human Infants." *Ann Nutr Metab* 70 (Suppl 3): 17–25.
Krebs, N. F., et al. 2023. "Infant Factors That Impact the Ecology of Human Milk Secretion and Composition – A Report from 'Breastmilk Ecology: Genesis of Infant Nutrition (BEGIN)' Working Group 3." *Am J Clin Nutr* 117 (Suppl 1): S43–S60.

343. **Researchers compared breastfed babies**
Disantis, K. I., et al. 2011. "Do Infants Fed Directly from the Breast Have Improved Appetite Regulation and Slower Growth During Early Childhood Compared with Infants Fed from a Bottle?" *Int J Behav Nutr Phys Act* 8: 89.
Li, R., et al. 2012. "Risk of Bottle-Feeding for Rapid Weight Gain During the First Year of Life." *Archives of Pediatrics and Adolescent Medicine* 166 (5): 431–36.

345. **Servings may be tiny**
Robinson, D. T. 2021. "Big Steps for Advising the Smallest Bites: Dietary Guidelines for Americans Address Feeding Infants and Toddlers." *J Perinatol* 41 (5): 926–27.
Roess, A. A., et al. 2018. "Food Consumption Patterns of Infants and Toddlers: Findings from the Feeding Infants and Toddlers Study (FITS) 2016." *J Nutr* 148 (Suppl 3): 1525S–1535S.

347. **you can assume it's ultraprocessed**
Monteiro, C. A., et al. 2019. "Ultra-Processed Foods: What They Are and How to Identify Them." *Public Health Nutr* 22 (5): 936–41.

347. **all kinds of health problems**
Pagliai, G., et al. 2021. "Consumption of Ultra-Processed Foods and Health Status: A Systematic Review and Meta-Analysis." *Br J Nutr* 125 (3): 308–18.
Wang, Z., et al. 2024. "Consumption of Ultra-Processed Foods and Multiple Health Outcomes: An Umbrella Study of Meta-Analyses." *Food Chem* 434: 137460.

350. **only 1 to 3 percent of the world's population**
Andrén Aronsson, C., et al. 2019. "Association of Gluten Intake During the First 5 Years of Life with Incidence of Celiac Disease Autoimmunity and Celiac Disease Among Children at Increased Risk." *JAMA* 322 (6): 514–23.
Martín-Masot, R., et al. 2020. "The Role of Early Programming and Early Nutrition on the Development and Progression of Celiac Disease: A Review." *Nutrients* 12 (11): 3427.

351. **early and late introduction of allergenic foods**
Comberiati, P., et al. 2019. "Prevention of Food Allergy: The Significance of Early Introduction." *Medicina (Kaunas)* 55 (7): 323.

De Silva, D., et al. 2020. "Preventing Food Allergy in Infancy and Childhood: Systematic Review of Randomised Controlled Trials." *Pediatr Allergy Immunol* 31 (7): 813–26.

Domínguez, O., et al. 2020. "Relationship Between Atopic Dermatitis and Food Allergy." *Curr Pediatr Rev* 16 (2): 115–22.

Ferraro, V., et al. 2019. "Timing of Food Introduction and the Risk of Food Allergy." *Nutrients* 11 (5): 1131.

Fleischer, D. M., et al. 2021. "A Consensus Approach to the Primary Prevention of Food Allergy Through Nutrition: Guidance from the American Academy of Allergy, Asthma, and Immunology; American College of Allergy, Asthma, and Immunology; and the Canadian Society for Allergy and Clinical Immunology." *J J Allergy Clin Immunol Pract* 9 (1): 22–43.e4.

Halken, S., et al. 2021. "EAACI Guideline: Preventing the Development of Food Allergy in Infants and Young Children (2020 Update)." *Pediatr Allergy Immunol* 32 (5): 843–58.

Heine, R. G. 2018. "Food Allergy Prevention and Treatment by Targeted Nutrition." *Ann Nutr Metab* 72 (Suppl 3): 33–45.

Järvinen, K. M., et al. 2019. "Immunomodulatory Effects of Breast Milk on Food Allergy." *Ann Allergy Asthma Immunol* 123 (2): 133–43.

Krawiec, M., et al. 2021. "Overview of Oral Tolerance Induction for Prevention of Food Allergy – Where Are We Now?" *Allergy* 76 (9): 2684–98.

Sampath, V., et al. 2021. "Food Allergy Across the Globe." *J Allergy Clin Immunol* 148 (6): 1347–64.

354. **The Power of Family Meals**

Frankel, L. A., et al. 2018. "The Relationship Between Structure-Related Food Parenting Practices and Children's Heightened Levels of Self-Regulation in Eating." *Child Obes* 14 (2): 81–88.

Hammons, A. J., and B. H. Fiese. 2011. "Is Frequency of Shared Family Meals Related to the Nutritional Health of Children and Adolescents?" *Pediatrics* 127 (6): e1565–e1574.

Harrison, M. E., et al. 2015. "Systematic Review of the Effects of Family Meal Frequency on Psychosocial Outcomes in Youth." *Canadian Family Physician/Médecin de famille canadien* 61 (2): e96–e106.

354. **Individual differences may also be important**

Lelakowska, G., et al. 2019. "Toddlers' Impulsivity, Inhibitory Control, and Maternal Eating-Related Supervision in Relation to Toddler Body Mass Index: Direct and Interactive Effects." *Appetite* 142: 104343.

355. **If you have any choices for caregivers**

McIsaac, J. D., et al. 2022. "Responsive Feeding Environments in Childcare Settings: A Scoping Review of the Factors Influencing Implementation and Sustainability." *Int J Environ Res Public Health* 19 (19): 11870.

355 **Cow's milk can cause tiny amounts of bleeding**

Ehrlich, J. M., et al. 2022. "The Effect of Consumption of Animal Milk Compared to Infant Formula for Non-Breastfed/Mixed-Fed Infants 6-11 Months of Age: A Systematic Review and Meta-Analysis." *Nutrients* 14 (3): 488.

356. **be cautious about ultraprocessed foods**

Lustig, R. H. 2020. "Ultraprocessed Food: Addictive, Toxic, and Ready for Regulation." *Nutrients* 12 (11): 3401.

Moreira, P. R., et al. 2022. "Complementary Feeding Methods and Introduction of Ultra-Processed Foods: A Randomized Clinical Trial." *Front Nutr* 9: 1043400.

Chapter 14: When You're Away from Your Baby

363. **having a longer leave *after* birth enables longer breastfeeding**
De Lauzon-Guillain, B., et al. 2019. "Maternity or Parental Leave and Breastfeeding Duration: Results from the ELFE Cohort." *Matern Child Nutr* 15 (4): e12872.
Navarro-Rosenblatt, D., and M. L. Garmendia. 2018. "Maternity Leave and Its Impact on Breastfeeding: A Review of the Literature." *Breastfeed Med* 13 (9): 589–97.

363. **those who start their leave a few weeks *before* birth are less likely**
Kwegyir-Afful, E. 2018. "Maternity Leave Duration and Adverse Pregnancy Outcomes: An International Country-Level Comparison." *Scand J Public Health* 46 (8): 798–804.

364. **thrive best in a home setting**
Im, Y., and T. J. Vanderweele. 2018. "Role of First-Year Maternal Employment and Paternal Involvement in Behavioral and Cognitive Development of Young Children." *Infant Ment Health J* 39 (4): 449–65.
Sluiter, R.M.V., et al. 2023. "Comparing Center-Based with Home-Based Child Care: Type of Care Moderates the Association Between Process Quality and Child Functioning." *Early Childhood Res Quart* 62: 102–14.
Stein, A., et al. 2013. "The Influence of Different Forms of Early Childcare on Children's Emotional and Behavioural Development at School Entry." *Child Care Health Dev* 39 (5): 676–87.

365. **not all settings of the same type are equal**
Vermeer, H. J., et al. 2016. "Quality of Child Care Using the Environment Rating Scales: A Meta-Analysis of International Studies." *Int J Early Childhood* 48: 33–60.

365. **The outcomes for babies who spend a few hours in nursery**
Gialamas, A., et al. 2015. "Time Spent in Different Types of Childcare and Children's Development at School Entry: An Australian Longitudinal Study." *Arch Dis Child* 100 (3): 226–32.
Huston, A. C., et al. 2015. "Time Spent in Child Care: How and Why Does It Affect Social Development?" *Develop Psych* 51 (5): 621–34.

365. **raised levels of the stress hormone cortisol**
Lumian, D. S., et al. 2016. "The Impact of Program Structure on Cortisol Patterning in Children Attending Out-of-Home Child Care." *Early Childhood Res Quart* 34: 92–103.
Vermeer, H. J., and M. G. Groeneveld. 2017. "Children's Physiological Responses to Childcare." *Curr Opin Psychol*: 201–6.

365. **Higher levels of behaviour problems**
Baker, M., et al. 2019. "The Long-Run Impacts of a Universal Child Care Program." *Amer Econ J: Econ Pol* 11 (3): 1–26.
Vandell, D. L., et al. 2021. "From Early Care and Education to Adult Problem Behaviors: A Prevention Pathway Through After-School Organized Activities." *Dev Psychopathol* 33 (2): 658–69.

365. **Long-term studies show increased risk of overweight in children**
Costa, S., et al. 2020. "Associations of Childcare Type, Age at Start, and Intensity with Body Mass Index Trajectories from 10 to 42 Years of Age in the 1970 British Cohort Study." *Pediatr Obes* 15 (9): e12644.

366. **importance of good early care**

HM Government (UK). 2021. *The Best Start for Life: A Vision for the 1,001 Critical Days: The Early Years Healthy Development Review Report.* March. https://assets.publishing.service.gov.uk/government/uploads/system/uploads/attachment_data/file/973085/Early_Years_Report.pdf.

366. **"Breastfeeding is work. It takes time, effort and skill,"**
Baker, P. Quoted in World Health Organization. 2023. "Launch of the 2023 Lancet Series on Breastfeeding." Video recording. www.who.int/news-room/events/detail/2023/02/08/default-calendar/launch-of-the-2023-lancet-series-on-breastfeeding – including-the-influence-of-commercial-milk-formula-marketing.

367. **how children cope with separation**
Belsky, J., et al. 2022. "Differential Susceptibility 2.0: Are the Same Children Affected by Different Experiences and Exposures?" *Develop Psychopathology* 34 (3): 1025–33.

379. **fewer days off work to care for a sick child**
Abdulwadud, O. A., and M. E. Snow. 2012. "Interventions in the Workplace to Support Breastfeeding for Women in Employment." *Cochrane Database Syst Rev* 10 (10): CD006177.

379. **the interest of the organisation**
Morris, L., et al. 2019. "How Companies Can Support Breastfeeding Employees." *Harvard Bus Rev.* April 30. www.hbr.org.
Whitley, M. D., et al. 2019. "Workplace Breastfeeding Support and Job Satisfaction Among Working Mothers in the United States." *Am J Ind Med* 62 (8): 716–26.

383. **Health professionals recommend that all babies**
Bably, M. B., et al. 2022. "Age of Bottle Cessation and BMI-for-Age Percentile Among Children Aged Thirty-Six Months Participating in WIC." *Child Obes* 18 (3): 197–205.

386. **peak milk intake is usually reached**
Geddes, D. T., et al. 2021. "25 Years of Research in Human Lactation: From Discovery to Translation." *Nutrients* 13 (9): 3071.

Chapter 15: Milk to Go

399. **How much you get now *doesn't* predict**
Moorhead, A. M., et al. 2022. "'Is There Any Point in Me Doing This?': Views and Experiences of Women in the Diabetes and Antenatal Milk Expressing (DAME) Trial." *Matern Child Nutr* 18 (2): e13307.

400. **your milk is a living fluid**
Fogleman, A. D., et al. 2018. "Storage of Unfed and Leftover Mothers' Own Milk." *Breastfeed Med* 13 (1): 42–49.

413. **What to Store Milk In**
Academy of Breastfeeding Medicine. 2017. "ABM Clinical Protocol #8: Human Milk Storage Information for Home Use for Full-Term Infants, Revised 2017." *Breastfeed Med* 12 (7): 390–95. Erratum in: *Breastfeed Med* 2018; 13 (6): 459.
Johnson, M. C., et al. 2019. "Nutritional Impact of Storage Containers on Macronutrient Integrity of Breastmilk." *J Breastfeed Biol* 1 (1): 29–37.
Trasande, L., et al. 2018. "Food Additives and Child Health." *Pediatrics* 142 (2): e20181410.

416. **Storage of Fresh Human Milk for Healthy Full-Term Babies**

Lactation Education Accreditation and Approval Review Committee (LEAARC). 2022. *Core Curriculum for Interdisciplinary Lactation Care, 2nd edition.* Burlington, Mass.: Jones & Bartlett Learning.

Mohrbacher, N. 2020. *Breastfeeding Answers: A Guide for Helping Families, 2nd edition.* Nancy Mohrbacher Solutions, Inc.

418. **milk that smells soapy**
Lawrence, R. A., and Lawrence, R. M. 2022. *Breastfeeding: A Guide for the Medical Profession, 9th edition.* Philadelphia: Elsevier.

419. **Real-World Milk Handling**
Scott, H., et al. 2020. "Expressed Breastmilk Handling and Storage Guidelines Available to Mothers in the Community: A Scoping Review." *Women Birth* 33 (5): 426–32.

Chapter 16: Everybody Weans

424. **most common weaning age**
Sellen, D. 2001. "Comparison of Infant Feeding Patterns Reported for Nonindustrial Populations with Current Recommendations." *J Nutrition* 131 (10): 2707–15.

Tsutaya, T., and M. Yoneda. 2013. "Quantitative Reconstruction of Weaning Ages in Archaeological Human Populations Using Bone Collagen Nitrogen Isotope Ratios and Approximate Bayesian Computation." *PLoS One* 8 (8): e72327. Erratum in: *PLoS One* 2015; 10 (3): e0119778.

424. **nursing often disappears from public view**
Brockway, M., and L. Venturato. 2016. "Breastfeeding Beyond Infancy: A Concept Analysis." *J Adv Nurs* 72 (9): 2003–15.

425. **recommend breastfeeding for *at least* two years**
World Health Organization. 2023. "Exclusive Breastfeeding for Optimal Growth, Development, and Health of Infants." August 9. www.who.int/tools/elena/interventions/exclusive-breastfeeding.

425. ***less* secure and independent**
Oddy, W. H., et al. 2010. "The Long-Term Effects of Breastfeeding on Child and Adolescent Mental Health: A Pregnancy Cohort Study Followed for 14 Years." *J Pediatr* 156 (4): 568–74.

Villar, J., et al. 2020. "Late Weaning and Maternal Closeness, Associated with Advanced Motor and Visual Maturation, Reinforce Autonomy in Healthy, 2-Year-Old Children." *Sci Rep* 10 (1): 5251.

Weaver, J. M., et al. 2018. "Breastfeeding Duration Predicts Greater Maternal Sensitivity over the Next Decade." *Dev Psychol* 54 (2): 220–27.

427. **Nursing calms us, too**
Ohmura, N., et al. 2023. "Maternal Physiological Calming Responses to Infant Suckling at the Breast." *J Physiol Sci* 73 (1): 3.

427. **Illnesses tend to be milder**
Frank, N. M., et al. 2019. "The Relationship Between Breastfeeding and Reported Respiratory and Gastrointestinal Infection Rates in Young Children." *BMC Pediatrics* 19 (1): 339.

428. **Breastfeeding helps protect us**
Del Ciampo, L. A., and I.R.L. Del Ciampo. 2018. "Breastfeeding and the Benefits

of Lactation for Women's Health. Aleitamento materno e seus benefícios para a saúde da mulher." *Rev Bras Ginecol Obstet* 40 (6): 354–59.

Pérez-Escamilla, R., et al. 2023. "Breastfeeding: Crucially Important, but Increasingly Challenged in a Market-Driven World." *Lancet* 401 (10375): 472–85.

431. **Nursing, when it's going well**
Yuen, M., et al. 2022. "The Effects of Breastfeeding on Maternal Mental Health: A Systematic Review." *J Womens Health (Larchmt)* 31 (6): 787–807.

433. **nipple tenderness or pain in early pregnancy**
Flower, H. 2019. *Adventures in Tandem Nursing: Breastfeeding During Pregnancy and Beyond*, 2nd edition. CreateSpace Independent Publishing Platform.

434. **necessary to wean to maintain a pregnancy**
López-Fernández, G., et al. 2017. "Breastfeeding During Pregnancy: A Systematic Review." *Women Birth* 30 (6): e292–e300.

435. **pregnancies are very closely spaced**
Molitoris, J. 2019. "Breast-Feeding During Pregnancy and the Risk of Miscarriage." *Perspect Sex Reprod Health* 51 (3): 153–63.

436. **a good two years for a woman's body**
World Health Organization. 2007. *Report of a WHO Technical Consultation on Birth Spacing, Geneva, Switzerland, 13–15 June 2005*. Geneva: World Health Organization.

445. **single spoonful of your own milk**
Mane, S., et al. 2022. "Study of Stem Cells in Human Milk." *Cureus* 14 (3): e23701.
Witkowska-Zimny, M., and E. Kaminska-El-Hassan. 2017. "Cells of Human Breast Milk." *Cell Mol Biol Lett* J22: 11.

446. **"Breastmilk is the ideal food"**
World Health Organization. n.d. "Breastfeeding." www.who.int/health-topics/breastfeeding#tab=tab_1.

446. **"Over 820,000 children's lives"**
World Health Organization. 2023. "Infant and Young Child Feeding." December 20. www.who.int/news-room/fact-sheets/detail/infant-and-young-child-feeding.

457. **experienced depression or anxiety before**
Ystrom, E. 2012. "Breastfeeding Cessation and Symptoms of Anxiety and Depression: A Longitudinal Cohort Study." *BMC Pregnancy Childbirth* 12: 36.

Chapter 17: Alternate Routes

463. **"mechanics" of feeding are different**
Cudziło, D., et al. 2018. "Infant and Baby Feeding and the Development of the Maxillofacial Complex Based on Own Observations and the Literature." *Dev Period Med* 22 (3): 255–59.

463. **immune system "messages" pass between baby and breast**
Camacho-Morales, A., et al. 2021. "Breastfeeding Contributes to Physiological Immune Programming in the Newborn." *Front Pediatr* 9: 744104.

466. **babies are warmer, calmer, and more stable**
Pados, B. F., and F. Hess. 2020. "Systematic Review of the Effects of Skin-to-Skin

Care on Short-Term Physiologic Stress Outcomes in Preterm Infants in the Neonatal Intensive Care Unit." *Adv Neonatal Care* 20 (1): 48–58.

466. **evidence that babies do best in Kangaroo Care**
Lode-Kolz, K., et al. 2023. "Immediate Skin-to-Skin Contact After Birth Ensures Stable Thermoregulation in Very Preterm Infants in High-Resource Settings." *Acta Paediatr* 112 (5): 934–41.
Narciso, L. M., et al. 2022. "The Effectiveness of Kangaroo Mother Care in Hospitalization Period of Preterm and Low Birth Weight Infants: Systematic Review and Meta-Analysis." *J Pediatr (Rio J)* 98 (2): 117–25.
WHO Immediate KMC Study Group. 2021. "Immediate 'Kangaroo Mother Care' and Survival of Infants with Low Birth Weight." *N Engl J Med* 384 (21): 2028–38.

468. **your milk will be different from milk produced**
Caba-Flores, M. D., et al. 2022. "Breast Milk and the Importance of Chrononutrition." *Front Nutr* 9: 867507.

468. **formula, increases the risk of damage**
Altobelli, E., et al. 2020. "The Impact of Human Milk on Necrotizing Enterocolitis: A Systematic Review and Meta-Analysis." *Nutrients* 12 (5): 1322.

468. **cow-milk-based fortifiers added to their expressed milk**
Brown, J. V., et al. 2020. "Multi-Nutrient Fortification of Human Milk for Preterm Infants." *Cochrane Database Syst Rev* 6 (6): CD000343.
Thanigainathan, S., and T. Abiramalatha. 2020. "Early Fortification of Human Milk Versus Late Fortification to Promote Growth in Preterm Infants." *Cochrane Database Syst Rev* 7 (7): CD013392.

469. **Breastfeeding is *less* stressful for a preemie**
Lin, S. C. 2013. [Breast- and Bottle-Feeding in Preterm Infants: A Comparison of Behavioral Cues] *Hu Li Za Zhi* 60 (6): 27–34. Chinese.

469. **thin pieces of shaped silicone**
Meier, P. P., et al. 2000. "Nipple Shields for Preterm Infants: Effect on Milk Transfer and Duration of Breastfeeding." *J Hum Lact* 16 (2): 106–31.

488. **Milk produced by inducing lactation or relactation**
Ballard, O., and A. L. Morrow. 2013. "Human Milk Composition: Nutrients and Bioactive Factors." *Pediatr Clin North Am* 60 (1): 49–74.

489. **parents with disabilities and chronic health conditions**
Andrews, E. E., et al. 2021. "Experiences of Breastfeeding Among Disabled Women." *Women's Health Issues* 31 (1): 82–89.
Johnson, C., et al. 2022. "Supporting Women with Learning Disabilities in Infant Feeding Decisions: A Scoping Review." *Matern Child Nutr* 18 (2): e13318.
Powell, R. M., et al. 2018. "Breastfeeding Among Women with Physical Disabilities in the United States." *Journal of Human Lactation* 34 (2): 253–61.
Rosetti, L., et al. 2022. "The Availability and Quality of Breastfeeding Guidelines for Women with Spinal Cord Injury: A Narrative Review." *Spinal Cord* 60 (9): 837–42.

489. **working around spinal cord injuries**
Cowley, K. C. 2005. "Psychogenic and Pharmacologic Induction of the Let-Down Reflex Can Facilitate Breastfeeding by Tetraplegic Women: A Report of 3 Cases." *Arch Phys Med Rehabil* 86 (6): 1261–64.

490. **hormonal and metabolic shifts of pregnancy and lactation**
Desai, M. K., and R. D. Brinton. 2019. "Autoimmune Disease in Women:

Endocrine Transition and Risk Across the Lifespan." *Front Endocrinol (Lausanne)* 10: 265.

Fragoso, Y. D., et al. 2018. "Practical Evidence-Based Recommendations for Patients with Multiple Sclerosis Who Want to Have Children." *Neurol Ther* 7 (2): 207–32.

Ghiasian, M., et al. 2020. "Effect of Pregnancy and Exclusive Breastfeeding on Multiple Sclerosis Relapse Rate and Degree of Disability within Two Years After Delivery." *Clin Neurol Neurosurg* 194: 105829.

Williams, D., et al. 2019. " 'Nobody Knows, or Seems to Know How Rheumatology and Breastfeeding Works': Women's Experiences of Breastfeeding whilst Managing a Long-Term Limiting Condition – A Qualitative Visual Methods Study." *Midwifery* 78: 91–96.

490. **Many medications and treatments used for chronic conditions**
Hale, T., and K. Krutsch. 2022. *Hale's Medications and Mothers' Milk 2023: A Manual of Lactational Pharmacology*, 20th edition. New York: Springer Publishing.

496. **believe that formula is as good**
Nelson, J. M., et al. 2016. "Public Opinions About Infant Feeding in the United States." *Birth* 43 (4): 313–19.

Pereira-Kotze, C., et al. 2022. "Conflicts of Interest Are Harming Maternal and Child Health: Time for Scientific Journals to End Relationships with Manufacturers of Breast-Milk Substitutes." *BMJ Global Health* 7 (2): e008002.

496. **marketed primarily to make profits for shareholders**
Rollins, N., et al. 2023. "Marketing of Commercial Milk Formula: A System to Capture Parents, Communities, Science, and Policy." *Lancet* 401 (10375): 486–502.

Chapter 18: A–Z "Tech Support" Tool Kit

508. **Blebs (Milk Blisters)**
Academy of Breastfeeding Medicine. 2022. "ABM Clinical Protocol #36: The Mastitis Spectrum, Revised 2022." *Breastfeed Med* 17 (5): 360–76. Erratum in: *Breastfeed Med* 2022; 17 (11): 977–78.

Betts, R. C., et al. 2021. "It's Not Yeast: Retrospective Cohort Study of Lactating Women with Persistent Nipple and Breast Pain." *Breastfeed Med* 16 (4): 318–24.

Obermeyer, S., and S. Shiehzadegan. 2022. "Case Report of the Management of Milk Blebs." *J Obstet Gynecol Neonatal Nurs* 51 (1): 83–88.

509. **Breast Lumps**
Academy of Breastfeeding Medicine. 2020. "ABM Clinical Protocol #34: Breast Cancer and Breastfeeding." *Breastfeed Med* 15 (7): 429–34.

Academy of Breastfeeding Medicine. 2019. "ABM Clinical Protocol #30: Breast Masses, Breast Complaints, and Diagnostic Breast Imaging in the Lactating Woman." *Breastfeed Med* 14 (4): 208–14.

Carmichael, H., et al. 2017. "Breast Cancer Screening of Pregnant and Breastfeeding Women with BRCA Mutations." *Breast Cancer Res Treat* 162 (2): 225–30.

Expert Panel on Breast Imaging, et al. 2018. "ACR Appropriateness Criteria® Breast Imaging of Pregnant and Lactating Women." *J Am Coll Radiol* 15 (11S): S263–S275.

Tayyab, S. J., et al. 2018. "A Pictorial Review: Multimodality Imaging of Benign and Suspicious Features of Fat Necrosis in the Breast." *Br J Radiol* 91 (1092): 20180213.

510. **Breast Tissue Insufficiency (Hypoplasia/IGT)**

Burt Solorzano, C. M., and C. R. McCartney. 2010. "Obesity and the Pubertal Transition in Girls and Boys." *Reproduction* 140 (3): 399–410.

Centers for Disease Control and Prevention (CDC). 2023. "Breastfeeding and Special Circumstances." April 17. www.cdc.gov/breastfeeding/breastfeeding-special-circumstances.

Kam, R. L., et al. 2021a. "Is There an Association Between Breast Hypoplasia and Breastfeeding Outcomes? A Systematic Review." *Breastfeed Med* 16 (8): 594–602.

Kam, R. L., et al. 2021b. "Modern, Exogenous Exposures Associated with Altered Mammary Gland Development: A Systematic Review." *Early Hum Dev* 156: 105342.

Lo, A. C., et al. 2021. "Breast Hypoplasia and Decreased Lactation from Radiation Therapy in Survivors of Pediatric Malignancy: A PENTEC Comprehensive Review." *Int J Radiat Oncol Biol Phys* S0360-3016 (21)02725-5.

Thorley V. 2005. "Breast Hypoplasia and Breastfeeding: A Case History." *Breastfeed Rev* 13 (2): 13–16.

512. **Colds and Minor Illnesses**

Goldman, A. S., and S. Chheda. 2021. "The Immune System in Human Milk: A Historic Perspective." *Ann Nutr Metab* 77 (4): 189–96.

Hassiotou, F., et al. 2013. "Maternal and Infant Infections Stimulate a Rapid Leukocyte Response in Breastmilk." *Clin Transl Immunology* 2 (4): e3.

Hassiotou, F., and D. T. Geddes. 2015. "Immune Cell-Mediated Protection of the Mammary Gland and the Infant During Breastfeeding." *Adv Nutr* 6 (3): 267–75.

Ladomenou, F., et al. 2010. "Protective Effect of Exclusive Breastfeeding Against Infections During Infancy: A Prospective Study." *Arch Dis Child* 95 (12): 1004–8.

Lokossou, G.A.G., et al. 2022. "Human Breast Milk: From Food to Active Immune Response with Disease Protection in Infants and Mothers." *Front Immunol* 13: 849012.

513. **Crying and Colic**

Cabana, M. D., et al. 2021. "Newborn Daily Crying Time Duration." *J Pediatr Nurs* 56: 35–37.

Etherton, H., et al. 2016. "Discussion of Extinction-Based Behavioral Sleep Interventions for Young Children and Reasons Why Parents May Find Them Difficult." *J Clin Sleep Med* 12 (11): 1535–43.

Halpern, R., and R. Coelho. 2016. "Excessive Crying in Infants." *J Pediatr (Rio J)* 92 (3 Suppl 1): S40–S45.

Little, E. E., et al. 2018. "Mother-Infant Physical Contact Predicts Responsive Feeding Among U.S. Breastfeeding Mothers." *Nutrients* 10 (9): 1251.

Mai, T., et al. 2018. "Infantile Colic: New Insights into an Old Problem." *Gastroenterol Clin North Am* 47 (4): 829–44.

Matijasic, N., and Z. Plesa Premilovac. 2019. "Inconsolable Crying in Infants: Differential Diagnosis in the Pediatric Emergency Department." *Clin Pediatr (Phila)* 58 (2): 133–39.

Oldbury, S., and K. Adams. 2015. "The Impact of Infant Crying on the Parent-Infant Relationship." *Community Pract* 88 (3): 29–34.

Scott-Jupp, R. 2018. "Why Do Babies Cry?" *Arch Dis Child* 103 (11): 1077–79.

Wiley, M., et al. 2020. "Parents' Perceptions of Infant Crying: A Possible Path to Preventing Abusive Head Trauma." *Acad Pediatr* 20 (4): 448–54.

Wolke, D., et al. 2017. "Systematic Review and Meta-Analysis: Fussing and Crying Durations and Prevalence of Colic in Infants." *J Pediatr* 185: 55–61.e4.

515. **Diet and Weight (Yours)**

Guzmán-Mercado, E., et al. 2021. "Full Breastfeeding Modifies Anthropometric and Body Composition Indicators in Nursing Mothers." *Breastfeed Med* 16 (3): 264–71.

Hart, T. L., et al. 2022. "Nutrition Recommendations for a Healthy Pregnancy and Lactation in Women with Overweight and Obesity – Strategies for Weight Loss Before and After Pregnancy." *Fertil Steril* 118 (3): 434–46.

Karcz, K., and B. Królak-Olejnik. 2021. "Vegan or Vegetarian Diet and Breast Milk Composition – A Systematic Review." *Crit Rev Food Sci Nutr* 61 (7): 1081–98.

MacMillan Uribe, A. L., and B. H. Olson. 2019. "Exploring Healthy Eating and Exercise Behaviors Among Low-Income Breastfeeding Mothers." *J Hum Lact* 35 (1): 59–70.

McAuliffe, F. M., et al. 2020. "Management of Prepregnancy, Pregnancy, and Postpartum Obesity from the FIGO Pregnancy and Non-Communicable Diseases Committee: A FIGO (International Federation of Gynecology and Obstetrics) Guideline." *Int J Gynaecol Obstet* 151 (Suppl 1): 16–36.

Most, J., et al. 2020. "Increased Energy Intake After Pregnancy Determines Postpartum Weight Retention in Women with Obesity." *J Clin Endocrinol Metab* 105 (4): e1601–e1611.

Nnodum, B. N., et al. 2019. "Ketogenic Diet-Induced Severe Ketoacidosis in a Lactating Woman: A Case Report and Review of the Literature." *Case Rep Nephrol* 2019: 1214208.

Ringholm, L., et al. 2022. "Dietary Advice to Support Glycaemic Control and Weight Management in Women with Type 1 Diabetes During Pregnancy and Breastfeeding." *Nutrients* 14 (22): 4867.

516. **Dysphoric Milk Ejection Reflex (D-MER)**

Deif, R., et al. 2021. "Dysphoric Milk Ejection Reflex: The Psychoneurobiology of the Breastfeeding Experience." *Front Glob Womens Health* 2: 669826.

Frawley, T., and D. McGuinness. 2023. "Dysphoric Milk Ejection Reflex (D-MER) and Its Implications for Mental Health Nursing." *Int J Ment Health Nurs* 32 (2): 620–26.

Ureño, T. L., et al. 2019. "Dysphoric Milk Ejection Reflex: A Descriptive Study." *Breastfeed Med* 14 (9): 666–73.

517. **Engorgement (Full, Swollen Breasts)**

Academy of Breastfeeding Medicine. 2016. "ABM Clinical Protocol #20: Engorgement, Revised 2016." *Breastfeed Med* 11 (4): 159–63.

Academy of Breastfeeding Medicine. 2022. "ABM Clinical Protocol #36: The Mastitis Spectrum, Revised 2022." *Breastfeed Med* 17 (5): 360–76. Erratum in: *Breastfeed Med* 2022; 17 (11): 977–78.

Ozkaya, M., and O. Korukcu. 2023. "Effect of Cold Cabbage Leaf Application on Breast Engorgement and Pain in the Postpartum Period: A Systematic Review and Meta-Analysis." *Health Care Women Int* 44 (3): 328–44.

Zakarija-Grkovic, I., and F. Stewart. 2020. "Treatments for Breast Engorgement During Lactation." *Cochrane Database Syst Rev* 9 (9): CD006946.

519. **Feeding in Emergencies**

Emergency Nutrition Network. 2024. "Operational Guidance on Infant Feeding in Emergencies (OG-IFE) version 3.0." January 23. www.ennonline.net/operationalguidance-v3-2017.

Ratnayake Mudiyanselage, S., et al. 2022. "Infant and Young Child Feeding During Natural Disasters: A Systematic Integrative Literature Review." *Women Birth* 35 (6): 524–31.

522. **Hospitalisation or Surgery, Your Child's or Yours**

Academy of Breastfeeding Medicine. 2021. "ABM Clinical Protocol #35: Supporting Breastfeeding During Maternal or Child Hospitalization." *Breastfeed Med* 16 (9): 664–74. Erratum in: *Breastfeed Med* 2021; 16 (11): 928.

Demirci, J., et al. 2018. "Winging It: Maternal Perspectives and Experiences of Breastfeeding Newborns with Complex Congenital Surgical Anomalies." *J Perinatol* 38 (6): 708–17.

Elgersma, K. M., et al. 2021. "Feeding Infants with Complex Congenital Heart Disease: A Modified Delphi Survey to Examine Potential Research and Practice Gaps." *Cardiol Young* 31 (4): 577–88.

Foligno, S., et al. 2020. "Evaluation of Mother's Stress During Hospitalization Can Influence the Breastfeeding Rate. Experience in Intensive and Non Intensive Departments." *Int J Environ Res Public Health* 17 (4): 1298.

Hookway, L., et al. 2021. "The Challenges of Medically Complex Breastfed Children and Their Families: A Systematic Review." *Matern Child Nutr* 17 (4): e13182.

Salvatori, G., et al. 2018. "The Experience of Breastfeeding Infants Affected by Congenital Diaphragmatic Hernia or Esophageal Atresia." *Ital J Pediatr* 44 (1): 75.

522. **Hypoglycaemia (Low Blood Sugar in Your Baby)**

Academy of Breastfeeding Medicine. 2021. "ABM Clinical Protocol #1: Guidelines for Glucose Monitoring and Treatment of Hypoglycemia in Term and Late Preterm Neonates, Revised 2021." *Breastfeed Med* 16 (5): 353–65.

Doughty, K. N., and S. N. Taylor. 2021. "Barriers and Benefits to Breastfeeding with Gestational Diabetes." *Semin Perinatol* 45 (2): 151385.

Hubbard, E. M., and W. W. Hay Jr. 2021. "The Term Newborn: Hypoglycemia." *Clin Perinatol* 48 (3): 665–79.

Roberts, L., et al. 2023. "Oral Dextrose Gel to Prevent Hypoglycaemia in At-Risk Neonates." *Cochrane Database Syst Rev* 11 (11): CD012152.

Rozance, P. J., and J. I. Wolfsdorf. 2019. "Hypoglycemia in the Newborn." *Pediatr Clin North Am* 66 (2): 333–42.

524. **Hypothermia**

Academy of Breastfeeding Medicine. 2016. "ABM Clinical Protocol #10: Breastfeeding the Late Preterm (34–36 6/7 Weeks of Gestation) and Early Term Infants (37–38 6/7 Weeks of Gestation), Second Revision 2016." *Breastfeed Med* 11: 494–500.

Kardum, D., et al. 2022. "Duration of Skin-to-Skin Care and Rectal Temperatures in Late Preterm and Term Infants." *BMC Pregnancy Childbirth* 22 (1): 655.

Lode-Kolz, K., et al. 2023. "Immediate Skin-to-Skin Contact After Birth Ensures Stable Thermoregulation in Very Preterm Infants in High-Resource

Settings." *Acta Paediatr* 112 (5): 934–41.

524. **Jaundice, or Hyperbilirubinemia (Too Much Bilirubin)**
Academy of Breastfeeding Medicine. 2017. "ABM Clinical Protocol #22: Guidelines for Management of Jaundice in the Breastfeeding Infant 35 Weeks or More of Gestation-Revised 2017." *Breastfeed Med* 12 (5): 250–57.
Altuntaş, N. 2020. "Is There Any Effect of Hyperbilirubinemia on Breastfeeding? If Any, At Which Level?" *Breastfeed Med* 15 (1): 29–34.
Boskabadi, H., et al. 2020. "Evaluation of Maternal Risk Factors in Neonatal Hyperbilirubinemia." *Arch Iran Med* 23 (2): 128–40.
Fujiwara, R., et al. 2018. "Systemic Regulation of Bilirubin Homeostasis: Potential Benefits of Hyperbilirubinemia." *Hepatology* 67 (4): 1609–19.
Hanin, E. A., et al. 2022. "Breastfeeding and Readmission for Hyperbilirubinemia in Late Preterm and Term Infants in Beirut, Lebanon." *Indian Pediatr* 59 (3): 218–21.
Hassan, B., and M. Zakerihamidi. 2018. "The Correlation Between Frequency and Duration of Breastfeeding and the Severity of Neonatal Hyperbilirubinemia." *J Matern Fetal Neonatal Med* 31 (4): 457–63.
Mitra, S., and J. Rennie. 2017. "Neonatal Jaundice: Aetiology, Diagnosis, and Treatment." *Br J Hosp Med (Lond)* 78 (12): 699–704.
Prameela, K. K. 2019. "Breastfeeding During Breast Milk Jaundice – A Pathophysiological Perspective." *Med J Malaysia* 74 (6): 527–33.

526. **Low Milk Supply**
Farah, E., et al. 2021. "Impaired Lactation: Review of Delayed Lactogenesis and Insufficient Lactation." *J Midwifery Womens Health* 66 (5): 631–40.
Foong, S. C., et al. 2020. "Oral Galactagogues (Natural Therapies or Drugs) for Increasing Breast Milk Production in Mothers of Non-Hospitalised Term Infants." *Cochrane Database Syst Rev* 5 (5): CD011505.
Nommsen-Rivers, L. A., et al. 2022. "Measures of Maternal Metabolic Health as Predictors of Severely Low Milk Production." *Breastfeed Med* (7): 566–76.
Shen, Q., et al. 2021. "Efficacy and Safety of Domperidone and Metoclopramide in Breastfeeding: A Systematic Review and Meta-Analysis." *Breastfeed Med* 16 (7): 516–29.
Stuebe, A. M. 2015. "Does Breastfeeding Prevent the Metabolic Syndrome, or Does the Metabolic Syndrome Prevent Breastfeeding?" *Semin Perinatol* 39 (4): 290–95.
Whipps, M. D., and J. R. Demirci. 2021. "The Sleeper Effect of Perceived Insufficient Milk Supply in US Mothers." *Public Health Nutr* 24 (5): 935–41.

530. **Mastitis and Blocked Ducts**
Academy of Breastfeeding Medicine. 2022. "ABM Clinical Protocol #36: The Mastitis Spectrum, Revised 2022." *Breastfeed Med* 17 (5): 360–76. Erratum in: *Breastfeed Med* 2022; 17 (11): 977–78.
Baeza, C., et al. 2022. "Re: 'Academy of Breastfeeding Medicine Clinical Protocol #36: The Mastitis Spectrum, Revised 2022' by Mitchell et al." *Breastfeed Med* 17 (11): 970–71.
Douglas, P. 2022. "Re-Thinking Benign Inflammation of the Lactating Breast: Classification, Prevention, and Management." *Womens Health (Lond)* 18: 17455057221091349. Erratum in: *Womens Health (Lond)* 2023; 19:

17455057231157916.

Wilson, E., et al. 2020. "Incidence of and Risk Factors for Lactational Mastitis: A Systematic Review." *J Hum Lact* 36 (4): 673–86.

533. **Medications**

Allegaert, K. 2022. "Pharmacotherapy During Pregnancy, Childbirth, and Lactation." *Int J Environ Res Public Health* 19 (18): 11336.

Anderson, P. O. 2018. "Drugs in Lactation." *Pharm Res* 35 (3): 45.

Caritis, S. N., and R. Venkataramanan. 2021. "Obstetrical, Fetal, and Lactation Pharmacology – A Crisis That Can No Longer Be Ignored." *Am J Obstet Gynecol* 225 (1): 10–20.

Eyal, S. 2018. "Use of Therapeutics in Pregnancy and Lactation." *Pharm Res* 35 (5): 107.

Hale, T., and K. Krutsch. 2023. *Hale's Medications and Mothers' Milk 2023: A Manual of Lactational Pharmacology, 20th Edition*. New York: Springer Publishing Co.

Newman, M. 2018. "Drug Companies Are Incentivised to Profit Not to Improve Health, Says Report." *BMJ* 363: k4351.

Nice, F. J. 2023. *The Breastfeeding Family's Guide to Nonprescription Drugs and Everyday Products*. Washington, D.C.: Platypus Media.

Stuebe, A. 2009. "The Risks of Not Breastfeeding for Mothers and Infants." *Rev Obstet Gynecol* 2 (4): 222–31.

Verstegen, R.H.J., and S. Ito. 2019. "Drugs in Lactation." *J Obstet Gynaecol Res* 45 (3): 522–31.

535. **Milk Sharing**

Akre, J. E., et al. 2011. "Milk Sharing: From Private Practice to Public Pursuit." *Int Breastfeed J* 6: 8.

Baumgartel, K. L., et al. 2016. "From Royal Wet Nurses to Facebook: The Evolution of Breastmilk Sharing." *Breastfeed Rev* 24 (3): 25–32.

Cassar-Uhl, D., and P. Liberatos. 2018. "Use of Shared Milk Among Breastfeeding Mothers with Lactation Insufficiency." *Matern Child Nutr* 14 (Suppl 6): e12594.

Doherty, T., et al. 2022. "They Push Their Products Through Me: Health Professionals' Perspectives on and Exposure to Marketing of Commercial Milk Formula in Cape Town and Johannesburg, South Africa – A Qualitative Study." *BMJ Open* 12 (4): e055872.

Hosseini, M., et al. 2021. "Short-Term Outcomes of Launching Mother's Milk Bank in Neonatal Intensive Care Unit: A Retrospective Study." *Arch Iran Med* 24 (5): 397–404.

Jung, J., et al. 2023. "The Curious Case of Baby Formula in the United States in 2022: Cries for Urgent Action Months After Silence in the Midst of Alarm Bells." *Food Ethics* 8 (1): 4.

Kullmann, K. C., et al. 2022. "Human Milk Sharing in the United States: A Scoping Review." *Breastfeed Med* 17 (9): 723–35.

Langland, V. 2019. "Expressing Motherhood: Wet Nursing and Human Milk Banking in Brazil." *J Hum Lact* 35 (2): 354–61.

Lucas, A. 1987. "AIDS and Human Milk Bank Closures." *Lancet* 1 (8541): 1092–93.

Norsyamlina, C.A.R., et al. 2021. "A Cross-Sectional Study on the Practice of Wet Nursing Among Muslim Mothers." *BMC Pregnancy Childbirth* 21 (1): 68.

Obeng, C., et al. 2022. "Human Milk for Vulnerable Infants: Breastfeeding and

Milk Sharing Practice Among Ghanaian Women." *Intl Jnl Env Res Public Health* 19 (24): 16560.

Palmquist, A.E.L., et al. 2022. "Racial Disparities in Donor Human Milk Feedings: A Study Using Electronic Medical Records." *Health Equity* 6 (1): 798–808.

Peregoy, J. A., et al. 2022. "Human Milk-Sharing Practices and Infant-Feeding Behaviours: A Comparison of Donors and Recipients." *Matern Child Nutr* 18 (4): e13389.

Pérez-Escamilla, R., et al. 2023. "Breastfeeding: Crucially Important, but Increasingly Challenged in a Market-Driven World." *Lancet* 401 (10375): 472–85.

Pitino, M. A., et al. 2021. "The Impact of Thermal Pasteurization on Viral Load and Detectable Live Viruses in Human Milk and Other Matrices: A Rapid Review." *Appl Physiol Nutr Metab* 46 (1): 10–26.

Subudhi, S., and N. Sriraman. 2021. "Islamic Beliefs About Milk Kinship and Donor Human Milk in the United States." *Pediatrics* 147 (2): e20200441.

Wesolowska, A., et al. 2019. "Innovative Techniques of Processing Human Milk to Preserve Key Components." *Nutrients* 11 (5): 1169.

538. **Nipple Diversity**

Mimouni, G., et al. 2022. "Nipple/Areola Dimensions in Early Breastfeeding." *Breastfeed Med* 17 (6): 506–10.

Puapornpong, P., et al. 2013. "Nipple Length and Its Relation to Success in Breastfeeding." *J Med Assoc Thai* 96 (Suppl 1): S1–S4.

Thanaboonyawat, I., et al. 2013. "Pilot Study of Normal Development of Nipples During Pregnancy." *J Hum Lact* 29 (4): 480–83.

Ventura, A. K., et al. 2021. "Associations Between Variations in Breast Anatomy and Early Breastfeeding Challenges." *J Hum Lact* 37 (2): 403–13.

Wang, Z., et al. 2021. "The Effectiveness of the Laid-Back Position on Lactation-Related Nipple Problems and Comfort: A Meta-Analysis." *BMC Pregnancy Childbirth* 21 (1): 248.

540. **Nipple Shields**

Coentro, V. S., et al. 2021. "Nipple Shield Use Does Not Impact Sucking Dynamics in Breastfeeding Infants of Mothers with Nipple Pain." *Eur J Pediatr* 180 (5): 1537–43.

Chow S., et al. 2015. The Use of Nipple Shields: A Review. *Front Public Health* 3: 236.

543. **Nursing Strike (Breast Refusal)**

Jalali, F., et al. 2021. "Nursing Strikes Among Infants and Its Affecting Factors in Rafsanjan City." *J Med Life* 14 (1): 56–60.

Nayyeri, F., et al. 2015. "Frequency of 'Nursing Strike' Among 6-Month-Old Infants, at East Tehran Health Center and Contributing Factors." *J Family Reprod Health* 9 (3): 137–40.

Winchell, K. 1992. "Nursing Strike: Misunderstood Feelings." *J Hum Lact* 8 (4): 217–19.

545. **Oversupply (Too Much Milk)**

Academy of Breastfeeding Medicine. 2020. "ABM Clinical Protocol #32: Management of Hyperlactation." *Breastfeed Med* 15 (3): 129–34.

547. **Postnatal Mood Disorders (Depression, Anxiety, Obsessive-Compulsive Disorder)**

Bye, E., et al. 2022. "Parental Postpartum Depression Among Medical Residents." *Arch Womens Ment Health* 25: 1–7.

Dagnaw, F. T., et al. 2022. "Determinants of Postpartum Depression Among Mothers in Debre Tabor Town, North-Central, Ethiopia: Community-Based Unmatched Case-Control Study." *Front Glob Womens Health* 3: 910506.

Galbally, M., et al. 2023. "Rurality as a Predictor of Perinatal Mental Health and Well-Being in an Australian Cohort." *Aust J Rural Health* 31 (2): 182–95.

Howard, K., et al. 2022. "Modifiable Maternal Factors and Their Relationship to Postpartum Depression." *Int J Environ Res Public Health* 19 (19): 12393.

Lin, Y. H., et al. 2022. "Risk and Protective Factors Related to Immediate Postpartum Depression in a Baby-Friendly Hospital of Taiwan." *Taiwan J Obstet Gynecol* 61 (6): 977–83.

Mohd Shukri, N. H., et al. 2022. "The Associations of Breastfeeding and Postnatal Experiences with Postpartum Depression Among Mothers of Hospitalized Infants in Tertiary Hospitals." *Cureus* 14 (9): e29425.

Nicolás-López, M., et al. 2022. "Maternal Mental Health and Breastfeeding amidst the Covid-19 Pandemic: Cross-Sectional Study in Catalonia (Spain)." *BMC Pregnancy Childbirth* 22 (1): 733.

Strahm, A. M., et al. 2022. "Repetitive Negative Thinking During Pregnancy and Postpartum: Associations with Mental Health, Inflammation, and Breastfeeding." *J Affect Disord* 319: 497–506.

Tucker, Z., and C. O'Malley. 2022. "Mental Health Benefits of Breastfeeding: A Literature Review." *Cureus* 14 (9): e29199.

Van Sieleghem, S., et al. 2022. "Childbirth Related PTSD and Its Association with Infant Outcome: A Systematic Review." *Early Hum Dev* 174: 105667.

Wang, Z., et al. 2021. "Mapping Global Prevalence of Depression Among Postpartum Women." *Transl Psychiatry* 11: 543.

551. **Reflux**

Curien-Chotard, M., and P. Jantchou. 2020. "Natural History of Gastroesophageal Reflux in Infancy: New Data from a Prospective Cohort." *BMC Pediatr* 20 (1): 152.

Djeddi, D., et al. 2018. "Effects of Smoking Exposure in Infants on Gastroesophageal Reflux as a Function of the Sleep-Wakefulness State." *J Pediatr* 201: 147–53.

Kim, S. 2017. "Gastroesophageal Reflux in Neurologically Impaired Children: What Are the Risk Factors?" *Gut Liver* 11 (2): 232–36.

Li, A., and H. Bhurawala. 2021. "Pyloric Stenosis in an Infant." *Aust J Gen Pract* 50 (10): 744–46.

Loots, C., et al. 2014. "Body Positioning and Medical Therapy for Infantile Gastroesophageal Reflux Symptoms." *J Pediatr Gastroenterol Nutr* 59 (2): 237–43.

Michalak, Z., et al. 2022. "Does Feeding Modification Strategies Help Improve Reflux Symptoms in NICU Infants?" *J Perinatol* 42 (2): 286–88.

Rosen, R., et al. 2018. "Pediatric Gastroesophageal Reflux Clinical Practice Guidelines: Joint Recommendations of the North American Society for Pediatric Gastroenterology, Hepatology, and Nutrition and the European Society for Pediatric Gastroenterology, Hepatology, and Nutrition." *J Pediatr Gastroenterol Nutr* 66 (3): 516–54.

Tighe, M. P., et al. 2023. "Pharmacological Treatment of Gastro-Oesophageal

Reflux in Children." *Cochrane Database Syst Rev* 8 (8): CD008550.

553. **Sore Nipples**
American College of Obstetricians and Gynecologists (ACOG). 2021. "Breastfeeding Challenges: ACOG Committee Opinion Summary, Number 820." *Gynecol Obstet* 137 (2): 394–95.
Amir, L. H., et al. 2021. "Identifying the Cause of Breast and Nipple Pain During Lactation." *BMJ* 374: n1628.
Betts, R. C., et al. 2021. "It's Not Yeast: Retrospective Cohort Study of Lactating Women with Persistent Nipple and Breast Pain." *Breastfeed Med* 16 (4): 318–24.
Coca, K. P., et al. 2019. "Measurement Tools and Intensity of Nipple Pain Among Women with or without Damaged Nipples: A Quantitative Systematic Review." *J Adv Nurs* 75 (6): 1162–72.
Coentro, V. S., et al. 2021. "Impact of Nipple Shield Use on Milk Transfer and Maternal Nipple Pain." *Breastfeed Med* 16 (3): 222–29.
Cornejo-Del Río, E., et al. 2022. "Preventing Nipple Pain/Trauma in Breastfeeding Women: A Best Practice Implementation Project at the Marqués de Valdecilla University Hospital (Spain)." *JBI Evid Implement* 20 (4): 374–84.
Dennis, C. L., et al. 2014. "Interventions for Treating Painful Nipples Among Breastfeeding Women." *Cochrane Database Syst Rev* 12: CD007366.
Douglas, P. 2022. "Re-Thinking Lactation-Related Nipple Pain and Damage." *Womens Health (Lond)* 18: 17455057221087865.
Gianni, M. L., et al. 2019. "Breastfeeding Difficulties and Risk for Early Breastfeeding Cessation." *Nutrients* 11 (10): 2266.
Jackson, K. T., et al. 2019. "Moving Toward a Better Understanding of the Experience and Measurement of Breastfeeding-Related Pain." *J Psychosom Obstet Gynaecol* 40 (4): 318–25.
Jiménez Gómez, M. I., et al. 2021. "Prevalence of Nipple Soreness at 48 Hours Postpartum." *Breastfeed Med* 16 (4): 325–31.
Laageide, L., et al. 2021. "Postpartum Nipple Symptoms: Risk Factors and Dermatologic Characterization." *Breastfeed Med* 16 (3): 215–21.
Marrazzu, A., et al. 2015. "Evaluation of the Effectiveness of a Silver-Impregnated Medical Cap for Topical Treatment of Nipple Fissure of Breastfeeding Mothers." *Breastfeed Med* 10 (5): 232–38.
Nakamura, M., et al. 2018. "Nipple Skin Trauma in Breastfeeding Women During Postpartum Week One." *Breastfeed Med* 13 (7): 479–84.
Niazi, A., et al. 2018. "A Systematic Review on Prevention and Treatment of Nipple Pain and Fissure: Are They Curable?" *J Pharmacopuncture* 21 (3): 139–50.
Wang, Z., et al. 2021. "The Effectiveness of the Laid-Back Position on Lactation-Related Nipple Problems and Comfort: A Meta-Analysis." *BMC Pregnancy Childbirth* 221 (1): 248.

556. **Supplementing (Giving Extra Milk)**
Academy of Breastfeeding Medicine. 2017. "ABM Clinical Protocol #3: Supplementary Feedings in the Healthy Term Breastfed Neonate, Revised 2017." *Breastfeed Med* 12: 188–98.
Allen, E., et al. 2021. "Avoidance of Bottles During the Establishment of Breastfeeds in Preterm Infants." *Cochrane Database Syst Rev* 10: CD005252.
Azad, M. B., et al. 2018. "Infant Feeding and Weight Gain: Separating Breast Milk from Breastfeeding and Formula from Food." *Pediatrics* 142 (4): e20181092.

Biggs, K. V., et al. 2018. "Formula Milk Supplementation on the Postnatal Ward: A Cross-Sectional Analytical Study." *Nutrients* 10 (5): 608.

Cheung, K. Y., et al. 2023. "Health and Nutrition Claims for Infant Formula: International Cross Sectional Survey." *BMJ Clinical Research* 380: e071075.

Mildon, A., et al. 2022. "High Levels of Breastmilk Feeding Despite a Low Rate of Exclusive Breastfeeding for 6 Months in a Cohort of Vulnerable Women in Toronto, Canada." *Matern Child Nutr* 18 (1): e13260.

Park, J., et al. 2018. "Systematic Review: What Is the Evidence for the Side-Lying Position for Feeding Preterm Infants?" *Adv Neonatal Care* 18 (4): 285–94.

Raczyńska, A., and E. Gulczyńska. 2019. "The Impact of Positioning on Bottle-Feeding in Preterm Infants (≤34 GA). A Comparative Study of the Semi-Elevated and the Side-Lying Position – A Pilot Study." *Dev Period Med* 23 (2): 117–24.

World Health Organization. 2017. *Guidance on Ending the Inappropriate Promotion of Foods for Infants and Young Children: Implementation Manual.* Geneva: World Health Organization.

562. **Tongue-Tie**

Bruney, T. L., et al. 2022. "Systematic Review of the Evidence for Resolution of Common Breastfeeding Problems-Ankyloglossia (Tongue Tie)." *Acta Paediatr* 111 (5): 940–47.

Cordray, H., et al. 2023. "Severity and Prevalence of Ankyloglossia-Associated Breastfeeding Symptoms: A Systematic Review and Meta-Analysis." *Acta Paediatr* 112 (3): 347–57.

Cruz, P. V., et al. 2022. "Prevalence of Ankyloglossia According to Different Assessment Tools: A Meta-Analysis." *J Am Dent Assoc* 153 (11): 1026–40.e31.

Kelly, Z., and C. J. Yang. 2022. "Ankyloglossia." *Pediatr Rev* 43 (8): 473–75.

Talmor, G., and C. L. Caloway. "Ankyloglossia and Tethered Oral Tissue: An Evidence-Based Review." *Pediatr Clin North Am* 69 (2): 235–45.

563. **Vasospasm**

Anderson, J. E., et al. 2004. "Raynaud's Phenomenon of the Nipple: A Treatable Cause of Painful Breastfeeding." *Pediatrics* 113 (4): e360–e364.

Betts, R. C., et al. 2021. "It's Not Yeast: Retrospective Cohort Study of Lactating Women with Persistent Nipple and Breast Pain." *Breastfeed Med* 16 (4): 318–24.

Buck, M. L., et al. 2014. "Nipple Pain, Damage, and Vasospasm in the First 8 Weeks Postpartum." *Breastfeed Med* 9 (2): 56–62.

Douglas, P. 2022. "Re-Thinking Lactation-Related Nipple Pain and Damage." *Womens Health (Lond)* 18: 17455057221087865.

Kent, J. C., et al. 2015. "Nipple Pain in Breastfeeding Mothers: Incidence, Causes, and Treatments." *Int J Environ Res Public Health* 12 (10): 12247–63.

Perrella, S. L., et al. 2015. "Case Report of Nipple Shield Trauma Associated with Breastfeeding an Infant with High Intra-Oral Vacuum." *BMC Pregnancy Childbirth* 15: 155.

Rosin, S. I. 2019. "A Case Study of Biological Nurturing." *J Hum Lact* 35 (2): 318–22.

National Institute of Arthritis and Musculoskeletal and Skin Diseases (NIAMS). "Raynaud's Phenomenon." U.S. Department of Health and Human Services (USDHHS), May 2021. www.niams.nih.gov/health-topics/raynauds-phenomenon.

Wu, M., et al. 2012. "Raynaud's Phenomenon of the Nipple." *Obstet Gynecol* 119 (2 Pt 2): 447–49.

565. **Weight Gain Worries**
Appleton, J., et al. 2018. "Infant Formula Feeding Practices Associated with Rapid Weight Gain: A Systematic Review." *Matern Child Nutr* 14 (3): e12602.
Askari, M., et al. 2020. "Ultra-Processed Food and the Risk of Overweight and Obesity: A Systematic Review and Meta-Analysis of Observational Studies." *Int J Obes (Lond)* 44 (10): 2080–91.
Azad, M. B., et al. 2018. "Infant Feeding and Weight Gain: Separating Breast Milk from Breastfeeding and Formula from Food." *Pediatrics* 142 (4): e20181092.
Brown, J.V.E., et al. 2019. "Formula versus Maternal Breast Milk for Feeding Preterm or Low Birth Weight Infants." *Cochrane Database Syst Rev* 8 (8): CD002972.
Galloway, C., and J. Howells. 2015. "Harnessing Breastmilk Composition to Improve a Preterm Infant's Growth Rate – A Case Study." *Breastfeed Rev* 23 (1): 17–21.
Gomez, M. S., et al. 2020. "Baby-Led Weaning, An Overview of the New Approach to Food Introduction: Integrative Literature Review." *Rev Paul Pediatr* 38: e2018084.
Gribble, K., et al. 2017. "Volume Marker Inaccuracies: A Cross-Sectional Survey of Infant Feeding Bottles." *Matern Child Nutr* 13 (3): e12388.
Hails, K. A., et al. 2021. "Breastfeeding and Responsive Parenting as Predictors of Infant Weight Change in the First Year." *J Pediatr Psychol* 46 (7): 768–78.
Horta, B. L., et al. 2015. "Long-Term Consequences of Breastfeeding on Cholesterol, Obesity, Systolic Blood Pressure and Type 2 Diabetes: A Systematic Review and Meta-Analysis." *Acta Paediatr* 104 (467): 30–37.
Huang, S. K., and M. H. Chih. 2020. "Increased Breastfeeding Frequency Enhances Milk Production and Infant Weight Gain: Correlation with the Basal Maternal Prolactin Level." *Breastfeed Med* 15 (10): 639–45.
Isganaitis, E., et al. 2019. "Maternal Obesity and the Human Milk Metabolome: Associations with Infant Body Composition and Postnatal Weight Gain." *Am J Clin Nutr* 110 (1): 111–20.
Kramer, M. S., and R. Kakuma. 2012. "Optimal Duration of Exclusive Breastfeeding." *Cochrane Database Syst Rev* (8): CD003517.
Larqué, E., et al. 2019. "From Conception to Infancy – Early Risk Factors for Childhood Obesity." *Nat Rev Endocrinol* 15 (8): 456–78.
Li, H. T., et al. 2013. "The Impact of Cesarean Section on Offspring Overweight and Obesity: A Systematic Review and Meta-Analysis." *Int J Obes* 37: 893–99.
Ortega-García, J. A., et al. 2018. "Full Breastfeeding and Obesity in Children: A Prospective Study from Birth to 6 Years." *Child Obes* 14 (5): 327–37.
Pagliai, G., et al. 2021. "Consumption of Ultra-Processed Foods and Health Status: A Systematic Review and Meta-Analysis." *Br J Nutr* 125 (3): 308–18.
Prado, E. L., and K. G. Dewey. 2014. "Nutrition and Brain Development in Early Life." *Nutr Rev* 72 (4): 267–84.
Quigley, M., et al. 2019. "Formula Versus Donor Breast Milk for Feeding Preterm or Low Birth Weight Infants." *Cochrane Database Syst Rev* 7 (7): CD002971.
Rana, R., et al. 2020. "Feeding Interventions for Infants with Growth Failure in the First Six Months of Life: A Systematic Review." *Nutrients* 12 (7): 2044.
Victora, C. G., et al. 2016. "Breastfeeding in the 21st Century: Epidemiology,

Mechanisms, and Lifelong Effect." *Lancet* 387 (10017): 475–90.

Westland, S., and H. Crawley. 2018. "Fruit and Vegetable Based Purées in Pouches for Infants and Young Children. Report from First Steps Nutrition Trust (UK)." www.firststepsnutrition.org/s/Fruit__veg_pouches_report_for_web_Oct_2019.pdf.

Wood, C. T., et al. 2016. "Bottle Size and Weight Gain in Formula-Fed Infants." *Pediatrics* 138 (1): e20154538.

Wood, C. T., et al. 2021. "Effects of Breastfeeding, Formula Feeding, and Complementary Feeding on Rapid Weight Gain in the First Year of Life." *Acad Pediatr* 21 (2): 288–96.

Zhang, S., et al. 2022. "Effect of Elective Cesarean Section on Children's Obesity from Birth to Adolescence: A Systematic Review and Meta-Analysis." *Front Pediatr* 9: 793400.

570. **Yeast (Thrush/Candida Infections)**

Plachouri, K. M., et al. 2022. "Nipple Candidiasis and Painful Lactation: An Updated Overview." *Postepy Dermatol Alergol* 39 (4): 651–55.

PICTURE CREDITS

Illustrations

Laura Surentu, pages 78, 79, 84, 89, 151, 315, 401, 415, 471, 541
Brigitte Sparnaaij, pages 72, 75, 81, 83, 109, 137, 476, 477, 511, 518, 538, 562
Jessica de Jong, pages 115, 446

Photographs

We are delighted to include photos from around the world! With thanks to
    Evelina García, page xii
    Sophia Koutsou, page 2
    Jenny García, Evelina García, Marielena Fañas, Yennifer Gómez, page 20
    Breea Seward, page 38
    Anna Swisher, page 70
    Itzul Bayardo, pages 96, 506
    Nikoesi Lisane, page 130
    Kim Moreau, page 166
    Jennifer Hanratty, page 204
    Paola Prince, page 236
    Alisha Jobe, page 262
    Elsa and Winy, page 282
    Rhiannon Cooper, page 302
    Justine Fieth, page 336
    Pirat Aurélie, page 360
    Laura Merryweather, page 396
    Aylin Ebe Gaziantep, page 422
    Sandra Diosdado, page 460
    Leaders of La Leche League Greece, page 572

INDEX

A

abscesses, 530
across-the-chest hold, 81
ADHD (attention deficit hyperactivity disorder), 490, 535
adoption, 3, 6, 25, 141, 219, 269–270, 430, 436, 478, 480–482, 484–485. *See also* induced lactation; relactation
Adri, 437–438
ages and stages
  first few days, 97–128
  four to fourteen days, 131–164
  four to nine months, 237–261
  nine to eighteen months, 263–281
  six weeks to four months, 205–234
  toddlers and beyond, 283–301
  two to six weeks, 167–203
Akiko, 375
alcohol use, 316, 393
Alejandra, 446
Alexa, 225
Alexis, 441
Ali, 12, 63–64, 211
Alison, 8
allergies, food, 158, 287, 351–353
Allison, 100, 241–242, 304, 308–309, 320, 332, 379, 384, 462

Alma, 114, 425
Alquizareña, Guajirita, 39, 53, 55, 71, 98, 174, 225, 255, 256, 263, 277, 353, 389–390
alveoli, 6
Amanda, 124
American Academy of Pediatrics, 157, 315, 446
amniotic sac, 52
amount of milk. *See* quantity of milk
anaesthesia, 52
anaphylaxis/anaphylactic shock, 352–353
Andrea, 94, 171, 372
Angi, 142
animal milks, 158, 266, 355–356
Anita, 54, 87, 174, 228
Anna, 203, 288, 333–334, 341
Annabé, 194
Annalee, 87, 325
antibiotics, 533
antibodies, 214, 288, 512
antidepressants, 550
anti-inflammatory medication, 518, 531–532
anxiety, 148, 193–194, 226–227, 548
Apgar score, 44

apps
  feeding tracking, 162
  sleep tracking, 162
  support networks, 33
ASD (autism spectrum disorders), 74, 274, 298, 357, 425–426, 478
Aphrodite, 392
Asia, 185–186, 281, 310
at-breast supplementers, 220, 479, 483, 484–485, 559. *See also* supplementation
Audrey, 28, 62, 63, 190, 252–253, 329, 372, 380, 443, 444
Aurelia, 67–68, 103, 167, 203
Ausilia, 24, 364, 370, 377, 379, 383, 384, 387
autism, 74, 274, 298, 357, 425–426, 478
aversion to nursing, 270–271
Avery, 492–493

B

babbling, 207
baby blues, 102, 147, 194
baby bounce, 151
baby monitors, 320
Baby Friendly Hospital Initiative, 46
babymoon, 168
babywearing, 18, 29, 150, 220–221, 273, 448, 472, 482, 489–490
Baker, Phillip, 367
banked milk (donor milk, milk sharing), 25–27, 114, 504–505, 535–538
Barbara, 206
bariatric surgery, 5
bassinets, 306, 311, 313
baths, 29, 53–54, 65
bedding-in, 109
bed-sharing, 306, 309, 311, 314–319, 325–326

bedtime. *See* sleeping
bereavement/loss, 125–126, 501–505
Beth, 295
Betsy, 488–489
bililights, 526
Biological Nurturing. *See* laid-back breastfeeding
birth, 39–69
  caregivers, 46–48
  cutting the umbilical cord, 58, 217
  difficult and high-risk births, 63–69
  drying the baby, 61
  epidurals, 52
  first nursing, 51–54, 60
  labour and delivery, 55–60
  medical interventions, 51–54, 55–60, 90–91
  preparing for, 40–43
  settings, 48–54
  warming the baby, 54–55, 61
birth centres, 50
birth control, 182, 231–232, 244, 254
birth trauma, 65–67, 227
bisphenol-A (BPA), 413
biting, 249–251, 278–279
B.J., 56, 240–241, 258–259, 260–261, 269, 286, 294, 387, 439–440, 452
bladder issues, 100
blebs, 280, 508–509, 531
blisters, 280, 508–509, 531
blocked ducts, 530–533
bottle-feeding
  baby won't take bottle, 384–386
  frequency, 464–465
  paced bottle-feeding, 184–185, 560
  preterm/premature infants, 469–470
  side-lying bottle-feeding, 560–562
  supplementation, 559

two to six weeks, 175, 184–185, 197–198
weaning, 442
working parents, 383–386
bowel movements. *See* poo
brain growth
four to nine months, 243
six weeks to four months, 206
toddlers and beyond, 285
bras
blocked ducts, 532
exercise, 212
hands-free pumping bra, 405–406
night nursing, 324
nursing bras, 16–17
breaking suction, 107
breast augmentation surgery, 5, 491–494
breast binding (during weaning), 453, 504
breast compressions, 124, 137–138, 150
breast hypoplasia (insufficient glandular tissue), 510–512
breast lumps, 509–510
breast pads, 17, 213
breast pumps, 17, 403–404. *See also* pumping
breast reduction surgery, 491–494
breast sandwich technique, 77–78, 89
breast size and shape
engorgement, 57, 108, 517–519
induced labour, 57
insufficient glandular tissue, 142
nipple diversity, 538–540
positions for nursing, 85–86
during pregnancy, 4–5
softness, 178–179
tissue insufficiency, 510–512
breast surgeries, 5, 491–494
breast tissue insufficiency (hypoplasia), 510–512

breastfeeding (as term), xv
breathing, 79, 80
Brenda, 136–137
brick dust (urate crystals), 115, 137
Brie, 467, 469, 470, 471
burping, 159, 323
bus travel, 221

C

caffeine, 158
calcium, 215
calm/alert babies, 223
calming a baby. *See* soothing
Camilla, 117
cancer, 215
Candida, 185, 570
car travel, 218–219
caregivers. *See* childcare; doulas; healthcare providers
cavities, 251, 323–324, 454
Cecily, 268, 284, 313, 326, 333, 440, 451–452, 457
Centers for Disease Control, 512–513
cervical dilation, 52
caesarean sections, 58–60, 61–63, 85, 101–102
chestfeeding, xiv–xv
Chetana, 436, 480–481, 482, 483, 484
child visitation, 441–442
childbirth. *See* birth
childcare, 363–371
adjustment, 387–389
milk storage, 368
milk supply, 369–371
sensitive babies, 225–226
choking risks, 344–345, 350
Chris, 198
Christina, 41, 50, 177–178, 280, 427, 428

Christine, 311, 312
chronic conditions and illnesses, 490–491
chronotypes, 246
Cindy, 56
circumcision, 149
Claire, 206
Clare, 32, 40, 42, 43, 50, 86, 102, 131, 132, 177, 178–179, 191, 199, 200, 228–229, 299–300, 393, 427, 440
Claudia, 98–99
cleft lip or palate, 499
clothing, 16–17, 196, 324–325, 383
cluster feeding, 174
clutch hold, 81–82, 477
coeliac disease, 350–351
cold compresses, 519, 532
colds, 443, 512–513
colic, 152, 513–514
colic hold, 151, 552
colour of milk, 416
colostrum, 5–6, 91, 92, 99, 139, 399–400, 487–488
Colson, Suzanne, 73
communication skills. *See* feeding signals/cues
  babbling, 207
  building trust, 201–203
  conversational nursing, 176, 207, 238–239, 375
  touching, 240
community, 31–33
co-mothers, 31, 35, 56, 146–147, 162, 202, 258–259, 260–261, 269, 372, 435. *See also* co-nursing; partners
constipation, 101, 116, 210–211
consumer-grade pumps, 403–404
contraception, 182, 231–232, 244, 254
contractions, 52, 99

co-nursing, 26, 30, 31, 146–147, 202, 372, 435, 488
conversational nursing, 176, 207, 238–239, 375
cortisol levels, 365
co-sleeping, 109, 306, 311, 313–314, 453
cow milk, 158, 266, 355–356
cradle hold, 80
crawling, 271
cream, 416
cribs, 306, 311, 312
criticism, 257–261, 280–281, 439–441
cross-cradle hold, 81
crying, 152, 190–192, 513–514
cups, 250, 559
Cyndel, 31, 147, 202, 372, 435

D

dairy products, 158
dads, 21, 26, 28, 30, 45, 63, 67, 132, 190, 193, 198, 202, 257, 303, 327, 329, 385, 406, 486, 491–492, 548. *See also* partners
Dan, 303
Dawn, 49, 223, 471
daycare. *See* childcare
Deaf/deaf, 45
delayed milk release, 184
Denise, 101–102, 182–183
dental problems. *See* teeth
depression, 102, 146–147, 230, 547–548
detachment, 227
developmental stages. *See* ages and stages
diabetes, 5
Diane, 33, 106, 122, 289, 291, 294
  nappy changes, 324
diet and weight (of mother), 213, 515–516

difficult births, 40, 63–69
disabilities, 488–490. *See also* special needs babies; special needs toddlers
discipline, 241–242, 249–250, 278, 299–301
disease, 185, 512–513
   cancer, 215
   chronic conditions, 490–491
   coeliac disease, 350–351
   rickets, 215
distractibility, 208–209, 239–240, 244, 339–340
diversity in families, xiv–xv
donor milk, 25–27, 114, 504–505, 535–538
doulas, 25, 43–45
Down syndrome, 499
drugs. *See* medications
duration of breastfeeding, 15, 424–425
dyschezia ("grunting baby syndrome"), 211
dysphoric milk ejection reflex (D-MER), 133, 194, 516

E

ear infections, 249, 443
eating disorders, 208, 354, 511
ear piercing, 149
Ecobavila, 489
eczema, 279
electric pumps, 403
Eliana, 298
Eline, 181–182
emergency situations, 519–522
Emily, 144, 426
Emma, 68–69, 104, 438, 500
emotions. *See* baby blues
engorgement, 57, 108, 517–519
enticing baby to breast, 480–484
environmental impact of formula-feeding, 9
environmental pollutants, 213–214
epidurals, 52, 57–58
episiotomies, 84, 101–102
Esmaralda, 397
exclusive pumping, 188, 462–465
exercise, 212–213, 391–392
exhaustion, 270–271, 319–320, 327–330
expressing milk. *See* hand expression; pumping
eyedroppers, 483

F

Faith, 461
family beds, 312–313, 333
family diversity, xiv–xv
family doctors, 47
family foods. *See* solid foods
family meals, 354
fathers. *See* dads; partners
Fatmata, 63, 114, 173, 364
Fee, 499
feeding signals/cues
   calm babies, 223
   crying, 157, 223–224
   first few days, 110
   fists, 156
   four to fourteen days, 136–137, 153–154, 156–157
   rooting, 157, 464
   six weeks to four months, 208
   two to six weeks, 173–174
Fernanda, 285
fertility, 231–232, 267–268, 436–437
fertility treatment, 269, 437
finger-feeding, 92, 559
first few days, 18–19, 97–128
   cramps and bleeding, 99
   nappy changes, 114–116
   emotions/baby blues, 102–103
   feeding signals, 110

first few days (*cont.*)
   formula, 111–113
   health impacts of breastfeeding, 447
   hormones, 100
   hunger, 99
   leaking, 100
   love, 103
   meconium, 99
   nighttime, 104
   nipple pain, 107, 122–123
   nursing patterns, 104–108
   parenting instincts, 117–118
   poo and wee, 101, 114–116
   SIDS (crib death), 122
   skin-to-skin contact, 104
   sleep, 108–111
   support for breastfeeding, 106
   swaddling, 121–122
   swallowing, 123
   visitors, 100, 127
   waking the baby for feeding, 107, 120–121
   weight changes, 116–117
fists, 156
flange size, 404–405
flat nipples, 538–539
flipple, 89
fluttery sucks, 123–124
food. *See* nutrition; solid foods
food allergies, 158, 287, 351–353
football hold, 81–82
footstools, 90
forceps, 44
foremilk, 156
formula, 9–10, 11, 27, 111–113, 265–266
   contaminants, 214
   early recipes, 337–338
   environmental impact, 9
   iron, 216
   jaundice, 526
   premature infants, 468
   SIDS risks, 314–316

four to fourteen days, 131–164
   burping, 159
   dummies, 160–161
   emotions/baby blues, 146–148
   feeding signals/cues, 136–137, 153–154, 156–157
   fussiness, 140, 149–152
   gas, 158–159
   milk production, 132, 138–143, 150
   mothers' food intake, 143–144
   naps and sleep, 144–146, 149–150
   nighttime, 146, 149–150
   nursing for pain relief, 148–149
   nursing patterns, 132–135, 152–157, 162–163
   nursing schedules, 161–162
   poo and wee, 136–137
   SIDS (crib death), 160
   slings, 150
   spitting up, 159–160
   spoiling the baby, 163–164
   weight gain, 134, 154–155
four to nine months, 237–261
   activities, 256–257
   biting, 249–251
   brain growth, 243
   common questions, 242
   criticism, 257–261
   distractions, 239–240
   fidgeting, 240–242
   independence, 255–256
   liquids, 247
   milk production, 244
   naps, 245–246
   night feeding, 251
   nursing patterns, 238–243
   nursing in public, 252–253
   nursing schedules, 245
   pregnancy protection, 254
   separation anxiety, 239
   solid foods, 244, 247
   teething, 247–248

travelling, 253–254
weaning, 244–245
frequency days (growth spurts), 180–181, 206, 221, 339, 386–387
frozen milk, 414, 417
   power outages, 417–418
   stockpiling, 370
   thawing, 418
fruit juices, 266
fullness. *See* engorgement
furniture, 17
fussiness. *See* sensitive babies

G

Gabriela, 46
gagging, 344, 350
galactagogues, 469, 486, 529
galactoceles, 509–510
gas, 158–159
gastroesophageal reflux, 551–553
general practice physicians, 47
Georgie, 272, 378, 433
Ginny, 430, 485, 486
Gisel, 21, 48, 58, 175, 273, 287, 425
glass bottles, 413
Glenda, 473
Glenys, 313
going out, 198–199
   nursing in public, 195–197, 252–253
   travel, 218–220, 253–254, 392–393, 420–421
"golden hour", 71
grandparents, xv, 27, 32, 199, 257, 258, 259, 264–265, 275, 292, 294, 296, 333–334, 338, 348, 364–365, 441
gravity, 54, 73–74
growth spurts (frequency days), 180–181, 206, 221, 339, 386–387

"grunting baby syndrome" (dyschezia), 211
guilt, 494–495
gynaecologists, 48

H

hair loss, 217–218
hand expression, 5–6, 92, 398–402, 518
hands-free pumping, 403, 405–406
Hannah, 307–308, 371, 438, 490
Hansen, Keith, 9
hard palate development, 285
Haydee, 360, 457
health impact of breastfeeding, 7–9, 426–428, 446–448, 496
   immunological impact, 8–9, 214, 285, 427–428, 512–513
healthcare providers, 34–35, 194, 330
hearing impaired, 45
Heather, 433
Hedi, 398–399
Helen, 11, 195, 494
Helena, 300–301, 439
help with breastfeeding. *See* support networks
Heranush, 21, 224
high needs babies. *See* sensitive babies
hindmilk, 156
Hitomi, 111–112
holds. *See* positions for nursing
home births, 40, 49–50, 114
hormones, 6, 176, 224, 254. *See also* oxytocin
   breastfeeding, 8
   fertility, 436–437
   first few days after childbirth, 100
   induced lactation, 486–487
   pregnancy, 6
   during sex, 229

hospital births, 51–54
  bedding-in, 109
  co-sleeping, 110
  medical interventions, 55–60
  nurseries, 109
  rooming-in, 109
hospital-grade pumps, 403. *See also* consumer-grade pumps
hospitalisations, 197, 326, 393–394, 522
human milk. *See also* milk production
  antibodies, 214
  colostrum, 5–6, 91, 92, 99, 139, 487–488
  donor milk, 25–27, 114, 504–505, 535–538
  environmental pollutants, 213–214
  foremilk, 156
  fortifiers, 468
  hindmilk, 156
  induced lactation, 484–488
  iron, 216–217
  nutritional content, 266
hunger. *See* feeding signals
hydrogels, 555
hyperbilirubinemia (jaundice), 524–526
hyperlactation, 183. *See also* oversupply
hypoglycaemia (low blood sugar), 119, 522–524
hypoplasia (insufficient breast tissue), 142, 510–512
hypothermia (baby too cold), 119, 524

I

Ilana, 381
illness. *See* disease
immunizations. *See* vaccinations
immunological impact, 8–9, 214, 285, 427–428, 512–513

Imogen, 219, 220
implants, 491–494
Indigenous parents, 24, 26, 45, 72–73, 168, 190–191, 424, 468
induced labour, 56–57
induced lactation, 482, 484–488
infant death, 125–126, 501–505. *See also* miscarriage; stillbirth; sudden infant death syndrome (SIDS)
infertility, 5
information. *See* resources
instinct, 10–12, 13–14, 71–72
instrumental delivery, 44
insufficient glandular tissue (IGT) (breast hypoplasia), 142, 510–512
International Board Certified Lactation Consultants (IBCLC), 5, 34, 94, 432
International Labor Organization, 363
intrauterine device (IUD), 182, 232
inverted nipples, 539–540
IQ/intelligence, 10
iron, 216–217, 355–356
IV (intravenous) fluids, 57, 116
Ivannia, 7, 27–28, 448

J

Janedy, 170, 280, 378, 440, 450
jaundice (hyperbilirubinemia), 119, 474, 524–526
jaw development, 285
jaw room, 77
Jayne, 245–246
J.D., 319
Jeanie, 13
Jessalyn, 435
Jo, 187
Joan, 257

juice drinks, 266
Julie, 97, 171–172, 193, 224, 237

K

Kallyn, 500
Kangaroo Care, 466–467, 482
Kara, 21, 66–67
Karina, 36
Karla's son, 290
Kat, 108, 285, 293, 435–436
Kate, 237, 275–276
Keiko, 45–46
Kia, 376
Kirsten, 3, 286
Kristin, 68

L

La Leche League
   founding, xiii
   meetings, 36–37, 43
   online support, 34, 36
   as support network, 5, 10–12, 35–37, 64, 93–94, 127, 170, 187, 200–201, 243, 280–281, 328, 432–433
labour. *See also* birth
   doulas, 43–45
   epidurals, 57–58
   induced, 56–57
   medical interventions, 55–60
   movement, 53
   pushing, 53–54
   vaginal exams, 53
labour support persons. *See* doulas
lactational amenorrhea method (LAM) of contraception, 231–232, 254
lactoferrin, 216
laid-back breastfeeding, 71–72, 73–75, 145, 170, 184, 470, 474, 476, 482, 555

lanolin, 555
Lara, 30, 314
latching, 71–95
   adaptations, 84–85
   baby needs, 76–80
   breast manipulation, 77–78, 79, 80, 88–89
   difficult births, 40, 64–65
   engorged breasts, 518
   hand movements, 82
   holds and positions, 80–84
   instinct, 13–14
   laid-back breastfeeding, 170
   nipple pain, 15
   pain, 86–90
   readiness for, 90–91
   tongue-tie, 87–88
   two to six weeks, 169
late-premature and early-term babies, 473–475
Laura, 47, 119, 160–161, 274, 284, 430–431, 439, 478
Lauren, 95, 105, 143, 205
Leah, 291, 293, 369, 450, 497, 498
leaking, 100, 179, 213, 223
lesbian mums. *See* LGBTQIA+ families
letdown (milk ejection reflex, milk release), 133, 184, 267
LGBTQIA+ families, 31, 35, 45, 56, 146–147, 162, 202, 258–259, 260–261, 269, 372, 435. *See also* trans/transgender parents
Lieke, 133, 189
Liesanne, 264–265
Lindsay, 283–284, 333
Linett, 62, 113–114, 432
lipase enzymes, 418, 419
Lisa, 301
Lisa (Teresa's daughter), 290
Liz, 102, 270, 366, 447–448, 451
Lizzeth, 64, 234

lochia, 99
Lola, 42, 73, 207
loss/bereavement, 125–126, 501–505
Louise, 40, 239, 369, 374, 394–395
low blood sugar (hypoglycemia), 474, 522–524
low supply, 140–143, 494–498, 526–529
lower jaws, 77
Luisa, 89, 178, 191, 195, 238, 337, 502, 505
lumps, 509–510
luteal phase, 437
lymphatic drainage, 532
Lynett, 206
Lynn, 177, 213, 264, 383

M

Magic Baby Hold (colic hold), 151, 552
Mandy, 41
manual pumps, 403–404
Maria, 117–118
Mariana, 85, 466
Mariatu, 169
Marina, 467, 481, 482, 495
Marisela, 465, 497
Mary, 34, 61, 112, 116, 122, 258
mastitis, 530–533
maternity leave, 363
meconium, 99
medications, 437–439, 489, 490–491, 533–535
  ADHD, 490, 534
  anaesthesia, 52
  antibiotics, 533
  anti-inflammatories, 518, 531–532
  epidurals, 52, 57–58
  fertility treatment, 269
  galactagogues, 469, 486, 529
  milk suppression, 453, 503–504

pain relief, 102
postnatal depression, 550
Megan, 288
melatonin, 309
Melissa, 202, 298, 462, 472
membranes, 52
menstruation (periods), 254–255, 267–268, 270–271, 279, 437
microbes, 59
microbreaks, 391–392
midwives, 47
military mothers, 381–382
milk. *See* animal milks; human milk; plant-based milks
milk banks, 504–505, 536
milk blisters, 280, 508–509, 531
milk ejection reflex (letdown, milk release), 133, 184, 267
milk production
  abrupt discontinuation, 448–449
  discarding milk, 419
  exercise, 212–213
  flavor, 212
  flow, 133, 184, 267
  four to fourteen days, 132
  four to nine months, 244
  galactagogues, 469
  increasing, 155, 521
  induced lactation, 482, 484–488
  during menstruation, 267–268
  milk suppression, 453–454
  miscarriage, 501–502
  mothers' diet, 99, 143–144, 157–158
  multiple births, 475–476
  nine to eighteen months, 267
  oversupply, 143, 182–184, 222–223, 323, 545–547
  during pregnancy, 268–269, 433–434
  pumping, 402
  quantity, 140–143
  relactation, 478–480, 482

supply and demand, 12–13, 91–92,
   104–106, 138–140, 150,
   170–172, 178–184, 222–223,
   311–312
suppression, 502–504
surgeries, 491–494
breast tissue insufficiency, 510–512
for toddlers and beyond, 285
low supply, 140–143, 494–498,
   526–529
milk release (milk ejection reflex,
   letdown), 133, 184, 267
milk sharing (donor milk, milk
   banks), 25–27, 114, 505,
   535–538
Mimi, 219
minerals. *See* vitamin and mineral
   supplements
minibreaks, 392–394
miscarriage, 434–435, 501–505
Missy, 496
Monica, 301, 314, 317–318, 367
Monique, 269–270
Montoya, 112, 381–382
Montserrat, 14, 444
Morrison, Toni, 22
mouth development, 285
multiple births, 90, 475–478

N

naps, 245–246, 275–277, 321–322,
   451
Natalie, 35, 60, 162
Natalie G., 108, 283, 456
natural breastfeeding. *See* laid-back
   breastfeeding
natural disasters, 519–522
natural family planning, 254
natural weaning, 428–429
necrotizing enterocolitis (NEC),
   468
negotiated nursing, 289–290, 428

neonatal intensive care unit (NICU)
   care, 49, 465–473
networks. *see* support networks
neurodiversity, xvi. *See also* ADHD;
   ASD; autism; sensory
   processing disorder
Nicola, 445
Nicole, 202, 365
nicotine, 316, 568
night feedings, 251, 309–310,
   311–312
night waking, 285, 340
night weaning, 451, 454–456
Nikki, 476
nine to eighteen months, 263–281
   biting, 278–279
   criticism, 280–281
   health impact of breastfeeding, 447
   liquids, 265–267
   milk production, 267
   mobility, 271
   naps, 275–277
   nipple fiddling, 274–275
   nipple pain, 279–280
   nursing aversion, 270–271
   nursing patterns, 264–265,
      273–274, 278
   shyness, 275
   solid foods, 265
   weaning, 271–273
   weight gain, 267
nipple shields, 14, 93, 469, 483, 539,
   540–543
nipples
   blebs, 280, 508–509, 531
   creams and gels, 555
   flange size, 404–405
   flat nipples, 538–539
   flipple, 89
   inverted nipples, 539–540
   kneading and fiddling, 240,
      274–275
   mastitis, 530–533

nipples (*cont.*)
  menstruation, 279
  pain and sensitivity, 14–15, 86–90, 107, 122–123, 169, 279–280, 553–556
  pregnancy, 433
  pumping, 404–405, 412–413
  rashes, 279–280
  size, 14, 540
  teething babies, 212
  thrush, 279
  tilting, 88–89
  vasospasm, 563–565
  wound care, 250–251, 555–556
  yeast infections, 570
Noémie, 97, 351–352
nursing (as term), xv, 291–292
nursing patterns. *See* schedules for nursing
  breast compressions, 137–138, 150
  cluster feeding, 174
  distractibility, 208–209, 339–340
  first few days, 104–108
  four to fourteen days, 132–135, 152–157, 162–163
  four to nine months, 238–243
  frequency, 105–106, 107–108, 134, 152–154
  latching, 71–95, 170
  nine to eighteen months, 264–265
  nursing too fast, 155
  six weeks to four months, 206–209
  switching breasts, 107, 155
  toddlers and beyond, 286–292
  two to six weeks, 169–172, 180
nursing pillows, 89–90, 476
nursing strikes, 251–252, 272, 443–444, 543–544
nutrition. *See also* weight gain (baby)
  baby's needs, 7, 266
  mothers' needs, 143–144

O

obsessive-compulsive disorder (OCD), 548–550
obstetricians, 47
oestrogen, 182, 232
Olivia, 36, 224, 233, 263, 304, 394, 398
one year
  health impact of breastfeeding, 447
  weaning six months to one year, 450
  weaning twelve months or older, 450–452
online information, 23, 25, 33–34
overfeeding, 464
oversupply, 143, 182–184, 222–223, 323, 545–547
ovulation, 267, 268, 437
oxytocin, 8, 52, 176, 200, 434–435

P

paced bottle-feeding, 184–185, 560
pacifiers, 160–161, 219, 250, 320, 386, 442
pads, 17, 213
pain, 14–15
parental leave, 363
partners, 27–31
  bottle-feeding, 197–198
  co-mothers, 31, 35, 56, 146–147, 162, 258–259, 260–261, 269, 372, 435
  co-nursing, 26, 30, 31, 146–147, 372, 435, 488
  dads, 21, 26, 28, 30, 45, 63, 67, 132, 190, 193, 198, 202, 257, 303, 327, 329, 385, 406, 486, 491–492, 548
  during first days, 125, 127
  helping mum get rest/dealing with exhaustion, 325, 329

parental leave, 363
sex and intimacy, 199–200, 227–231
support from, 150–151
use of term, xv
Peggy, 93
periods (menstruation), 254–255, 267–268, 270–271, 279, 437
personalities (temperament), 192–193
physical challenges, 488–490
the pill, 182, 232
pillows, 89–90, 476
pincer grip, 339
placenta, 105, 139
plane travel, 219–220
plant-based milks, 266
polycystic ovary syndrome (PCOS), 5
polypropylene containers, 413
Pomme, 322
poop (stool, bowel movements)
colour, 135–136
constipation, 116, 210–211
first few days, 101, 115–116
four to fourteen days, 135–136, 137
meconium, 99
six weeks to four months, 210–211
smell, 136
positions for nursing
across-the-chest hold, 81
adaptations, 62, 84–85
blocked ducts, 532–533
breast size and shape, 85–86
clutch hold, 81–82, 477
cradle hold, 80
footstools, 90
laid-back breastfeeding, 71–72, 73–75, 145, 170, 184, 470, 474, 476, 482, 555
lying down, 328

pillows, 89–90
side-lying, 82–83, 184, 314, 315
sitting up, 17, 75–76
standing, 84
supportive, 76–77
postnatal depression, 102, 146–147, 193–194, 230, 547–548
postnatal mood disorders, 102, 146–147, 193–194, 226–227, 230, 547–550
postnatal psychosis, 147, 549
post-traumatic stress disorder (PTSD), 65–67, 227, 550
Praveena, 118, 183
pre-birth leave, 363
pregnancy. *See also* birth
breast size and shape, 4–5
breast tenderness, 433
hormones, 6
milk production, 268–269, 433–434
prevention, 231–232, 254
weaning, 433–434
preterm/premature babies
bottle-feeding, 469–470
digestive systems, 468
Kangaroo (skin-to-skin) Care, 466–467
laid-back breastfeeding, 470
latching, 90–91
late-premature and early-term babies, 473–475
milk fortifiers, 468
milk supplies, 468–469
nutritional needs, 217
stress, 468
sucking coordination, 471
two to six weeks, 185–187
progesterone, 182, 232
prolactin, 8, 437
props for nursing, 17, 90
public nursing, 195–197, 252–253, 294–295

pumping, 369–371, 373–380, 397–421
  after breastfeeding, 410
  bottle-feeding, 383–386
  cleanup, 419
  common problems, 387, 411–413
  exclusive pumping, 188, 462–465
  flange size, 404–405
  frequency, 408
  growth spurts, 386–387
  hands-free pumping, 403, 405–406
  hygiene, 414–415
  induced lactation, 485–486
  milk storage, 368, 380, 413–414
  pain, 412–413
  premature babies, 468–469
  relactation, 479
  supply challenges, 464
  techniques, 407–408
  types of pumps, 403–404
  weaning, 444–445

Q

quantity of milk. *See also* milk production
  four to fourteen days, 132
  four to nine months, 244
  oversupply, 143, 182–184, 222–223, 323, 545–547
  separations, 370–371
  supply and demand, 12–13, 91–92, 104–106, 138–140, 170–172, 178–184, 222–223, 311–312
  support networks, 150

R

race, racism, 44, 278, 382, 535
Rae, 188, 366–367
Rafaela, 16, 170
Raquel, 200–201, 205

rashes, 248
reflexes, 72–74
reflux, 551–553
refrigerated milk, 414, 415–416
refusal to nurse, 394
relactation, 478–480, 482, 521–522
rental-grade pumps, 403. *See also* consumer-grade pumps
resources
  breastfeeding, 94
  medications, 535
  "tech support" tool kit, 507–570
responsive feeding, 175–176, 343–344
reverse pressure softening, 518
rickets, 215
Rieko, 243
room sharing. *See* co-sleeping
rooming-in, 109
rooting, 157, 464
Rosie, 103, 133, 145, 362, 369, 377
Roxana, 168
rugby hold, 81–82

S

Safe Sleep Seven guidelines, 306, 307, 316–317
Sam, 504
Samantha, 77, 169, 174, 234, 253, 381, 434, 457
Sandra, 66, 67, 141
sandwich technique, 77–78, 89
Santi Sebas, Caro, 101
Sara Diana, 51–52, 249, 287, 376, 406
Sara Edith, 19, 294
Sarah, 292, 297–298
schedules for nursing
  four to fourteen days, 161–162
  two to six weeks, 172–176
self-care, 277–278
sensory processing disorder, 171–172, 224

separation anxiety, 239
separations, 198–199, 361–395. *See also* bottle-feeding; working parents
  expressing milk, 369–371, 373–380
  hospitalisations, 393–394, 522
  microbreaks, 391–392
  missing your baby, 387–390
  six weeks to four months, 232–234
  travel and vacations, 392–393
sepsis, 530
sex and intimacy
  bed-sharing arrangements, 326–327
  during pregnancy, 434
  six weeks to four months, 227–231
  two to six weeks, 199–200
Shanna, 93, 207, 458
Shoko, 55, 59, 84, 88, 110, 189, 217, 268, 300, 345, 377
showers, 53–54
sidecars, 306, 311, 313
side-lying, 82–83, 560–562
side-lying position, 184
SIDS (crib death). *See* sudden infant death syndrome (SIDS)
Sien, 185, 281
sign language, 292
silicone containers, 413
single parenting, 25
sitting up, 17, 75–76
six months
  health impact of breastfeeding, 447
  weaning six months to one year, 450
  weaning under six months, 449
six weeks to four months, 205–234
  brain growth, 206
  calm babies, 223
  constipation, 210–211
  conversational nursing, 207
  distractibility, 208–209, 339–340
  exercise, 212–213
  frequency days, 206
  going out, 218–220
  health impact of breastfeeding, 447
  love, 227
  nursing patterns, 206–209
  nursing schedules, 220–221
  pregnancy protection, 231–232
  sensitive babies, 206, 223–226
  separations, 232–234
  sex and intimacy, 227–231
  sleep, 209–210, 221
  solid foods, 217
  teething, 211–212
  travelling, 218–220
  vaccinations, 214
  vitamin and mineral supplements, 215–217
  working parents, 222
skin-to-skin contact, 54–55, 59, 61–63, 65, 71–72, 92–93, 104, 121, 385, 466–467, 482
sleeping
  apps for tracking, 310
  bed-sharing, 306, 309, 311, 314–319, 325–326
  co-sleeping, 110, 306, 311, 313–314
  "cuddle curl" position, 314, 315
  family beds, 312–313, 333
  first few days, 108–111
  four to fourteen days, 144–146
  nap nursing, 321–322
  naps, 245–246, 275–277
  night feeding, 309–310, 311–312
  night waking, 285, 340
  normal amounts, 305
  nursing to fall asleep, 276–277, 278, 320–322, 372–374
  Safe Sleep Seven guidelines, 306, 307, 316–317
  separate rooms, 305, 308, 320, 331–333

sidecars, 306, 311, 313
SIDS (crib death), 210, 306, 311, 320, 330
six weeks to four months, 209–210
sleep training, 221, 330–331
sleeping through the night, 221, 304–305
solid foods, 338
tracking sleep hours, 309–310
weaning, 451, 454–456
working parents, 372–374
slings, 18, 150, 220–221, 389, 472, 482, 489–490
smell of milk, 418–419
smiling, 169, 207
Smillie, Christina, 15
smoking, 74, 316, 568
soap and water, 400, 555
soapy smelling milk, 418, 419
solid foods, 337–358
    baby-led beginnings, 340–341
    bedtime, 331
    breastfeeding approach to, 343–344
    cautious eaters, 349–350, 357
    cavities, 324
    choking, 350
    food allergies, 287, 351–353
    food prep, 348–349
    four to nine months, 244, 247
    gagging, 344, 350
    gluten, 350–351
    healthy foods on a budget, 348
    indigestion, 337
    iron, 355–356
    messiness, 353–354
    nine to eighteen months, 265
    parent-controlled feedings, 345–346
    preterm/premature babies, 217
    readiness for, 338–340, 350
    salt and spices, 346
    spoon feeding, 341
    starter foods, 342–344
    ultraprocessed foods, 346–348, 356–357
    vegan diets, 343
    weaning, 356
Sonja, 433–434, 456
soothing, 76, 150–152, 157
Sorrel, 384
special needs babies, 498–501
    cleft lip or palate, 499
    Down syndrome, 499
special needs toddlers, 298
spitting up, 159–160
spoiling the baby, 163–164, 173–174, 176
spoon feeding, 92, 341, 483
standing, 84
Stephanie, 24, 26, 45, 72–73, 168, 190–191, 424, 468
stepping reflex, 77
stillbirth, 501–505
stool. *See* poop
storing milk, 368, 380
    colostrum, 400
    containers, 413–414
    freshness, 415, 416
    heating and reheating, 415–416, 419
    stockpiling, 370
    thawed milk, 419
stress, 194, 365, 387–388, 520–521, 531
stuffy noses, 185, 249, 443
sucking
    breaking suction, 107
    fluttery sucks, 123–124
    late-premature and early-term babies, 474
    preterm/premature babies, 471
    swallowing sounds, 123, 134
    tongue-tie, 140
sudden infant death syndrome (SIDS), 122, 160, 210, 306, 311, 314–317, 330

sudden unexpected postnatal
    collapse (SUPC), 74
sunlight, 215
sunscreen, 215
supplementation, 479, 487, 556–559.
    See also bottle-feeding
  at-breast supplementers, 220, 479,
      483, 484–485, 559
  four to nine months, 242
  milk sharing, 114
  nursing supplementers, 220, 479,
      483, 484–485, 559
  paced bottle-feeding, 560
  side-lying bottle-feeding, 530–562
  wet nursing, 113–114
supply and demand, 12–13, 91–92,
      104–106, 138–140, 150,
      170–172, 178–184, 222–223,
      244, 521, 545–547
support networks
  community, 31–33
  doulas, 43–45
  exhaustion, 328–329
  first few days, 18–19
  healthcare providers, 34–35, 330
  importance of, 21–24
  La Leche League, 5, 10–12, 35–37,
      64, 93–94, 127, 170, 187,
      200–201, 243, 328, 432–433
  late-premature and early-term
      babies, 474–475
  low supply, 497–498
  mothers' groups, 170
  NICU, 472–473
  online information, 23, 25, 33–34
  paid help, 330
  partners, 27–31, 150–151, 325, 329
  physical challenges and
      disabilities, 490
  postnatal depression, 194
surrogacy, 3, 6, 141, 488. *See also*
      induced lactation; relactation
suppression

milk production, 453–454,
    503–504
  physiological, 502–503
Susana, 62, 290
swaddling, 121–122, 322–323
swallowing, 123, 134
Sweet Sleep (LLL), 198, 314, 316
swinging, 151–152
switching breasts, 107, 155
synthetic oxytocin, 52

T
tandem nursing, 269–270, 292–293,
      435–436
Tatjana, 34–35
teeth
  brushing, 323–324
  cavities, 251, 323–324, 454
  chips, 279
  first tooth, 248
  teething, 211–212, 247–248
temperament, 99, 192–193
Teresa, 18, 164, 209, 291, 310–311,
      356, 423
terms for nursing, xiv–xv, 291–292
Theresa, 48, 168
Three Keeps, 91–94
thrush, 185, 279, 570
thyroid problems, 5, 184, 528, 548
timeframe for breastfeeding, 424–425
Tina, 306, 318, 331–332
tobacco use, 316, 568
toddlers and beyond, 283–301
  brain growth, 285
  common questions, 294–298
  emotional needs, 298–299
  negotiation and compromise,
      289–290, 428
  nursing patterns, 286–292
  nursing in public, 294–295
  parenting, 297–298
  play nursing, 289

reassurance, 284
setting limits, 295–297
sick or stressed toddlers, 285, 288
special needs, 299
talking, 290
tandem nursing, 292–293, 435–436
terms for nursing, 291–292
working parents, 293
tongue-tie, 87–88, 140, 562–563
train travel, 221
Tran, Uyen, 290, 292
trans/transgender parents, xv, 5, 44, 45, 132, 141, 462, 486, 491–492, 493, 498. *See also* LGBTQIA+ families
travelling, 218–220, 253–254, 392–393, 420–421
Trevor, 5, 132, 486, 491–492, 493, 498
triplets, 475–478
twins, 90, 475–478
two to six weeks, 167–203
   bottle-feeding, 175, 184–185, 197–198
   conversational nursing, 176
   disinterest in nursing, 171–172, 184–190
   feelings, 177
   frequency days, 180–181
   health impact of breastfeeding, 447
   nursing patterns, 169–172, 180
   nursing in public, 195–197
   nursing schedules, 172–176
   personalities, 192–193
   premature infants, 185–187
   separations, 198–199
   sex and intimacy, 199–200
   sensitive babies, 188–192
   weight gain (baby), 171, 172, 173–175
   working parents, 197

U

umbilical cord, 58, 217
underarm hold, 81–82
United Nations Children's Fund (UNICEF), 35, 111, 425, 446
urate crystals, 115, 137
urine, 101, 115, 139
U.S. Food and Drug Administration, 248

V

vaccinations, 214
vacuum extraction, 44
vaginal bleeding, 52, 99
vaginal exams, 53
vaginal seeding, 59
Vanesa, 290
Vanessa, 22, 456
vasospasm, 563–565
vegan diets, 216, 343
Verena, 186
Verity, 125–126, 503
Verity-Rose, 197
visitors, 100, 127
vitamin and mineral supplements, 216–217
   iron, 216–217, 355–356
   vitamin B_{12}, 216
   vitamin D, 215–216

W

waking the baby for feeding, 107, 120–121
walking, 271
warm compresses, 532
warming chilled milk, 415–416
water, 247, 265
water breaking, 52
weaning, 356, 423–458
   abrupt weaning, 448–449
   child visitation, 441–442

child-led, 445–448
criticism, 439–441
duration of breastfeeding, 424–425
early weaning, 442–443, 449–450
emergency weaning, 452–454
feelings, 429–431, 451–452, 454, 456–457
four to nine months, 244–245
medical indications, 437–439
natural weaning, 428–429
new pregnancies, 268–269, 293, 436–437
night weaning, 451, 454–456
nine to eighteen months, 271–273
nursing impatience, 428–429
partial weaning, 430
returning to work or school, 437
sudden refusal to nurse, 443–444, 543–544
weaning parties, 452
weaning window, 284
wee, 101, 115, 136
weight gain (baby), 565–569
first few days, 116–117
four to fourteen days, 134, 154–155
four to nine months, 257
growth spurts, 339, 387
multiple births, 475–476
night weaning, 454
nine to eighteen months, 267
rapid growth, 567–569
slow growth, 565–567
supplementation, 557–558
two to six weeks, 171, 172, 173–175
weight loss (mother), 7–8, 213, 515–516
Wendy, 48

wet nursing, 26–27, 113–114
whim nursing, 170
Widström, Ann Marie, 71
working parents, 362–390
bottle-feeding, 383–386
career changes, 389–390
childcare, 363–371
expressing milk, 370–371, 373–380
flexible schedules, 375–378
maternity leave, 363, 382
military mothers, 381–382
missing your baby, 387–390
quitting your job, 389–390
six weeks to four months, 222
solid foods, 355
toddler nursing, 293
two to six weeks, 197
weaning, 437
working from home, 377
World Health Organization, 111, 141, 231, 338, 436, 512–513
breastfeeding recommendations, 271, 286, 338, 425, 446, 568
formula recommendations, 266
International Code on the Marketing of Breastmilk Substitutes, 35

X
Xiang, 287

Y
yeast infections, 185, 279, 570

Z
Zoe, 252

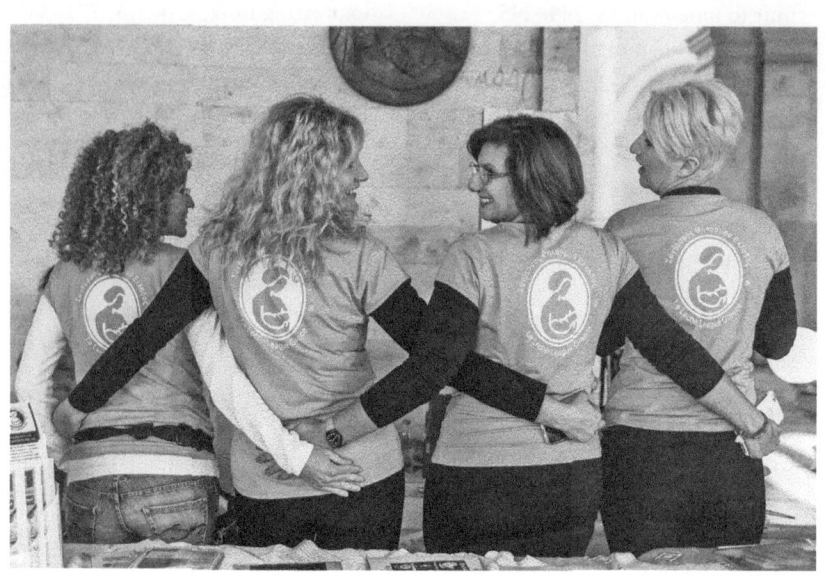

ABOUT LA LECHE LEAGUE

LA LECHE LEAGUE, founded in 1956, is the world's largest mother-to-mother, parent-to-parent breastfeeding support organisation, active in over eighty countries worldwide. Visit www.llli.org to find out how LLL can support you.

ABOUT THE TYPE

The text of this book was set in Janson, a typeface designed about 1690 by Nicholas Kis (1650–1702), a Hungarian living in Amsterdam, and for many years mistakenly attributed to the Dutch printer Anton Janson. In 1919, the matrices became the property of the Stempel Foundry in Frankfurt. It is an old-style book face of excellent clarity and sharpness. Janson serifs are concave and splayed; the contrast between thick and thin strokes is marked.